CLINICAL ACUPUNCTURE

(Revised Edition 2001)

ANTON JAYASURIYA

M.B.B.S. (Cey.), D. Phys. Med, R.C.P. (Lond.), & R.C.S, (Eng.).
M.Ac.F. (Sri Lanka), Ph.D., F.Ac.F. (India), D.Litt.,
Diploma in Acupuncture (Peking),
Member of the International Institute of Homoeopathy,
Member of the Acupuncture Foundation (Canada),
Diploma of the Homoeopathy Research Institute of Canada
and New York Academy of Homoeopathic Medicine,
Fellow of the Australian Medical Acupuncture Society,
Fellow of the Scandinavian Acupuncture Foundation,
Fellow of Medical Acupuncture Association (Bratislava),
Fellow of the Korean Acupuncture Association,
Fellow of the British Acupuncture Association,
Vice-President of the
British & European Osteopathic Association,
Fellow of the Royal Society of Medicine (England),
Member of the American Association of Natural Medicine,
Honorary Presedent,
Atlantic College of Medical Homoeopathy, Republic of Columbia,
Senior Consultant Rheumatologist, Ministry of Health, Sri Lanka,
Chief Acupuncturist, Institute of Acupuncture, Lasertherapy & Homoeopuncture,
Colombo, South Government General Hospital, Kalubowila,
W.H.O. Fellow in Acupuncture (China 1974),
Laureate United Nations Dag Hammarskjoid Award for Medicine (1984),
Chairman, Medicine Alternativa
(Author of 19 books on Acupuncture, Homoeopathy, Oriental Philosophy and Neurophysiology in 7 languages)

B. Jain Publishers (P) Ltd

New Delhi

Note

Any information given in this book is not intended to be taken as a replacement for medical advice. Any person with a condition requiring medical attention should consult a qualified practitioner or therapist.

Revised edition : 2002

Price: Rs. 275.00

Published by:
Kuldeep Jain
For
B. Jain Publishers (P) Ltd
1921, Street No.10, Chuna Mandi
Paharganj, New Delhi-110 055 (INDIA)
Phones: 3670430, 3670572, 3683200, 3683300
FAX : 011-3610471 & 3683400
Email : bjain@vsnl.com
Website : www.bjainbooks.com

Printed in India by:
Unisons Techno Financial Consultants (P) Ltd.
522, FIE, Patparganj, Delhi-110 092

ISBN : 81-7021-348-7
BOOK CODE : BS-2602

Dedicated

to

My Parents

"If you cannot be the king,
be a healer".

(Ancient Sinhala aphorism from
an ola manuscript of 500 B.C.)

CONTENTS

A Brief History 1
Modern Scientific Views 19
Materials and Techniques 35
Precautions 65
Anatomy of Acupuncture 87
The System of Channels and Collaterals 115
Lung Channel (Lu.) 117
Large Intestine Channel (L.I.) 133
Stomach Channel (St.) 143
Spleen Channel (Sp.) 161
Heart Channel (H.) 169
Small Intestine
Channel (S.I.) 177
Urinary Bladder
Channel (U.B.) 187
Kidney Channel (K.) 207
Pericardium Channel (P.) 215
Sanjiao Channel (S.J.) 223
Gall Bladder Channel (G.B.) 233
Liver Channel (Liv.) 249
Du Channel (Du)1 255
Ren Channel (Ren.)1 271
The Extraordinary Points (Ex.) 283
The Un-numbered Extraordinary Points (U.Ex.) 297
Philosophical Concepts 301
Traditional Chinese Diagnosis 357
The Circulation of Vital Energy (Qi) 415
The Principles of Acupuncture Point Selection 435
Stematic Therapy 473
Diseases of the Nervous System 477
Respiratory Disorders 501

Cardiovascular Disorders 513
Blood Disorders 523
Disorders of the Gastrointestinal System 525
Hepatic, Biliary, Splenic And Pancreatic Disorders 541
Genitourinary Disorders 551
Disorders of Women 559
Locomotor Disorders—Diseases of Soft Tissues, Muscles,
Bones and Joints 571
Skin Disorders 589
Ear Disorders 601
Eye Disorders 607
Endocrine Disorders 615
Psychiatric Disorders 621
Disorders of Children 629
Acute Disorders 635
Traditional Chinese Therapeutics 645
The Ancillary Techniques Of Acupuncture 757
Acupuncture Analgesia In Childbirth 817
Prognosis of Disease with Acupuncture 827
Auriculotherapy 835
Scalp Acupuncture 861
Locations of All Acupuncture Points of the 14 Channels 869
Glossary of Common Terms used in Acupuncture Practice 915
Appendix on Complications 931
Tai Yun – The Great 60 Year Chinese Calendar 939
Some Common Western Medical (Allopathic) Disorders
with their Traditional Chinese and Homoeopathic
Equivalents 964
The Chinese Language 1023
Some Common Ideograms and their Meanings 1026
Correspondense of the 5 Elements 1031
Nature 1032
Health Care/Medicine 1033
Numbers 1034

PREFACE TO THE SEVENTH EDITION

It is indeed always a pleasant thought to be asked to preface a book–one's mind wanders over all the facets which the book itself deals with, and also into the byways which lead from the particular into the wider scene. After several long years of exposure to the practice of acupuncture, both the writer and the author have explored in detail the subject itself, and have thus wandered, somethimes unwittingly, into the broader scene of communication with colleagues, students, patients, and the community at large—both national and international. Mainly these contacts are enormously rewarding—but even the occasional rebuffs have the benefit of making us look at ourselves critically at what we are doing.

After many years what has been learned and achieved? Modern theories about the physiology of acupuncture have been expounded, trialled, and accepted as probable mechanisms for some physiological actions of acupuncture. Apart from the Gate Control Theory of Melzack and Wall, the neurotransmitter theories certainly have suggested that acupuncture triggers central neurological mechanisms, which cause alterations in a wide spectrum of neurotransmitter substances, which in turn may set the scene for a return to normal physiology within the body i.e. homeostasis. However, as yet, no one definitive theory explains all the observed and varied phenomena.

On the other side of the story, years of clinical practice have positively identified that acupuncture has a definite place in the health care of all peoples of the world, both in the East and the West, and that it can be integrated successfully with modern medical practice. In properly trained hands it is inexpensive, harmless—but essentially effective over a large range of common disorders, and can be used, together with modern diagnostic methods, to help reduce the increasing upsurge of side effects (some serious) produced by so many of our potent modern chemotherapeutic agents.

"New methods of stimulating the Acupunture points have been devised including ultrasound and laser therapy. Laser therapy in particular has been shown to be safe and effective, and where Hepatitis B and AIDS are a risk with needle puncture, laser therapy is a viable alternative. This is surely a marriage of modern technology and an ancient art, using the best of the old and the new together for the benefit of all, looking towards health care for all people by the year 2000."

The new edition of **Clinical Acupuncture,** *now translated to five languages, again flowing from the voluminous and seemingly never ending pen of Professor Anton Jayasuriya, is a further meaningful step in keeping students of this ancient art up to date with clear, concise information which should help them develop, with time, as well-qualifiied acupuncturists. In doing so, Professor Jayasuriya is making available to the world at large valuable material for the benefit of the whole of mankind.*

G.M. GREENBAUM*
M.B.B.S., F.R.A.C.G.P., F.Ac.F.,
Past President and Chief Examiner,
Australian Medical Acupuncture Association,
Chairman of the Board, Victorian Academy for
General Practice,
Director, Medicina Alternativa.

---

* Dr G.M. Greenbaum is the first practitioner to have carried out acupuncture anaesthesia for major surgery in Australia, in 1977 — Author.

FOREWORD

(to the First Edition)

Three to four thousand years after the Yellow Emperor's Canon on Acupuncture, modern doctors are now rediscovering acupuncture. While China leads the world today, it is important that centres outside China replicate their results; the essence of the scientific method is replication. Moreover, sceptics outside China will only accept their results if they are repeated in other countries. Hence the experience of healers in Sri Lanka, as summarized in this book, is an important contribution to the scientific world.

This book has been written with the experience of treating over 250,000 patients in Sri Lanka with methods learned in China, and of teaching over six thousand acupuncturists from many countries. I have spent several months at the 'Colombo South General Hospital', Kalubowila, and have observed over 500 patients a day being treated with acupuncture alone. I also saw many local and foreign students being trained in acupuncture therapy. It was evident that the training program was an excellent one, deriving from two factors: the huge patient load, and the superb training methods of Professor Anton Jayasuriya. Sri Lanka has, no doubt, the best acupuncture teaching centre in the world.

Of particular interest to me, of course, was the performing of surgery using acupuncture analgesia. The methodology of acupuncture analgesia, I saw done in Colombo seems to be more acceptable to the West, than what I was shown in The People's Republic of China.

In Colombo, some of the results of acupuncture therapy were truly amazing. For example, I saw 6 severe cases of acute bronchial asthma restored to normal breathing within 10 minutes; acupuncture was used, instead of noradrenaline. I observed a case of frozen shoulder of 8 month's duration completely cured within 15 minutes (far more effective than steroids). I saw a severely wasted leg of a polio victim (of 15 years duration), completely restored to normal after 80 days of acupuncture (a cure unheard of in Western medicine). The "cure" rate, anecdotally, seemed very high (more than 60% of cases) in many diseases such as asthma, psoriasis, migraine and backache. In other diseases such as epilepsy, neuromuscular disorders and mental disorders there were cures, but the frequency of cure was somewhat lower. In China I was shown similar results, but I could not verify their claims because of the language barrier; in Sri Lanka a majority of the patients spoke English.

As I stated, the evidence I observed was only anecdotal. Although many controlled studies have been done to validate acupuncture analgesia in many research laboratories throughout the world, much work is needed to verify scientifically the effectiveness of acupuncture in curing disease. I have no doubt that this book will serve to inspire clinicians and scientists to study acupuncture therapy of disease in controlled experiments.

It domes not worry me much, if acupuncture yet defies scientific explanation; after all, Einstein's discoveries were made by studying the exceptions to Maxwell's equations. If acupuncture is an exception to the Western medical model, all the better; perhaps this will be the chance for a major breakthrough in the further understanding of the human body complex.

BRUCE POMERANZ*
M.D. (McGill), Ph.D. (Harvard), F.Ac.F.,
Professor of Neurobiology,
University of Toronto (Ontario), Canada,
Dean, International College of Acupuncture,
Medicina Alternativa.

* Professor Bruce Pomeranz is one of the pioneer scientific workers on the endorphin mechanism of acupuncture analgesia.

INTRODUCTION

The barefoot doctor system still forms the backbone of the medical services in rural China. In many backward areas of the world such as countries in Asia, Africa and Latin America, and even in the affluent countries with large rural areas cut off from the population centres, the barefoot doctor experiment could be adopted with a certain degree of success. A very large part of the world's population lives, in fact, in rural and sometimes inaccessible areas where Western medicine, due to the constraints of its sophistication, cannot easily be made available. The most potent therapeutic weapon of the barefoot doctor is the acupuncture needle. It is safe, simple, effective and economical, and can be used by personnel after a short period of training. Acupuncture, therefore, is the short term, as well as the long term answer, to the health needs of the greater part of the Third World in many everyday illnesses.

This is not to say that acupuncture should be used only in the absence of Western medicine. Many people, even in the West, are becoming more aware of the manifold and horrendous complications of drug therapy, and are seeking alternative forms of therapy. But a large quantity of drugs is still consumed as home remedies in minor self-limiting illnesses like the common cold, tonsillitis, insomnia, constipation, headache and gastro-enteritis. It is incumbent for the cultured mind of today to have an elementary understanding of acupuncture and to employ it in such common disorders, before reaching for the bottle of pills.

Acupuncture is eminently applicable also in such modern situations as submarine missions, off-shore oil rigs, polar research missions and space travel*, where groups of workers are cut off from the rest of the world, for prolonged periods.

This elementary book is written mainly as a guide to the barefoot doctors of the world. It is hoped that it will also serve as a

---

* The Russian cosmonauts carry acupuncture needles on their space missions, they are prohibited to take any medications.

reference to every initiated person for methods of first aid in minor and uncomplicated disorders. It is also directed at the Western trained physician as a first step in understanding the methodology of acupuncture, which can be usefully combined with scientific medicine, to create a wide-spectrum weapon in the fight against disease. In modern China the approach today is to combine Western with traditional methods, both in diagnosis and therapy (and this in fact is the approach of the teachers at the Academy of Traditional Medicine in Beijing). The Western trained doctor will find this approach particularly meaningful as the diseases discussed in this book are in the terminology and semantics familiar to him.

This book is the synthesis of the experience of treating a very large number of patients daily at the Institute of Acupuncture of the Colombo South General Hospital, and the teachings of the great masters at the Academy of Traditional Medicine in Peking, the Institute of Physiology, Shanghai, and other centres in the People's Republic of China, where I had the privilege to study. This book, in fact, is a synopsis of the short teaching courses conducted by us at the Institute of Acupuncture, Sri Lanka*.

I wish to place on record my grateful thanks to the World Health Organization for the granting of a Fellowship in 1974 which resulted in my obtaining the Diploma in Acupuncture in Peking, and to the Foreign Office of the People's Republic of China for invitations in 1976, 1977 and again in 1979 to study the latest advances in acupuncture therapy and anaesthesia in China.

To Professor Zhang Xiang-Tung of the Institute of Physiology, Shanghai, a man for all seasons, who taught me the neurophysiology of acupuncture, my special thanks for many helpful criticisms.

ANTON JAYASURIYA

Chief Acupuncturist,
Institute of Acupuncture,
Homoeopuncture & Lasertherapy,
Colombo South General Hospital,
Kalubowila,
Sri Lanka.

Chairman
Medicina Alternativa

* Four week courses commence on the 1st day of each month.

CLINICAL ACUPUNCTURE

TABLE OF CHINESE DYNASTIES

	夏	HSIA kingdom (legendary?)		*c.* −2000 to *c.* −1520
	商	SHANG (YIN) kingdom		*c.* −1520 to *c.* −1030
	周	CHOU dynasty (Feudal Age)	Early Chou period	*c.* −1030 to −722
			Chhun Chhiu period 春秋	−722 to −480
			Warring States (Chan Kuo) period 戰國	−480 to −221
First Unification	秦	CHHIN dynasty		−221 to −207
	漢	HAN dynasty	Chhien Han (Earlier or Western)	−202 to +9
			Hsin interregnum	+9 to +23
			Hou Han (Later or Eastern)	+25 to +220
	三國	SAN KUO (Three Kingdoms period)		+221 to +265
First Partition	蜀	SHU (HAN)	+221 to +264	
	魏	WEI	+220 to +265	
	吳	WU	+222 to +280	
Second Unification	晉	CHIN dynasty:	Western	+265 to +317
			Eastern	+317 to +420
	劉宋	(Liu) SUNG dynasty		+420 to +479
Second Partition		Northern and Southern Dynasties (Nan Pei chhao)		
	齊	CHHI dynasty		+479 to +502
	梁	LIANG dynasty		+502 to +557
	陳	CHHEN dynasty		+557 to +589
	魏	Northern (Thopa) WEI dynasty		+386 to +535
		Western (Thopa) WEI dynasty		+535 to +556
		Eastern (Thopa) WEI dynasty		+534 to +550
	北齊	Northern CHHI dynasty		+550 to +577
	北周	Northern CHOU (Hsienpi) dynasty		+557 to +581
Third Unification	隋	SUI dynasty		+581 to +618
	唐	THANG dynasty		+618 to +906
Third Partition	五代	WU TAI (Five Dynasty period) (Later Liang, Later Thang (Turkic), Later Chin (Turkic), Later Han (Turkic) and Later Chou)		+907 to +960
	遼	LIAO (Chhitan Tartar) dynasty		+907 to +1124
		West LIAO dynasty (Qarā-Khiṭāi)		+1124 to +1211
	西夏	Hsi Hsia (Tangut Tibetan) state		+986 to +1227
Fourth Unification	宋	Northern SUNG dynasty		+960 to +1126
	宋	Southern SUNG dynasty		+1127 to +1279
	金	CHIN (Jurchen Tartar) dynasty		+1115 to +1234
	元	YÜAN (Mongol) dynasty		+1260 to +1368
	明	MING dynasty		+1368 to +1644
	清	CHHING (Manchu) dynasty		+1644 to +1911
	民國	Republic		+1912
		People's Republic		+1948

CLINICAL ACUPUNCTURE

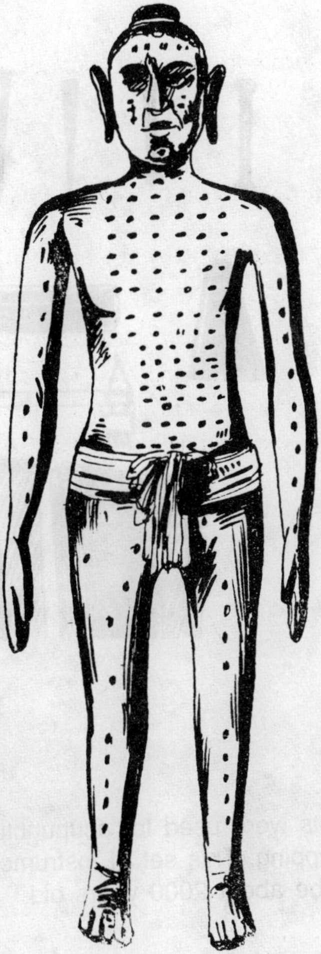

Photo — the author

This bronze figure showing acupuncture points is a reproduction of one cast in 1443 A.D., during the Ming Dynasty.

TRADITIONAL ACUPUNCTURE EQUIPMENT FROM SRI LANKA

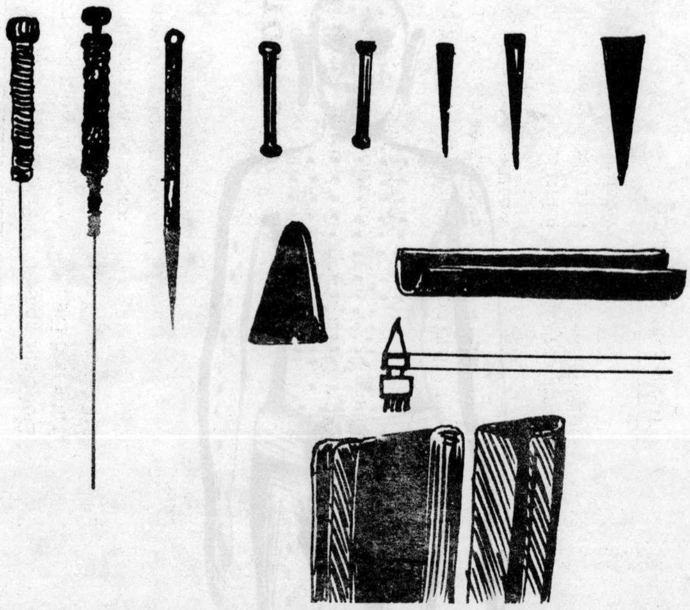

Photo — the author

These instruments were used for acupuncture, surgery, moxibustion and cupping. This set of instruments is believed to be about 2000 years old.

A BRIEF HISTORY

The beginnings of traditional Chinese medicine are obscure. It is believed, however, to have developed, like the Indian Ayurveda system, from folk medicine and, as in *Ayurveda,* there is no lack of mythical explanations. The three legendary Emperors, *Shen Nung, Huang Di* and *Fu Hsi* are traditionally believed to have been the originators of Chinese medicine. The classical book on traditional Chinese Medicine is the *Huang Di Nei Jing,* meaning 'The Yellow Emperor's Classic of Internal Medicine' and this work is ascribed to Huang Di (the Yellow Emperor), who is believed to have lived about 2697-2596 B.C. It is more likely, however, that it is a collective work written about the third century B.C. and antedated to enhance its value and to give it a stamp of authority. It is presented as a dialogue between the Yellow Emperor and his prime minister—physician, *Chi Po.* The book is in two sections, first *Su Wen,*[1] contains the principles of traditional Chinese medicine, and the second, *Ling Shu,*[2] describes the various therapeutic processes.

There are four basic therapeutic methods in traditional Chinese medicine.

a) *Herbal therapy.*

---

1 Su Wen = Simple Questions. Deals with preventive medicine.

2 Ling Shu= Magic Gate or Spiritual Pivot. Deals with therapeutics.

THE ACUPUNCTURE POINTS OF THE ASIAN ELEPHANT

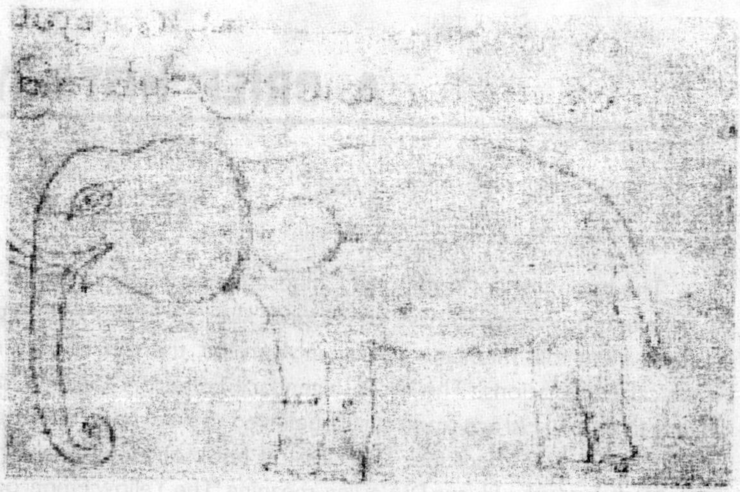

The Asiatic elephant (*Elephans maximus asiaticus)* has 89 charted acupuncture points. Above is a photograph of an ola manuscript of Sri Lanka (*circa* 500 A.D.) in the author's possession, depicting the points used for controlling the animal, in such tasks as lifting heavy logs or carrying riders. The Asiatic elephant has also been used very effectively in battle since ancient times. Control is obtained by jabbing specific points with a sharp prod and hook attached to the end of the long pole (known as the henduwa). Hannibal of Carthage used elephants to cross the Alps more than two thousand years ago. It is recorded that he used the Asiatic and not African elephants. Roman coins before the time of Christ, found at the sites of several ancient cities of Sri Lanka, is evidence that the elephants were taken to the West via the spice route. The African elephant cannot be tamed as its acupuncture points have not been ascertained. The same acupuncture techniques are still used by Asian elephant keepers (mahouts) both for controlling as well as for therapeutic purposes.

b) *Moxibustion.* i.e. heating or burning certain areas of the body with the powdered leaves of the moxa plant (Latin: *Artemesia vulgaris*).

c) *Acupuncture.* (Latin: *Acus*—needle; *punctura*—to penetrate) Acupuncture and Moxibustion (Zhen-Jue) are the most ancient and characteristic therapeutic techniques of Chinese Medicine.

d) *Surgery.* This method of treatment was used only as a last resort, as according to the Confucian[3] doctrine the human body was considered to be sacred. Surgery, however, was used extensively in treating war injuries and in a more traditional procedure, to produce eunuchs for the Imperial Court.

Acupuncture—Moxibustion (*Zhen—Jue*) is one of most ancient and characteristic therapeutic techniques of Chinese medicine. Very broadly speaking, the acupuncture technique was from ancient times onwards thought most valuable in both acute and chronic diseases, while moxa was more appropriate in chronic ones. The main components of traditional Chinese medicine originated in different geographical parts of China. At least two of the chapters of the Nei Ching enlarge on the theme that varying methods of treatment had been found appropriate for people living in the diverse conditions of the several provinces and the four quarters. Different environments gave rise to different incidences of endemic disease, hence the invention of different therapeutic methods. Thus, moxibustion came mainly from the North, materia medica and pharmacy from the West, and gymnastics, remedial exercises and massage from the Centre. But acupuncture originated in the East, where people suffered greatly from boils and carbuncles; while its elaboration (in the form of the nine needles) came from the South. As for apotropaics (exorcisms, magical spells, and sacrifices to the Gods and ancestors), this, it was considered, had been fairly universal from the earliest times. In part, it may be, this ancient proto-historical presentation was following the system of symbolic co-relations, five types of medical treatment

---

3. Confucius was a philosopher who lived about five centuries before Christ.

being analogised with the fivefold[4] classification and especially the five directions of space, but there may be rather more to it than that. For we know that ancient Chinese society was built upon, or greatly influenced by, a number of "local cultures", environing societies, which brought various distinguishable traits into the eventual common Sinic stock. In this case, acupuncture would have been associated with the south-eastern quasi-Indonesian aquatic element, while moxa would have come down to join it from the northern quasi-Tungusic nomadic element, and the pharmaceutical influence would have come from the Western Szechuanese and quasi-Tibetan element. Acupuncture is a system of therapy which has been in constant use throughout the Chinese culture-area[5] for some four and a half thousand years; and the labours of a multitude of devoted men and women, through the centuries, have given it a highly developed doctrine and a set of rules to carry out the clinical practice.

"In evaluating acupuncture through the works of representatives of the present day practitioners in the Western World some reserve should be exercised, for the following reasons; (a) very few of them have had reliable linguistic access to the voluminous Chinese sources of many different periods, (b) it is often not quite clear how far their training has given them direct continuity with the living Chinese clinical traditions, (c) the history in their works is liable to be minimal or unscholarly, (d) their familiarity of theory are generally very inadequate, (e) they tend to adopt a too simplistic assimilation of classical Chinese disease entities to those of modern-Western medicine, (f) the cardinal importance of sphygmology[6] in Chinese differential diagnosis is almost ignored, and (g) their works are naturally so much influenced by modern-Western concepts of disease

---

4 The Five Elements (Panchabhuta of Ayurveda).

5 Acupuncture and moxibustion have been used in many other regions of the world since pre-historic times. It was well developed in North India and in Sri Lanka, before the Christian era. Chinese travellers first came to Sri Lanka in 4th century A.D. Acupuncture and Moxibustion was practised before the Chinese travellers came to North Africa, Northern Europe and in several other regions of the World.

6 Pulse diagnosis

aetiology and pathology that they seem not to practise the classical Chinese methods of holistic classification and diagnosis. Not everyone with a modern-Western medical training can immediately perform all the traditional-Chinese therapeutic feats. Pulse diagnosis, for example, as well as a very organicist psychosomatic approach, is a fundamental feature of this traditional art, which after all depends on much subtle theorising, not of course in the modern style, but not nonsense either."[7]

In diagnosing an illness, traditional Chinese medicine places great stress on the physician's close observation of external signs of disease, the interpretation of the pulse, and the understanding of the symptoms associated with each disorder.

The main methods of diagnosis employed by the traditional Chinese physician may be described as follows:

a) *Looking.* i.e. examination especially of the eyes, tongue, lips, nose and ears (the Five Senses). Examination with special reference to colour (the Five Colours) and careful observation of the patient's hearing and disposition (the Five Emotions).

b) *Listening.* e.g. to the heart, the breathing and particularly the voice (the Five Vocal Expressions).

c) *Asking.* i.e. finding out by interrogation the history of the disorder and other factors such as sleep, dreams, bowel habits.

d) *Palpating*, specifically of points on the abdomen, thorax and on the Channels (Alarm points. *Ah-Shi points*).

e) *Taking the Pulses.* (Pulse diagnosis).

f) *Examining the Ear.* Using the principles of auriculotherapy.

g) *Tongue diagnosis.*

Today, however, it is more pragmatic to combine traditional methods with the methodology of modern scientific diagnosis. In this

7 Joseph Needham in "Celestial Lancets". Cambridge University, Press (1981)

THE NINE KINDS OF TRADITIONAL NEEDLES

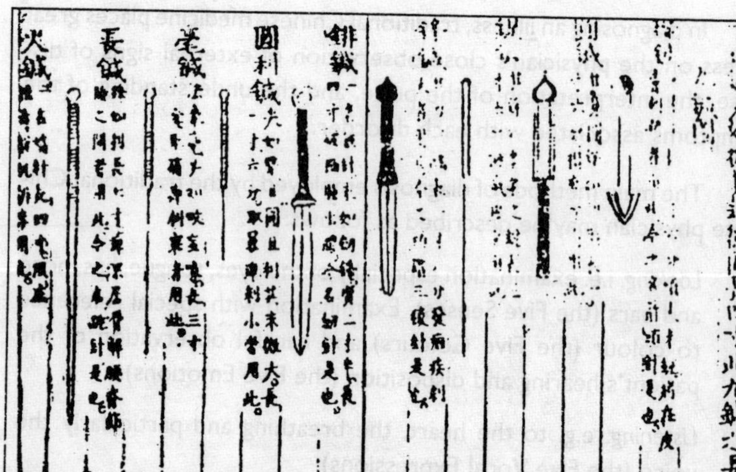

A page from the *Zhen Jiu Da Cheng* compiled in 1601 A.D.

respect the development of acupuncture anaesthesia may be taken as an example of the ideal combination of the two systems of medicine, and help to break down the artificial barriers between this traditional medicine and modern scientific medicine.

The theoretical concepts of the traditional medicine were based on the explanation of the cosmos in terms of the universalistic Chinese philosophy of *Yin* and *Yang*. According to this philosophy there is a constant struggle in the Universe between opposing and unifying forces. Man being part of the Universe, all laws that apply to the Universe must apply to him, and his health is determined by the fluctuations of these forces. Basically, it is an homoeostatic or regulatory concept of health and disease. In the healthy state when *Yin* and *Yang* are in balance, normal vital energy (or "Qi"[8]) which flows through the channels of the body) is produced. An excess or deficiency of Yin or Yang produces an imbalance of this vital energy which is disease.

The *Ling Shu* section of the Huang Di Nei Jing deals at length with the Channels and points on the body. It describe in detail the diseases which can be cured by acupuncture and the various methods of needling.

Acupuncture in China has a known history spread over some 5,000 years. In the earliest times stone needles were used. Later, needles made of bone and bamboo were developed. The use of metal needles had evolved by the times of the compilation of the Huang Di Nei Jing. A popular explanation offered for the discovery of acupuncture is the story of a warrior wounded by an arrow; the arrow was removed and the wound healed and then it was observed that a disease in an unrelated part of the body was cured. The story may be apocryphal, but it is evident that, over the years, a cause and effect relationship was worked out by observant physicians between the punctured point and the disease it cured, and then ultimately point and the disease it cured and then ultimately a whole series of points was charted. It was also realised that neither the size nor the depth

8 Pronounced "chee " as in "cheek"

HUANG DI NEI JING

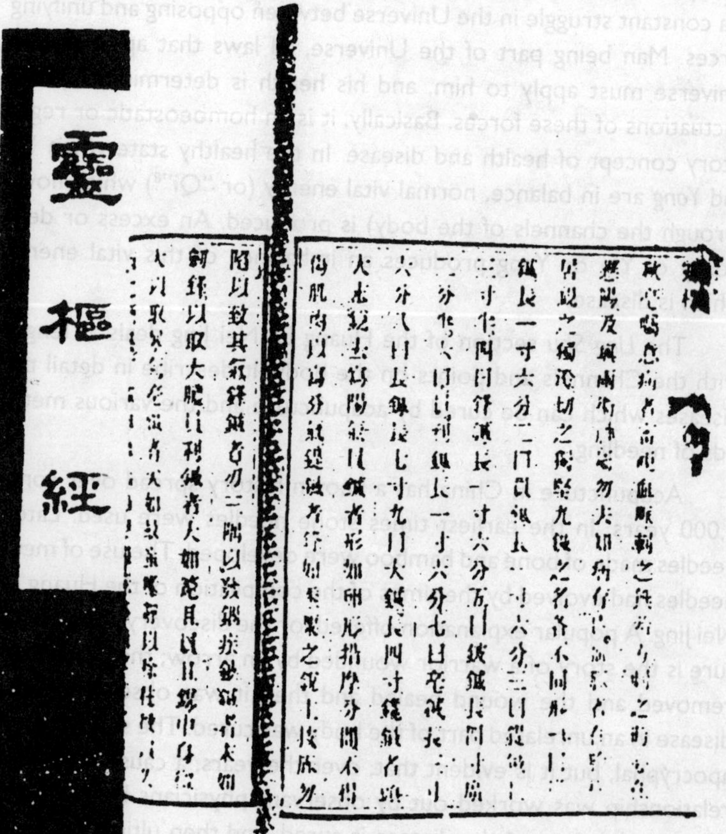

A page from the *Ling Shu* — describing the nine kinds of needles and their uses.

of the puncture was important but rather its exact location (i.e., the acupuncture point). The Channels or Meridians were formed by connecting together points with similar therapeutic properties.[9]

Traditional medicine served the Chinese people well into the 19th century. Thereafter China came into contact with Western medicine, which the British brought with them after the First Opium War of 1837 to 1842.

But there was a distrust of Western medicine among the people derived, perhaps, from the reason that it reached them after the Opium Wars. With the overthrow of the emperors, a new Republic was established in 1911 under President Sun Yat-Sen. In 1927 Chiang Kai-shek, the leader of the Kuomindang party became the National President, after a protracted civil war. The Kuomindang did not think very much of traditional medicine, calling it "unscientific quackery". President Chiang Kai-shek went so far as to propose a decree banning its practice, but had to retract when faced with strong protests from the public.

Mao-Zedong's People's Republic was established in 1949 after the overthrow of Chiang Kai-shek's government. Soon after their accession to power, the first National Hygiene Conference (1950) proclaimed a new set of medical principles which included the traditional methods of healing. One reason was the policy of Mao Zedong's government of preserving the national heritage; another was a more pragmatic policy of delivering adequate health care to the 650 million people at that time, with the available manpower and other resources. There were only 10,000 physicians trained in Western medicine to serve this entire population. To cope with this inadequacy, about half a million practitioners of traditional medicine were co-opted into the public health service.

At the time of the Revolution, according to some estimates, there were four million deaths annually from communicable diseases.

9 Recent archaeological excavations near Xian have discovered ancient manuscripts with channels, but no points. This discovery conflicts with the orthodox teaching.

THE HUANG DI NEI JING

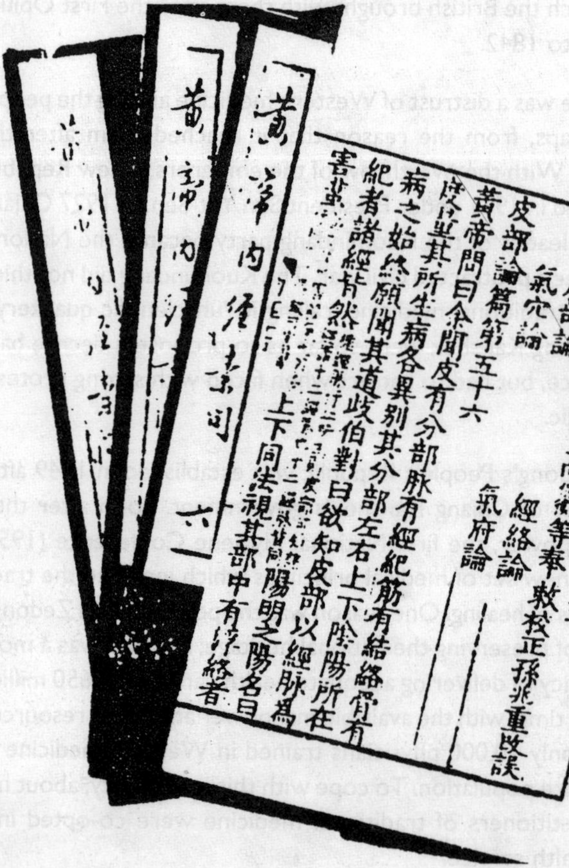

重廣補註黃帝內經素問卷第十五
啟玄子次注林億孫奇高保衡等奉敕校正孫兆重改誤
皮部論 經絡論
氣穴論 氣府論
皮部論篇第五十六
黃帝問曰余聞皮有分部脈有經紀筋有結絡骨有
度量其所生病各異別其分部左右上下陰陽所在
病之始終願聞其道岐伯對曰欲知皮部以經脈爲
紀者諸經皆然
陽明之陽名曰
害蜚
上下同法視其部中有浮絡者
六

Some pages from the *Su Wen*.

Starvation, drug addiction and prostitution were rampant. The infant mortality rate was over 200 per 1,000 in China[10].

The new government in 1949 organised the health services with four main objectives and, over the last four decades have made vast strides in its health service:

(1) To give priority for preventive work, on the following lines:

a) improving the physical health of the people;

b) eliminating the four pests, viz., rats, bed bugs, mosquitoes and flies;

c) popularising health knowledge, particularly preventive medicine.

(2) To improve environmental sanitation and personal hygiene.

(3) To ensure that no environmental pollution occurs from industry and agriculture.

(4) To carry out preventive innoculation programs.

In order to carry out these objectives the health service was organised according to the following four principles:

i) Serving the workers and peasants in the rural areas.

ii) Giving priority to prevention.

iii) Integrating the healers of traditional medicines and Western medicine.

iv) Integrating public health work with mass movement. (After the death of Mao Zedong intensive work on population control in China is being carried out).

It was as a result of these re-organisations that the "bare-foot doctor" evolved as a unique cadre of medical personnel created to suit the needs of rural China. As their picturesque name suggests, these practitioners were recruited at the local level for para-medical work in their native villages. In the post-cultural Revolution period,

10 The highest recorded in the world.

over two million bare-foot doctors were trained. Today, the majority of bare foot doctors work under the direction of the production brigades in the co-operative medical system.

While the bare-foot doctors work in their backward rural settings using local resources and materials, in the major hospitals and research centres of the country, the techniques of traditional medicine are being critically investigated on scientific lines in order to produce a true synthesis of traditional and modern medicine. Many foreign physicians visiting China have been impressed by the high quality of health care being administered today, to over one billion people who form about one fourth of the human race. The remarkable advances in health care over the past quarter century in the People's Republic of China have drawn the attention of the World Health Organisation to actively promote traditional medicine and to adopt the Chinese patterns of health care in many developing countries of the Third World.

With the spread of Chinese acupuncture to the West[11] while it gained a great degree of respect among its adherents an even greater degree of disbelief spread among its opponents, due probably to a lack of a proper scientific explanation. In as much as its adherents became evangelical in promoting it, its critics have consistently maintained that it lacks a proper scientific explanation and it cannot therefore be accepted.

The lack of an explanation regarding a phenomenon does not make it any the less likely that it exists. Modern medicine uses many empirical materials and methods. Aspirin[12] for example, the commonest drug in use today, does not have or need a scientific explana-

11 The main thrust of acupuncture to the West occurred after President Nixon's visit to China (1972). An article by the celebrated reporter James Reston in the **New York Times** woke up the Western medical Societies to the existence of this curious oriental healing art of acupuncture.

12 Reverend Edward Stone in 1757 discovered the bitter taste of bark of the white willow tree which reminded him of the bitter Cinchona bark while taking a walk near the meadows of Chipping Norton in Britain. He successfully treated 50 neighbours for fever with the bark extract. In 1899 Felix Hoffmann extracted the active principle and named it "Aspirin".

tion as it is empirically a very useful drug. Many procedures of Western medicine, for example physiotherapy, hypnotherapy and psychotherapy have doubtful scientific explanations, although they are used as part of the Western scientific therapeutic armamentarium.

A noteworthy feature of the past decade has been the curious tendency of many Western medical societies to take steps to ban traditional practitioners from practising acupuncture, while they themselves are enlarging on their acupuncture practices. This is proof positive that acupuncture works and highlights its growing popularity among the public, the world over.

At present, there are many theories to explain the many facets of acupuncture, but no integrated theory is as yet available to cover all its manifold aspects. Mindful of the fact that, even in the People's Republic of China, serious research into acupuncture commenced only after the Cultural Revolution, it is not surprising that more time will be needed to unravel such a complex neuro-physiological phenomenon as this. The discovery of the endorphin mechanism in the last decade appears to be a promising lead in explaining some effects of acupuncture. In the meantime, all critical observers will concede that acupuncture is useful in curing or alleviating the vast majority of disorders. The clinical results achieved are overwhelming, and the side effects are minimal. Of course, acupuncture is not a panacea for all human ills. But in the hands of a sensible person the needle does really work wonders. One-fourth of the human race has been employing acupuncture, even before history was written. There is no reason why we should not continue to use it, on an empirical basis, till a fuller explanation is discovered. With the upward surge of health costs the world over, there is little doubt that acupuncture and other forms of alternative medicines, will occupy an increasingly important place in the relief of human suffering. It is gratifying to see that the young practitioners of today are adopting an holistic approach to health, discarding the tunnel vision of an earlier generation of orthodox Western physicians in "scientific blinkers".

In the post-Mao Zedong era, with the policy of modernisation in the upswing, many aspects of life are undergoing sweeping changes in China. With Deng Xiaoping at the helm of policy making, a renewed interest in acupuncture is evident. The first National Symposium of Acupuncture and Moxibustion was held in 1979[13] in Peking. Representatives of all countries were invited and Chairman Hua personally met all the delegates from the different countries. The Symposium itself was a field day for the scientist, rather than the practitioner. This is an obvious effort on the part of China to establish acupuncture on a scientific footing rather than leave it as traditional medicine. It is evident in places like the Academy of Traditional Chinese Medicine and the Shanghai Institute of Physiology, that a new Scientific Acupuncture is being gestated by the scientists. A more pragmatic science will probably evolve in time that will be immensely acceptable to the practising Western trained physician, and the intellectual caucus who wish to see all healing structured on the Newtonian-Cartesian paradigm.

In the meantime many aspects of traditional acupuncture such as pulse diagnosis, the semantics of hot and cold, excess and deficiency will worry the modern practitioner till modern scientific equivalents for these traditional paradigms are formulated.

With the introduction of modern practices such as[14] *Electrotherapy, EAV, Ryodoraku, Lasertherapy, Magnetotherapy, Reflexotherapy* and so on, the face of traditional Chinese clinical medical practice has undergone sweeping changes, during the past few years. The discovery of a plethora of neurotransmitters, hormonal mechanisms, neural mechanisms, which are triggered by needling have swung the pen-

13 The Second National symposium was held in August 1984 in Beijing.

14 The combination of Acupuncture with Moxa (moxa-on-a-needle) is also a very popular form of therapy in China in Yin type of deficiency disorders. Modern innovations, such as the use of acupuncture with modern anaesthetics (Acuesthesia) for anaesthesia in surgery, and the combined use of acupuncture and homoeopathy on the needle (homoeopuncture) have also been carried by the present author with success at the Institute of Acupuncture, Kalubowila. See paper titled "Homoeopuncture" presented at 3rd European Acupuncture Symposium, Stockholm, Sweden (June, 1984).

dulum of credibility on acupuncture in one great leap forward from a folk medicine to a sophisticated finely tuned neuro-humoral mechanism, which probably it is.

The World Heath Organisation at the last Interregional Seminar, Beijing 1979, drew up the following provisional list of disorders that lend themselves to acupuncture treatment. The list is based on clinical experience (and not necessarily based on controlled research).

Upper Respiratory Tract:

Acute sinusitis

Acute rhinitis

Common cold

Acute tonsillitis

Respiratory System:

Acute bronchitis

Bronchial asthma (most effective in children and in patients without complicating diseases)

Disorders of the Eye:

Acute conjunctivitis

Central retinitis

Myopia (in children)

Cataract (without complications)

Disorders of the Mouth:

Toothache, post-extraction pain

Gingivitis

Acute and chronic pharyngitis

Gastro-intestinal Disorders:

Spasms of the oesophagus and cardia

Hiccough

Gastroptosis

Acute and chronic gastritis

Gastric hyperacidity

Chronic duodenal ulcer (pain relief)

Acute duodenal ulcer (without complications)

Acute and chronic colitis

Acute bacilliary dysentery

Constipation

Diarrhoea

Paralytic ileus

Neurological and Musculo-skeletal Disorders:

Headache and migraine

Trigeminal neuralgia

Facial palsy (early stage. i.e., within three to six months)

Paresis following a stroke

Peripheral neuropathies

Sequelae of poliomyelities (early stage i.e. within six months)

Meinere's disease

Neurogenic bladder dysfunction

Nocturnal enuresis

Intercostal neuralgia

Cervicobrachial syndrome

"Frozen shoulder", "tennis elbow"

Sciatica

Low-back pain

Osteoarthritis

The only criticism is that this list was drawn up by a panel of Western qualified clinicians. It would have been more gracious for the W.H.O. to have allowed a few traditional practioners to be on this committee and have this list of disorders set out in their traditional equivalents as well, in listing these disorders. The W.H.O. held another ill-advised meeting in Manila, Phillipines in 1983, to revise the names of acupuncture points. Such a hare-brained scheme was doomed to failure.

The traditional historical names of acupuncture points are followed by millenia of usage. To rename them or re-number them now, would be tantamount to sacrilege. Many such revisionist tendencies exist in the world of modern clinical practice. The odious, exhibitionist practice of some present day practitioners of naming acupuncture points by their own names must be ostracised in all serious journals and publications.

■

MODERN SCIENTIFIC VIEWS

"There are many things in heaven and earth, Horatio,

that are not dreamt of in your philosophy". Hamlet (Act I Sc. V)

Acupuncture, the ancient Chinese art of healing, has become popular the world over during the past few decades. Not only as an anaesthetic agent for surgical operations, but in many diseases, which are resistant to conventional forms of therapy, acupuncture has proved remarkably effective. Besides being free from the side effects commonly encountered in drug therapy, it is a simple, safe, effective and economical form of therapy. Therefore, slowly but surely, it is being integrated into the mainstream of modern medicine. Many prestigious hospitals, universities, and medical schools around the world have now established departments for acupuncture research, therapy and analgesia.[1]

Whether acupuncture works or not, is no longer the question today. The only question is "how does it work?" This in not an easy question, which can be fully answered in our present state of knowledge. After several decades of dedicated research we know very little of how the normal nervous system functions in health, let alone

1 The Karolinska Institute, Stockholm, Sweden; for instance, the ivory tower which awards Nobel Prizes annually in Western medicine and allied sciences, has established a Pain Clinic with acupuncture since 1982.

in disease. Serious research on acupuncture commenced only a few years ago, and such a short period of time has been insufficient to unravel all the mechanisms of the complicated neurophysiological phenomenon, which acupuncture evidently is. Part of the difficulty lies in the fact that acupuncture works in a great variety of disorders and its action must, therefore, be assumed to vary, to some extent, with each type of pathology. Nevertheless, many aspects of its action are now being understood in the light of recent research and these are now being pieced together in an attempt to solve this profound enigma.

The effects observed on needling are both subjective and objective. One of the subjective effects may be slight pain at the site of needling, but with the use of a proper technique by a trained acupuncturist this is usually negligible. Another important subjective effect is the appearance of a peculiar sensation, which is called "deqi" in Chinese. There is no exact equivalent for this term in English, but it is usually translated as "take". The deqi which the patient feels is a combinations of numbness, heaviness, slight soreness, and distension. Radiation of one or more of these sensations may also occur along the channel. For acupuncture analgesia to be successful it is essential that adequate "deqi" is elicited.[2]

As regards the objective effects produced by needling six different effects may be recognised. Of these the best known is the **analgesic (pain-relieving)** effect, which is achieved by the raising of the pain threshold. This is the physiological basis of acupuncture anaesthesia and also explains how acupuncture analgesia similarly produced, during therapy is able to relieve the pain of arthritis, toothache, headache, low backache and other similar painful disorders. Some acupuncture points are more effective, in this respect, than others. This

---

2 According to many authorities the eliciting of 'deqi' or acupuncture sensation is necessary in acupuncture anaesthesia, painful conditions and in acute disorders only.

is an example of the principle of "the specificity of acupuncture points".[3]

Secondly, the needling of certain specific acupuncture points results in **sedation.** Some people may even fall asleep during treatment, but wake up refreshed. It has been shown that there is a decrease in delta and theta wave activity on the electro-encephalogram during acupuncture treatment. These effect are utilised in the acupuncture treatment of insomnia, anxiety states, addictions, epilepsies, mental disorders and behavioural problems.

The third effect is very important; it is called the *homeostatic or regulatory* effect, which means adjustment of the internal environment of the body towards a state of normal balance. Generally, homeostasis is maintained by the balanced activity of the sympathetic and parasympathetic divisions of the autonomic nervous system and also by the endocrine system. In addition, there are numerous homeostatic mechanisms in the body for regulating the respiration, heart rate, blood pressure, urinary excretion, metabolic rate, sweating, temperature, ionic balance of the blood and many other vital parameters. These mechanisms are seriously deranged in many diseases, and in such cases, acupuncture has been very helpful in restoring the original state of equilibrium. Very often, the same set of points may be used for treating opposite disorders like high and low blood pressure, or diarrhoea and constipation. These are examples of the homeostatic or normalising action of acupuncture.

Fourthly, there is the *immune-enhancing* action of acupuncture, whereby body resistance to disease is strengthened. This has been shown to be due to an increase in the white corpuscles (leucocytosis), antibodies, gammaglobulins and other substances, which increase the resistive powers of the body. In many cases a two to four fold

3. Some authorities believe that acupuncture points do not exist. It is the myotome, dermatome or sclerotome of the disordered segment or segments that is important. Further, there are points which produce generalised effects probably mediated through the central nervous system, the autonomic nervous system or through neurotransmitters.

increase in antibody titre has been observed, presumably brought about by activation of the reticulo-endothelial system. Acupuncture is, therefore, very useful in combating infections. Where antibiotics may have to be used, the need for prolonged antibiotic therapy can be considerably reduced by the concurrent use of acupuncture. It is also indicated in case of resistance or hypersensitivity to antibiotics and in chronic infections where the antibiotics have failed or given rise to serious side-effects. In the People's Republic of China, it has been shown that acupuncture alone can be effective in infections, like appendicitis and tonsillitis. Here again, certain specific points have to be used to enhance the immunological effects.

(According to some workers, acupuncture may cause release of interferon and may be helpful in treating certain malignant disorders).[4]

The fifth objective effect of acupuncture is the *psychological effect*, which is a calming and tranquilizing action apart from mere sedation. This is believed to be due to an action on the mid-brain reticular formation and certain other specific areas of the brain. Measurable effects have also been reported on the metabolic chemistry of brain tissue. For instance, there is an increase in the dopamine content of brain after acupuncture. This may account for its effectiveness in certain mental disorders and in parkinsonism, where there is a depletion of the dopamine content of the brain.[5]

The psychlogical effect mentioned above should not be confused with hypnosis or autosuggestion. These effects follow (they do not precede) the use of acupuncture, and are, therefore, not a precondition of its success, as erroneously supposed by some critics. Hypnosis and suggestion are very different from acupuncture in many important respects. Hypnotism has been found to work only in 10 to 15 per cent of a population, whereas some degree of acupuncture

4 At the Institute of Acupuncture Kalubowila, certain malignant disorders have been treated with acupuncture successfully.

5 Several other neurotransmitters and hormones have been demonstrated to increase in brain tissue following acupuncture.

analgesia may be induced in any person or animal. Patients with low hypnotisability scores respond equally well to acupuncture as those with high scores, showing that suggestibility is by no means a requisite factor for success in acupuncture treatment. Also, prolonged training periods are required for hypnotic analgesia, whereas emergency surgery may also be performed under acupuncture analgesia. Spontaneity of movements, gestures and facial expressions are found in acupunctured patients unlike in hypnotised patients, who move around like robots. Further, injection, of local anaesthetic (procaine block) at acupuncture points, or injection of nalaxone have been found to nullify the analgesic effects of acupuncture, thus pointing to a non-hypnotic explanation.[6]

The sixth important effect of acupuncture is that it hastens *the motor recovery* in patients who have become paralysed from some cause or another. Even late cases of motor paralysis, respond well to acupuncture therapy, despite previous failure with other forms of therapy. The explanation, which is complex, apparently involves antidromic stimulation of the anterior horn cells and their re-activation through a bio-feedback mechanism, operating through the Renshaw and Cajal cells of the spinal cord, or their cranial equivalents. (*Motor Gate Theory:* Jayasuriya and Fernando, Paper presented at the Fifth World Congress on Acupuncture, Tokyo, 1977)

What has been discussed above are the physiological effects of needling. As regards the scientific explanation of these effects, numerous theories have been formulated in recent times. The earlier theories of simple reflex action[7] are insufficient, as the neurological pathways are complex. The situation has become further complicated by the demonstration that humoral (chemical) factors are also involved in acupuncture. As far as pain relief is concerned, the most

---

6 A good healer will of course, complement the physiological effects with appropriate psychological reinforcement.
The injection of local anaesthetic into acupuncture points is carried out in the discipline called 'neural-therapy'.

7 Somato-visceral reflexes – Segmental Theory – Embryological Theory.

THE MOTOR GATE THEORY

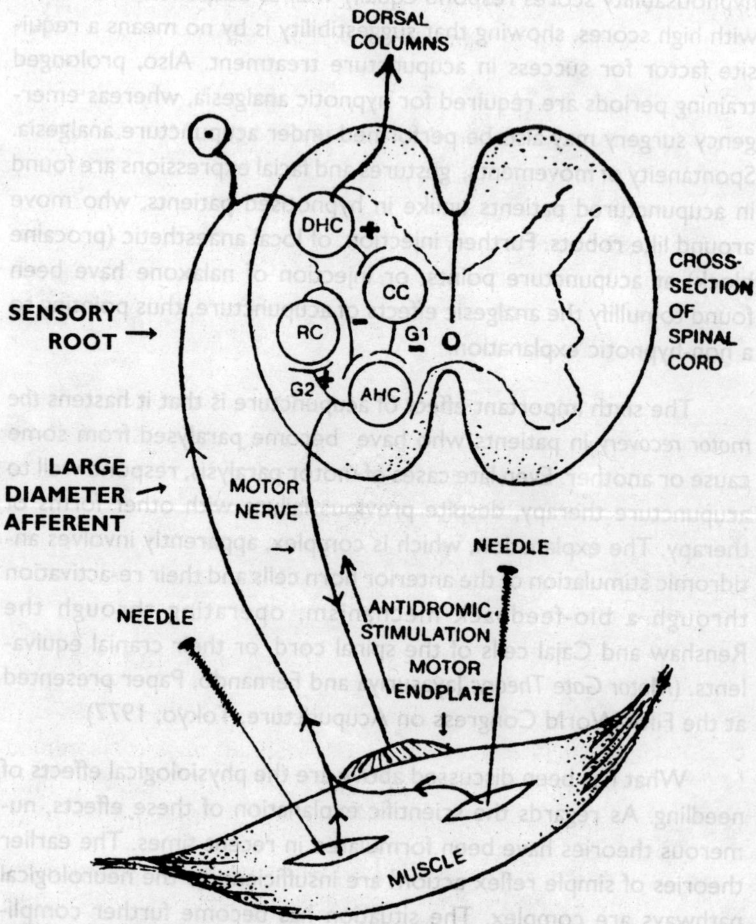

DHC = Dorsal Hom Cell
CC = Cajal Cell
AHC = Anterior Hom Cell
RC = Renshaw Cell
G1 = Gate I
G2 = Gate 2

Hypothesis to explain the mechanisms of motor recovery in paralytic conditions when acupuncture therapy is carried out. (From a paper read at the 5th World Congress of Acupuncture, Tpkhyo, October, 1977).

SCHEMATIC DIAGRAM OF THE GATE CONTROL THEORY OF PAIN (Melzack & Wall - 1965)

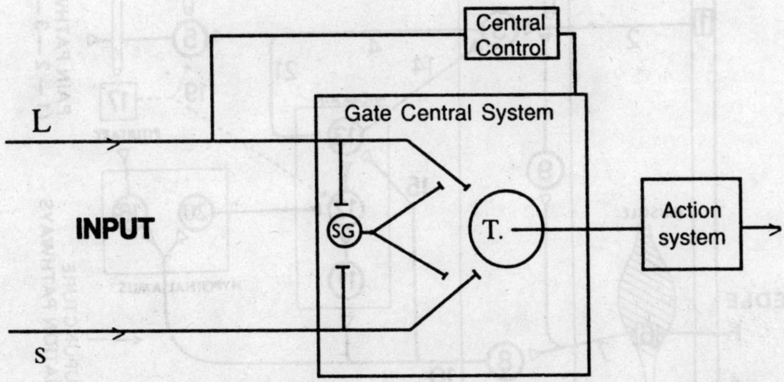

L.	= Large Diameter Fibres.
S.	= Small Diameter Fibres.
S.G.	= Substantia Gelatinosa.
T.	= First Central Transmission Cells

The main site of "the gate" is the substantia gelatinosa. The small fibres open the gate for pain; the large fibres close this physiological gate.

(Other workers have postulated multiple gates at higher levels of the central nervous system).

From Pain-Mechanism: A New Theory by R. Melzack and P.D. Wall, Science 150: 971- 979 (1965).

HOW ACUPUNCTURE SUPRESSES PAIN.

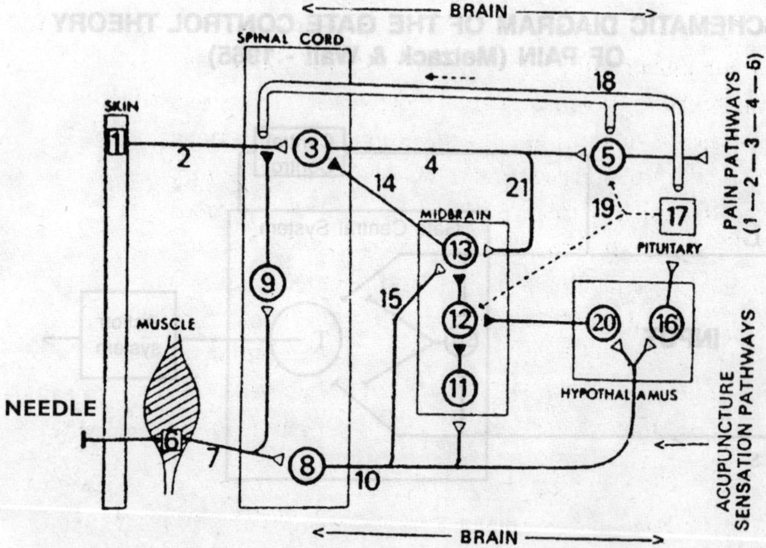

Pain pathway is 1--> 2 --> 3 --> 4 -->5

1. Skin—point of painful stimulation
2. Deeper tissues—`C' fibres carrying pain sensations to the spinal cord.
3. Spinal cord —the dorsal horn.
4. Spino-thalamic tract.
5. Thalamic & basal ganglia, limbic system.
6. Deep receptors of muscles (acupuncture point stimulated by needle)
7. `A' fibres carrying acupuncture sensations to the spinal cord.
8. Dorsal horn cell.
9. Gate Control Mechanism. Intra-segmental pain relief mechanism.
10. Ascending pathways to the brain.
11. Peri-aqueductal gray. } enkephalins proruced by low frequency stimulation.
12. Reticular formation }
13. Raphe system.
14. Dorso-lateral fibers (serotonin mechanism)
15. Direct stimulation of the raphe system to activate the serotonergic system. This occurs when high frequency lectro-stimulation (over 200 Hertz) is carried out.
16. Acupuncture sensation pathway through hypothalamus to the pituitary.
17. Pituitary.
18. Endorphins carried from pituitary in the cerebrospinal fluid to the thalamus and spinal cord (endorphins act as a hormone)
19. Endorphin flow from pituitary to the thalamus and reticular formation (endorphins act as a neurotransmitter).
20. Acupuncture sensation reaching the reticular formation through the hypothalamus.
21. Pathway --> 13--> 14 is a negative feed-back mechanism to the pain pathway.

The centre where pain is felt is unknown.

popular neurological explanation is based on the *"Gate Control Theory of Pain"* proposed by R. Melzack and P.D. Wall in 1965. According to this theory, our perception of pain is modulated by a functional gate (or gates) within the central nervous system. Under normal circumstances this gate is wide open and pain impulses (via the small diameter fibres) get through quite easily. But when acupuncture needling is carried out, a second stream of non-painful impulses is set up from the site of needling (via the large diameter fibres)[8]. The result is overcrowding or jamming at the gate causing it to close. In other words, there is competitive inhibition of the pain impulses and no pain (or less pain) is felt, even during a surgical operation. The autonomic nervous system is also believed to play an important role in acupuncture. There is experimental evidence to show that, it is along the sympathetic plexuses surrounding blood vessels that some of the acupuncture impulses travel to the spinal cord and brain.

Chemical or humoral mechanisms are also involved in acupuncture. For instance, if a rabbit is acupunctured its pain threshold is found to rise. If the cerebrospinal fluid from this animal is then circulated into a non-acupunctured rabbit, the pain threshold of the second animal also rises, showing that chemical transmitters are definitely involved in the mechanism of acupuncture. The exact nature of these chemical transmitters is still under investigation; however, the work of Bruce Pomeranz (Professor of Neurobiology, Toronto University) and his co-workers suggest that the naturally occuring endorphins play a prominent part. Pomeranz believes that, by binding on to the opiate receptors in the brain cells, the endorphins released by acupuncture could produce the analgesic effect.

Research carried out at Shanghai Institute of Physiology by Professor Chang Hsiang-Tung[9] and his co-workers indicate that 5 hydroxy tryptamine (serotonin) is also actively involved in the mechanism of acupuncture analgesia. Over 100 other neurotransmitters,

---

8 The deqi or acupuncture sensation.

9 Zhang-Xiang Tung in Pinyin.

GRAPHIC REPRESENTATION OF THE PATH OF PAIN BEING BLOCKED BY ENKEPHALIN

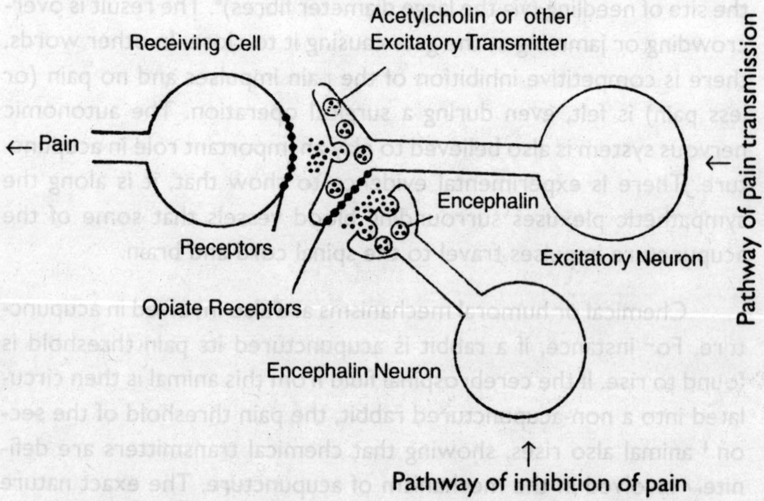

The phenomenon is known as pre-synaptic inhibition.

Different opiate neuro-transmitters are involved at different locations in the central nervous systems. Non-opiate neural mechanisms and hormonal mechanisms are also involved in the pain relief mechanism with acupuncture.

which may be possibly involved in the pain mechanism have now been described.[10]

The endorphins originate in the pituitary and the midbrain raphe mechanism; the latter chemicals are termed enkephalins. The pituitary endorphins are secreted as a part of a long chain molecule Beta-lipotropin. This molecule is a pituitary hormone 91 amino acids long, and has amino acid sequences with several distinct physiological functions. The peptide chain as a whole induces the metabolism of fat, as does the segment termed gamma-lipotropin (aminoacid units 1 through 58). The sequence 41 through 58 is that of the hormone beta-melanotropin, which plays a role in skin pigmentation. The sequence 61 through 91 is that of beta-endorphin, a pituitary peptide that has analgesic effects, when it is injected intravenously or is injected directly into the brain. A second pituitary peptide, designated alpha-endorphin (61 through 76) has similar but less potent effects. The beta-lipotropin sequence 61 through 65 is identical with that of methionine-enkephalin, a morphine like peptide found in the brain, the spinal cord and the intestines. The relation between the opiate-like peptides and beta-lipotropin is not known.

The mechanism of how enkephalin inhibits pain may be indirect. Instead of acting directly on the receiving nerve cell the substance may block the release of directly acting neurotransmitters such as acetylcholine and glutamate, thereby reducing the receiving cell's excitatory input. According to Bruce Pomeranz's model, enkephalin released from a neuron binds to the opiate receptors on the terminal of an excitatory neuron, partially depolarizing the terminal membrane and reducing the nett depolarization produced by the arrival of a nerve impulse. The amount of neurotransmitter released from the terminal is proportional to the nett depolarization, so that less excitatory transmitter is released. The receiving cell is then exposed to less excitatory stimulation and reduces its firing rate. This phenomenon is called *pre-synaptic inhibition.* Such an en-

---

10 A few neurotransmitters enhance or potentiate pain.

kephalin inhibitory system may also modulate the activity of the ascending pain pathways in the spinal cord and the brain. Opiate drugs would act by binding to unoccupied enkephalin receptors, thereby potentiating the effect of the system. Antipeptidases have a potentiating action on the analgesic effect by preventing the premature destruction of the enkephalin. Recently, several non-opiate pathways have also been demonstrated. These findings have been confirmed by several other workers. Promeranz (Canada), Lars Terenius (Sweden), Chapmen and Mayer (United States), are the leading workers on endorphins outside the People's Republic of China. Their work has strengthened the credibility of this millennia old science.

Today, the objective existence of acupuncture points is no longer in serious doubt. Biomedical engineers and research scientists have established, by painstaking investigations, they are, in fact, points of lowered electrical resistance on the skin. By making use of this principle they have been able to devise instruments called **"acupunctuscopes",** which can electronically detect the exact position of the points. The points detected by this modern method have been found to correspond very closely to those found on the ancient Chinese charts. Acupuncture points have also been found to display the phenomenon of bioluminescence when studied under high frequency radiation photography (Kirlian and Kirlian, 1939). As regards the channels, the evidence is less conclusive, but the recent work of Professor Robert O. Becker and his co-workers at the Department of Orthopaedic Surgery, Upstate Medical Centre, Syracuse, New York, suggests that the acupuncture points and channels represent a primitive transmitting and control system working by means of D.C. electronic signalling. According to Becker, the channels appear to be communication routes and the acupuncture points are "booster amplifiers" or power stations (booster transformers), which restore signal strength and maintain intelligibility of transmission over long distances. Also, certain isotopes injected subcutaneously seem to follow the pathways of the channels rather than the vascular, lymph or nervous pathways[11].

11 Many workers believe that neither the points nor channels exist peripherally. They may be a central neurological representation.

The effectiveness of certain specific acupuncture points, such as the distal points and the confluent points are explained on the *Thalamic Neuron Theory,* which postulates that the central representation of the acupuncture points in the thalamus[12] are minaturized into a foetal homonculus.

The ancient Chinese believed that disease ("dis-ease"[13]), was caused by the imbalance in the body of two principles, which they called *Yin* and *Yang:* By Yin they meant the negative or female principle, while Yang was the positive or male principle, both of which are universally present in all nature. In the healthy state, there was believed to be a harmonious balance between these opposite but mutually interacting principles—a state of affairs which today we would call "homeostasis". But when disease supervenes, it was believed that one or other principle becomes dominant at the expense of the other. Corrections of this imbalance was achieved by the needling of selected acupuncture points. While these ideas may look esoteric and irrational from today's stand-point, one must remember that they were man's first steps in logical thinking. To have formulated these ideas at a time when the rest of the world was living in caves and on tops of trees was, itself, a remarkable intellectual achievement of analytical thinking and penetrative insight.

Modern scientific medicine is built on the study of chemical changes in disease; the basis of traditional acupuncture is correction of the energy imbalances. What we know today of homeostatic bodily mechanisms has an unmistakable Yin-Yang paradigm. If a modern physician accepts this position, there is no contradiction in practising acupuncture, as no one who is familiar with this discipline has any doubts that it works, and not infrequently when all other modalities have failed.

Thus, obviously, there is no dearth of theories to account for the many aspects of acupuncture. What is really lacking, at the mo-

12 Or other sensory centre.

13 Lack of ease.

ment, is an integrated theory which covers all the known facets. The very fact that there is a multiplicity of theories is an admission that each theory by itself, is unable to explain all the innumerable facets of the acupuncture phenomenon. This is no reason, however, for the modern physician to be unduly disturbed. The lack of a complete scientific explanation regarding some phenomenon does not make it any less likely that the phenomenon exists, still less does it eliminate the possibility of putting it to practical use. If we look dispassionately at so-called "modern scientific medicine" we find only an empirical basis, or none at all, for many procedures that are carried out daily. For example, many high-powered procedures in physical medicine such as short-wave, micro-wave and iontophoresis, do not have much scientific basis for their medical applications. In fact, what little research that has been done on these methods has shown their value to be nil, or at the most equal to a hot water bottle! Similarly, it has not yet been shown in the long term therapy of rheumatic disorders that the administration of large doses of analgesics and steroids changes the natural history of the disease for the better, any more than the untreated case.[4]

It is against the backdrop of such present day practices and the spiralling incidence of iatrogenic (drug-induced) diseases, that the safety and efficacy of acupuncture should be judged. Theories, hypotheses, conjectures and speculations are interesting, and essential for scientific research to proceed, but they should not be regarded as immutable. Theories in medicine change from decade to decade. Books on Western pharmacology and therapeutics have changed face, almost completely, with each decade over the past century. In no other system, as in Western medical science, has one decade rejected so decisively the therapy of a previous decade, not only as useless, but as even being harmful. The precise action of many drugs such as Aspirin[15] are still obscure but we continue to use them be-

14 Many studies have highlighted the serious complications of using such therapy.

15 The symptomatic use of Aspirin for instance to treat fever is not logical, as the fever is a protective reaction of the organism. This is the commonest use of Aspirin in Western "scientific" medicine.

cause they are effective. Acupuncture is a simple safe, effective and an economical method of therapy. The scientific basis of its action is being clarified to a considerable extent by modern research and its value in clinical medicine is today beyond any reasonable doubt. There is every reason why we should use it in our daily medical practice either alone, or to supplement the deficiencies of other therapeutic methods.

With so many broadminded colleagues, the world over, who are now critically examining traditional healing methods, before long a holistic medicine is bound to emerge, which will serve mankind, even better, in the 21st century. Even though many theories are now current, the secret of acupuncture will not be easily solved. As it is a very complex phenomenon, it will remain a mystery inside, an enigma, surrounded by total darkness, for many more decades to come.

SUMMARY OF THE THEORIES TO EXPLAIN THE ACUPUNCTURE EFFECTS

A. NEUROLOGICAL THEORIES

1) Somato-Visceral Theory (Felix Mann 1960, Ishikawa 1949, 1962).

2) Gate Control Theory (Melzack and Wall, 1965).

3) Multiple Gate Theory (Zhang Xiangtong. 1970), (Man and Chen. 1972).

4) Thalamic Intergration Theory (Zhang Xiangtong 1972).

5) Thalamic Neuron Theory (Tsun-Nin Lee 1977, 1978).

6) Cortical Inhibitory Surround Theory (Neo-Pavlovian).

7) Motor Gate Theory (Jayasuriya and Fernando, 1977).

8) Autonomic Neuron Theory (Ionescu-Tirgoviste 1973).

B. HUMORAL THEORIES (Neurotransmitter Theories)

1) 5- Hydroxytryptamine (Serotonin), (Zhang Xiangtong, 1974, 1976).

2) Endorphin Release Theory (Bruce Pomeranz, 1976).

3) Other neurotransmitters, hormones.

C. BIOELECTRIC THEORIES

1) Kirlian and Kirlian (1939).

2) Becker et al. (1976).

D. EMBRYOLOGICAL THEORY (Segmental Theory) Felix Mann (1972).

E. DEFENCE MECHANISM AND TISSUE REGENERATION THEORY: Cracuim (1973) and others.

F. PSYCHOGENIC AND IDEOLOGICAL THEORY

Theory of Hoax or Hypnosis (Kroger et al. 1972).

G. PLACEBO EFFECT THEORY

American Medical Association (1972).

H. CATASTROPHIC THEORY R. Thom (1975).

I. TRADITIONAL CHINESE THEORIES OF ACUPUNCTURE

(Based on Taoistic Chinese philosophy)

MATERIALS AND TECHNIQUES

MATERIALS

1) THE ACUPUNCTURE NEEDLES

In ancient China, nine different types of needles were used for acupuncture. Although they were called needles, some of them were really in the form of small lances, while others had a small cutting edge. One type of needle had a ball point and was used for micromassage (acu-massage) at the acupuncture point.

The following is a description of the types of needless in common use today:

a) The filiform needles

The filiform needle comprises a handle or holder, and a shaft. The handle may be made of copper, bronze, aluminium, silver or stainless steel. Plastic handled disposable acupuncture needles are also now available. The shaft nowadays is always manufactured from stainless steel (astematic steel).

The length of these needles (i.e., the length of the shaft) varies from 0.5 inch to 8 inches or more. The calibre (diameter) may range

THE PARTS OF AN ACUPUNCTURE NEEDLE

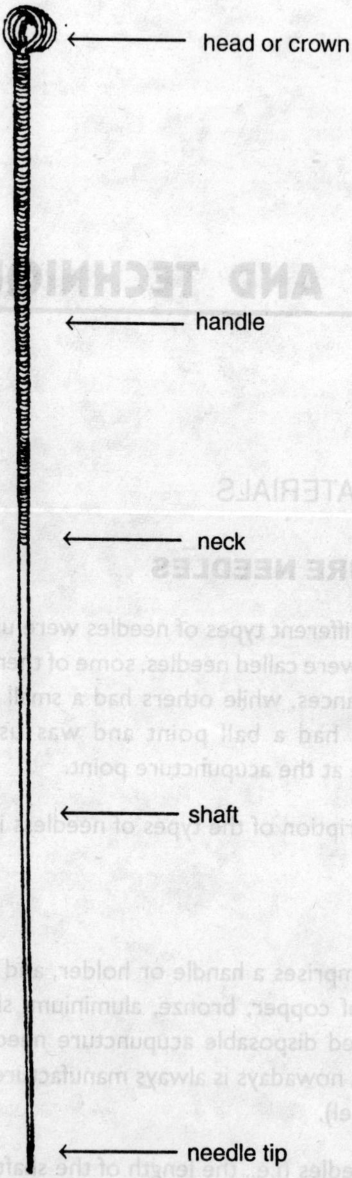

from gauge 26 to 34. The following table shows the standard sizes available:

Length

Inches (cuns[1]):	0.5	1.0	1.5	2.0	2.5	3.0	3.5	4.0	4.5	5.0	6.0
Millimetres:	15	25	40	50	65	75	90	100	115	125	150

Diameter

Standard Wire Gauge No.:........	26	28	30	32	34
Millimetres:	0.45	0.38	0.32	0.26	0.22

For general use the 1.0 inch or 1.5 inch long, No.28 or 30 needles are preferred. Gauge No. 30 (i.e., the thinner needles) are particularly recommended for points in the eye region, in children and for conditions where minimum stimulation is needed. The longer needles are used for areas where the muscular mass is thick. e.g. Huantiao (G.B. 30), and in the puncturing-through technique, where the needle is directed from one point through to another. The thicker needles, Gauge No. 26 and 28, are used in regions where relatively stronger stimulation is required.

b) The embedding needles

Also called the press needle and implanted needle, they come in several shapes, depending on their use.

i) **The thumbtack type:** This looks like a small thumbtack. The body of the needle is in the form of a small circle about 3 mm in diameter and its tip stands out at right angles to the circle. It penetrates to a depth of 2-3 mm. It is used more commonly in ear acupuncture.

1 Refers to the cun of an average adult

POSTURES FOR ACUPUNCTURE

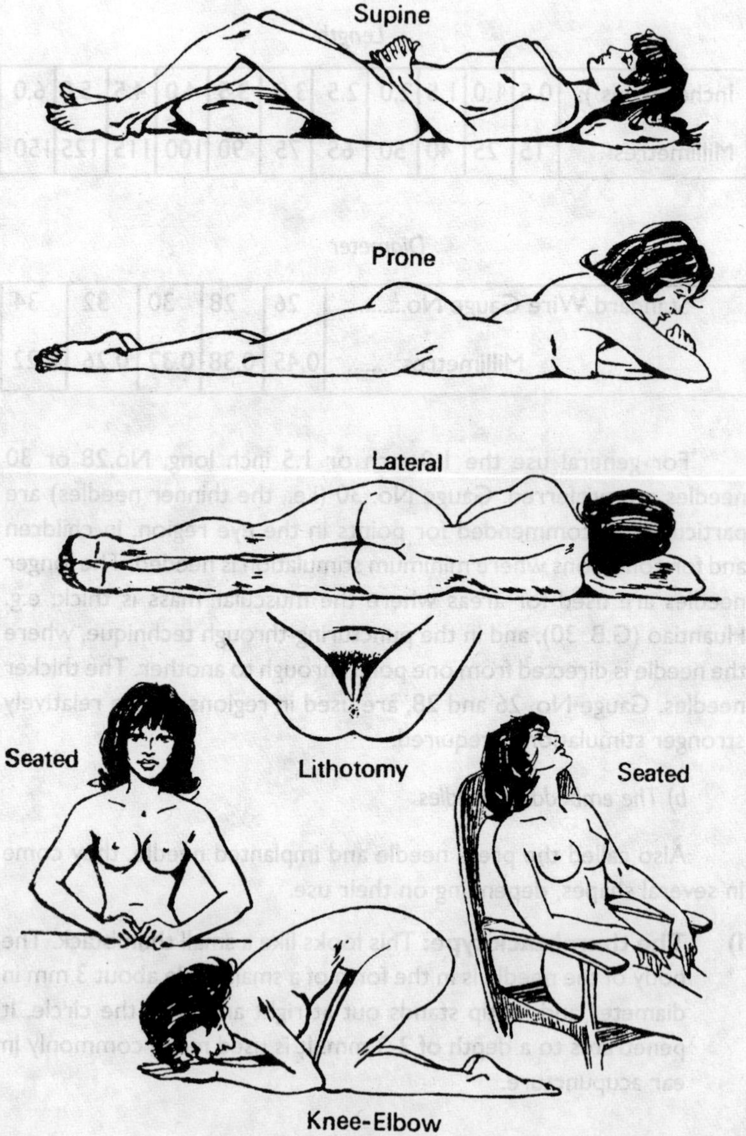

ii) **The "fish tail" type:** This is similar to the thumbtack type, except that its shaft lies at the same plane as its body. This needle is used on certain body acupuncture points for continuous stimulation. It is inserted horizontally under the skin, and then fixed with adhesive tape.

Both these types of needles are indicated in chronic conditions like bronchial asthma, epilepsy and in painful conditions like migraine. They may be kept in place for up to seven days and are, therefore, useful in providing mild stimulation of an acupuncture point between treatment sessions. In warm weather it is advisable to change the needle in about half this time.

iii) **The spherical press needle (ball bearing type):** This may also be used for the same purpose. This is becoming more popular nowadays, as it is safer because there is no chance of damage to cartilage and infection of the ear. It consists of a tiny stainless steel ball which is fixed on the skin at the acupuncture point with adhesive porous tape.[2]

iv) **The muscle embedding needle:** These are slighty longer than the fish tail type and are used to allay very intractable painful conditions like phantom limb pain and the pain of secondary cancer. The muscle embedding needle is left in situ at local painful points in the muscle (Ah-Shi point[3]) for a few days.

c) The "Plum Blossom" needle

This is also known as the "Five Star" or "Seven Star" needle. It is made up of 5 or 7 short filiform needles attached to a holder at the end of long handle. The plum blossom needle is used to tap on the skin along a channel or at specific points. It is indicated in children, in weak patients, in skin diseases and in those who dislike puncturing.

2 This author has been several cases of local skin allergy due to the adhesive tape.

3 Ah-Shi means "Oh Yes" in Chinese. These are painful points (not necessarily acupuncture points) "Oh Yes" is the reaction of the patient when these points are palpated and tenderness is felt.

FINGER MEASUREMENTS

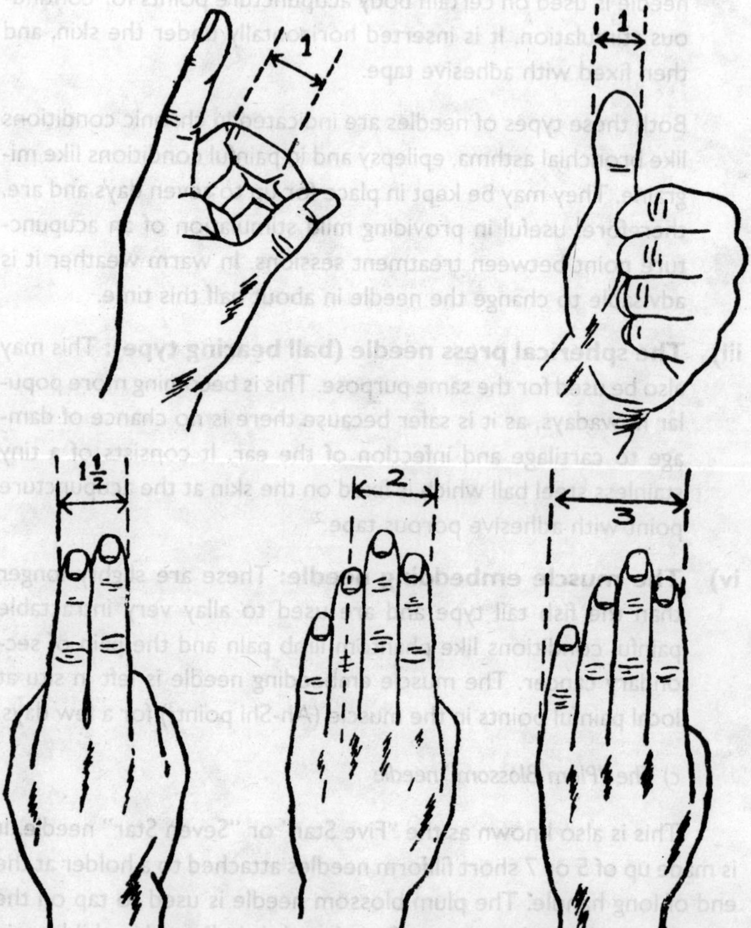

1 cun = 10 fen

2 cun = 2 1/3 finger breadths (of the patient).

5 cun = 6 ½ finger breadths (of the patient).

d) The three-edged (or prismatic) needle

This has a triangular point and is used to bleed certain areas in skin disorders, arthritis, and in acute emergencies. (In modern acupuncture a syringe and an intravenous needle are used for the same purpose)[4].

e) The hot needle

This is a special silver alloy needle which is heated and used to puncture certain superficial lumps, such as "ganglions" on the back of the wrist, thyroid adenomas and other benign tumours.

2) APPARATUS FOR THE ELECTRICAL STIMULATION OF ACUPUNCTURE POINTS VIA NEEDLES

Instead of manual stimulation the needles could also be stimulated by the use of electrical pulses. This is referred to as electro-acupuncture or electro-needle treatment, and was invented in China in 1954. Apart from the advantage of saving on the tedium of manual stimulation, it is possible to regulate precisely the amount of stimulation required. It is also possible to produce stronger stimulation, thus making it a convenient alternative method for acupuncture anaesthesia. There are many kinds of electro-acupuncture apparatus currently available. The type that is most favoured uses a biphasic spiked pulse.

3) APPARATUS FOR THE DETECTION OF ACUPUNCTURE POINTS (ACUPUNCTOSCOPE)

It could be shown that the electrical resistance of the skin at an acupuncture point is less than the resistance of the surrounding area. The acupuncture point detector is an instrument incorporating a

4 Re-injecting the blood at point Taner (U. Ex.) or at Xuehai (Sp. 10.) is also commonly carried out allergies, skin and lung disorders.

circuit which could register the exact point by means of an ammeter or a source of sound, which changes pitch as a suitable electric current passes through the acupuncture point area. There are many varieties of point detectors available. Often they are incorporated in one instrument with the electro-acupuncture stimulator.

The point detector is also useful in diagnosis and prognosis as the skin resistance of an acupuncture point is further lowered in disease. As the patient recovers, it progressively returns to its normal levels.

Electrical point detectors are mainly used in ear acupuncture as the location of the reactive points is important for diagnosis. In electroacupuncture according to Voll (EAV) various homoeopathic remedies can also be tested against the patient.[5]

4) STERILIZATION AND DISINFECTION OF NEEDLES

Sterilization implies the elimination of all living organisms.

Disinfection means the destruction or the removal of pathogenic organisms rendering the object relatively non-infective. It may not destroy all micro-organisms and hence certain bacteria, spores, and viruses may yet remain. However in many clinics in the Third World disinfection, rather than sterilization, is carried out due to economic reasons.

There are physical and chemical methods designed to prevent infection by acupuncture needles.

5 For similarity or isopathy.

A. Physical Methods

I. Heat

a) Dry Heat

i) Fire: A direct flame sterilizes metals at red heat. This principle is used to sterilize the acupuncture needle in hot needle therapy. The needle is held over a spirit lamp flame, till the shaft of the needle becomes red-hot. When the metal is at red heat, no organism thrives on it and, hence, it is a good method of sterilization.

ii) Hot air ovens: Hot air is maintained at 160°C for 1 hour, or 180°C for 20-30 minutes. At this temperature sterilization takes place.

iii) Infrared radiation: Here a temperature of 180°C is maintained for 10 minutes. This is a method employed for large scale sterilization.

iv) Glass bead sterilizer: This is also a dry heat method. Its shortcoming is that it is difficult to sterilize the entire needle.

v) Micro-wave and gamma rays: These methods are used by some needle manufacturers (see below under Radiation).

b) Moist Heat

i) Boiling in water: Boiling water at 100°C for 10-20 minutes destroys most vegetative organisms, but some spores may yet remain. Hence boiling, though a common method of disinfection; it does not guarantee the sterility of the needles.

ii) Autoclaving: An autoclave consists of a closed chamber in which objects are subjected to steam at pressures greater than that of the atmosphere, achieving temperatures of over 100°C. In high vacuum autoclaves, sterilization is possible in 3 minutes at a temperature of 143°C. In the downwards displacement type of autoclave, sterilization is possible in 15 minutes at a temperature of 121^{0}C.

II. Radiation

Ionizing radiation is used in the large scale sterilization of articles and needles. Since it does not destroy plastic materials, it may be used to sterilize the plum-blossom needles. Gamma radiation obtained from radioactive isotopes such as from Cobalt-60 are being used by the manufacturers on a large scale to sterilize surgical instruments.

B. Chemical Methods

Since Lister used "carbolic acid" or phenol, enlightening the world to the importance of antiseptic techniques there have been a vast number of chemicals used throughout the world. (In ancient times many herbal pastes such as saffron were used as disinfectants.)

The commonly used chemicals at the present time are:

a) Surgical spirits-70% alcohol.

b) Cetrimide (Cetavlon)).

c) Chlorhexidine (Hibitane).

d) Chloroxylenol (Dettol).

These chemical methods have only disinfecting propertes. There are many spores and viruses that withstand their action.

In clinics without sterilizing facilities in the Third World, disinfection may be resorted to, with adequate precautions. First, the needles should be boiled in water for 10-20 minutes at 100°C. Then the needles are submerged in 70% alcohol, and may be used 24 hours after such immersion.

Since sterilization eliminates all micro-organisms, it is undoubtedly the best method of preventing infection as there is no complete elimination of all micro-organisms with disinfection. Hepatitis virus may be transmitted through the skin, if the needles are only disinfected. (We sometimes treat painful leprosy neuritis in our clinic with acupuncture. Each such patient is allocated his or her own needles which are carried home by the patient and disinfected at home by boiling and then immersion in alcohol.)

The most important part of the aseptic procedure however is for the acupuncturist to wash his hands well with soap and water, using a nail brush. It is much more likely that an infection can be introduced with dirty hands than with unclean needles. The removal of rings and clipping of the nails of the acupuncturist should be routinely carried out before washing the hands.

Plastic plum-blosson needles cannot be sterilized in the usual manner. They should be washed well in soap and water.

5) CARE OF THE NEEDLES

The needles must be carefully examined regularly during use. Hooked, cracked, blunt, rusted or otherwise defective needles must be discarded. Needles which are bent after insertion can be straightened between the forefinger and the thumb (or by using a pair of wooden chopsticks). Each time after they have been used they must be washed in clean running water and then sterilized. When the tip of the needle gets blunt after repeated insertion it could be sharpened with sandpaper or on a jeweller's polishing stone. However, today needles are so cheap that this procedure is hardly worthwhile.[5]

5 Many substandard needles are available throughout the world. Several cases of broken needles, electrical burns, and other complications have been recently reported, from several countries. Certain medico-legal problems have occurred on account of these complications.

POSTURE OF THE PATIENT DURING ACUPUNCTURE

The posture of the patient during acupuncture depends on the area to be needled. At all times, the patient should be comfortable and needling should be carried out with the minimum of pain or discomfort to the patient. It is always preferable to have nervous, old and very ill people lying down, rather than seated, when administering acupuncture. The acupuncturist, too, should assume a comfortable position when needling. The common postures of the patient are as follows:

a) The sitting position:

i) With knee flexed and spine resting on the back of a chair.

ii) With elbow flexed, hands resting on a table in front.

iii) With hands on a table in front and head resting on hands.

b) The lying down position:

i) **Supine** (facing upwards).

ii) **Prone** (facing downwards).

iii) **Recumbent** (lying on a side, left or right recumbent, as convenient).

iv) **Lithotomy** (labour room position: lying down facing upwards, with hips and knees flexed).

v) **Genu-pectoral** or **knee-elbow position** (facing downwards, with the weight on the elbows and the knees).

The most comfortable position for each patient, compatible with the points selected, should be adopted.

In general, it would be preferable to treat patients in groups, as this tends to lesson the anxiety of apprehensive individuals. Discussion with each other of the progress of their illnesses also seem to reinforce the motivation for cure.

For surgery, a position compatible with the operative procedure is adopted.

METHODS OF LOCATING ACUPUNCTURE POINTS

There are many methods of locating acupuncture points. Each acupuncture point has its most convenient method and for some points, two or more methods may be applied with equal ease. Some of the more commonly used methods are described here.

1) Anatomical landmarks

Prominent anatomical markings of the body surface are made to serve as a basis for locating points. These include the body landmarks, felt or seen, on the surface, the sense organs, the eyebrows, the hairline, joint creases, the nipples, and the umbilicus. For example; Yintang (Ex. 1.), lies at the midpoint between the eyebrows. Weizhong (U.B. 40.), is situated in the middle of the posterior crease of the knee joint i.e., in the middle of the popliteal fossa.

2) Finger measurement

In this method, the Chinese "body inch" or "cun" is taken as the standard. When an acupuncture point is situated some distance away from anatomical landmarks, its position can be defined only by stating the distance from such landmarks. But, due to the wide variations of the body build of different persons, it is not realistic to use inches or centimetres, as units of measurement. The finger measurement of the patient is, therefore, taken as the criterion.[6]

a) When the tips of the thumb and the middle finger are brought together to form a circle, there are the two creases of the middle finger well outlined. The distance between these two creases in the extended middle finger is equal to one cun.

b) The breadth of the distal phalanx of the thumb at its widest point is also equal to one cun.

6 However, in Scalp Acupuncture the centimetre scale is being used to locate the areas (points).

PROPORTIONAL MEASUREMENTS

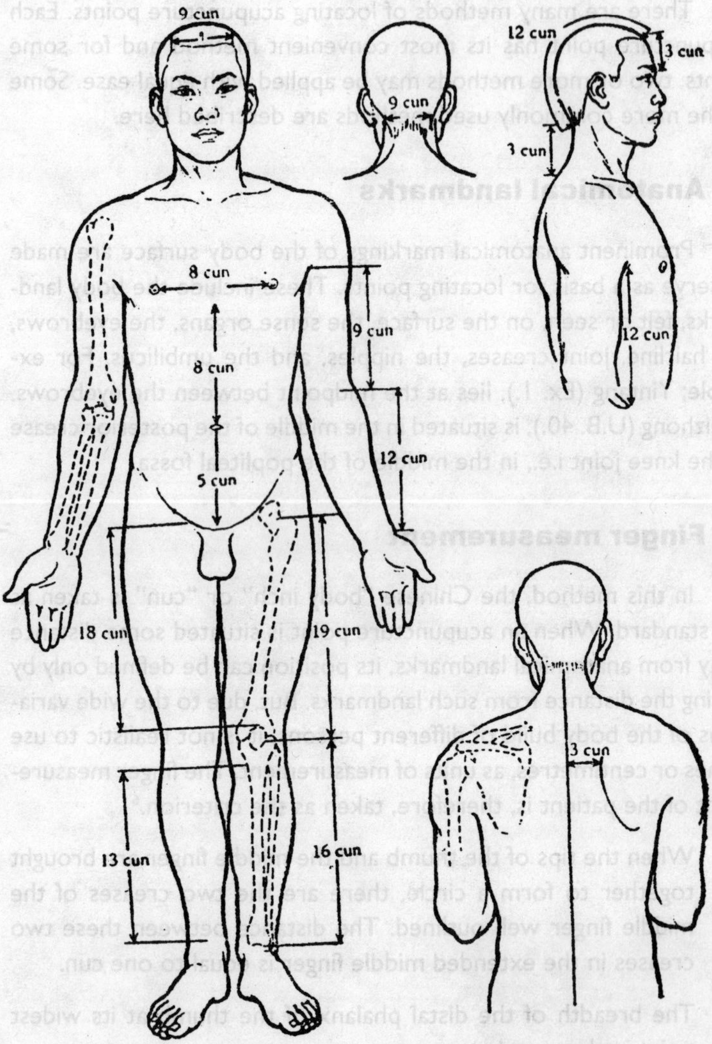

In an average person the different parts of the body are in proportion to each other.

(From "The Outline of Chinese Acupuncture" Beiling) 1965—Page 92).

c) The combined breadth of the four fingers at the level of the proximal interphalangeal joint of the little finger is equal to three cuns.

d) The combined breadth of the index finger and the middle finger is equal to 1.5 cuns.

If the patient's body build is about the same as that of the acupuncturist, then the acupuncturist would be able to locate the points using his own fingers. If the patient's size differs widely from that of the physician, or when treating a child, proportionate adjustments must be made when locating points with the physician's fingers. (A cunometer is a mechanical device, which makes accurate measurement of cuns possible).

3) Proportional measurement

This method takes as its basis that in an average person the various parts of the body are generally in relative proportion to each other. In "cun" measurement, therefore, there would be a constancy of lengths from person to person, regardless of body build. Based on this principle, the distances between certain important anatomical landmarks have been noted in order to facilitate the location of acupuncture points.

Head and neck area	*cuns*
The anterior hairline and the posterior hairline at their midpoints:	12
The anterior hairline and the eyebrow line:	3
The midpoint of the posterior hairline and the spinous process of 7th cervical vertebra:	3
The lateral corners of the anterior hairline	9
The tips of the mastoid processes:	9

Chest and abdomen area:

The two nipples:	8
Two ribs:	1
The inferior margin of the sternum and the umbilicus:	8
The umbilicus and the superior border of the pubic symphysis:	5

Back of the trunk:

The medial margins of the sacro-iliac joints:	3

Upper Limb:

Anterior or posterior axillary fold and the elbow crease:	9
The elbow crease and the wrist crease:	12[7]

Lower Limb:

The greater trochanter of the femur and the middle of the patella:	19
The middle of the patella and the tip of the lateral malleolus:	16

4) Location of points by using a posture

a) *The patient's posture:*

In this method, the patient is instructed to assume certain postures, which will help to identify the point.

The following are some examples of this method:

i) The point Hegu (L.I. 4.), may be located at the highest point of the muscle of the back of the hand, when the thumb and the forefinger are juxtaposed.

ii) The point Quchi (L.I. 11.), is located at the lateral end of the elbow crease, when the elbow is semiflexed.

---

7 Measured diagonally on the forearm.

iii) The point Fengshi (G.B. 31.), can be located by asking the patient to stand and hold his arms at full stretch down the side of his thighs, this point is located on the thigh at the tip of the middle finger.

b) *The acupuncturist's posture:*

Some examples of this method are:

i) For locating the point Xuehai (Sp.10.), the acupuncturist places his palm[8] over the patient's knee cap; the point lies at the tip of the acupuncturist's thumb.

ii) Similarly, the point Femur-Futu (St. 32.), is found at the tip of the acupuncturist's middle finger, when he places his palm[8] over the patient's knee cap with his fingers along the thigh of the patient.

Proportionate adjustments will, of course, have to be made if the patient's body build differs significantly from that of the acupuncturist.

5) Tender points (Locus dolenti)

Certain points of the body (which may or may not coincide with an acupuncture point) become tender to finger pressure in conditions of disease. The Chinese call them "Ah-Shi" points. The needle is inserted at the centre of the tender area. As the patient's condition improves it will be found that the tenderness progressively decreases, till it disappears altogether. Alarm points are also similarly located. Ah-Shi in Chinese means "O Yes", this being the verbal reaction of the patient, when tender points are palpated.[9]

6) Location of points with an acupunctoscope

This method depends on the fact that the skin at acupuncture points has high electrical conductivity due to lowered electrical re-

8 Contralateral palm e.g. left palm on right knee cap.

9 The fibrositic and trigger points also belong to this category.

sistance. Based on this principle, different types of electronic point detectors, called acupunctoscopes, have been devised. The patient is asked to grip one of the two electrodes (banana electrode) connected to the instrument and the acupuncturist uses the other (probing) electrode, which is equipped with a blunt point, to explore the body surface for reactive points. Correct location is signalled by the deflection of an ammeter needle, or the flickering of a source of light, or by a high "beep", produced by a sound amplifying device.

With this instrument, it is possible locate an acupuncture point very accurately. It has, however, the disadvantage that is a very time consuming procedure. The use of this device is more popular in ear acupuncture where the points are far more reactive and the area for exploration is restricted. Unless it is a very sensitive acupunctoscope, the body points may be very difficult to locate. A very moist or very dry skin may also make the detection of points difficult.

7) Location by reference to another point

Example of this method are

a) Sishencong (Ex. 6.), which is located by reference to Baihui (Du 20.);

b) Fenglong (St. 40.) and Tiaokou (St. 38), which are both located by reference to Zusanli (St. 36.).

8) Cunometer[10]

This is a specially designed pair of double callipers by which the patient's "cun" is directly measured, With this one measurement, the instrument could show multiples of cun. Nowadays, this method is generally used for the location of points in acupuncture anaesthesia for surgery, where a high degree of accuracy is required.

10 Invented in 1974 by the medical workers of the Institute of Acupuncture, Kalubowila, Sri Lanka. There is no patent on this instrument.

9) Skin Changes

This method is used in locating reactive acupuncture points in auriculotherapy.

10) Combination of two or more of the above methods

The location of the point Fenglong (St.40.), illustrates this method.

Measure 5 cun distally (cun measurement) from the point Zusanli (St. 36.) (reference to another point), and 2 finger breadths lateral (finger measurement) to the anterior border of the tibia (anatomical landmark).

11) Using a centimetre scale

In head needle therapy the acupuncture areas are located using a centimetre scale. This is, however, not a very satisfactory method as the shapes and sizes of heads vary.

12) Electronic point detector

In modern electrotherapy and laserbeam apparatus there are coloured indicators or computerized devices to signal the arrival of the probe over the acupuncture point. These indicators are quite accurate, except if the skin in too dry or too moist.

It must be understood that the location of acupuncture points is a clinical exercise and that, often it is not possible to be mathematically exact. However, it has been observed that the greater the degree of accuracy employed by the clinician the more it is likely that he would obtain better therapeutic results. (A rival school of thought on this matter maintains that acupuncture points, as traditionally described, do not in fact exist, and it is sufficient to needle the correct segment; dermatome sclerotome, or myotome).

THE TECHNIQUE OF ACUPUNCTURE NEEDLE INSERTION

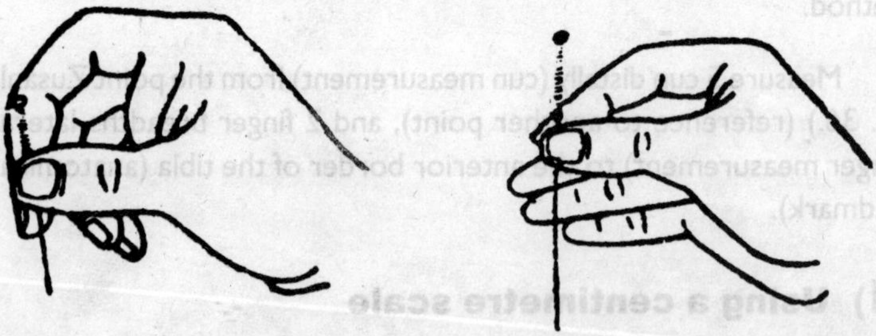

METHODS OF HOLDING THE NEEDLE

Note: It is mandatory that the needle tip should be on the palmar side of the hand.

When insertion of long needles such as at Huantiao (G.B. 30), are carried out, both hands may be used to hold the needle when inserting.

A page from the *Chen Jiu Da Cheng* compiled in 1601 A.D.

Particular care as to accuracy will have to be observed when treating patients who have any physical deformities.

METHODS OF PUNCTURE

Methods of needle insertion, called puncturing techniques, can be described with reference to the three main stages of the puncture 1) insertion 2) retention and 3) withdrawal of the needle.

Insertion of the needle

There are many ways in which a needle could be inserted, and the technique to be used for a particular acupuncture point depends upon the site of the point and the length of the needle. The most frequently employed are described here. In this description it is assumed that the acupuncturist is right handed.

a) Press the patient's skin beside the acupuncture point, with the tip of the thumb or forefinger of the left hand. Hold the handle of the needle with the right forefinger and thumb, with the middle finger and ring finger resting lightly on the upper part and lower part respectively of the needle. Exert a little more downward pressure with the tip of the index finger or thumb of the left hand and insert the needle rapidly into the skin at the acupuncture point The needle may, thereafter, be penetrated to its proper depth either fast or slow with a to and fro screwing movement. This technique is ideally suited for the short needle (1.5 cun or less)[11].

b) Grip the shaft of the needle with the thumb and forefinger of the right hand so that about 0.2 cun of the needle at its tip is exposed. Then aim at the point and insert the needle rapidly. Now hold the lower part of the shaft with the thumb and forefinger of the left hand, and the handle of the needle with the thumb and forefinger of the right hand. Push the needle slowly

11 In the method of fast insertion this is carried out in one swift to and fro stroke (like throwing a dart).

DIRECTIONS OF INSERTION

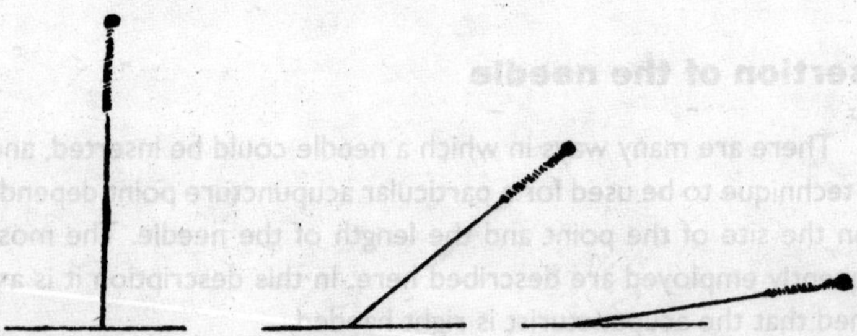

Perpendicular **Oblique** **Horizontal**

in, to its proper depth, using both hands together. Although this technique may be used satisfactorily at most acupuncture points, it is particularly recommended when using the longer needles, in areas where the muscular mass is thick, e.g., the point Huantiao (G.B. 30.).

c) Pinch the skin with the left forefinger and thumb and lift it up a little, with the acupuncture point exposed at the top. Then insert the needle with a quick movement of the right hand. This method is suitable for points of the face or where the muscular mass is thin, e.g., Yintang (Ex. 1.). Pinching the skin, however, makes patients nervous.

d) Stretch the skin beside the acupuncture point with the thumb and forefinger and insert the needle rapidly with the right hand. This method is useful where the skin lies over loose tissue such as on the abdomen, e.g., Tianshu (St. 25.).

e) Insertion through a needle guide: some acupuncturists find it convenient to insert the needle through a tiny cylinder made of glass or metal. The type of needles used in this method have a smooth cylindrical handle, that fits precisely inside the guide. This technique is popular in Japan, South Korea and in some Western countries. This method is time consuming[12].

f) In many clinics in Northern Europe, a no touch technique of insertion using a forceps is carried out.

In using any of the above puncturing methods what has to be borne in mind is that the puncturing must be performed so that the patient is made to feel the minimum of pain. The acupuncturist must ensure that the needle pass through the skin very quickly[13]. The student could start to learn these techniques by practising on a roll of toilet paper or a pillow. He is advised thereafter to practice needling on himself and on his fellow students, till he or she achieves proficiency.

12 If sterility is to be preserved the needle guide, also, must be changed with each insertion.

13 Swift insertion should *not* be carried out at dangerous points.

Depth and Direction

The depth and direction of needle insertion varies with each situation and disease.

The direction of insertion of the needle may be described in terms of the angle the needle makes with the skin surface. There are three directions of insertion[14]:

Perpendicular: 90° to the skin,
e.g., Hegu (L.I.4.), Zusanli (St.36).

Oblique: 45° to the skin,
e.g., Liangmen (St.21.), Zhongfu (Lu.1.)

Horizontal: 15° to the skin,
e.g., Baihui (Du 20.), Shanzhong (Ren 17.)

Perpendicular insertions are made when the underlying muscle is thick. Oblique insertions are made, usually, where an underlying structure has to be avoided. Horizontal insertions are made where the overlying tissue is very thin, e.g., all points in the scalp area.

Order of inserting and removing the needles

Acupuncture is no exception to the rule that one must be orderly in one's activities. In inserting the needles (as also in removing them, thereafter) it is of definite advantage to follow an orderly sequence. It ensures that all the points that the acupuncturist intends to puncture are so punctured, and afterwards that all the needles on the patient's body are duly removed. The order of the insertion and removal would, of course, vary according to the circumstances. Five possible methods are given below:

a) From above downwards

b) From proximal to distal

14 At points like Tiantu (Ren 22.) or Taivang (Ex. 2.) more than one direction of insertion may be carried out.

c) Away from or towards the acupuncturist

d) Less painful to the more painful points

e) To encircle a lesion such as a scar, ulcer or a skin eruption. This is known as "encircling the dragon"

When the acupuncturist has learnt to needle little children satisfactorily he or she can, indeed, then claim to have reached proficiency in the art of needling.

Retaining of the acupuncture needle

Usually the needle is retained in position for 15 to 30 minutes and removed. Treatment is carried out for 7 to 10 days daily, every other day, or every third day. Then a period of 5 to 7 days, rest is given to allow for further improvement and thereafter the patient is reviewed. In the case of patients who are found not able to tolerate the retention of needles, each needle may be rapidly stimulated after insertion and withdrawn immediately[15].

In acute diseases like diarrhoea, treatment may be carried out 3 or 4 times a day, if necessary.

In very painful disorders, like trigeminal neuralgia the needles may be retained up to one hour[16] during which period intermittent strong stimulation may be given manually, or where an electro-stimulator is available, continued densedisperse electrical stimulation may be given[17].

In very painful disorders such as trigeminal neuralgia, *causalgia,* Buerger's disease, the patient may be given an electro-stimulator and taught to carry out his or own therapy of electro-stimulation without needles, at home. If the patient is unable to do this, a relative may be taught to carry out this therapy.

15 This method of non-retention of the needle is suitable for treatment of infants, children and for adults, who are apt to faint.

16 Or more; combined high frequency and low frequency stimulation is often employed in very painful disorders.

17 Electro-acupuncture for prolonged periods up to 6 to 8 hours are applied in the treatment of addictions and during major surgery.

Removal of the acupuncture needle

The needle is removed at the end of the period of treatment, rapidly and gently. Any jerky movements may cause pain. The acupuncture point is then massaged with a dry sterile piece of cotton wool. This is done to prevent the entry of infection, or the escaping of vital energy.

Use of other types of needles

In inserting and removing press needles one has to take great care not to damage the cartilage of the ear. Adhesive plasters of inferior quality may cause an infective eczema.

Plum-blossom needle tapping should always be done gently, so as not to damage the skin.

A hot needle should be heated to red hot before insertion, otherwise infection or profuse bleeding may occur.

STIMULATION WITH THE NEEDLE

The stimulation of an acupuncture point with the needle is usually carried out in acute diseases, in paralytic conditions, for obtaining acupuncture anaesthesia, and (for a very short time) in the case of some patients who faint, if the needles are left in the body.

Stimulation is usually performed manually or electrically.

The following methods may be used in manual stimulation:

i) **Lifting and thrusting:** After insertion to the correct depth, hold the needle between the thumb and the forefinger, lift it a little and then thrust it back to the original depth. The amplitude of the movement should not be more than a few millimetres.

ii) **Rotation:** After insertion to the correct depth, rotate the needle clockwise and counter-clockwise at an amplitude of not more than 180°. If the amplitude is greater, fibrous tissue and nerve tissue may get entangled in the needle, causing undue pain to the patient. The needle is also liable to get stuck.[18].

iii) **Combination of the lifting and thrusting with rotation:** This method generally gives better results, but a good deal of practice is required to perfect the technique.

iv) **Scraping the handle:** The method may be fixed with the thumb and then the handle is scraped with the forefinger.

v) **Vibration of the needle:** The needle may be vibrated after insertion by gently tapping on the handle from one side.

Electrical stimulation is more convenient and has the added advantage that the degree of stimulation could be more precisely regulated. However electrical stimulation must be performed with great care, so that undue pain is not caused to the patient.

THE GREAT LAW OF BU-XIE

TONIFICATION & SEDATION

The Classical Procedures:

BU	XIE
1. Use a gold needle.	1. Silver needle.
2. Insert during inspiration.	2. Expiration.
3. Along the direction of the energy flow.	3. Against the direction.
4. Rotate anti-clockwise.	4. Clockwise.
5. With little force.	5. Forcefully.
6. Retain long period.	6. Short period.
7. Remove slowly.	7. Rapidly.
8. Close the hole.	8. Leave the hole open.
9. Massage after needling.	9. No massage.

18 In scalp acupuncture, however, three or four turns manually are carried out, in order to cause strong stimulation, usually this is carried out in paralytic disorders such as in stroke.

The classical procedures of stimulation as enunciated by the Great Law of Bu-Xie are, not anymore, routinely used in the classical manner in the People's Republic of China by modern acupuncturists. The routine evoking of deqi at every point is a dying practice today. The accent is on painless acupuncture, with non-invasive methods such as laserpuncture, electropuncture micro-wavepuncture, and sonopuncture becoming very popular.

The frequency of electrical stimulation used is generally from about 5 seconds up to about 50 times a second. Where electrical stimulation is used for acupuncture analgesia the frequency used may vary from about 5 Hertz[19] to about 2000 Hertz. (ultra high frequencies up to 30,000 Hertz are now being used in some centres).

Electrical stimulation should not be carried out at Baihui (Du 20.) or Neiguan (P. 6.). In the case of pregnant women, very little children, old and debilitated people and those with bleeding diathesis, it is wise not to stimulate any point as a rule.[20]

Manual stimulation should not be carried out at points close to vital organs, major blood vessels, special sense orga+ns, or at Dangerous points. When strong stimulation is carried out the patient must be carefully observed and the stimulation discontinued, as soon as adequate sensation is felt.

Mild stimulation (re-enforcing or "bu" method) is used in Yin disorders (deficient activity or "xu" disorders) to increase the vital energy. Strong stimulation (reducing or "xie" method) is used in Yang disorders, to reduce the vital energy. The former procedure is known as tonification (accumulation), and the later sedation (dispersion).

vi) **Acupressure:** Under manual stimulation may be included the use of acupuncture with the finger (acupressure) at points such as Renzhong (Du 26.) in emergencies.

19 Hertz = impulses per second.

20 Electro-stimulation is prohibited on patients wearing a cardiac pace-maker.

An acupuncture point may also be stimulated by means other than a needle such as with acupressure, electrostimulation, moxa or other forms of heat, cold, ultrasonics, laser-beam and other physical methods. Aquapuncture or point injection therapy whereby distilled water or certain kinds of drugs are injected into acupuncture points or Ah-Shi points, is an example of combining acupuncture and western methods. Here a prolonged needle sensation (deqi) is produced due to the combined physical and chemical stimulation. The addition of homoeopathic remedies on the needle which is used to puncture the specific point is used experimentaly (Homoeopuncture). This is not a traditional Chinese method.

NEEDLING SENSATIONS (DEQI)

The ancient Chinese physicians called the sensation felt on needling "deqi". They attached great importance to the producing of deqi as this was usually an indication of the needle having been inserted at the correct point and to the correct depth thus ensuring better therapeutic results[21].

The sensations felt by the patient are subjective and are described as:

a) numbness;

b) heaviness;

c) soreness;

d) distension.

Radiation of one or more of these sensations, usually along the Channel, may also be felt. This characteristic is referred to by modern acupuncturists as the P.S.C. phenomenon (Propagated Sensation along the Channel). P.S.C. can occur even in the missing part of a limb, thus the radiation is probably a central neurological happening.

---

21 This view is disputed by modern authorities. Deqi is now usually elicited in acute disorders, during surgery and in paralytic conditions.

Deqi may also be felt by the acupuncturist (referred to as the acupuncturist's deqi), as a sense of tightening felt through the needle handle, due to local muscle spasm.

It has been observed that different acupuncture points produce different qualities of sensations. Generally, when needling in areas where the muscular mass is thin the sensation is one of local distension, while in areas where the muscular mass is thick, it is one of numbness or soreness. When needling close to a nerve trunk, a sensation of "electric shock" may run down the path of the Channel (or nerve); for example, when needling the point Huantiao (G.B.30.), a sensation of electricity may run down the leg to the region of the ankle.

The sensation of deqi must be distinguished from pain or discomfort due to improper needling. ■

PRECAUTIONS

AREAS PROHIBITED FOR ACUPUNCTURE

Needling is absolutely prohibited at the following sites:

a) The scalp areas of infants before the fontanelles have closed.

b) The nipples and breast tissue. (The nipple is anatomically the point Ruzhong (St.17.).

Both acupuncture and moxibustion are prohibited at this point; it is used only as a landmark for locating other acupuncture points[1].

c) The umbilicus. Point Shenjue (Ren 8.). Although prohibited for acupuncture, it has excellent therapeutic value as a moxibustion point, mostly in Yin disorders.

d) The region of the external genitalia[2].

Lasertherapy is used, with good results, at all prohibited points. Laser can be used at all points on the body, not excluding the eye and orifices of the body.

---

1 This is a variable landmark in women and obese persons.

2 Genitalia are punctured sometimes in intractable cases of impotence.

(We have found good results in treating impotence and premature ejaculation in men by puncturing deep, four points at the base of the penis in the 12 o'clock, 3 o'clock, and 9 o'clock positions. These points have been named for convenience, as Penis 12, Penis 3, Penis 6 and Penis 9.

In treating oligospermia it is found that the sperm count rises significantly in a majority of cases, by puncturing two points on the front midline of the testicle. These points are one cun above and one cun below the midpoint of the front midline of the testicle. These points are punctured equally slanted, so that their tips will point to the centre of the testicle. These points are termed Testis one and Testis two (T1 & T 2).

Electro-acupuncture at these genital points is also found useful. Usually the stimulation is combined with Sanyinjiao (Sp. 6) or Taixi (K.3).

These local points are also very effective in genital herpes, together with lasertherapy on the affected areas).

DANGEROUS OR VULNERABLE ACUPUNCTURE POINTS

There are certain acupuncture points overlying vulnerable structures. These are useful points in the treatment of common disorders and are therefore used very frequently. It is advisable for the beginner to puncture these sites under the guidance of an experienced acupuncturist.

Following is a list of these points:

a) Points of needle insertion into the *orbit* of the eye:

i) Jingming (U.B.I.).

ii) Chengqi (St.I.).

iii) Qiuhou (Ex.4.).

b) Certain points in the *neck* area:

i) *Front* of neck: Tiantu (Ren 22.) (Superior mediastinum.).

ii) *Side* of neck: Neck-Futu (L.I.18.) (over the great vessels of the neck); Tianrong (S.I. 17.). (over the carotid body).

iii) *Back* of neck: Yamen (Du. 15.) (over the spinal cord).

Fengfu (Du. 15.) (over brain stem; introduction of a needle in the wrong direction may cause death by damaging the upper part of the spinal cord, or the lower part of the brain stem)[3].

c) Points over the *chest* unprotected by bone or cartilage, e.g., Zhongfu (Lu.1.), Jianjing (G.B.21.).[4]

d) The point Liangmen (St.21.) on the right side, as it *overlies the gall bladder area.* In order to prevent damage to the gall bladder, the needle at this point must be inserted superficially or obliquely, or the left side only may be punctured.

e) Points in close *proximity to the vessels:* Care must be taken to locate these points precisely, to avoid damage to the large vessels, e.g., Taiyuan (Lu.9.), Quze (P.3.) Neck-Futu (L.I.18.)[5].

f) The point Taichong (Liv.3.) can produce *overcorrection of certain physiological conditions.* In particular, hypertensive patients may suffer from too rapid lowering of blood pressure. Hypoglycaemia may occur in diabetics.

g) Ah-Shi points situated close to vulnerable structures.

A knowledge of anatomy is extremely important in carrying out acupuncture, in order to avoid untoward complications resulting from damage to vulnerable structures.

---

3 Deaths have in fact occurred, probably by injury to the vessels of this area.

4 The cheat includes the front, sides and back of chest, as well as the shoulder areas related to the apices of the lungs.

5 The neck vessels are particularly vulnerable to the hot needle.

It is best to avoid acupuncturing certain pathological sites, such as an area of varicosity of veins, or an inflammatory area of unhealthy skin.

Points in front of the tragus of the ear may be dangerous, if punctured perpendicularly and carelessly. A case of rupture of the eardrum has been reported by such puncture. The auricular points (ear acupuncture points) themselves are dangerous, in the area of the cartilage of the external ear, as they are prone to infection owing to the fact that the cartilage is avascular.

Points on the pathways of the main nerves such as the median and ulnar nerves, where they travel in confined spaces, must be punctured with care. Any bleeding or inflammatory reaction around them may give rise to pain, hyperaesthetic or paraesthetic phenomena.

CONTRAINDICATIONS TO ACUPUNCTURE THERAPY

There are some disorders which do not respond to, or are adversely affected, by acupuncture. In these conditions it is advisable to avoid acupuncture and recommend the patient to seek other appropriate remedies.

A summary of some of these contraindications are given below:

(1) **Cancer and other malignant diseases:** Acupuncture has no curative effect on malignant disorders.[6] However, secondary effects such as severe pain; loss of appetite, mental depression and lack of sleep can be effectively and safely managed with acupuncture.

(2) **Mechanical obstructions:** If there is a mechanical obstruction like a twisted loop of intestine, severed tendon, or some object stuck in the throat, these will have to be mechanically removed.

6 At the Institute of Acupuncture, Kalubowila selected cases of malignant disorders, have been treated with success during the past ten years.

(3) **Clear indications for surgery:** Fractured bone, a dislocated joint, a bleeding wound, congenital defects (like a hare-lip) are examples of this type of contraindication.

(4) **Fulminating infections:** Antibiotics are preferable in such cases. Acupuncture may however, be combined with drug therapy, especially to relieve symptoms. Where the infection is resistant or the patient is intolerant of the antibiotic, acupuncture may be used.

(5) **Pregnancy:** In the first three months and the last three months of pregnancy it is best to avoid acupuncture, as needling may cause abortion or premature delivery. This is only a relative contraindication. Vomiting of pregnancy has been effectively treated with acupuncture. Acupuncture is also effective as a means of relieving the pain of childbirth.[7]

Points which are especially likely to disturb a pregnancy are:

Hegu (L.I.4.).

Sanyinjiao (Sp.6.).

Zusanli (St.36.).

Taixi (K.3.).

Zhiyin (U.B.67.).

Points of the lower abdomen.

Ear (auriculotherapy) points related to the endocrine and the genito-urinary systems.

Scalp points: Genital and Foot Motor Sensory areas.

Strong manual stimulation or electrical pulse stimulation must be strictly avoided during pregnancy. (Acupuncture may be employed to relieve the pain of childbirth, or to carry out a caesarean section).

7 Acupuncture has also been used to carry out Caesarean section, forceps delivery and manual removal of the placenta.

(6) Drugs: Patients receiving drug treatment for certain diseases may suffer complications, due to the overcorrection of that condition, by the homoeostatic action of the needling. In this respect particular attention must be paid to patients suffering from high blood pressure and to diabetic patients[8].

a) An abrupt fall of blood pressure has been known to occur sometimes when patients suffering from very high blood pressure are needled at the point Taichong (Liv.3.). In hypertensive patients, therefore, the use of this point should be avoided. If this point is used in the treatment of hypertension itself, blood pressure levels should be watched during therapy. In all cases, it is advisable to have the patient recumbent when using this point.

b) In the case of diabetes, it is possible that a hypoglycaemic state may occur. This type of situation can be brought about by patient taking acupuncture treatment for some ailment other than diabetes mellitus and continuing to take antidiabetic medication. It is prudent, therefore, to ascertain whether a patient is on such medication before commencement of acupuncture. His glucose levels should be regularly determined during the course of treatment and the antidiabetic drug dosage adjusted accordingly.[9]

(7) Haemorrhagic diseases: In haemorrhagic diseases, needling must be done with care. Non-invasive methods such as lasertherapy are particularly useful in these types of cases.

(8) Miscellaneous conditions: Other conditions where acupuncture is contraindicated are:

a) Very old patients.

b) Debilitated and dying patients.

---

8 The actions of the acupuncture and the drug combined together, may cause overcorrection.

9 Acupuncture may also be used in the treatment of diabetes mellitus.

c) Patients who have just had an intensive emotional experience or a period of excitement.

d) Patients sweating profusely.

e) Patients under the influence of alcohol.

f) Immediately after a hot bath.

g) Immediately after sexual intercourse

The acupuncturist must use good judgement in selecting his or her cases for therapy: good judgement comes with experience and learning from one's mistakes, or even better, from other's mistakes. (A master acupuncturist is one who has already made all the mistakes!).

COMPLICATIONS DUE TO ACUPUNCTURE

Complications of acupuncture (also called acupuncture accidents) can occur from improper technique, lack of skill, or failure to observe certain guidelines.

The following are the more common complications of acupuncture:

1) Pain on insertion of the needle:

Causes of pain during needling:

a) Bad acupuncturist (unskillful insertion, clumsy stimulation, needle striking a sensitive structure).

b) Bad needle (blunt or hooked needle).

c) Bad posture (the patient is not correctly postured at the commencement of the needling).

d) Bad patient (e.g., tense and anxious patient).

Pain has to be elicited when using acupuncture or acupressure at Jing-Well points as a concomitant part of the treatment in acute emergencies. Some degree of pain will always occur when

COLLAPSE OF THE LUNG DUE TO ACUPUNCTURE NEEDLING AT DUSHU (U.B. 16)

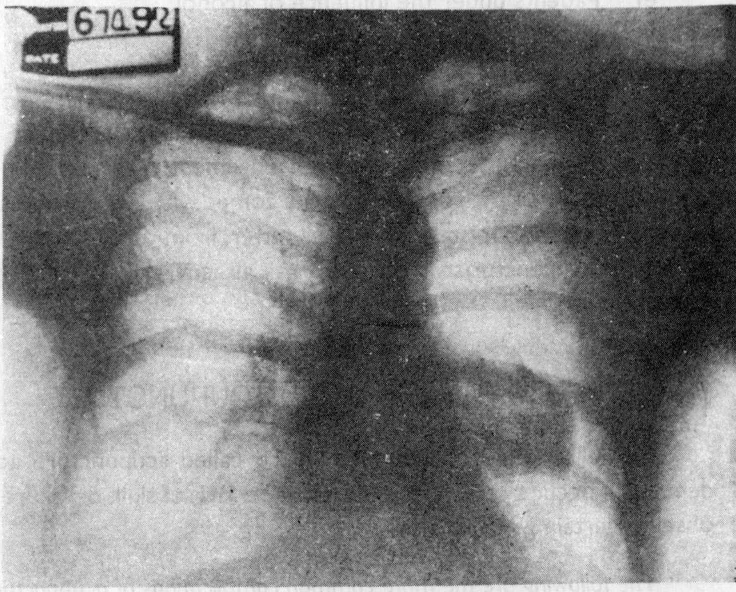

Patient—Male 36 years, X-ray showing complete collapse of the left lung after stimulating Dushu (U.B. 16), to relieve pruritus (March 1980 at The Institute of Acupuncture, Colombo South Government General Hospital, Sri Lanka).

Acupuncturist: (The author)

acupuncturing close to sense organs like the eyes, nose and ears. However, at the majority of other points needling should be relatively painless, if carried out expertly.

2) **Bleeding:** Bleeding sometimes occurs on withdrawal of the needle. This may be considered a benign complication. Bleeding can often be prevented by avoiding any visible veins in the area. If bleeding occurs, massaging the point with a dry cotton swab will stop the bleeding and seal the wound.

   Slight bruising and ecchymosis at the site of acupuncture is fairly common and has no dangerous implications.

3) **Fainting:** Common causes of fainting are nervous apprehension, tiredness, hunger, general weakness, as also painful insertion or excessive stimulation with the needles.

   Fainting can be avoided by explaining the procedure of acupuncture to the patient beforehand, to allay his anxiety. The anxious patient should preferably be treated in a recumbent position. Fainting can be alarming to the patient and the onlooker alike. However, it has been observed that the patient who faints will be found to respond very well to acupuncture treatment. This should be explained to the patient and his relatives. On the patient's first visit, it is best to insert only one or two needles. Afterwards, the number of needles at each sitting should not generally exceed 12 to 15.

   When fainting occurs, remove the needles immediately. Place the patient in a recumbent position, and perform acupressure at the point Renzhong (Du 26.), or needle Yongquan (K.1.) or other Jing-Well points. Keep the airway clear. After the patient has recovered he may be given a hot drink and allowed to rest.

   It is not very unusual to have a patient fainting at his first sitting. However, if fainting occurs at subsequent sittings the technique of quick insertion, stimulation and immediate withdrawal should be practiced. This procedure is known as the non-retention

COLLAPSE OF THE LUNG DUE TO ACUPUNCTURE NEEDLING AT DUSHU (U.B.16).

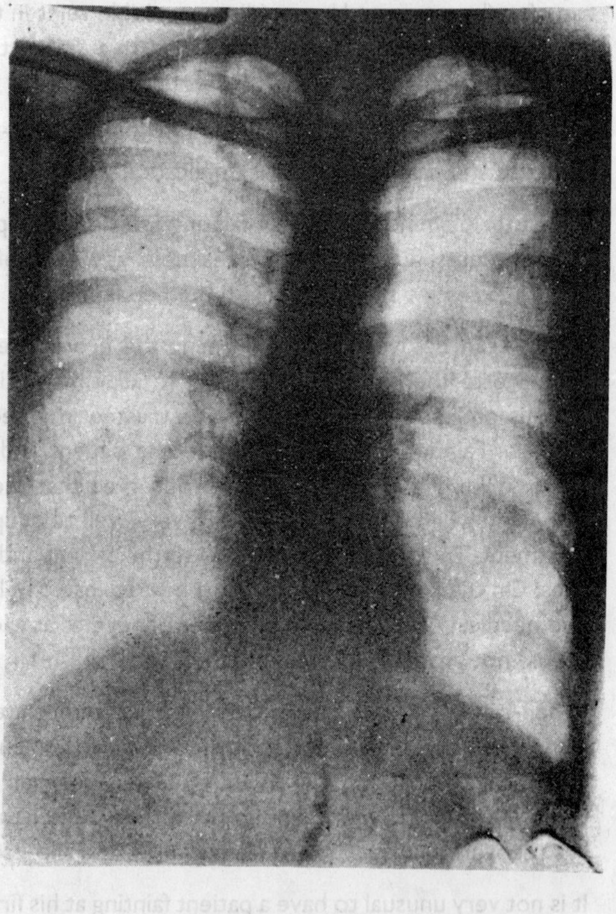

X-ray after 16 days of conservative treatment showing complete expansion of the lung.

Acupuncturist: (The author)

method of needling. If not, a non-invasive acupuncture method may be used.[10]

Patients who take treatment in a seated position should be closely watched at the initial sittings. The needles should be immediately removed, if any untoward feeling is complained of by the patient.

Patients with an empty stomach should not be needled (execpt for surgery).

4) **The forgotten needle:** Failure to remove all needles inserted is a common error, in a busy clinic (no less, the forgotten patient!).

The following are the less common complications of acupuncture:

5) **Bent, broken or stuck needle:** The bending of a needle after it has been inserted, may occur from too forcible insertion of the needle or may be due to the patient changing his posture after insertion. The angulation may be visible at the skin surface or it may be at a deeper level. The patient should be restored to his original posture and the needle should then be withdrawn following the angulation. Efforts at forcible withdrawal may result in a broken or stuck needle and considerable tissue damage.

The breaking of a needle and the impaction of the broken end at the site of needling, can be an alarming complication to the patient, (no less to the acupuncturist!). It can be caused by the use of an old and rusted needle or by any of the reasons which causes a needle to bend or get stuck. When this complication arises, it is important to instruct the patient to refrain from moving, as the broken part might sink still further. If the broken part is visible above the skin surface it can easily be removed with the fingers or with a pair of forceps. If it lies at a deeper level, efforts may be made to manipulate it towards the site of

10 Such as moxa or lasertherapy.

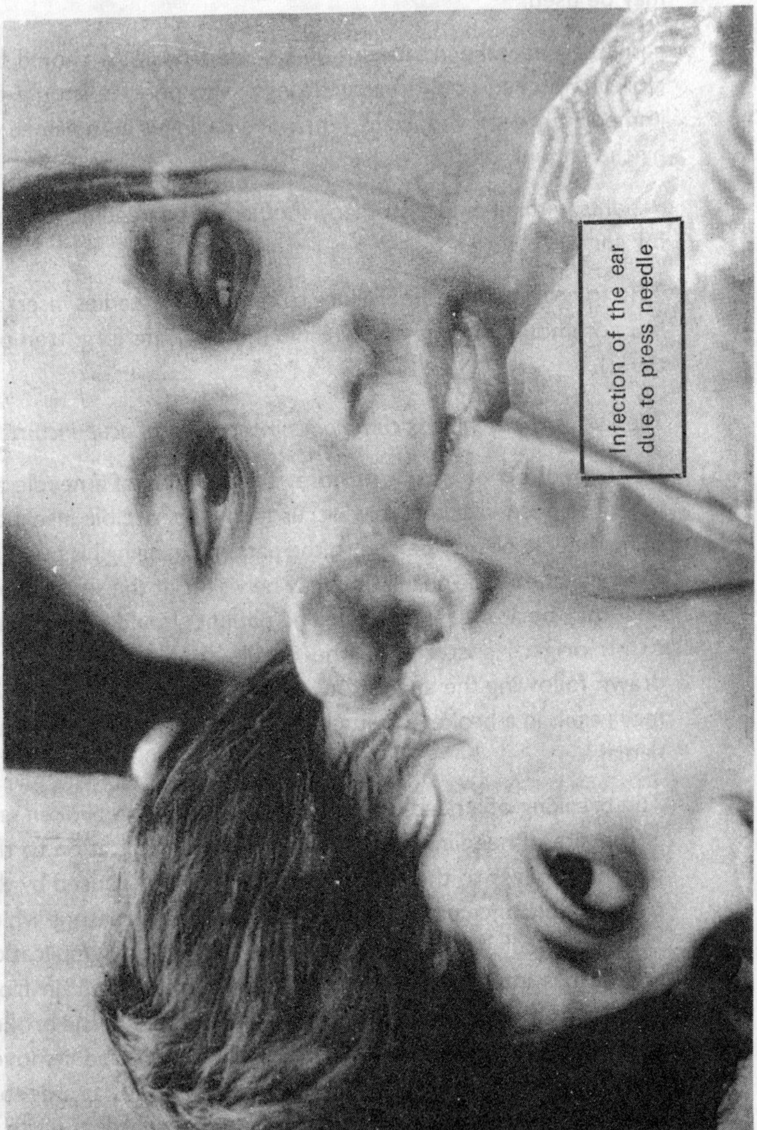

Infection of the ear due to press needle

the puncture. Failure will necessitate surgical removal, if it causes symptoms.[11]

A stuck needle is caused by the impaction of the needle in the surrounding tissues, making it difficult, if not impossible, to remove. It may be due to muscular spasm, or the entanglement of the needle in fibrous tissue during stimulation, or the patient having changed position after the insertion. The management of this complication consists of allaying the patient's apprehensiveness, relaxing his muscles or changing his posture slightly, after which gentle removal of the needle should be attempted. Application of light massage around the area of the stuck needle, or insertion of two needles may help in obtaining better relaxation of the muscles. If the needle is entangled in fibrous tissue, it should be gently rotated in a direction opposite to the original direction of rotation, until it becomes disentangled.

6) **Infection:** Theoretically one would expect a high incidence of infective complications with acupuncture, since it is doubtful whether ideal conditions of asepsis are ever attained, especially as regards the sterilization of the skin. It is, therefore, strange to note that complications like abscess formation or systemic infection are hardly ever reported, and this has also been the experience in our clinic. The reason for this is not clearly understood, but it may possibly be due to the leucocytosis and increase of immune responses associated with acupuncture. Nevertheless, every attempt should be made to maintain asepsis. In particular, precaution must be taken to prevent the transmission of infective hepatitis by the needles. Aseptic precautions must also be particularly observed in ear acupuncture as the cartilage of the ear, being avascular, is very resistant to treatment. However, in treating over 10,000 patients with ear acupuncture in our clinic, we have experienced only two infections, that being due to damage to the cartilage of the ear.[12]

---

11 The use of inferior quality of steel may cause fracture of the needle.

12 We have also reported damage of the ear by sensitivity to the adhesive plaster used for fixing the press needle.

7) **Injury to internal organs or vital structures:** This subject has been dealt with under Dangerous or Vulnerable points. However points like Tiantu (Ren. 22.), Fengfu (Du. 16.), Yamen (Du. 15.) and all points on the intercostal spaces must be needled with special care.

We have had a case of collapse of one lung due to needling points of the chest. Deaths have been reported, from other centres, due to bilateral collapse of the lungs.

8) **Overcorrection of certain physiological parameters, especially if the patient is also on drug therapy:**

a) Fall of blood sugar below the normal level (hypoglycaemia) in a diabetic patient, who is on antidiabetic drugs.

b) The too rapid fall of blood pressure in a hypertensive patient.

This has been dicussed under "Dangerous or Vulnerable points".

9) **Abortion or premature delivery in pregnancy:** This has been discussed under "Contraindications to Acupuncture Therapy".[13]

10) **Complications arising out of acupuncture anaesthesia:** In a series of 3900 major surgical cases operated under acupuncture anaesthesia we have documented a large series of acupuncture complications. About 10% failure of acupuncture anaesthesia in our hands is due to these complications. A similar failure rate has been reported in about 2 million cases over a twenty year period, in the People's Republic of China.

11) **Drug withdrawal:** The withdrawal of certain drugs, like steroids, may cause profound complications.

12) **Complications from electro-acupuncture:** In general, these complications arise from the use of unreliable or makeshift ap-

13 Two cases of inadvertent abortion have occurred in our practice due to needling young mothers. He-Ne Lasertherapy is safe in pregnant mothers.

paratus and where the operating instructions are not properly followed. Beginners are well advised to familiarise themselves in the operation of the controls of the apparatus, preferable by starting with the simpler models which are easier to operate. While ensuring that no undue discomfort is caused to the patient by overstimulation, the acupuncturist must be aware of the possibilities of the following specific complications:

a) Electrocution due to short-circuiting or transformer breakdown. Nowadays, most apparatus are battery operated and this is, therefore, a rare complication.

b) Electrical burns. This is more likely to occur when electro-acupuncture is carried out without needles. In needle-less electro-acupuncture electro-pads are used, which necessitate the use of high levels of current. Burns are likely when the current exceeds 10 mA. or when needles of inferior quality are used.

c) Ventricular fibrillation or cardiac arrest may occur from exposure to current of high intensity (over 100 mA). Generally the current used for electroacupuncture should not exceed 0.5 mA, and this level should be reached gradually from zero setting. However, even at low intensities of current the point Neiguan (P.6.) may cause fibrillation on account of its influence over circulatory functions. It is therefore best to observe the rule that this particular point is forbidden for electro-acupuncture, with or without needles. It should also be noted that if the needle is inadvertently inserted directly into a blood vessel, by reason of the higher conductivity of the blood, cardiac and circulatory problems may be caused.

d) Interference of cardiac pace-makers. Extreme caution is advised in the case of a patient fitted with pacemakers. DC or low frequency AC currents may interfere with the pace-maker operation.[14]

14 Lasertherapy in the area of implantation of a pace-maker is reported to cause extra-systoles.

13. **Addiction to acupuncture:** Every practising acupuncturist experiences the patient who keeps returning for treatment, even after the original complaint has been successfully dealt with. It is known that acupuncture causes a significant euphoria probably due to the secretion of endorphins, which for this reason is sometimes referred to as the "happiness hormone". This phenomenon is also called "the addiction to the hormone within". This is a complication which is best left to the individual acupuncturist to deal with, in his own way, depending on the demands of each such patient. Many patients who are cured with acupuncture enjoy regular needling to serve as a preventive. This is common in cases of patient who have been cured of diseases like bronchial asthma and trigeminal neuralgia.

Some Rarer Complications Reported:

a) *Nerve Damage:* This is possible as many of the effective points are in close proximity to the peripheral nerves. At our Institute we have encountered on many occasions traumatic polyneuropathy of the median nerve due to inexpert needling at Neiguan (P. 6.). The symptoms are similar to those of median carpal compression and they often subside after a few weeks' rest .

b) *Arterial or Venous Damage:* This may result from manipulating needles inserted too close to arteries. Jingqu (Lu. 8.), the Horary point of the Lung Channel is a potentially dangerous point in this respect. Care must also be taken in needling at Ah-Shi point over the great vessels.

c) *External and Middle Ear Damage:* This may result from a perpendicular insertion at the preauricular points. (Acupuncture—A Report to the National Health and Medical Research Council, Canberra, Australia, 1974).

d) *Penetration of Joints:* Escape of synovial fluid may occur, particularly if thick needles have been used around the synovial joints.

e) *Penetration of the Uterus:* This has occurred in one of our cases, where the incisional needles in a Caesarean section under acupuncture anaesthesia penetrated the buttock of the foetus. He[15] received 2000 Hz stimulation for about 25 minutes before delivery. No ill-effects occurred.

f) *Penetration of the Urinary Bladder:* This may occur, particularly if it is not empty, from needling of the lower abdomen points in the treatment of genito-urinary disorders and paraplegia.

g) *Generalised Convulsions:* One case has been reported by H. L. Wen at the K'Wong Wah Hospital, Hong Kong.

h) *Paralytic Ileus:* This occurred in one drug addict when electrical stimulation was inadvertently continued all night during therapy for the drug withdrawal symptoms. This complication is also reported by H.L. Wen at the K'Wong Wah Hospital, Hong Kong.

i) *Foreign Body Granuloma:* The broken ends of acupuncture needles have been found in a foreign body granuloma in a case reported by K. Asano of Tokyo, Japan, K. Fukuda, T. Kiriyama and T. Kashiwagl of Kyoto, Japan, have reported a broken acupuncture needle in a kidney causing a renal stone.

j) *Cardiac Tamponade:* A fatality due to acupuncture has been reported by A. F. Schiff in 1965 in the Medical Times (London) U.K. This was due to penetration of the 5th left intercostal space. Persistent bradycardia has occurred in another case when the left triangle of auscultation had been penetrated (personal communication from Sweden).

k) *Microelectrocution:* J. J. Bischko of Vienna, Austria has discussed the occurrence of cardiac arrhythmias during electrical stimulation. This is liable to occur when electro-stimu-

15 The male child delivered.

lation is carried out across the points of the chest or the upper abdomen. We have had two cases of cardiac arrest due to bilateral stimulation of the neck points, during the induction period for thyroid surgery. Both patients were resuscitated without any later complications. This may happen probably due to over-stimulation of the vagus sympathetics of the baro-receptors of the neck.

l) *The Hyperstimulation Syndrome:* P.J. Pontinen of the Department of Physiology of Kuopio and Pain Clinic, Tampere, Finland has described what is known as the "Hyperstimulation Syndrome" as follows:

"The hyperstimulation syndrome is a hyper-reactive response to stimulation-produced analgesia, mainly occurring in myofascial disorders. Reactions to stimulation-produced analgesia may be divided into: 1) normal reaction, slight increase of pain, less than 24 hours after the first or second treatment: 2) exaggerated reaction, intensive pain lasting longer than 24 hours: 3) prolonged reaction, increase of pain after three or more subsequent treatments: hyperstimulation syndrome (inverted reaction to stimulation produced analgesia), cumulative increase of pain after repeated treatments. Patients with highly sensitive vegetative nervous systems are the most prone to hyperstimulation syndrome[16]. Other factors leading to hyperstimulation syndrome are repeated "locus dolendi" stimulations in acute myofascial disorders and electric stimulation of trigger points during reactive periods to previous treatment. The normal response to stimulation-produced analgesia can often be regained by interrupting all treatment for 3 or 4 days. Patients who react to stimulation-produced analgesia with an increase of pain are better treated with trigger point blockade, until continuous pain is relieved. Patients with a highly sensitive autonomic ner-

16 Often seen in trigeminal neuralgia.

vous system seem to be those most liable to the hyper-stimulation syndrome."

m) *Burns*: This has occurred by (i) electroacupuncture using substandard needles, (ii) Careless moxibustion.

n) *Acupuncture needles as a cause of bacterial endocarditis*: D.B. Jefferys, et al. British Medical Journal Vol.287, 30th July 1983 (see addenda).

Apart from complications of acupuncture therapy and acupuncture anaesthesia described above, a phenomenon that is often observed is the metamorphosis of the symptoms of a disease into a totally different set of symptoms, when acupuncture therapy is being carried out. Some common examples are as follows:

i) A lung disorder such as bronchial asthma presenting as a skin disorder or a rhinitis. The reverse process is also common.

ii) A patient with a heart disorder such as angina pectoris, displaying symptoms of euphoria when treated with acupuncture. This is a particularly dangerous situation as we have seen two deaths by such heart patients over-exerting themselves in their euphoric state.

iii) Liver disease when treated may give rise to muscle weakness.

iv) When migraine is treated impotence may result. (Christain Bay, Switzerland, has reported this).[17]

v) Cases of bronchial asthma after successful therapy may end up with problems of Fire (insomnia, anxiety), Earth (diabetes mellitus) Water (sexual problems, tinnitus, vertigo, joint disorders).[18]

---

17 Water-Fire imbalance

18 With all medical therapies do we exchange one set of symptoms for another.

The use of the wrong polarity of stimulation may aggravate the manifest symptoms. This complication is often seen when migrainous headaches are being treated with pulse diagnosis. The wrong polarity of stimulation may also cause disease in the coupled Organ, the son Organ or related Organ in the Ko cycle.

The present day acupuncturist has often the problem of managing various drug withdrawal effects, seen when acupuncture therapy is commenced and the administration of drugs is withheld or tailed off. This is particularly important when steroids have been administered in the long term therapy of diseases like rheumatoid arthritis or bronchial asthma. The curtailment of anti-epileptic drugs may sometimes cause severe withdrawal problems such as status epilepticus. The acupuncturist must make himself well aware of the clinical problems that may arise by the withdrawal of drugs, to which the patient has become habituated. The withdrawal of anti-hypertensive and anti-diabetic drugs, in particular, require the daily follow-up of the patient.

Note: It has been repeatedly observed in our clinical practice that in a few patients severe pain at the site of needling may occur *immediately after* the removal of the needles. This phenomenon, known as *"the post needling pain syndrome,"* sometimes results in almost unbearable pain at certain needle sites only. Left alone, this may develop in a few hours into exquisite pain, for which the patient may seek drastic drug remedies from other practitioners, who have often misdiagnosed this as an infection at the site of the needling. It has been our experience that needling with strong stimulation at the contralateral points, almost invariably, relieves these symptoms immediately.

Usually, this pain arises at or near the regions of the motor points of the voluntary muscles. Some clinicians believe that the post-needling pain syndrome is due to local muscle spasm following the local tissue injury of needling.

Complications of Ancilliary Methods

Moxibustion: Burns due to careless treatment.

Lasertherapy:[19]

1) Headache due to over-exposure. Nausea in some cases has been reported.

2) Co-carcinogenesis from surface ointments.

3) Fainting, sweating.

4) Tachycardia if used in the region of a cardiac pacemaker.

5) Burns from infra-red lasers.

References

Asano, K., (1969) *Foreign Body Granuloma caused by a broken silver needle of acupuncture,* Otolalaryngology (Tokyo **41**: 289-291.).

Bischko, J.J., (1973) *Letters to the Editor,* American Journal of Chinese Medicine, **1**: 375-378.

Fukuda, K., Kiriyama, T., Kishlwagi T., et al. (1969) *Foreign Bodies (acupuncture needles) in the kidney combined with a stone:* Report of a case. Acta Urologica Japonica (Kyoto) **15**: 223-6.

Goldberg, I., (1973) *Pneumonthorax Associated with Acupuncture,* Medica Journal of Australia, **L**: 941-2.

Kao, F.F., (translator) (1973) *Acupuncture therapeutics for deafmutism.* American Journal of Chinese Medicine, **1**; 361-364.

Leiwis-Driver, D. J., (1973) *Pneumothorax Associated with Acupuncture,* Medical Journal of Australia, **2**: 296-7.

19 Although damage to the eyes is a much discussed complication, the author uses the Helium Neon Laser of 632.8 nanometers directly on the eye, to treat chronic eye disorders, with significantly good results. No complications have occurred. Early cataract seems to resolve with use of laser directly on the eye.

Lowe, W. C., (1973) *Introduction of Acupuncture Anaesthesia,* Medica Examination Publishing Co., New York, pp. 27-28.

Schiff, A.F., (1965) *A fatality due to acupuncture,* Medical Times (London). **93**; 630-631.

Tan, L.T., Tan, M.Y.C. and Veith, I., (1973) *Acupuncture Therapy.* Temple University Press, Philadelphia, p.61. pp. 94-95.

Wen, H.L., (1973) *Personal Communication* (Reported in Commonwealth of Australia Publication No. ISBM 0640 005184) (November 5. K'Wong Wah Hospital, Hong Kong).

ANATOMY OF ACUPUNCTURE

In pre-historic times, the Chinese discovered that there were certain points of the body, which if massaged, punctured, heated or burned, relieved pain or had a beneficial effect on certain disorders. Through the passage of time, many such points were discovered and it was found that by the stimulation of widely separated points it was possible to influence the functioning of a specific internal Organ. These points were then systematically arranged on the basis of the pertaining Organ, over which it was perceived they had an influence. The series of points which had an effect of a particular Organ were connected to form a Channel. This is the basis of the theory of Jing-Luo, leading in time, to the finely evolved system of causal interrelationship between points in a Channel, and between the Channels themselves, which were described in the ancient classic, **Huang Di Nei Jing.**

There are twelve Regular Channels, called the Twelve Paired Channels, and eight extra Channels, called the Eight Extraordinary Channels.[1]

Each of the Twelve paired Channels relates to one of the twelve internal Organs. Like the internal Organs, therefore, six Channels

1 Several other Channels such as Luo Channels, Muscular or Reticular Channels, Divergent Channels and several others have been described.

are Yin and six are Yang. The Yin and Yang Channels, thus, follow the coupling of the Zang and Fu[2] Organs and, for this reason, they are referred to as Paired Channels and are said to have an "interior-exterior relationship" with each other. Because of other direct connections to the twelve internal Organs, they are also called the Organ Channels, and the Channel is named after the Organ to which it is connected.

Of the eight Extraordinary Channels, two run on the midline one in front (the Ren Channel) and the other in the back (the Du Channel). These two channels have their own acupuncture points. The other six Extraordinary. Channels do not have their separate points, but are formed by the interconnection of points of the Twelve Paired Channels and the Two Midline Channels. The Eight Extraordinary Channels are not connected to any pertaining Organ.

Since only the Ren and Du Channels of the Eight Extraordinary Channels possess their own points, they are regularly used like the Twelve Paired Channels and together, they the known as "the Fourteen Channels".

This network of Channels connects the internal Organs and the exterior of man, the microcosm, with the Universe, the macrocosm, to establish a Universal Harmony. For example, when the body is attacked by such external factors as wind, cold, heat, humidity, dryness and fire (also called "exogenous factors") disease may be caused as these factors affect the balance of Qi (vital energy) in their pertaining Organs. On the other hand, disease may be caused by emotional factors such as joy, anger, melancholy, obsession, sorrow, horror, surprise and shock. These diseases first occur in the internal Organs and then affect the Channels via the connections of the internal Organ with the Channels. The ancient Chinese discovered that it was possible to cause a change in the body by skillfully influencing the Qi (vital energy) at the surface level, and this is the prime objective of acupuncture therapy.

2 Zang=Solid organs; Fu=Hollow organs.
In Chinese: Zang=to store; Fu= to receive.

Modern scientists puzzle why acupuncture points exist on the body surface. They were certainly not evolved for acupuncturists to insert needles! According to some modern workers the points, probably, form "windows" on the body surface for exchange of cosmic energies, so that the body can remain in energy balance with the rest of the Universe (Macrocosm).

Of the Twelve Paired, Channels, six traverse the arm. Of the six Channels serving the arm, three are Yin and run on the anterior aspect of the upper limb Centrifugally "The Three Yin Channels of Hand"; three are Yang and run centripetally on the poserior aspect of the upper limb "The Three Yang Channels of Hand". Likewise, of the six Channels serving the lower limb, three are Yin and run centripetally on the medial aspect of the leg. "The Three Yin Channels of Foot"; three are Yang and run centrifugally on the anterior, lateral, and posterior aspects of the lower limb "The Three Yang Channels of Foot".

The Three Yin Channels of Hand commence from the chest and flow to the Hand where they meet with the Three Yang Channels of Hand near the nails.

The Three Yang Channels of Hand commence from the hand, ascend to the head where they meet three Yang Channels of Foot.

The Three Yang Channels of Foot commence from the head, run towards the foot and there meet the three Yin Channels of foot.

The Three Yin Channels of Foot commence from the foot ascend to the chest and meet the three Yin Channels of Hand.

A change of polarity of energy takes place from Yin to Yang at the wrist, and vice versa at the ankle.

When a standing man raises his hands above his head and worships the father, the sun above in heaven the originator of all Yang energy, then the Yang energy of heaven flows (to the Yin of the mother earth) via the "outer" side of his upper and lower limbs. The

Yin energy ascends in the reverse direction from the earth to the heaven above on the "inner" side of his limbs, thus, completing the macrocosmic circulation. Man is the son of heaven and earth.

All Organs above the diaphragm are Yin. These are the Lung, Heart, and Pericardium.[3] They are connected to the three Yin channels of Hand. All solid Organs below the diaphragm are Yin. These are the Spleen, Kidney[4] and Liver. They are connected to the Three Yin Channels of Foot.

Of the Yang Organs, three are connected to the Three Yang Channels of Hand. These are the Large Intestine, the Small Intestine, and the Sanjiao (or the Three Body Cavities). The other three Yang Organs are connected to the Three Yang Channels of foot. They are the stomach, Urinary Bladder and the Gall Bladder.

The ancient Chinese postulated that Qi-vital energy flowed in the Twelve Paired Channels in a precise cyclic sequence. The following table illustrates the sequence of this flow of Qi (vital energy):

Channel	Abbreviation	Qi Flow	Polarity	Limb
1. Lung	Lu.	Centrifugal	Yin	Arm
2. Large Intestine	L.I.	Centripetal	Yang	Arm
3. Stomach	St.	Centrifugal	Yang	Leg
4. Spleen	Sp.	Centripetal	Yin.	Leg
5. Heart	H.	Centrifugal	Yin	Arm
6. Small Intestine	S.I.	Centripetal	Yang	Arm
7. Urinary Bladder	U.B.	Centrifugal	Yang	Leg
8. Kidney	K.	Centripetal	Yin	Leg

3 Pericardium, is the potector of the Heart functionally, they form one internat Organ.

4 The Kidney has a Yin and a Yang aspect.

9.	Pericardium	P.	Centrifugal	Yin	Arm
10.	[5]Saniao	S.J.	Centripetal	Yang	Arm
11.	Gall Bladder	G.B.	Centrifugal	Yang	Leg
12.	Liver	Liv.	Centripetal	Yin	Leg

The twelfth Channel is connected to the first Channel, so that there is a continuous circulation of Qi (vital energy) in the Twelve Paired, Visceral or Organ Channels.

We have outlined above the relationship of Points, Channels and Organs. The Organs also have special relationships with other tissues according to traditional Chinese medicine, and these relationships are considered to be important for purposes of treatment. According to the *Zang-Fu Theory* there are 5 Zang and 6 Fu Organs (the Heart and Pericardium being considered as one Organ). They have the following functions and relationship:

THE FIVE ZANG ORGANS[6]

The five Zang Organs store the vital essences of the body.

Heart (H.)—Pericardium (P.): The Chinese term for this organ complex refers to the heart and the cerebrum.

1) Regulates circulation of the blood.
2) Controls mental acitivity.
3) Heart opens to the tongue. The tongue colour denotes whether heart is functioning properly (cyanosis, anaemia etc.).
4) Heart governs the blood vessels.
5) Heart couples with the Small Intestine.

5 Sanjiao = The three body cavities.

6 Manfred porket refers to Organs as Orbs, meaning the orbit of influence, rather than the concept of an anatomical organ.

Lung (Lu.):

1) Regulates respiration.
2) All blood travels to the Lung and then circulates.[7]
3) "Opens to" the nose.
4) Lung governs the skin and body hair.
5) Lung couples with the large Intestine.

Spleen (Sp.):

1) Regulates digestion.
2) Controls water metabolism.
3) Controls the circulation of the blood.
4) Spleen governs muscle (soft tissues) and the four extremities (limbs).
5) Supplies nutrition to the tongue and the lips.
6) "Opens to" the mouth.
7) Spleen couples with the Stomach.

Liver (Liv.):

1) Stores and regulates the blood.
2) Secretes bile.
3) Liver governs the tendons and endocrines.
4) Transports blood, bile and endocrines.
5) "Opens to" the eye.
6) Liver couples with the Gall bladder.

Kidney (K.): The concept of "Kidney" in traditional Chinese medicine includes the genital functions.

7 The point of origin of the circulation of Blood and Qi is the Lung (not the Heart)

1) Regulates bone growth and teeth.

2) Kidney governs bones, cartilage and head hair.

3) Generates vital essences— a) congenital.

b) acquired

(Vital essence is that component of Qi or vital energy that is directly concerned with the reproductive mechanisms. Congenital vital essence refers to the genetic meterial in the sperm and ovum one obtains at conception; while acquired vital essence refers to the secondary sexual characteristics exhibited by the individual after puberty.)

4) Promotes new life ("Kidneys" as an extension of the genital functions).

5) "Opens to" the ear.

6) Kidney couples with the Urinary Bladder.

(**Note**—Kidney governs the head hair, Lung governs the body hair.)

THE SIX FU ORGANS

The Fu Organs digest and absorb food and excrete the wastes.

Stomach (St.):

1) Ingestion of food and water (fluids).

2) Digestion of food and water (fluids).

3) Transport of food and water (fluids).

Small Intestine (S.I.): Separates the essence from the waste of food and transports the latter to the Large Intestine.

Large Intestine (L.I.): Excretes the wastes.

Gall Bladder (G.B.):

1) Stores bile.

2) Controls the mental activities.

3) Maintains the integrity of muscles.

Urinary Bladder (U.B.): Controls water (fluid) circulation.

Sanjiao (S.J.): Preserves the homoeostasis of the body.

Zang Organs support each other; *Fu* Organs control each other. The *Zang* and *Fu* Organs have a coupled relationship with each other. Although the different Organs have separate functions, they work in co-ordination with each other, to preserve the unity of the organism and to carry out its vital functions.

THE ZANG—FU FUNCTIONS

All the *Zang-Fu* Organs are connected to the special sense organs and tissues as follows:

Tissues:

1) Heart governs blood vessels.

2) Lung governs skin and body hair.

3) Spleen governs soft tissue ("flesh") and the four extremities.

4) Liver governs metabolism, muscles and tendons.

5) Kidney governs bones, cartilage, teeth and head hair.[8]

(**Note:** Muscles and tendons are governed by both Spleen and Liver).

8 Also nails according to some authorities.

Sense Organs:

1) Heart "opens to" to tongue.

2) Lung "opens to" the nose.

3) Spleen "opens to" the mouth.

4) Liver "opens to" the eye.

5) Kidney "opens to" the ear.

Colors:

Head hair is supported by the essences of the kidney (sex), of the liver and of the blood. The colours of various structures are important in making a diagnosis, according to traditional Chinese medicine:

1) Colour of the mouth (tongue)-shows the condition of the Heart and Pericardium.

2) Colour of the skin–shows the essence of the Lung.

3) Colour of the lips–shows the essence of the Spleen.

4) Colour of the nails–shows the essence of the Liver.

5) Colour of the ears–shows the essence of the Kidney.

All features must be taken together when making a diagnosis, as the body acts as an organic whole.

THE EXTRAORDINARY ORGANS

The following six Organs are known as Extraordinary Organs in traditional Chinese medicine:

(1) Brain:

The "*Shen*" or the room of the spirit[9] was located in the brain by ancient Chinese philosophers and physicians.

9 The Chakra located superior most.

a) Also called the "Sea of Marrow,"—According to traditional Chinese medicine, it helps in the formation of vital marrow.

b) Mental activity—The Heart, Pericardium and Brain act as one functional unit. In treating brain disorders, the Heart and Pericardium Channels may be used in addition to the Channels that pass over the brain area i.e., the Du, Gall Bladder and Urinary Bladder Channels.[10]

2) Uterus or male sex organs:

a) Menstruation.

b) Procreation:

i) Uterus.

ii) Associated male or female sex organs.

3) Marrow (located in the bone).

4) Bones (Joints and Cartilage).

5) Meninges

6) The Flesh—Muscles, tendons and other soft tissues.

7) Gall Bladder—The Gall Bladder is a Fu Organ, which is also an Extraordinary Organ.[11]

The conceptualization of the human body by the traditional Chinese physician varies greatly from that of the concepts of anatomy, physiology and pathology of Western medicine. The overall relationships of points, Channels, Internal Organs, etc., as outlined in this description is the complex manner in which the human body is looked at by the traditional Chinese physician. These relationships are further geared to the relationships of the Five Elements to each other. The concept of an internal Organ in Traditional Chinese medicine differs, therefore, from the concept of an organ in Western medi-

10 Also the Stomach channel e.g. point Fenglong (St, 40.), in treating epilepsy.

11 The Liver and Gall Bladder are also involved in mental functions.

cine. For example, the liver in Western medicine means the anatomical entity lying in the upper abdomen. In traditional Chinese medicine "The Liver" means the Internal Organ Liver, its connections to the sense organs and tissues, the Channels, the points of the Liver Channel and the functions of the liver in health and in disease. Headaches, eye disease, muscle and tendon disorders may occur as a result of Liver disease. The liver of traditional Chinese medicine, lies in the Lower *Jia* (lower body cavity). The liver of Western medicine lies under the diaphragm. The Spleen means all the functions of the spleen and pancreas. The genital organs belong to the Organ Kidney. The concept of an Organ and a Channel, therefore, in traditional Chinese medicine is an abstract, conceptual functional entity.

For example, the concept of Kidney in traditional Chinese medicine includes:

a) Hearing

b) Balance (equilibrium of the body)

c) The functions of joints. The integrity of the bones-locomotion[12]

d) Reproduction. Secondary sexual characteristics[13]

e) Excretory functions

f) Head hair

g) Genetic and Hereditary aspects

h) Stress mechanisms

i) Water balance

j) Conservation of vital materials

k) Nails (also related to the Liver and Lungs)

i) The Kidneys store the Essences

m) Regulates blood pressure

12 Spleen and Liver are involved in locomotion, according to traditional Chinese medicine, as they preserve the integrity of the muscles.

13 (According to the teachings of Yoga kundalini energy originates in the Kidney).

ZANG - FU RELATIONSHIPS

YIN 5 ZANG Organs and their related	Connected	Connected Sense Organ	Colour reference for diagnosis	YANG 6 Coupled FU Organs and their related functions
HEART (PERICARDIUM) Blood circulation, Mental activity	Blood vessels. Brain (nervous system)	Tongue.	Mouth.	SMALL INTESTINE Separation of essence from food and transport of waste to the Large Intestine (SANJIAO) (Maintains the homoeostasis of the body).
LUNG Respiration.	Skin and Body hair.	Nose.	Skin.	LARGE INTESTINE Excretion of wastes
SPLEEN Digestion. Water metabolism. Blood circulation.	Soft tissues, Flesh i.e., muscles tendons, fascae, ligaments, fat Four Extremities (limbs).	Mouth.	Lips.	STOMACH Ingestion, digestion, and transport of food and water.
LIVER Bile secretion and transport. Regulation, storage and transport of blood. Control of tendons. Control of endocrines.	Muscles and Tendons	Eyes.	Fingernails and Toenails.	GALL BLADDER Storage of bile. Control of mental activity.

KIDNEY Regulation of blood pressure. Promotes growth of bone, teeth and head-hair. Promotes 'new life' as an extension of genital function.	Bone Cartilage, Teeth and Head hair	Ears.	Medial side of the forearm.	URINARY BLADDER Water circulation.

(This table illustrates the Zang-Fu theory)

Note: I. Heart and Pericardium are considered as one internal Organ. Therefore there are 5 Zang and 6 Fu Organs (5 viscera and 6 entrails).

II. The muscles and tendons are related to both the Spleen and the Liver.

III. Although the tongue is connected to the Heart, the colours of different tongue areas are used in the differential diagnosis of disorders of several other internal Organs.

THE ZANG—FU FUNCTIONS

The concept of the Internal Organs (also called the Viscera) in Chinese medicine is radically different from that of contemporary Western medicine. Understanding this difference is very important because the physiology of the Organs are fundamental to the understanding and treatment of diseases. Because the meanings of the terms Organ Liver, Heart, and so on in Chinese medicine are very different from their Western equivalents (we have capitalized them throughout this text). Assuming that treatments which are regarded by Chinese as beneficial to the Liver will automatically be useful against Western-defined hepatic disorders, is incorrect.

The salient characteristic of the Chinese conception of the Organs (to an allopath[14]) is the lack of emphasis on the anatomical structure. Although many of the terms for the Organs are similar in Western semantics they do not refer to the specific tissue, but rather to semiabstract concepts, which are complexes of closely interelated functions. These functions, which are fully described in traditional texts, are not based on histological discoveries, but on clinical observations of patients over many centuries. This lack of concreteness has many explanations: the principal one being the relative lack of emphasis placed on the physical structure. Although a traditional physician believes most Organs have some kind of physical presence in the body, one Organ, the *Sanjiao,* has no anatomical representation at all. Instead, it is rather the total manifestation of the complexes that are integrated to produce homeostasis of all other Organs.

The Organs are divided into two principal groups, the Yin (Zang) and Yang (Fu) Organs. The five Yin Organs, which are the core of the entire system, are the Lungs, Heart, Liver, Spleen and kidneys. (In discussions of the channels a sixth Organ, the Pericardium, exists, but, otherwise it is an adjunct of the Heart). The six Yang Organs are the Gall Bladder, Stomach, Small Intestine, Large Intestine, Urinary Bladder and *Sanjiao.*

The Yin Organs are described in the ancient literature more fully than the Yang Organs. They are said to "store and not drain," meaning that their functions are directed towards sustaining homeostasis. The Yang Organs are said to "drain and not store," referring to their role in the transformation of food and disposal of wastes. All the Yang Organs receive food or products of food and pass it along. Each Yang Organ is associated with 3 Yin Organs by a special Yin/Yang relationship. Pairs of Yin and Yang Organs, so linked, belong to

14 Western medical physician.

the same Element, their channels are sequential to each other in the circulation of Jing Qi[15]; their functions are closely linked, and disease in one usually affects the other (conversely, excess in one may cause deficiency in the other).

The central thesis of traditional Chinese medicine—the patterns of disease may now be discussed. The classification of disorders and the rationale of treatment in Chinese medicine is based on pathological patterns of disease in the various Organs. The ideogram that the Chinese use for notating the disorders of the Organs is *zheng*, which means *'emblem'*. This is an example of the abstract in Chinese medicine, in that the signs and symptoms of disease are grouped into 'emblems' or syndromes, which represent the state of health of the patient as a whole. The main purpose of Chinese is to diagnose the syndrome and institute specific treatment for the whole patient, to re-establish the harmony.

Because the focus of diagnosis and the conceptualization of the body in Chinese medicine differ much from Western medicine, the fact that a Western-defined disease may have more than one corresponding Chinese pattern, or one Chinese pattern may appear under different Western defined diagnostic terms should be borne in mind. To practitioners of Western medicine, the patterns described here will be regarded merely as syndromes or groups of symptoms. In the context of Western medicine this would be true, where most cases are diagnosed generally speaking from the inside to outside, i.e., with a blood test, scan, X-ray etc., because that some kind of information from inside the body is necessary to name a disease with accuracy. But Chinese medicine approaches patients from the outside in.[16] The senses of the physician and patient are used to gather information which the physician can synthesize into a total picture of how the patient is functioning at that time. To physicians of Chinese medicine, this is the only way to get at the core of the problem. They view Western physicians as basically providing only symptomatic treat-

15 Jing Qi Energy in the Channels.

16 From above downwards (mental to physical) in a holistic manner.

ment; exactly how Western physicians view their traditional counterparts!

It should be understood that each of the vital Organs is responsible, as well, for a variety of disorders that appear along the path of its associated channel sense organ, tissues and vice versa.

Lungs and Large Intestines

These Organs[17] correspond to Metal, the westerly direction, the season of autumn, the dry climatic condition, the colour white the emotion of melancholy, the pungent taste, the rank odour, and the sound of crying. Their opening is the nose (and anus). They govern the skin.

The Lungs are responsible for absorbing Qi from the air[18], and for the energy state of this Qi in the body. They also control that part of the fluid metabolism which distributes the fluids to the skin.

The Lung is called the delicate Organ because it is often the first to be attacked by exogenous disease. Such disease also causes what is called the Non-spreading of the Lung Qi. The primary symptom associated with the Lung is coughing. This is a 'Rebellious Qi', since the Lung Qi normally flows downwards. When coughing is accompanied by lassitude, shortness of breath, light foamy phlegm, and weakness in the voice, it is called Deficient Lung Qi. When the cough is very dry with little phlegm, parched throat and mouth, and Deficient Yin symptoms such as night sweating, low grade fever and red cheeks, the condition is referred to as Deficient Lung Yin.

The Large Intestine is considered important in the metabolism of water and excretion of wastes. The Large Intestine extracts water from the waste materials it receives from the Small Intestine (and transmits it on to the Bladder), excreting the solid materials as stools.

17 Authorities such as Manfred Porket use the term "Orb" instead of "Organ". This clearly underlines the orbit of influence, rather than an anatomical structure.

18 Qi from inspired air = Ta Qi (or Oxygen).

However, many disorders affecting this Organ are associated with Spleen and Stomach syndromes. Certain varieties of abdominal pain are regarded as manifestations of a blockage of Qi or Blood, in the Large Intestines.

Spleen and Stomach (Spleen = Spleen + Pancreas)

These Organs correspond to the Earth, the central direction, the season of the late summer (the end of summer), climatic condition of dampness, the colour yellow, the emotion of pensiveness, the taste of sweetness, fragrant odour and the sound of singing. Their opening is the mouth. They control the flesh and the limbs (extremities).

The Spleen is the principal Organ of digestion. It transports nutrients. It produces and regulates the Blood (regulates in the sense of keeping it circulating within the channels). It is responsible for the transformation of foods for nourishment. The relationship between the Spleen and the Stomach is a particularly important example of the Yin/Yang relationship between Organs. The Stomach receives food; the Spleen transports nutrients. The Stomach moves materials downwards; the Spleen upwards. The Stomach has an affinity for dampness; the Spleen dryness (i.e., the Stomach, being Yang, easily copes with Dampness (Yin) but produces disorders with Dryness (Yang).

When the Spleen is Weak,[19] the body is unable to use[20] the nourishment in the food. This leads to general lassitude and fatigue, and a pale complexion. The upper abdomen is the region of the Spleen, and Deficient Spleen Qi is marked by a sense of malaise or fullness in that area. Because the transportation function requires that the spleen distributes its Qi upwards, weakness in the Spleen is usually accompanied by diarrhoea. The Spleen Qi is also referred to as the Middle Qi, responsible for holding the viscera in place. Insuffi-

19 Deficient,

20 Digest or metabolise.

ciency of the Middle Qi causes prolapsed stomach, or kidneys. In more severe cases, the Spleen Yang Qi is Deficient. This pattern is manifested as diarrhoea, cold limbs, and abdominal pain that can be soothed by the warmth of frequent hot drink, friction massage or moxibustion.

When many of the above aymptoms are accompanied by bleeding, specially from the digestive tract or uterus, the syndrome is called "Spleen Not Controlling the Blood".

Cold and Dampness Harassing the Spleen is a frequent syndrome characterized by a pent-up feeling in the chest and a bloated sensation in the abdomen, lassitude, lack of appetite and taste, a feeling of cold in the limbs, a dark yellowish hue of the skin, some oedema and diarrhoea with watery stool. The Cold and Dampness prevent the Spleen from performing its transforming and transporting functions This leads to a severe disturbance in water metabolism and is one of the origins of phlegm, oedema, ascites and muscular weakness.

While there are some Deficiency disorders of the Stomach (Many of these originate in the Spleen), most Stomach disorders are an Excess. Stomach, Fire is a painful, burning sensation in the Stomach, unusual hunger, bleeding from the gums, constipation, and halitosis. Rebellious Stomach Qi may produce acute gastro-intestinal symptoms.

Heart and Small Intestines

These Organs correspond to the Fire phase, the southerly directions, the summer season, the climatic condition of heat, the colour red, the emotion of laughter, the taste of bitterness, the odour of burning. Their point of entry is the tongue. The Heart controls the blood vessels and circulation; their functions are reflected in the face.

The Heart controls the blood vessels and is responsible for circulating the blood through them. It also stores the Spirit, and is therefore the organ most frequently associated with mental processes.[21] The Small Intestine separates the waste material from the nutritious elements which are distributed throughout the body, while the waste is sent down to the Large Intestine for elimination.

Almost all the disorders of the Heart are those of weakness namely Deficient Heart Yang, Deficient Heart Blood, and Deficient Heart Yin.

The principal functions of the Heart are associated with the circulation and mental activity. Thus certain symptoms, e.g., emotional distress, dizziness, palpitations, shortness of breath, and lack of vitality in the face are common to all the Heart disease patterns. Deficient Qi in this Organ is marked by general lassitude, panting with shallow breathing, and excessive sweating. When the face is swollen and ashen grey or bluish-green, and the limbs are cold, the condition is called Deficient Heart Yang. Restlessness, irritability, dizziness, poor memory and insomnia are typical symptoms of Deficient Heart Blood. In more advanced cases, Deficient Heart Yin develops with a flushed appearance of the palms and face, low-grade fever, and sweating.

Excess Fire of the Heart is marked by fever, sometimes accompanied by delirium, a racking pulse, intense restlessness, insomnia or frequent nightmares, a bright red face, a red or blistered and painful tongue, and often a burning sensation during urination. The latter symptom is considered to be the result of Heat being transferred from the Heart to the Small Intestine, interfering with the Small Intestine's functions of metabolism and of water balance.

Kidneys and Urinary Bladder

These Organs correspond to water, the winter season, the cold climatic conditions, the southerly direction, the colour black, the emotion fear, the taste of salt, a rotten smell, and the sound of groan-

21 To a lesser extent, the extraordinary function of the Gall Bladder is mentation. Many forms of headaches, such as due to migraine or anxiety are due to Gall Bladder problems.

ing. Their sensory organ is the ear. Their openings are the urethra and vagina. They control the bones, marrow and cartilage, and their health is reflected in the hair of the head.

The Kidneys store Essence and are thus responsible for growth, development, and the reproductive functions. They assume the primary role in water metabolism and control of the body fluids. They also hoted the body's most fundamental Yin and Yang the Bladder transforms fluids into urine and excretes it from the body.

The Kidneys are the repositories of the congenital Yin and Yang of the body. Therefore, any disorder, if sufficiently chronic, will involve the Kidneys. Furthermore, a disease of the Kidneys will usually lead to problems in other Organs.[22] Strengthening the Kidneys is therefore done to increase or maintain vitality and health. The symptoms of Deficient Kidney Yang or Yin are classic symptoms that may appear in Deficient Yang or Yin disorders of any other Organ.

The symptoms of Deficient Kidney Yin are as follows. The lower back is weak and sore, there is ringing in the ears and loss of hearing acuity, the face is ashen or dark, especially under the eyes. Dizziness, thirst, night sweats and low grade fevers are common. Men have less semen and tend towards premature ejaculation, while women have scanty menstruation or may be frigid.

Deficient Kidney Yang symptoms are generally associated with loss of energy or warmth. As with Deficient Kidney Yin, there is ringing in the ears, dizziness, and soreness in the lower back. However, the soreness is characterized by a sensitivity to cold. There is lassitude fatigue and a feeling of coldness. There is a significant weakness in the legs. In men, there may be a tendency towards impotence, and in both sexes clear and voluminous urine or incontinence may be present.

Most frequently Deficient Kidney Yin produces similar disorders in the Heart and Liver, while Deficient Kidney Yang disturbs the

22 Tonification.

functions of the Spleen and Lungs. The disorder associated with the Lungs is called Kidney Not Receiving Qi, which is a type of wheezing characterised by difficult breathing, primarily during inhalation[23]. In addition to the Deficient Kidney Yang symptoms, this condition is also diagnosed by a faint voice, coughing puffiness of the face and spontaneous sweating.

The Kidneys perform important functions in the metabolism of water. When these functions are disorganized, the condition of Deficient Kidneys leading to Spreading Water occurs[24]. Several other Organs are also concerned with water metabolism.

Pericardium and Sanjiao

These two Organs are said to correspond to the "Ministerial Fire" as distinguished from the "Sovereign Fire" of the Heart and Small Intestine. The Pericardium Organ has no separate physiological functions, although it is mentioned as causing delirium induced by high fevers. At least as far back as the 3rd century Classic of Difficulties, the Sanjiao was described as "having a name, but no form". In the Inner Classic, the Sanjiao was regarded as an Organ that coordinated all the functions of water metabolism. In other traditions, the Sanjiao means the three regions of the body that are used to group the Organs. The Upper body Cavity includes the chest, neck, head and the functions of the Heart and Lungs. The Middle Cavity spans the region between the chest and the umbilicus and includes the functions of the Stomach and Spleen. The Lower Cavity refers to the lower abdomen and the functions of the Kidneys and Bladder (and usually the Liver which, however, is sometimes placed in the Middle Cavity). As such, the Upper body Cavity has been compared to a mist which spreads the Blood and Qi, the Middle body Cavity is like a foam which churns up the food in the process of digestion, and the Lower Body Cavity is likened to a swamp, where all impure substances are excreted from.

---

23 The clinical picture may be similar to Bronchial Asthma.

24 Generalized oedema or ascites.

FROM AN ANCIENT OLA* MANUSCRIPT (SRI LANKA) circa 500 B.C.

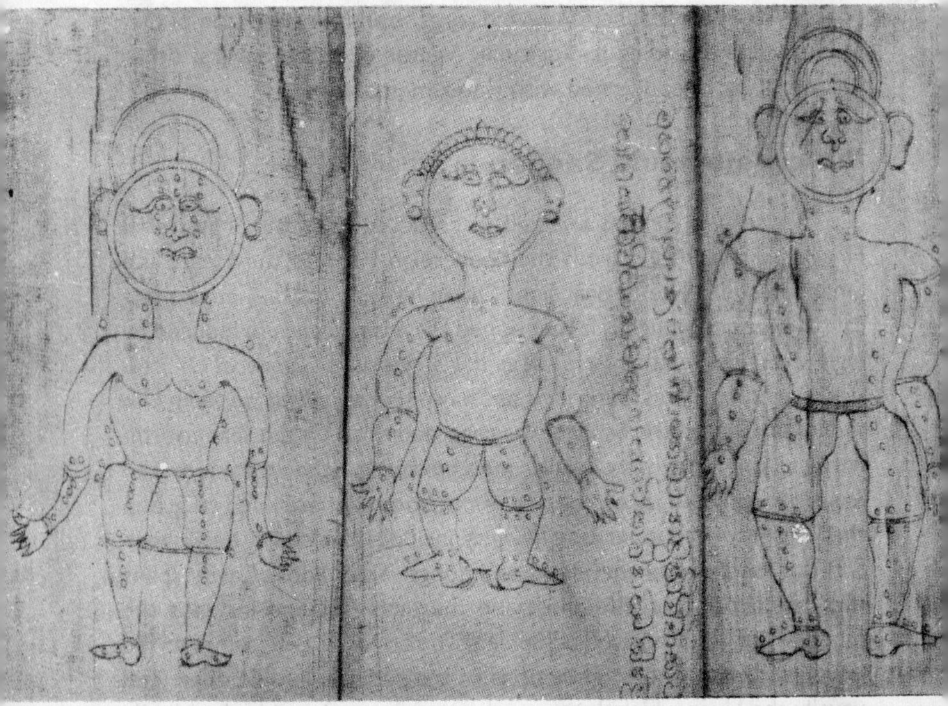

Acupuncture points on the human being

25 Ola= Dried leaf of a palm used in ancient times as writing material before paper was invented
(Manuscript in the possession of the author)

Liver and Gall Bladder

These Organs correspond to Wood, the direction east, the spring season, the climatic condition of wind, the colour of green, the emotion of anger, the sound of shouting. The point of entry is the eyes. They control the sinews (muscle tendons, joints) in the nail.

The Liver is the Organ that is responsible for circulation and regulating the Qi throughout the body. Its character is flowing and free. Thus, depression or frustration can disturb its functions. It is also responsible for storing Blood, when the body is at rest. This characteristic, combined with its control over the lower abdomen, makes it an important Organ with regard to women's menstrual cycle and sexuality. Depression of the Liver Qi is often the main cause of many gynaecological disorders, including menstrual irregularities, swollen and painful breasts. The gall bladder stores and excretes bile, which is produced by the Liver. Together with the Heart, the Gall Bladder is responsible for decision-making (both are connected to the Brain).

Depression or long-term frustration can upset the Liver's circulating functions and result in continuing depression, a bad temper and a painful, swollen feeling in the chest and sides. If it worsens, it may lead to disharmony between the Liver, the Stomach and the Spleen. This disorder is charachterized by the "rebellion" of Qi in the last two Organs, whereby the bad Qi moves in the opposite direction to normal. In the case of the Stomach, whose Qi normally descends, rebellious Qi means hiccoughing, nausea and vomiting. The Qi of the Spleen, on the other hand, is ordinarily directed upwards rebellious Qi in this Organ causes diarrhoea.

One of the Liver's most important functions is storage of Blood with the attendant emphasis upon nourishing and energising. When the Liver Blood is deficient (more severe cases are called Deficient Liver Yin), the Liver is incapable of storage. This is manifested as dry, painful eyes with a weak vision, lack of suppleness or pain on moving the joints, dry skin, dizziness (lack of Blood in the head), and infre-

CONCEPTUALIZATION OF THE 12 VISCERA

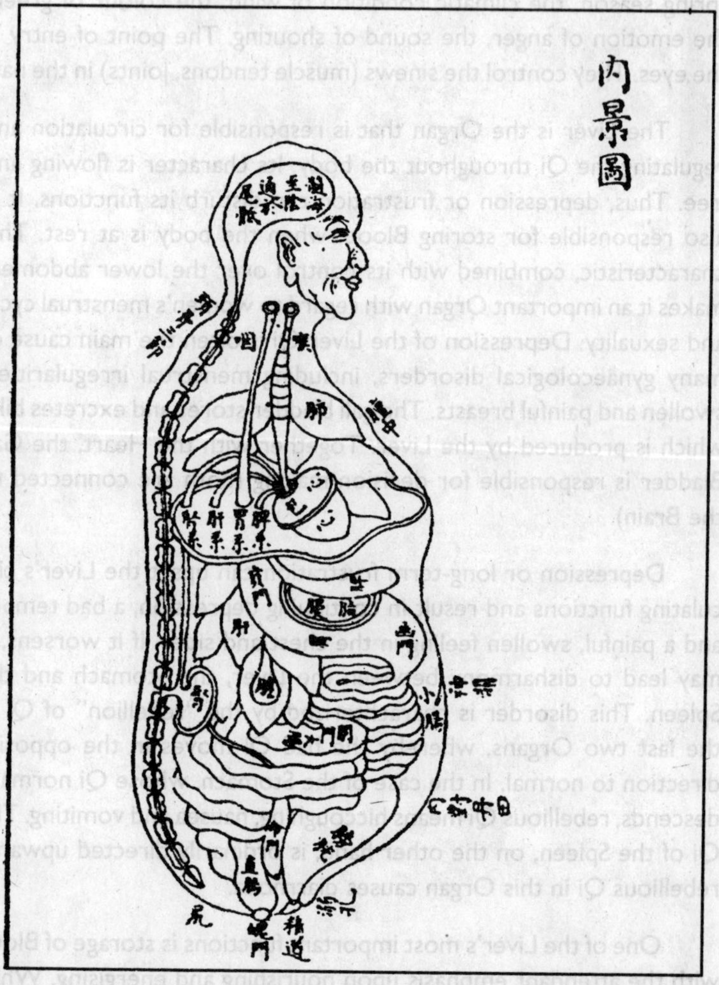

Traditional drawing of the twelve viscera, from the *Lei Ching* of Chang Chieh-Pin, 1624 A.D.

quent or scanty menstruation. When the Deficient Liver Yin reaches a certain degree of severity the disorders Rising Liver Fire or Hyper Liver Yang Ascending occur. These conditions are accompanied by an ill-temper, restlessness, headache, vertigo, flushed face and eyes and a parched mouth. They result when the Liver Yin is so deficient as to be incapable of securing the Liver Yang which rises uncontrollably in the head. While many of the symptoms appear as disorders of the head, a weakness in the lower limb joints may also be observed.

There are various meanings conveyed by the word 'Wind' in traditional. Chinese medicine, However, it is necessary here to discuss Liver Wind, or the syndrome of Interior Movement of the Liver Wind. This pattern often appears as a progression in the development of the condition Liver Fire, or Liver Yang Rising in Excess. Movement of the Interior Wind is evidenced by sudden onset of the symptoms: dizziness on locomotion, spasms, paralysis, difficulty in movement or severe vertigo. These symptoms represent the transitory, disorienting, and ultimately disassociative functions of "Wind".

The principal disease associated with the Gall Bladder is a disorder affecting the flow of bile caused by Dampness and Heat. This is manifested by pain in the region of the Liver, an oppressive sensation of fullness in the abdomen and yellowish eyes, skin, urine and tongue.

Functional Inter-relationships among the Zang-Fu

Some examples of the functional Inter-relationships among the Organs are described below.

The Spleen, Liver and Heart are three Organs that have the most direct relationship with the Blood. The Spleen creates it, and the Heart circulates it. Any disorder associated with the Blood will involve at least one of these Organs.

The Liver and the Kidneys are closely related. Their channels cross in many locations. The Liver stores Blood; the Kidneys store

THE PROXIMAL TARGET AREAS TREATED WITH THE FREQUENTLY USED SIX DISTAL POINTS

Proximal area treated by:

FRONT

Hegu (L.I.4.)

Neiguan (P. 6.)

Zusanli (St. 36.)

Proximal area treated by:

BACK

Lieque (Lu.7.)

Weizhong (U.B.40)

Sanyinjiao (Sp. 6.)

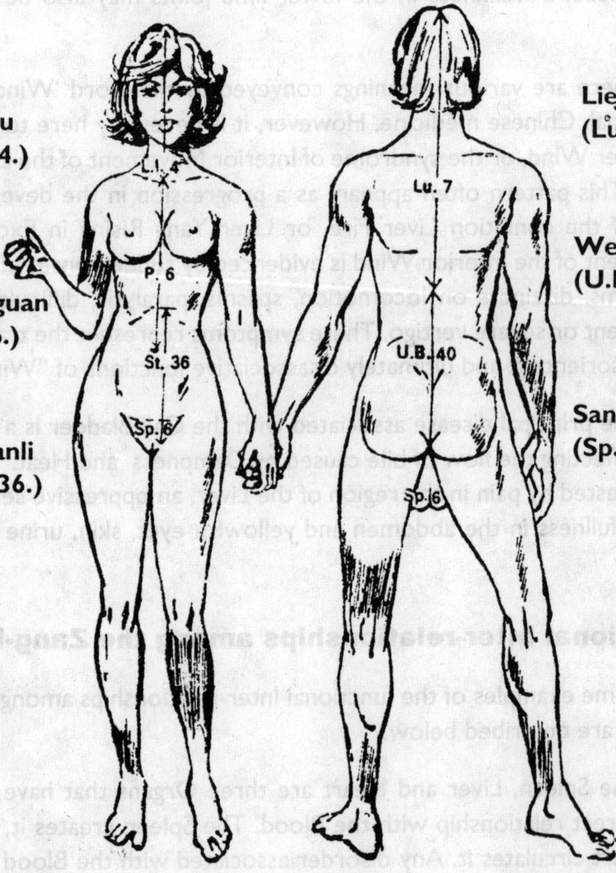

Essences. These substances, both of which are Yin, have a considerable influence on the reproductive functions.

The Heart (Upper Cavity, Fire) and the Kidneys (Lower Cavity, Water) keep each other in check and are dependent upon one another. The Spirit of the Heart and the Essence of the Kidneys cooperate in establishing and maintaining of consciousness.

The Spleen's digestive functions are associated with the distributive function of the Liver. Disharmony between these two Organs results in various digestive disorders. The transportive and digestive functions of the Spleen (also called the Middle Qi) depend upon the strength of the Kidney Yang.

Although the Lungs govern the Qi, the Qi from the Lungs must mix with the Essence from the Kidneys before Source Qi is produced. The Lungs govern the Qi, the Liver spreads it, and the Kidneys provide its basis.

These relationships are conceptual and metaphysical.

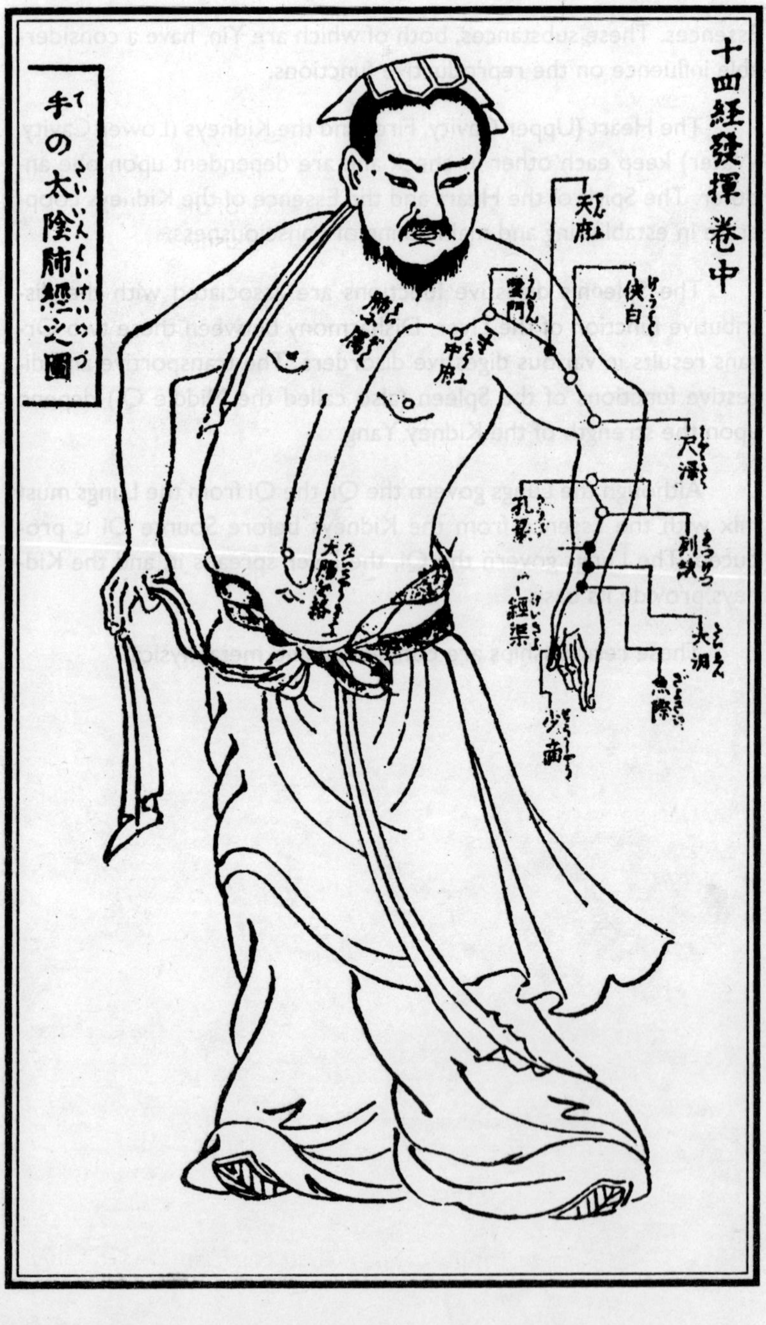
十四經發揮卷中
手の太陰肺經之圖
天府
俠白
雲門
中府
尺澤
孔冣
列缺
經渠
太淵
魚際
少商

THE SYSTEM OF CHANNELS AND COLLATERALS

I. SUPERFICIAL CHANNELS

A. Twelve Regular Channels.

The Lung Channel of Hand-Taiyin (Arm Greater Yin).

The Large Intestine Channel of Hand-Yangming (Arm Bright Yang).

The Stomach Channel of Foot-Yangming (Leg Bright Yang).

The Spleen Channel of Foot-Taiyin (Leg Greater Yin).

The Heart Channel of Hand-Shaoyin (Arm Lesser Yin).

The Small Intestine Channel of Hand-Taiyang (Arm-Greater Yang).

The Urinary Bladder Channel of Foot-Taiyang (Leg Greater Yang).

The Kidney Channel of Foot-Shaoyin (Leg Lesser Yin).

The Pericardium Channel of Hand-Jueyin (Arm Absolute Yin).

The Sanjiao Channel of Hand-Shaoyang (Arm Lesser Yang).

The Gall Bladder of Foot-Shaoyang (Leg Lesser Yang).

The Liver Channel of Foot-Jueyin (Leg Absolute Yin).

B. The Eight Extra Channels.

The Du Channel (Governing). These 2, together with the 12 regular Channels form the 14 Channels.

The Ren Channel (Conception).

The Chong Channel (Penetrating).

The Dai Channel (Girdle).

The Yangqiao Channel (Yang Heel).

The YInqiao Channel (Yin Heel).

The Yangwei Channel (Yang Linking).

The Yinwei Channel (Yin Linking).

C. The Fifteen Collaterals.

The collaterals of the fourteen Channels plus the major collateral of the Spleen.

II. INTERMEDIATE CHANNELS

Muscular Channels (Meridians) – a reticular network in the muscle, tendon, bone, cartilage and fascia layers.

III. DIVERGENT CHANNELS

IV. DEEP CHANNELS

— Connections between and with the internal Organs.

LUNG CHANNEL (LU.)

"Man's breathing connects the Qi of heaven and earth

in order to form the true Qi of the body."

— *Zangshi, Leijing*

— Polarity: Yin.

— Number of points 11.

— Pertaining organ - Lung

— Pertaining Channel: Large Intestine Channel (L. I.).

— Element: Metal.

— Energy flow: Centrifugal.

— Course:

The Lung Channel originates its superficial course in the upper part of the chest. It runs distally on the anterior and lateral aspect of the upper arm and forearm to reach the wrist, where it lies lateral to the radial pulse. Then it runs near the lateral border of the palm to end near the lateral edge of the base of the nail of the thumb.[1]

---

1 The energy from here reaches the deeper tissues reticular (network) of muscular channels.

THE LUNG CHANNEL

Lu. 1. Zhongfu
Lu. 5. Chize
Lu. 6. Kongzui
Lu. 7. Lieque
Lu. 9. Taiyuan
Lu. 11. Shaoshang

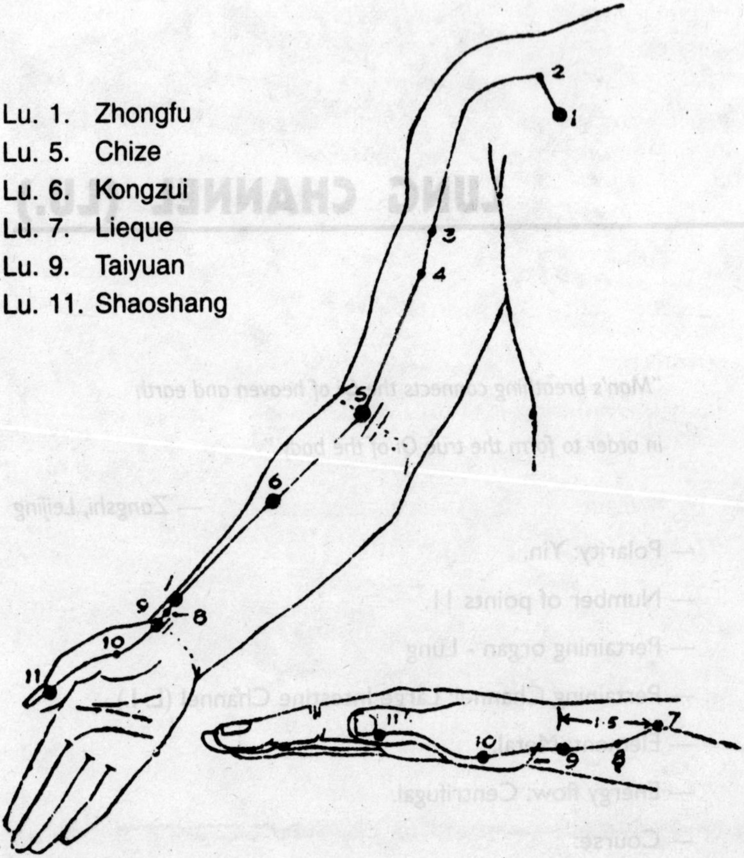

Note: Jingqu (Lu. 8.) is the Metal point (Element point of this (Metal channel. It is also known as the Horary point. Modern acupuncturists do not generally employ this point, as it is situated directly over the radial artery. In traditional acupuncture it was used at the appropriate time on the Organ clock (3 a.m. — 5 a.m.) to treat insufficiency or excess of the Lung respectively. Tonification (Bu) was carried out for insufficiency at 3 a.m. Sedation (Xie) was carried out for excess at 5 p.m.

Note: There are 3 Yin Channels which originate their superficial course in the chest and course distally more or less parallel to each other on the anterior aspect of the arm. On the medial border of the arm runs the Heart Channel (H); on the lateral border the Lung Channel and in between runs the Pericardium Channel (P). These 3 Yin Channels have as their pertaining Organs the three *Zang* ('solid') Organs which are situated above the diaphragm, viz: Heart, Lung and Pericardium. ("*Zang*" in Chinese means to store).

Connections with the Large Intestine Channel:

Yuan-Source point: Taiyuan (Lu.9.)

Luo-Connecting point: Lieque (Lu. 7.).

Clinical uses:

1) Disorders along the Lung Channel.

2) Disorders of the respiratory system.

3) Skin disorders (Lung is connected to the tissue, skin).

4) Vascular disorders.

5) Disorders of the Large Intestine (the related Yang Organ).

6) Neck disorders.

Commonly used acupuncture points:

Chest	:	Lu.	1.	
Elbow	:	Lu.	5.	
Forearm	:	Lu.	6,	Lu. 7.
Wrist	:	Lu.	9.	
Thumb	:	Lu.	11.	

Description of the commonly used points:

Zhongfu *(Lu. 1.)*. *(Chungfu)*. Alarm (Mu Front point of the Lung. Dangerous points.

TWO METHODS OF LOCATING LIEQUE (Lu. 7.)

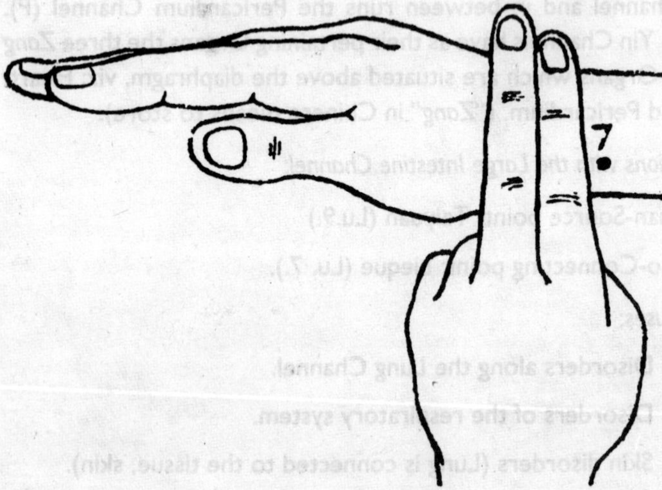

The above is the preferred method as it is more accurate.

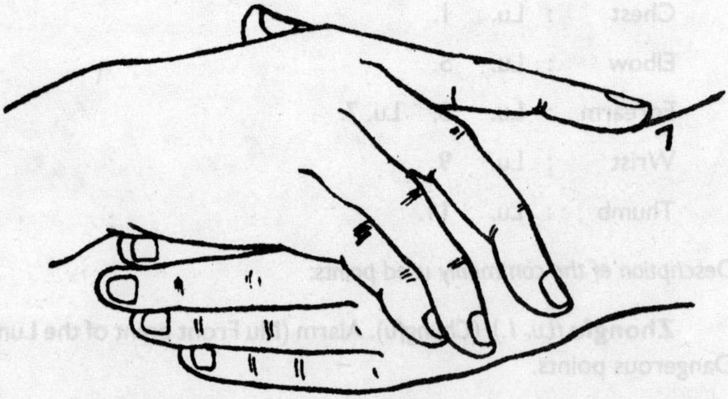

Location: (1) At the level of the interspace between the 1st and 2nd ribs 6 cun lateral to the midline.

(2) In the infracavicular fossa 1.5 cun below the midpoint of the clavicle.

Indications: Cough, pain in the chest and shoulder area, diseases of the lung, bronchial asthma, bronchitis.

Puncture: 0.5 cun laterally and horizontally. Moxa is applicable.[2]

Note: a) As the lung lies underneath this point, it is a *Dangerous point.* Inserting the needle perpendicularly may cause collapse of the lung. The beginner must be careful, if this point is used, to insert it in the correct direction. It is advisable for the beginner to use the point Shanzhong (Ren. 17.) for the same indications.

b) This is the *Front Alarm point*[3] *of the Lung.* In disorder of the Lung this point becomes tender (painful to pressure). (An Alarm point is a specific acupuncture point which becomes tender when there is disease of the related Organ).

c) This point illustrates a fundamental principle of acupuncture that *all* acupuncture points treat diseases of the local and adjacent areas.

(Recent research has shown that the local points are generally the most effective points in the treatment of most disorders).

Chize (*Lu. 5.*). (*Chihtse*). Water point. Son point.

Location: At the level of the elbow crease, on the lateral (radial) border of the tendon of the biceps muscle. (This tendon is better felt when the elbow is slightly flexed).

2 Moxibustion is used in Yin disorders such as chronic bronchial asthma.

3 Front Alarm Point = Mu point.

THE THREE FREQUENTLY USED DISTAL POINTS OF THE UPPER LIMB

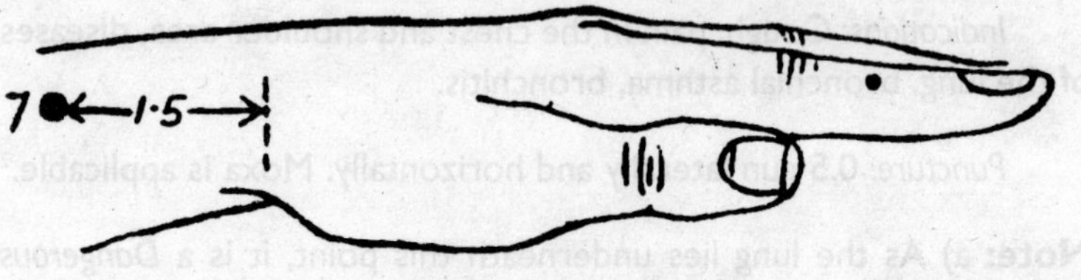

Lieque (Lu. 7.)

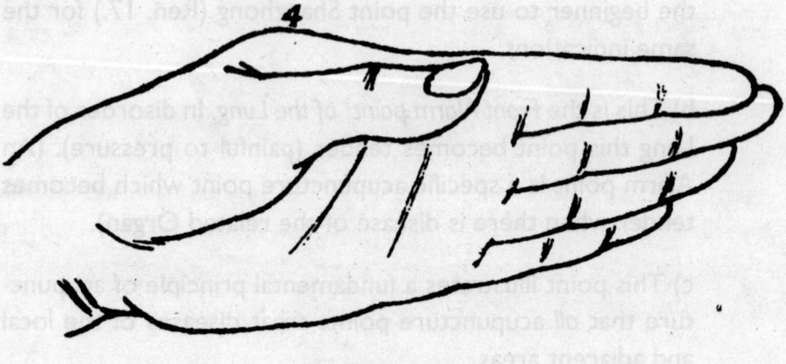

Hegu (L.I. 4.)

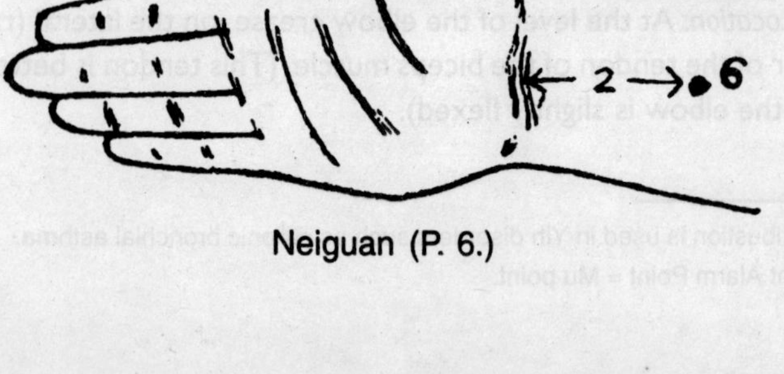

Neiguan (P. 6.)

Indications: Pain and swelling of the elbow, arthritis of the elbow, skin diseases.

Puncture: 0.5 cun perpendicularly. Bleeding at this point is carried out for skin disorders.[4] This is a very effective therapy for psoriasis and for eczema, especially with pruritus.

Kongzui (*Lu. 6.*). (*Kungtsui*). Xi-Cleft point.

Location: 5 cun distal to Chize (Lu. 5.), on the path of the Channel. It is located on the medial border of the radius.

Note: 5 cun = 6½ finger breadths.

Indications: Used in acute respiratory diseases, e.g., an acute attack of asthma, tonsillitis, acute cough, acute rhinitis, pruritus.

Puncture: 0.5 cun perpendicularly. Strong manual stimuiation is carried out.

Note: In each Channel there is a point for treating acute disorders of the pertaining Organ. This point is known as the *Xi-Cleft point.* For treating acute disorders of the Lung, for example in acute bleeding from the lung (haemoptysis), this point may be used until specialized medical treatment becomes available. It is very effective in the treatment of acute asthmatic attacks.

Lieque (*Lu. 7.*). (*Liehchueh*). Luo-Connecting point. One of the six important Distal points. Confluent point of the Ren Channel.[5]

Location: When the index fingers and the thumbs of both hands of the patient are crossed, this point is under the tip of the upper index finger. However, the better method of locating this point is by measuring 1.5 cun proximally from the wrist joint crease on the outer, radial or lateral border of the forearm. (1.5 cun=2 finger breadths).

---

4 One drop of blood is taken out from the ante-cubial vein and injected into another specific point such as Xuehai (Sp. 10.) or Dazhui (Du 14.).

5 There is a confluent point for each of the 8 Extraordinary Channels. This point is the main focus of energy.

THE THREE FREQUENTLY USED DISTAL POINTS OF THE LOWER LIMB

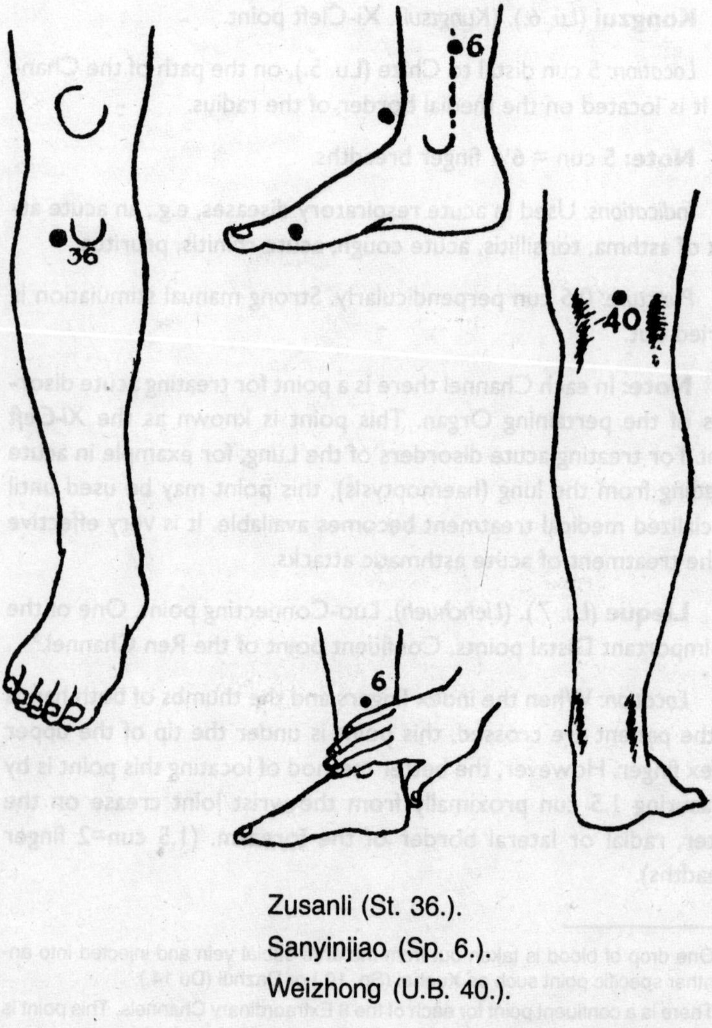

Zusanli (St. 36.).

Sanyinjiao (Sp. 6.).

Weizhong (U.B. 40.).

Indications: Headache on the back of the head (occipital headache), stiff neck, cervical spondylosis, pain along the back of the chest, lung disorders such as bronchial asthma, bronchitis, skin disorders.

Puncture: 0.5 cun horizontally. The needle is directed proximally in proximal disorders. i.e., where it is used as a Distal point. In disorders such as arthritis of the wrist the needle is inserted distally. Local moxibustion is carried out in De Quervain's disease.

Note: All points distal to the elbow and distal to the knee also treat proximal disorders. There are six commonly used Distal points. Of these, 3 are situated in the arm and 3 in the leg:-

Distal Point	Proximal Areas of Influence
Arm:	
Lieque (LU. 7.).	Back of the head and neck. Lung diseases, disorders of the upper half of the spine.
Hegu (L.I. 4.)	Front of head and neck, face and special sense organs. (This is the most potent analgesic) point of the body).
Neiguan (P. 6.).	Front of chest and upper half of abdomen (above the umbilicus), and the internal organs in these regions.
Leg	
Zusanli (St. 36.).	Abdomen, including the internal abdominal organs. (This is also a general Tonification point).
Weizhong (U.B. 40.).	Low backache, sciatica, genitourinary dis orders.
Sanyinjiao (Sp. 6.)	Pelvic disorders, external genitalia, perineal area. (This is also a Tonification point).

THE LUNG CHANNEL

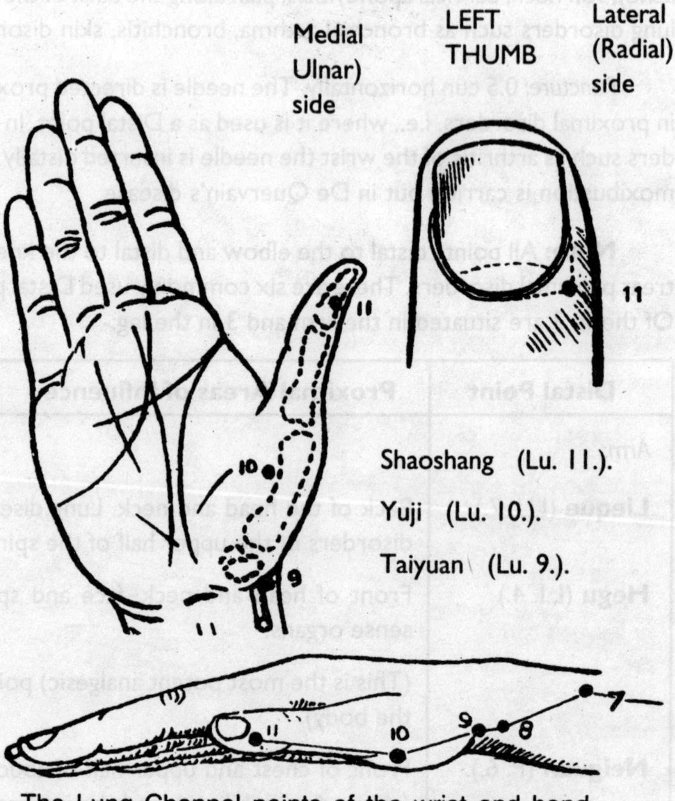

The Lung Channel points of the wrist and hand.

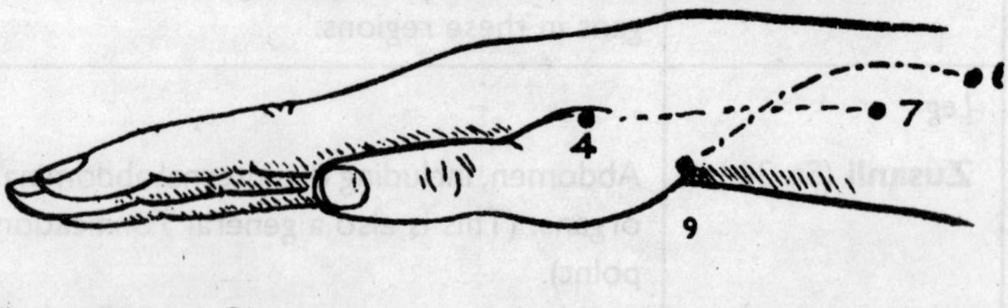

The collateral Channels connecting the Yuan-Source and Luo-Connecting points of the Lu. and L.I. Channels. (Use Luo-Connecting point of the deficient side)

Taiyuan (*Lu. 9.*) (*Taiyuan*). Yuan-Source point, Influential point for vascular disorders. Earth point. Mother point.

Location. At the outer end of the wrist crease, on the lateral side of the radial artery.

Indications: Diseases of the wrist joint, arteriosclerosis and other vascular disorders.

Puncture: 0.3 cun perpendicularly (avoiding the radial artery).

Note: An Influential point is an acupuncture point used to treat specific tissue disorders. According to traditional Chinese medicine there are 8 such specific tissues, and therefore 8 named Influential points.

Shaoshang (*Lu. 11.*) (*Shaoshang*). Jing-Well point.

Location: 0.1 cun proximal to the outer (lateral or radial) corner of the nail of the thumb.

Indications: Hysterical attack, fainting, epileptic attack convulsions, high fever, cardiac arrest, drowning, respiratory arrest, and other acute emergencies, Resuscitation of the newborn.

Puncture: 0.1 cun perpendicularly to cause bleeding, or strong acupressure to cause intense pain.

Note: a) The distal-most point of each of the 12 Channels is known as a *Jing-Well* point. These points are used to treat acute emergencies such as coma, severe pain, high fever and shock. The point Yongquan (K.I.) is generally considered the most responsive point. However, the point Renzhong (Du 26.) is used more often in practice due to its easier accessibility and its responsiveness even to finger-pressure. This is the Yang-most point in the body, there are 3 Yang Channels crossing here.

b) *A Yuan* Source point is a point at which the energy accumulates. From here the Yin energy is converted to yang energy, or *vice versa,* before it is transferred to the Paired

Channel *via* the Luo-Connecting point of the latter Channel. A Yuan-Source point may be specifically used in treating subacute and chronic disorders of the pertaining Organ. Where there is an imbalance of energy between two Paired Channels of their respective Organs, a combination of the relevant Yuan-Source and Luo-Connecting points may be used to re-establish the balance (or the Luo-Connecting point of the deficient Channel or Organ only may be needled).

c) The Lung Channel and the Large Intestine Channel (as also the other Paired Channels) have points called *Luo-Connecting*[6] points which serve the function of connecting the Yin and Yang Channels which are paired thereby obtaining a balancing of the vital energy. This connection is achieved by collateral Luo channels connecting the Yuan-Source point and Luo-Connecting point of the Paired Channels, thus:

Yuan-Source Point		*Luo-Connecting Point.*
Taiyuan (Lu. 9.)	—and—	Pianli (L.I. 6).
Hegu (L.I. 4)	—and—	Lieque (Lu. 7.).

Each of the Fourteen Channels has a Luo-Connecting point, with an extra point possessed by the Spleen Channel, making a total of 15. They are used for treating diseases involving both Paired Chinnels caused by an imbalance of vital energy between them. Energy may flow in either direction in the Luo channels. When an imbalance occurs in the coupled Organs or channels, the Luo-Connecting point of the deficient Organ or channel is needled.

6 Luo in Chinese means the door through which vital energy enters.

List of all the acupuncture points of the Lung Channel:

Lu. 1 : **Zhongfu** - Alarm point (MU-Font) of the Lung, Dangerous point.

Lu. 2 : **Yunmen**

Lu. 3 : **Tianfu**

Lu. 4 : **Xiabal**

Lu. 5 : **Chize** - Water point, Son point.[7]

Lu. 6 : **Kongzui** - Xi-Cleft point.

Lu. 7 : **Lieque** - Luo-Connecting point, one of the 6 im portant Distal points. Confluent point.

Lu. 8. : **Jingqu** - Metal point (Element point), Horary point.

Lu. 9. : **Taiyuan** - Yuan-Source point, Influential point, Earth point. Mother point.[8]

Lu. 10 : **Yuji** - Motor point, Fire point.

Lu. 11. : **Shaoshang** - Jing-Well point, Wood point.

Note I: There are 12 Paired Channels on each side (6 Yin and 6 Yang). Each Yin channel is coupled to a Yang Channel. Thus, there are 6 pairs coupled as follows:

Lu.-L.I., St.-Sp., H.-SI., U.B.-K., P.-S.J., G.B.-Liv. Vital energy flows sequentially in this order. From the Liver Channel the energy flows to the Lung Channel again, to complete the cycle.

The maximum flow of energy takes a period of two hours in each of the Twelve Channels thus completing a full cycle within a 24 hour period. In the Lung Channel the cycle commences at 3.00 a.m. and ends at 5.00 a.m. The use of the appropriate time of the day using the Horary (Element) point to treat an Organ disorder is known

7 Son point Reducing or Sedation point.

8 Mother point — Reinforcing or Tonification point. Earth is the mother of Metal.

as the Noon-Midnight Law (also called Midday-Midnight Law or the Organ Clock), the Phenomenon of circadian rhythm or biorhythm.

Note II: All acupuncture points treat disorders along the Channel, related sense organ (e.g., Lung Channel: the nose), and related tissue (e.g., Lung Channel: the skin).

THE CIRCULATION OF ENERGY IN THE LUNG

The Lung Channel of Hand-Taiyin originates internally in the middle (Zhong) body cavity (Jiao). Here it connects with the Organ Large Intestine. It ascends upwards along the oesophageal hiatus of the diaphragm to enter the upper body cavity (Zhang Jiao) where it communicates with Lung, its pertaining organ. From the Lung it ascends up the neck to the nose to the nose and occiput. From the occiput the internal channel descends to give rise to the superficial channel which commences at Zhongfu (Lu. 1.).

The main communications along the superficial course of the Lung Channel are as follows:

(a) From Lieque (Lu. 7.) a branch communicates with Shangyang (L.I. 1.).

(b) Communications with the Large Intestine Channel occur at the Yuan Source point Taiyuan (Lu. 9.) and the Luo-connecting points (Lieque Lu. 7).

(c) At the Yuan Source point a direct internal communication exists with the Lung Organ.

(d) The energy which escapes from the superficial Channel at the terminal (Jing-Well) point Shaoshang (Lu. 11.), fills the intricate network of muscular channels (meridians) and travels proximally, mainly in the soft tissues, deeper to the superficial Lung Channel and communicates with the Lung Organ and the origin of the channel in the middle body cavity. The superficial channel carries mainly yin energy while the intricate muscular merdian network is filled with mainly yang energy.

THE SYNDROMES OF THE LUNG

A. **The Lung Channel.** Cough, fullness of chest, bronchial asthma, haemoptysis: pharyngitis, pain along the superficial course of the channel.

B. **The Organ Lung.** Diseases of the lung are described according to traditional Chinese medicine under four main clinical syndromes.

1) **Deficient Yin.** This occurs in chronic lung disorders. The clinical manifestations are dry cough, scanty sputum, evening temperature, night sweating, red tongue, thready and rapid pulse.

2) **Invasion of the Lung by pathogenic wind.** Difficulty of breathing is pronounced. Cough and nasal obstruction occur accompanied by copious sputum and watery nasal discharge. If the wind is accompanied by cold, a white coated tongue occurs. If the wind is accompanied by heat, then tongue coating is yellow and the sputum is purulent.

3) **Damp-phlegm in the Lung.** The damp-phlegm blocks the passage of the vital energy pathways.

The clinical manifestations are cough, dyspnoea and expectoration of copious white frothy sputum. The tongue coating is white.

4) **Phlegm-heat in the Lung.** This is caused by the invasion of endogenous factors which produces heat in the Lung.

The clinical manifestations are those of bronchial asthma.
Foul smelling purulent sputum may be expectorated. The sputum may be blood-stained. A red tongue with a yellow coating and a rapid pulse may be present.

■

手の陽明大腸経之圖

て瞀此臂厥と爲。是肺を主る。所生の病ハ咳嗽。上氣喘喝煩心胷満

の内前廉痛掌中熱氣盛に餘有。則肩背痛風寒汗出。中風

便數小而欠し虚する則ハ肩背痛。寒少氣以て息に足不。溺色變し。卒

遺失爲を度無盛なる者ハ。寸口大なること人迎に三倍と。虚する者ハ寸口反

迎より小也

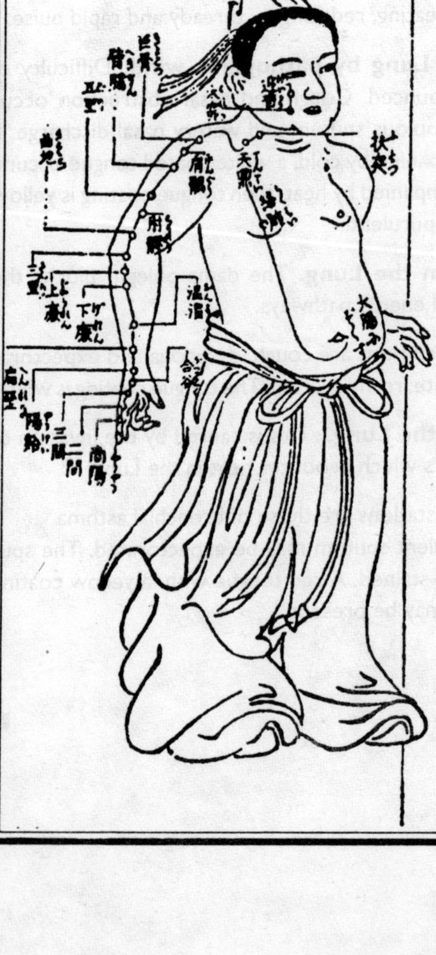

LARGE INTESTINE CHANNEL (L.I.)

"The Large Intestine transmits and drains the wastes".

— *Su Wen*

— Polarity: Yang.

— Number of points: 20.

— Pertaining Organ: Large Intestine.

— Related Channel: Lung Channel (Lu.)

— Element: Metal

— Energy flow: Centripetal.

— Course:

The Large Intestine Channel originates its superficial course near the lateral edge of the base of the nail of the forefinger. It travels up (proximally) to the opposite side of the face, along the posterior and lateral aspect of the arm and the side of the neck, to end lateral to the nostril of the opposite side. The Channels of the two sides cross each other on the upper lip.

Connections with the Lung Channel

Yuan-Source point: Hegu (L.I. 4.)

THE LARGE INTESTINE CHANNEL
Du 26. Renzhong (Also called Shigou)

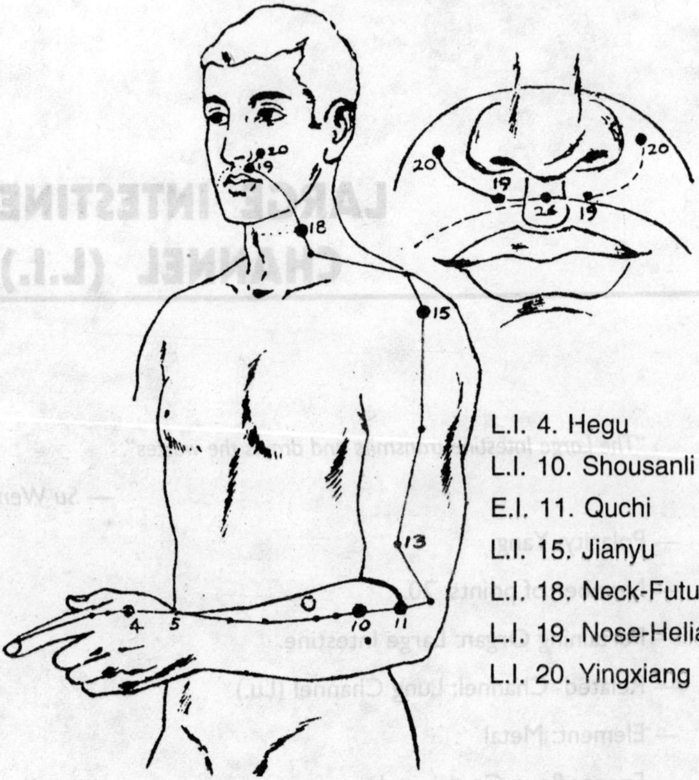

L.I. 4. Hegu

L.I. 10. Shousanli

E.I. 11. Quchi

L.I. 15. Jianyu

L.I. 18. Neck-Futu

L.I. 19. Nose-Heliao

L.I. 20. Yingxiang

Note: 1. The left Channel crosses to the right side and vice versa.

Nose - Heliao (L.I. 19.) and Yingxiang (L.I. 20.) are located on the opposite side after the crossing has occurred. However, according to some authorities, the former point is located before the crossing.

2. Renzhong (Du. 26.) is the crossing point of three yang channels. Therefore it is a useful point to be used in acute emergencies caused by an excess of yin (e.g. fainting).

Luo-Connecting point: Pianli (L.I. 6.).

Clinical uses:

1) Relief of pain. The point Hegu (L.I. 4.) is the best analgesic point in the body.

2) Diseases along the Channel, e.g., paralysis of the upper limb, frozen shoulder.

3) Respiratory disorders, e.g., rhinitis, pharyngitis.

4) Fever.

5) High blood pressure.

6) Skin disorders.

7) Therapy and surgery of thyroid gland disorders.

Commonly used acupuncture points:

Hand	:	L.I. 4.
Forearm	:	L.I. 10.
Elbow	:	L.I. 11.
Shoulder	:	L.I. 14.
Neck	:	L.I. 18.
Face	:	L.I. 19. L.I. 20.

Description of the commonly used points:

Hegu (L.I. 4.) (*Hoku*). Yuan-Source point. (In Chinese "Heagu" means "the great eliminator" One of the six important Distal points.

Location: It is situated in the web between the forefinger and thumb on the dorsal (posterior) aspect of the hand, and may be located by one of 4 methods:

a) When the forefinger and the thumb are adducted, at the highest point of the muscles on the back of the hand.

b) At the midpoint of line drawn from the junction of the 1st and 2nd metacarpal bones to the middle point of the border of the web.

c) Place the distal-most crease of one thumb against the web between the opposite thumb and forefinger. Where the tip of the former thumb (when it is flexed) then rests, is the point Hegu (L.I. 4). of the latter hand.

d) At the middle of the 2nd metacarpal bone, on the radial aspect (The acupuncture point falls more medially by this method. This is the method commonly used in acupuncture anaesthesia.)

Note: The 2 locations described by these methods lie in relation to the motor points of the adductor pollicis and of the first dorsal interosseous muscles respectively.

Indications:

a) Disorders of the thumb, forefinger and wrist joint.

b) The best analgesic point of the body both for therapy and anaesthesia.

c) Distal point for front of the head, face, special sense organs, and front of neck.

d) Disorders of the large intestine, e.g., acute intestinal colic.

e) Disorders of the lung.

Puncture: 0.5 to 0.1 cun perpendicularly, or towards Laogong (P.8.).

Note: There are 5 important physiological effects of needling. This point exhibits all effects well, although its principal effect is the analgesic effect. There is likewise a specificity of effect at certain acupuncture points, i.e. these 5 physiological effects are found to be more pronounced at certain points. These points are summarised as follows:

Effect	Acupuncture Points
1) Analgesic	Hegu (L.I. 4.), Neiting (St. 44.).
2) Sedative	Baihui (Du 20.), Shenmen, (H. 7.), Shenmai (U.B. 62.).
3) Homeostatic (regulatory)	Quchi (L.I. 11.) Zusanli (St. 36.), Sanyinjiao (Sp. 6.).
4) Immune-enhancing, anti-inflammatory	Dazhui (Du 14.), Quchi. (L.I. 11.), Sanyinjiao (Sp. 6.).
5) Motor recovery	Acupuncture points situated over the motor points of the affected muscles, e.g., Femur-Futu (St. 32.).

Shousanli (*L.I. 10*). (*Shousanli*). Shiatsu point to relieve pain.

Location: On the lateral aspect of the forearm, 2 cun below[1] Quchi (L.I, 11.). Motor point of the brachio-radiolis muscle.

Indications: Tennis elbow, arthritis of the elbow, pain tremor or paralysis of the forearm as in stroke, paraesthesia.

Puncture: 1.0-1.5 cun perpendicularly. Acupressure to relieve pain.[2]

Quchi (*L.I. 11.*). (*Chuchih*). Homoeostatic point.

Location: a) At the outer end of the elbow crease when the elbow is semiflexed.

b) Midway between Chize (Lu. 5) and the lateral epicondyle of the humerus, when the elbow is semiflexed.

Indications: Disorders of the elbow, tennis elbow paralysis of the arm, high blood pressure, skin diseases. This is the best homoeostatic point of the body.

---

1 Distal to

2 A popular Shiatsu (Japanese art of acupressure) point.

Puncture: 1.0 to 1.5. cun perpendiculary. Moxibustion may be used in deficiency disorder.

Jianya (*L.I. 15*). (*Chienyu*). In Chinese *"Jian"* mean shoulder.

Location: At the anterior depression lateral to the tip of the acromion process.

Indications: Disorders of the shoulder joint and the surrounding tissues, e.g., periarthritis of the shoulder (frozen shoulder). Paralysis of the arm.

Puncture: 0.5 to 10 cun perpendicularly.

Note: This point is commonly used for disorders of the shoulder joint in combination with Jianliao (S.J. 14.) and Jianzhen (S.I. 9.). When pain is present, the Distal point Hegu (L.I. 4.) may be added for very effective results. A frozen shoulder responds quicker to acupuncture than to any other form of treatment (Refer also to point Tiaokou St. 38.).

Neck-Futu (*L.I. 18*). (*Futu*) Endocrine point.

Location: 3 cun lateral to the prominence of the thyroid cartilage, (the Adam's apple).

Indications: Cough, excessive sputum, sore throat, thyroid enlargement, insufficiency of the thyroid gland, diabetes mellitus. This point is commonly used as the local point in thyroid surgery.

Puncture: 0.5 cun perpendicularly.

Note: This is a *Dangerous point* (vulnerable point) as the great vessels of the neck, vagus nerve, sympathetic trunk and the baro-receptors are situated in this area. This point is used mainly for thyroid surgery.

Nose-Heliao (*L.I. 19*). (*Heliao*).

Location: 0.5 cun lateral to point Renzhong (Du 26.), after the channel has crossed the midline.

Indications: Bleeding from the nose (epistaxis), nasal obstruction, facial paralysis, trigeminal neuralgia, toothache.

Puncture: 0.3 to 0.5 cun obliquely, directed medially.

Yingxiang (*L.I. 20*) (*Yinghsiang*). In Chinese "Yingxiang" means welcome fragrance.

Location: In the horizontal line drawn from on the outermost point of the ala nasi on the naso-labial groove.

Indications: Rhinitis, nose bleeding (epistaxis), blocking of the nose due to an inflammation, sinusitis, facial paralysis, trigeminal neuralgia, toothache.

Puncture: 0.3 to 0.5 cun obliquely and directed medially

List of all the acupuncture points of the Large Intestine Channel

L.I. 1. : **Shangyang** - Jing-Well points, Metal point.

L.I. 2. : **Erjian** - Water point.

L.I. 3. : **Sanjian** - Wood point.

L.I. 4. : **Hegu** - Yuan-Source point, the best analgesic point of the body, one of the 6 important Distal points.

L.I. 5. : **Yangxi** - Fire point.

L.I. 6. : **Pianli** - Luo-Connecting point.

L.I. 7. : **Wenliu** - Xi-Cleft point.

L.I. 8. : **Xialian**

L.I. 9. : **Shanglian**

L.I. 10. : **Shousanli**

L.I. 11. : **Quchi** - Best homoeostatic point of the body, immune enhancing point, Earth point.

L.I. 12. : **Zouliao**

L.I. 13. : **Wuli**

L.I. 14. : **Binao**

L.I. 15. : **Jianyu**

L.I. 16. : **Jugu**

L.I. 17. : **Tianding**

L.I. 18. : **Neck-Futu** - Dangerous point.

L.I. 19. : **Nose-Heliao**

L.I. 20. : **Yingxiang**

From Yingxiang (L.I. 20.) the Yang vital energy flows on to Chengqi (St. I.). The Large Intestine channel is therefore the mother of the Stomach channel, which is the son channel.

Note: The Lung and the Large Intestine are related to the skin and also to the body hair. These two Organs are also connected to the nose. Every Organ is similarly connected to specific tissues and to a special sense organ. The Large Intestine Channel is not usually used in treating chronic disorders of the Large Intestine.

CIRCULATION OF ENERGY IN THE LARGE INTESTINE

The Large Intestine Channel of Hand-Yangming, while traversing its superficial course, sends a communicating branch to the depression below the vertebra prominens (Dazhui, Du 14.).

The internal channel commences at the supraclavicular fossa and passes through the Organ Lung and then through the diaphragm to enter the Large Inestine, its pertaining Organ.

The Organ Large Intestine is also connected to the Stomach Channel at the point Shangiuxu (St. 37.), its lower or inferior He-Sea point.

SYNDROMES OF THE LARGE INTESTINE

A. **The Large Intestine Channel** - Pain along the Channel, frozen shoulder, pharyngitis, toothache, epistaxis, rhinitis.

B. **The Large Intestine Organ** - Diseases of the Large Intestine Organ are described under three main clinical syndromes.

1) **Stasis of the Large Intestine.** This is caused by eating unclean foods. The clinical manifestations are constipation, or diarrhoea distension of the abdomen, abdominal tenderness aggra-

vated on palpation. The tongue is white and sticky. A *shi* type of pulse is present.

2) **Damp-heat in the Large Intestine.** This is caused by unsuitable food. The clinical manifestations are diarrhoea, often with blood-stained mucus and tenesmus. The stools are very offensive smelling. The tongue is red with a yellow coating. The pulse is rapid and 'rolling'.

3) **Stagnation of blood and heat in the Large Intestine.** This syndrome is due to climatic or geographical changes. The clinical manifestations are lower abdominal pain, constipation. A red tongue with a yellow sticky coating may be present.

■

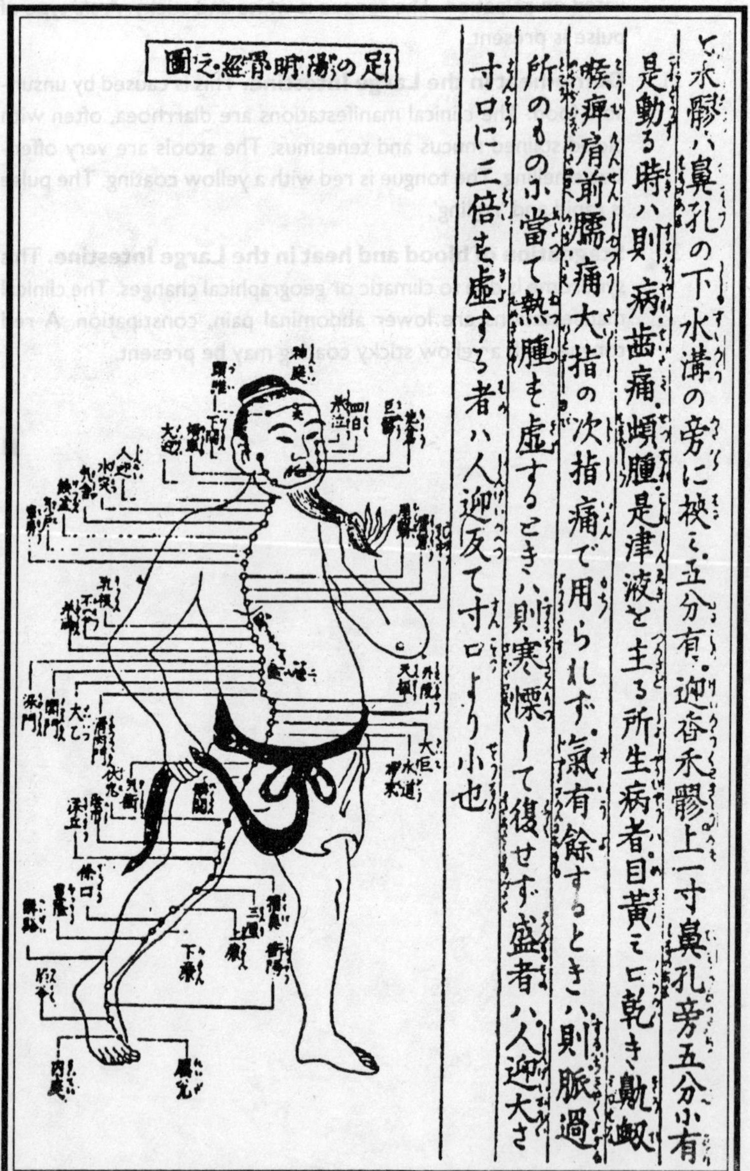
足の陽明胃経之図
水髎ハ鼻孔の下水溝の旁に挾こ五分有。迎香禾髎上一寸鼻孔旁五分ニ有
是動る時ハ則病歯痛。頄腫。是津液を主る所生病者目黄て口乾き鼽衄
喉痹肩前臑痛大指の次指痛で用られず。氣有餘するときハ則脈過
所のものニ當て熱腫を虚するときハ則寒慄して復せず盛者ハ人迎大さ
寸口に三倍を虚する者ハ人迎反て寸口より小也

STOMACH CHANNEL (ST.)

"Liquid and solid enter the Stomach. The five zang and six Fu organs are replensihed with Qi from the Stomach"

— Ling Shu

— Polarity: Yang.

— Number of points: 45.

— Pertaining Organ: Stomach.

— Related Channel: Spleen Channel (Sp).

— Element: Earth.

— Energy flow: Centrifugal.

— Course:

Orginates its superficial course below the eye and makes a U-turn outwards on the face. It continues from the lowest point of the "U" downwards, 4 cun lateral to the midline along the nipple line. In the abdomen it travels downwards 2 cun lateral to the midline. Then it runs along the anterior aspect of the lower limb, to end at the base of the nail of the 2nd toe.

Connections with the Spleen Channel:

Yuan-Source point: Chongyang (St. 42.).

Luo-Connecting point: Fenglong (St. 40.).

THE STOMACH CHANNEL
— Face Area —

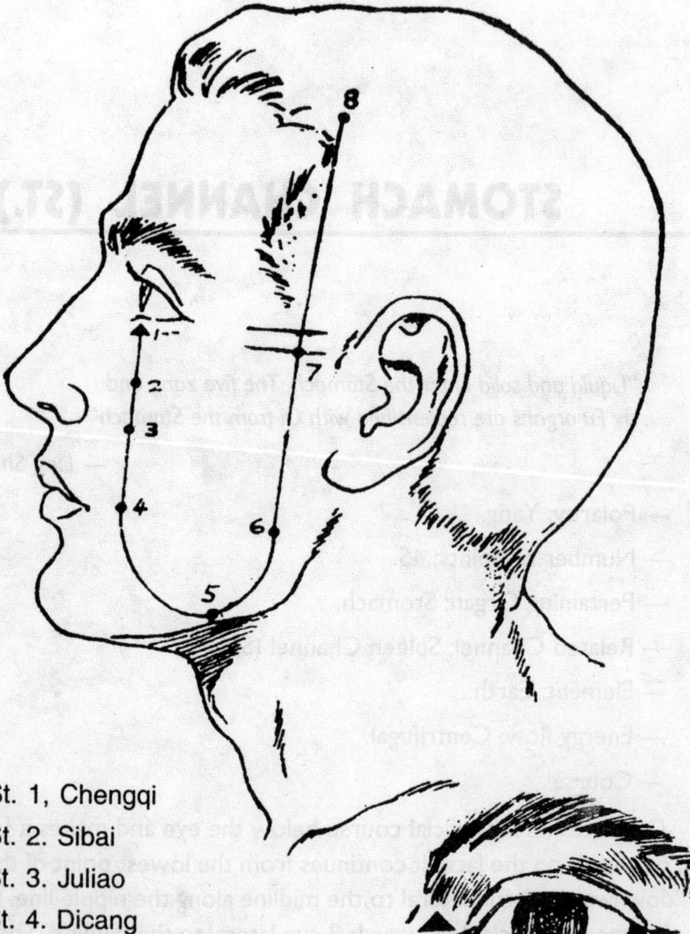

St. 1, Chengqi
St. 2. Sibai
St. 3. Juliao
St. 4. Dicang
St. 5. Daying
St. 6. Jiache
St. 7. Xiaguan
St. 8. Touwei

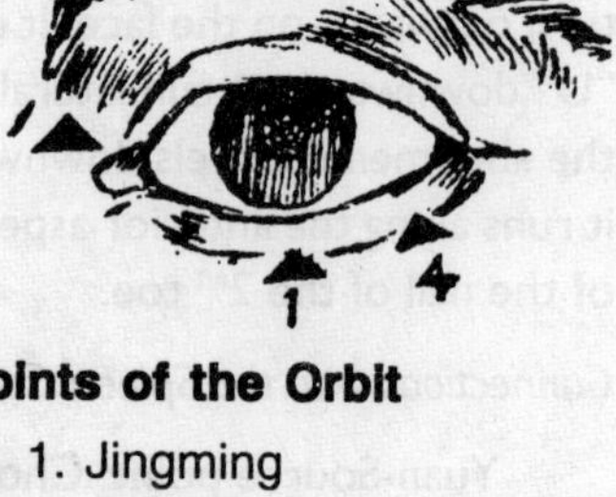

Dangerous Points of the Orbit

U.B.	1. Jingming
St.	1. Chengqi
Extra	4. Qiuhou

Clinical uses:

1) Disorders of the stomach, spleen and other abdominal organs.

2) Disorders along the Channel:

   a) face area, e.g., trigeminal neuralgia toothache, facial paralysis, sinusitis;

   b) chest diseases;

   c) breast disorders;

   d) abdomen, e.g., gastro-intestinal disorders, menstrual disorders;

   e) lower limb, e.g., paralysis of the lower limb, disorders of the joints of the lower limb.

Commonly used acupuncture points:

Face : St. 1 to St. 8.

Chest : St. 17-Prohibited point, St. 18.

Abdomen : St. 21, St. 25, St. 29.

Leg : St. 31 St. 32, St. 34, St. 35, St. 36, St. 37, St. 38, St. 39, St. 40. St. 41, St. 43, and St. 44.

Description of the commonly used points:

Chengqi (*St. 1.*). *Chengchi*).

Location: Below the eyeball at the midpoint of the lower margin of the orbit.

Indications: Disorders of the eyes and eye-lids.

Puncture: 0.3 to 0.5 cun perpendicularly. Insert the needle along the floor of the orbit, with the patient's eyeball turned upwards.

Note: a) All points located in the orbit are *Dangerous points:* i.e., Chengqi (St. 1.). Jingming (U.B. 1.), Qiuhou (Extra 4.). Great care and good sterilization of the needles must be ensured when needling these points. No force must be applied during insertion. No stimulation should be carried out at these points.

THE STOMACH CHANNEL

St. 1. Chengqi

St. 2. Sibai

St. 3. Juliao

St. 4. Dicang

St. 5. Daying

St. 6. Jiache

St. 7. Xiaguan

St. 8. Touwei

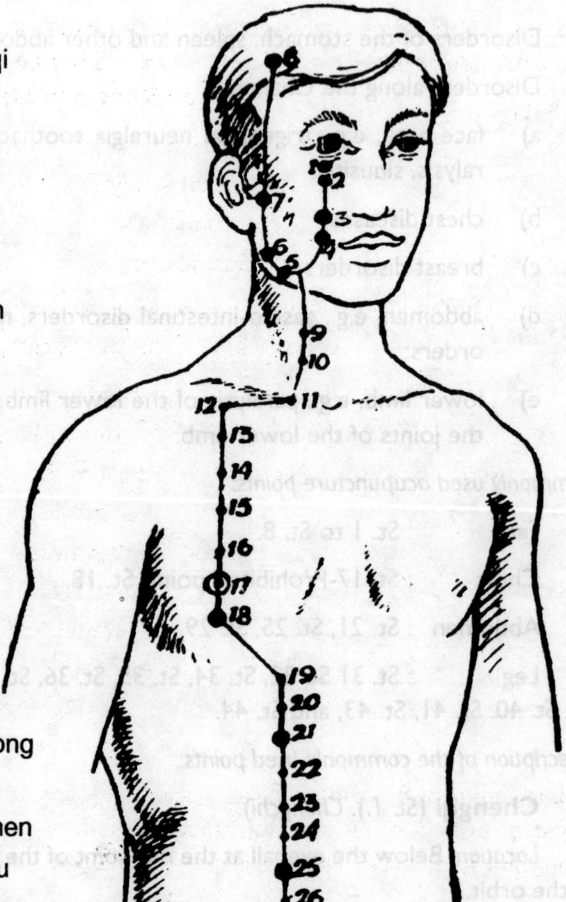

*St. 17. Ruzhong

St. 18. Rugen

St. 21. Liangmen

St. 25. Tianshu

St. 29. Guilai

Note: Liangmen (St. 21.) on the right side is a dangerous point, as it overlies the gall bladder.

* Prohibited point

b) The first 4 points of the Stomach Channel are in a straight line drawn vertically downwards on the face from Chengqi (St. 1.) This is called the mid-pupillary line.

Sibai (*St. 2.*). (*Szupai*).

Location: 0.7 cun below Chengqi (St. 1.) in the infraorbital foramen.

Indictions: Eye disease, facial paralysis trigeminal neuragia,

Puncture: 0.3 cun perpendicularly into the infra-orbital foramen.

Juliao (*St. 3.*). (*Chuliao*).

Location: Directly below Sibai (St. 2.), at the level of the lower border of the ala nasi.

Indications: Facial paralysis, trigeminal neuralgia, rhinitis, toothache.

Puncture: 0.3 to 0.5 cun obliquely.

Dicang (*St. 4.*). (*Titsang*).

Location: 0.4 cun lateral to the corner or the mouth.

Indications: Facial paralysis, trigeminal neuralgia, excessive salivation, cheilosis, speech difficulties, mutism, disorders of upper teeth, anaesthesia for extraction of upper teeth.

Puncture: 0.5 inch obliquely, or 2.0-3.0 cun horizontal insertion towards Jiache (St. 6.).

Daying (*St. 5.*). (*Taying*).

Locations: At the lowest point of the anterior border of the masseter muscle.

Indications: Facial paralysis, trigeminal neuralgia, toothache, parotitis; swelling of the cheek, trismus.

Puncture: 0.5 cun perpendicularly or obliquely.

Jiache (*St. 6.*). (*Chiache*).

Location: At the most prominent point of the masseter muscle, felt on clenching the jaws. This is a motor point.

Indications: Facial paralysis, trigeminal neuralgia, toothache, parotitis, spasm of the masseter muscle, trismus.

Puncture: 0.3 cun perpendicularly or horizontally towards Dicang (St. 4.).

Xiaguan (*St.* 7.). (Hsiakuan).

Location: In the depression on the lower border of the zygomatic arch.

Indications: Facial paralysis, trigeminal neuralgia, toothache, arthritis of the mandibular joint.

Puncture: 0.5 cun perpendicularly.

Touwei (*St.* 8.). (*Touwei*).

Location: 0.5 cun lateral to the corner (lateral end) of the anterior hairline.

Indications: Migraine, ophthalmoplegia, increased lacrimation.

Puncture: 0.5 inch horizontally, directed posteriorly for headache, anteriorly for eye disorders.

Note: a) At all points of the scalp the needles are inserted horizontally, because there is no fleshy mass of muscle under the skin to stabilise the needle.

b) If the patient has a receding hairline, then locate the hairline at 3 cun above the eyebrows or glabella. It extends 4.5 cun on either side from the midline.

c) The distance between the two points of each side is 9 cun.

Ruzhong (*St.* 17.). (*Juchung*). (The Nipple).

This is a *Prohibited point for acupuncture and moxibustion.* It is used only as a landmark. The anatomical location of the nipple is the level of the 4th intercostal space, 4 cun lateral to the midline.

Rugen (*St.* 18). (*Juken*).

Location: On the nipple-line, in the 5th intercostal space.

Indications: Mastitis, deficient lactation, chest pain, cough, dyspnoea, angina pectoris and other heart disorders.

Puncture: 0.5 cun obliquely or horizontally outwards.

Note: This is a Dangerous point, as it is situated in an intercostal space. No stimulation should be carried out.

Liangmen (*St. 21.*). (*Liangmen*).

Location: 4 cun vertically above Tianshu (St. 25) and 2 cun lateral to Zhongwan (Ren 12.).

Indications: Acute and chronic gastritis, peptic ulcer, nausea, vomiting, (i.e., upper abdominal disorders).

Puncture: 0.5 –1.0 cun perpendicularly on the left side or obliquely on the right side as it is over the gall bladder.

Note: This point on the patient's right side is a Dangerous point, as it overlies the gall-bladder. A distended gall bladder is liable to be punctured.

Tianshu (*St. 25.*). (*Tienshu*). Alarm point (MU-Front of the Large Intestine).

Location: 2 cun lateral to the umbilicus.

Indications: Acute and chronic gastro-enteritis, diarrhoea constipation, acute appendicitis, intertinal paralysis (Paralytic ileus), paralysis of the muscles of the abdominal wall (i.e., all abdominal disorders).

Puncture: 0.5 – 1.0 cun perpendicularly

Guilai (*St. 29.*). See page 150.

Biguan (*St. 31.*). (*Pikuan*).

Location: The meeting points of the vertical line from the anterior superior iliac spine and the horizontal line from the lower border of the pubtic symphysis.

Indications: Paralysis of the lower limb as in hemiplegia, osteoarthritis of the hip, sensory disorders of the lower limb.

Puncture: 1.5 cun perpendicularly.

STOMACH CHANNEL IN THE ABDOMEN

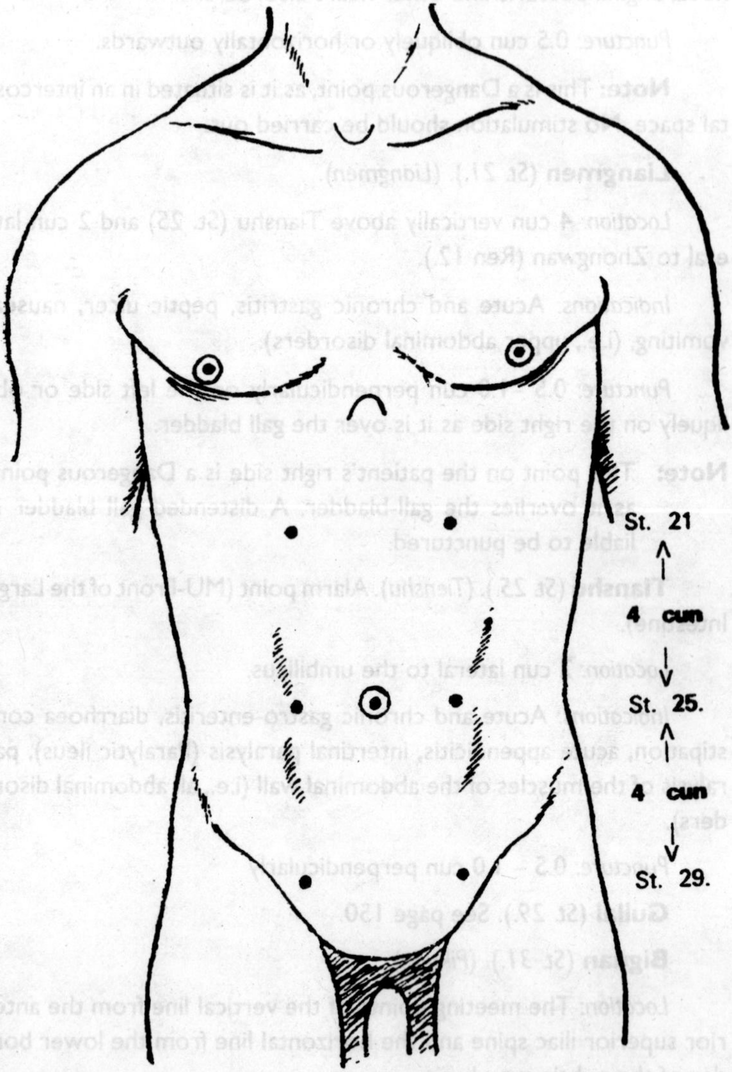

St. 21. Liangmen St. 25. Tianshu St. Guilai . The first two are the frequently used points of Stomach Channel on the abdomen

Note: In the treatment of hemiplegia, the commonly selected points are those of the Large Intestine Channel in the upper limb and Stomach Channel in the lower limb together with Yanglingquan (G.B. 34.), the Influential points for muscles and tendons.

Femur-Futu (*St. 32.*) (*Futu*).

Location: a) 6 cun above the supero-lateral point of the patella.

b) With the patient seated, place the contralateral wrist crease of the acupuncturist, on the middle of the patient's knee-cap with the fingers along his thigh. This point is located at the tip of the middle finger of the acupuncturist.

Indications: Paralysis of lower extremities, arthritis of the knee, wasting and weakness of the quadriceps. This is a motor point.

Puncture: 1.5 cun perpendicularly directed towards the lateral border of the femur, or 2.0 – 3.0 cun obliquely in a proximal direction.

Liangqiu (*St. 34*). (*Liangchiu*). Xi-Cleft point.

Location: 2 cun above the lateral end of the upper border of the patella.

Indication: Disorders of the knee, acute gastro-intestinal disroders.

Puncture: 1.0 cun perpendicularly.

Note: This is the Xi-Cleft point of the Stomach Channel. In acute gastric and intestinal disorders the pain and colic are rapidly relieved with strong stimulation (sedation) of this point.

Dubi (*St. 35.*). (*Tupi*). (Also known as Lateral-Xiyan.).

Location: This is in the depression (below the patella) on the lateral side of the ligamentum patellae. It is best located with the knee slightly bent (flexed).

Indications: Arthritis of the knee, sprain and strain of the knee.

Puncture: 0.5 cun obliquely and medially.

THE STOMACH CHANNEL
— Lower Limb —

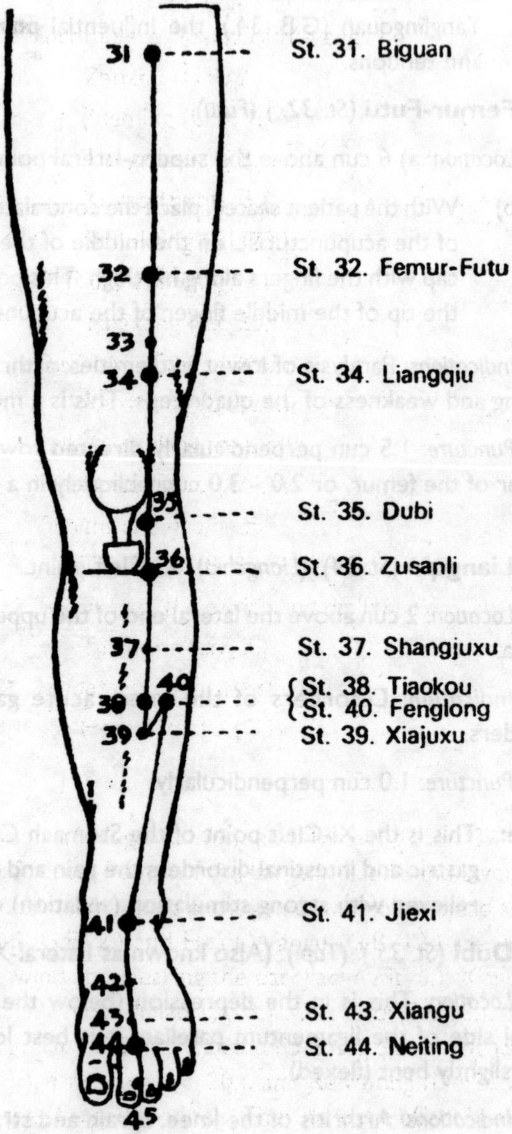

Note: There are two depressions on either side of the ligamentum patellae. The medial depression is the point Xiyan (Ex.32.)[1]. These two points and Heding (Ex. 31.) treat disorders of the knee. "Dubi" in Chinese means means the "nose of the calf".

Zusanli (*St. 36.*). (*Tsusanli*). One of the six important Distal points. General Tonification point.

Location: One finger breadth lateral to the inferior (distal) end of the tibial tuberosity.

Indications: Gastritis, nausea, vomiting, enteritis, diarrhoea, obesity, constipation, appendicitis and other diseases of the digestive tract, paralysis of lower limb, polyneuropathy of the lower limb, *This is also a general Tonification point and a Homoeostatic point.*

Puncture: 1.5 cun perpendicularly.

Note: a)The Stomach Channel runs one finger breadth lateral to the anterior border of the tibia.

b) The general Tonifications points are:

Zusanli (St. 36.).

Sanyinjiao (Sp. 6.).

Qihai (Ren. 6.).

c) Many acupuncturists find this point a good analgesic point for the lower half of the trunk and lower limbs, particularly in anaesthesia for abdominal surgery.

Shangjuxu (*St. 37.*). (*Shangchushu*). Lower He-Sea point of the Large Intestine.

Location: 3 cun distal to Zusanli (St. 36.). One finger breadth lateral to the anterior margin of the tibia.

Indications: Acute appendicitis, paralysis of the lower limb. Large Intestine disorders.

Puncture: 1.5 cun perpendicularly.

---

1 Ex- Extraordinary point.

THE STOMACH CHANNEL

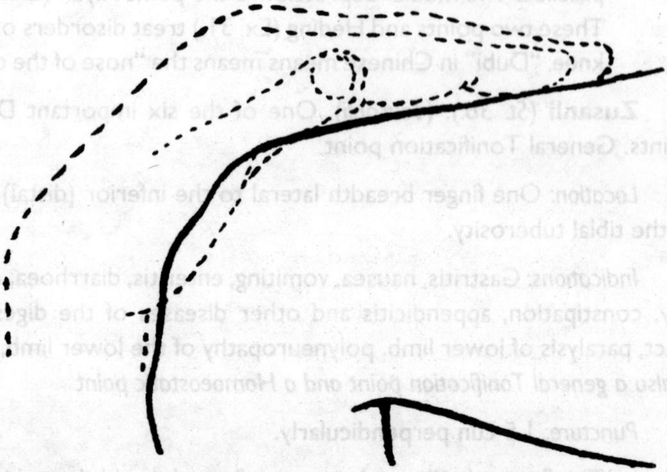

Femur-Futu (St. 32.) - Left side

ACUPUNCTURE POINTS AROUND THE RIGHT PATELLA
The point of the "nose of the calf"

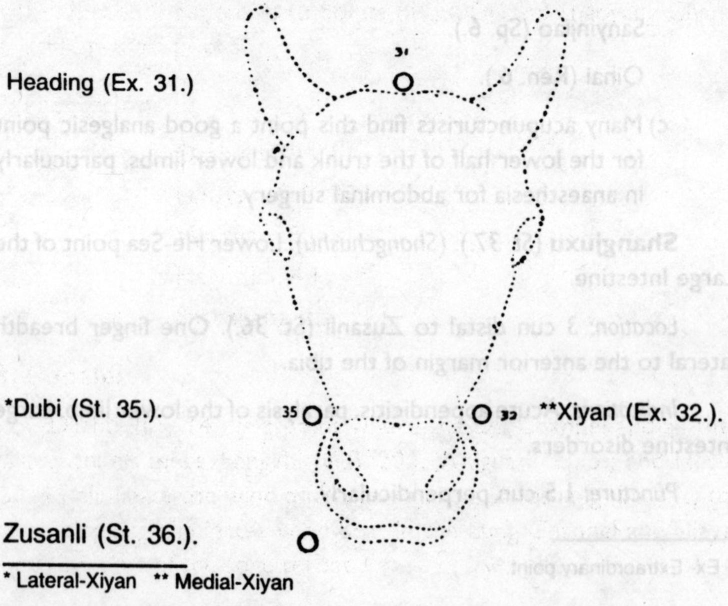

* Lateral-Xiyan ** Medial-Xiyan

Note: *Lanwei* (Ex. 33.), however, is the most effective point for acute appendicitis. It is situated on the Stomach Channel 2 cun below Zusanli (St. 36.). It is an *Alarm point,* becoming tender in diseases of the appendix. This point therefore may be used to diagnose diseases of the vermiform appendix.

Tiaolou (*St. 38.*). (*Tiaokou*).

Location: 5 cun below Zusanli (St. 36.), one finger breadth lateral to the anterior border of the tibia.

Indication: Frozen shoulder.

Puncture: 1.5 cun perpendicularly or penetrate through to Chengshan (U.B.57.).

Note: In a frozen shoulder this point could be manually stimulated while the patient mobilizes the shoulder joint to obtain an increased range of movement. (A significant improvement in the range of movement may be obtained with the first treatment in about 75% of **cases).**

Xiajuxu (*St. 39.*). (*Hsiachuhsu*). Lower He-Sea point of the Small Intestine.

Location: 3 cun distal to Shangjuxu (St. 37.).

Indications: Paralysis of the lower limb. Small Intestine disorders.

Puncture: 1.0 cun perpendicularly.

Fenglong (*St. 40.*). (*Fenglung*). Luo-Connecting point.

Location: One finger breadth lateral to Tiaokou (St. 38.).

Indications: Cough, excessive sputum, epilepsy.

Note: According to traditional Chinese medicine, epilepsy and excessive sputum are related.

Puncture: 1.5 cun perpendicularly.

Jiexi (*St. 41.*). (*Chiehhsi*).

Location: On the front ankle crease, midway between the tips of the malleoli, between the extensor digitorum longus and extensor hallucis longus tendons.

Indications: Disorders of the ankle joint and soft tissues of the area, paralysis of the leg, foot drop, hemiplegia, varicose veins, chronic ulcers of the ankle area.

Puncture: 0.5 cun perpendicularly.

Xiangu (*St. 43.*). (*Hsienku*).

Location: In the depression between the bases of the 2nd and 3rd metatarsals.

Indications: Mainly used as an analgesic point of the leg in surgery of the lower limb and of the brain. Local or facial oedema.

Puncture: 0.5 cun perpendicularly. Strong stimulation is used during surgery.

Neiting (*St. 44.*). (*Neiting*). Analgesic point.

Location: 0.5 cun proximal to the web margin between the 2nd and 3rd toes.

Indications: Distal point for toothache, headache, best analgesic point of lower limb and can be used for relief of pain in the lower limbs, in arthritis of joints of toes and feet. Abdominal pain.

Puncture: 0.3 cun perpendicularly or obliquely.

Note: This is the best analgesic point of the leg for therapy. It also one of the Bafeng (Ex. 36.) points.

List of all the acupuncture points of the Stomach Channel

St. 1 : **Chengqi** - Dangerous point.

St. 2 : **Sibai**

St. 3 : **Juliao**

St. 4 : **Dicang**

St. 5 : **Daying**

St. 6 : **Jiache**

St. 7 : **Xiaguan**

St. 8 : **Touwei**

St.	9	: **Renying**	
St.	10	: **Shuitu**	
St.	11	: **Qishe**	
St.	12	: **Quepen**	
St.	13	: **Qihu**	
St.	14	: **Kufang**	
St.	15	: **Wuyi**	
St.	16	: **Yingchuang**	
St.	17	: **Ruzhong**	- Forbidden point.
St.	18	: **Rugen**	
St.	19	: **Burong**	
St.	20	: **Chengman**	
St.	21	: **Liangmen**	- The point on the right side is a Dangerous point as it lies directly over the gall bladder.
St.	22	: **Guanmen**	
St.	23	: **Taiyi**	
St.	24	: **Huaroumen**	
St.	25	: **Tianshu**	- Alarm point. (Mu—Front) of the Large Intestine.
St.	26	: **Wailing**	
St.	27	: **Daju**	
St.	28	: **Shuidao**	
St.	29	: **Guilal***	
St.	30	: **Quichong**	
St.	31	: **Biguan**	
St.	32	: **Femur-Futu**	- Motor point.
St.	33	: **Yinshi**	
St.	34	: **Liangqiu**	- Xi-Cleft point.

* Guilal (*St. 29.*). (*Kuilal*). The lower points of the Ren channel are preferred in lower abdominal and pelvic disorders.

St.	35 :	**Dubi**	
St.	36 :	**Zusanli**	- Tonification point; one of the 6 important Distal points. Earth point.
St.	37 :	**Shangjuxu**	- Lower He-Sea point (L.I.).
St.	38 :	**Tiaokou**	
St.	39 :	**Xiajuxu**	- Lower He-Sea point (S.I.).
St.	40 :	**Fenglong**	- Luo-Connecting point.
St.	41 :	**Jiezi**	- Fire point.
St.	42 :	**Chongyang**	- Yuan Source point.
St.	43 :	**Xiangu**	- Wood point.
St.	44 :	**Neiting**	- Water point, Analgesic point.
St.	45 :	**Lidui**	- Metal point.

Note: St. 36 - Distal point for abdominal disorders.

St. 38 - Distal point for shoulder disorders.

St. 40 - Distal point for chest disorders.

St.43/St.44 - Distal points for painful conditions of the face and head area respectively.

It will be observed from this example that points further distal on a Channel treat disorders which are more proximal. This phenomenon is explained on the Thalamic Neuron Theory.

THE CIRCULATION OF ENERGY IN THE STOMACH

The Stomach Channel of Foot-Yangming originates its deep course at the supraclavicular fossa and descends in the abdominal cavity to communicate with its pertaining Organ the Stomach and also the Spleen. This deep part of the channel then runs downwards and rejoins the superficial channel in the lower part of the abdomen.

SYNDROMES OF THE STOMACH

A. The Stomach Channel –Mental disturbances, deviation of the eyes and mouth, sore throat, pain in the chest and abdomen, pain and paralysis of the anterior aspect of the lower limb and dorsum of the foot.

B. The Organ Stomach – Disorders of the stomach are described under three main clinical syndromes.

1) **Retention of fluid in the stomach.** This occurs due to overeating. The clinical manifestations are distention, pain in the epigastric region, belching, regurgitation and sometimes vomiting. The tongue shows a thick, sticky coating.

2) **Retention of fluid in the stomach due to cold.** This syndrome follows exposure to cold or rain. It may also occur due to excessive ingestion of cold or unsuitable raw foods (e.g. infected salads).

   The clinical manifestations are dull pain in the epigastric region and vomiting of watery fluid. A white sticky tongue coating with a thready or slow pulse may occur.

3) **Hyperactivity of the fire of the stomach.** This is due to over-eating of rich and spicy foods.

   The clinical manifestations are burning epigastric pain nausea and vomiting. A red tongue with a dry, yellowish coating may be present.

■

是動則病灑〻然〻而振寒善で伸數欠顔黒病至則人火と悪ㇺ音と聞バ惕然と而驚心動と欲獨戸牖を閉而處甚則高ホ上て歌衣を棄走賁嚮為と欲腹脹是骭厥を是血主所生病ハ狂瘧温淫汗出鼽衄口㖞唇胗頸腫喉痺大腹水腫膝臏腫痛膺乳氣街股伏兎骭外廉足の跗上を循皆痛中指用れぞ氣盛なるときハ身以前皆熱其胃に餘有則ハ穀を消し善飢溺の色黄也氣不足なる則ハ身の以前寒慄して胃中寒する則ハ脹滿を盛るる者ハ人迎大なるを寸口ホ三倍も虚なる者ハ人迎反て寸口より小也

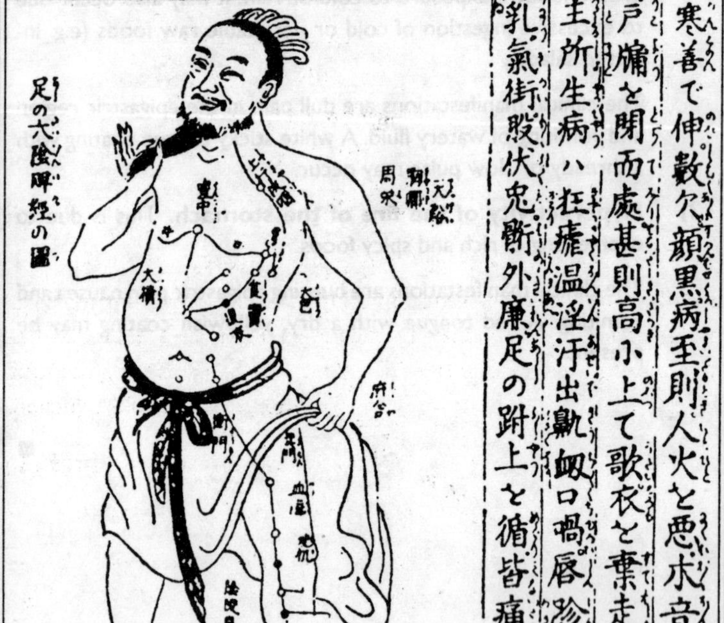

SPLEEN CHANNEL (SP.)

"The Spleen controls the movement of the fluids in the Stomach".

— *Su Wen*

— Polarity : Yin.

— Number of point: 21.

— Pertaining Organ: Spleen.

— Related Channel : Stomach Channel (St.).

— Element : Earth.

— Energy flow: Centripetal.

— Course:

The Spleen Channel originates its superficial course on the medial side of the big toe. It runs proximally up the medial side of the leg and the front the abdomen to end on the side of the chest in the mid-axillary line.

Connections with the Stomach Channel:

Yuan — Source point: Taibai (Sp. 3.).

Luo – Connecting points: Gongsun (Sp. 4.) and Dabao (Sp. 21.).

THE SPLEEN CHANNEL

Ren 8. Shenjue*
(Umbilicus)
St. 25. Tianshu
Sp. 15. Daheng

Sp. 10. Xuehai

Sp. 9. Yinlingquan

Sp. 6. Sanyinjiao

Sp. 4. Gongsun

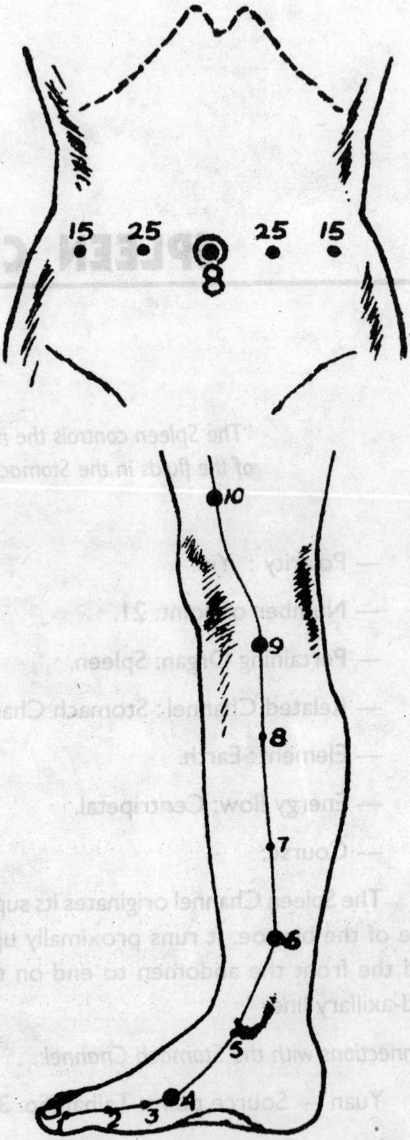

*Also spelt Shengue

Note: The Spleen Channel has 2 Luo-Connecting points. Dabao (Sp. 21.) is known as the Major. Luo point and is considered to have an influence over all other Luo-Connecting points of the body.

Clinical uses:

1) Diseases along the Channel, e.g., genital disorders.
2) Disorders of the spleen, pancreas and digestive disorders.
3) Metabolic disorders and immune mechanism disorders.
4) Skin disorders.
5) Oedema and ascites.
6) Perineal, external genital and pelvic disorders.
7) Disorders, of soft tissue (e.g. muscle and tendon), lips and mouth cavity.

Commonly used acupuncture points:

Leg: Sp. 4, Sp. 6, Sp. 9, Sp. 10.

Abdomen: Sp. 15.

Description of the commonly used points:

Note: This channel is related to the digestive, metabolic and immune mechanisms in the body. According to some authorities the Spleen Channel represents the splenopancreatic functions as well as reticulo-endothelial mechanisms.

Gongsun (*Sp. 4.*). (*Kungsun*). Luo-Connecting point. Confluent point.

Location: On the medial side of the foot in the depression below the base of the 1st metatarsal bone, at the junction of the two colours of the skin on the medial border of the foot.

Indications: Very acute diarrhoea.

Puncture: 0.5 cun perpendicularly, using strong manual stimulation.

THE SPLEEN CHANNEL

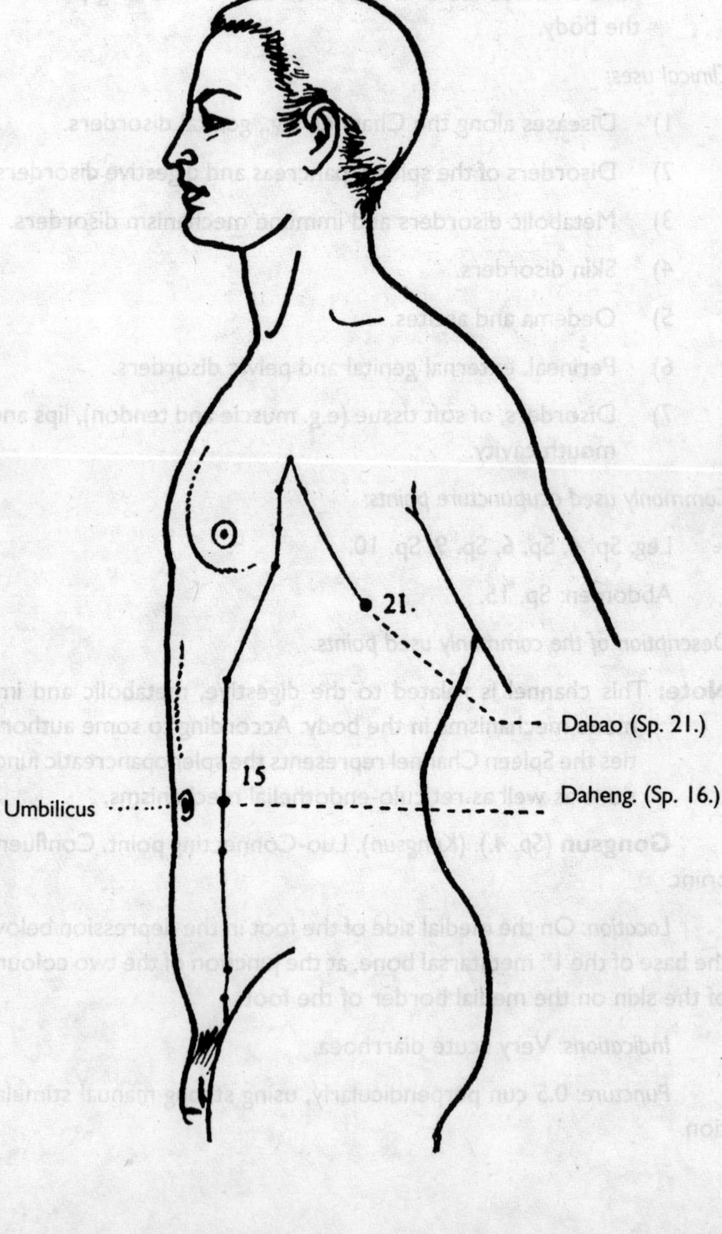

Note: Gongsun is a very painful point as it is situated close to the sole of the foot and is therefore generally used in *very acute conditions* only.

Sanyinjiao (*Sp. 6.*). (*Sanyinchiao*). One of the six important Distal points. General Tonification point.

Location: 3 cun above the tip of medial malleolus on the medial border of the tibia.

Indications: Gastro-intestinal disorders, genito-urinary disorders, lower limb disorders, muscle disorders, skin disorders, mouth disorders. General Tonification point.

All three Yin Channels of the leg meet at this point and it is therefore used in disorders of the Liver, Spleen and Kidney.

Puncture: 1.0 cun perpendicularly.

Note: a) "San"=3, "Jiao"=Junction. Sanyinjiao in Chinese therefore means "The junction of the three Yin Channels".

b)The main General Tonification point of the body are:

Zusanli (St. 36.).

Sanyinjiao (Sp. 6.).

Qihai (Ren 6.).

Yinlingquan (*Sp. 9.*). (*Yinlingchuan*)

Location: At the level of the lower border of the tibial tuberosity, in the depression below the lower border of the medial condyle.

Indications: Oedema and ascites. (Spleen is connected to soft tissues).

Puncture: 1.5 cun perpendicularly.

Note: Combination of points that may be used in oedema and ascites:

Yinlingquan (Sp. 9.).

Shimen (Ren 5.).

Shuifen Ren 9.).

Pishu (U.B. 20.).

Xiangu (St. 43.)—especially in oedema of the face and feet.

Xuehai (*Sp. 10.*). (*Hsuehhai*). Xuehai in Chinese means "the sea of blood".

Location:

a) At the highest point of the prominence of the vastus medialis muscle.

b) 2 cun above the medial end of the upper border of the patella.

c) Have the patient seated with his knees bent at right angles. The acupuncturist then places his right hand on the patient's left patella with the centre of his palm on the middle of the patella and his thumb resting on the inner surface of the thigh. The thumb should be held in a position midway between adduction and full abduction. The point will then lie at the tip of the thumb. This method is only valid if acupuncturist's and the patient's hands have similar proportions.

Indications:

a) Urticaria, allergies, skin disorders.

b) Dysmenorrhoea, functional uterine bleeding, irregular menstruation.

Puncture: 1.5 cun perpendicularly. Strong stimulation is carried out in allergies and to allay pruritus. Moxibustion is also very effective in allergies of extrinsic origin.

Daheng (*Sp. 15.*). (*Taheng*).

Location: 4 cun lateral to the umblicus (on the nippleline).

Indications: Constipation, diarrhoea, intestinal paralysis (paralytic ileus), intestinal parasitosis, dyspepsia, abdominal distention.

Puncture: 1.0 cun perpendicularly.

List of all the acupuncture points of the Spleen Channel:

Sp. 1	: **Yinbai**	- Wood point.
Sp. 2	: **Dadu**	- Fire point.
Sp. 3	: **Taibai**	- Yuan-Source point; Earth point.
Sp. 4	: **Gongsun**	- First (Minor) Luo-Connecting point.
Sp. 5	: **Shangqiu**	- Metal point.
Sp. 6	: **Sanyinjiao**	- Tonification point: one of the six important Distal points; "the meeting point of the three Yin Channels".
Sp. 7	: **Lougu**	
Sp. 8	: **Diji**	- Xi-Cleft point.
Sp. 9	: **Yinlingquan**	- Water point.
Sp. 10	: **Xuehai**	- Anti-allergic and antipruritic point.
Sp. 11	: **Jimen**	
Sp. 12	: **Chongmen**	
Sp. 13	: **Fushe**	
Sp. 14	: **Fujie**	
Sp. 15	: **Daheng**	
Sp. 16	: **Fuai**	
Sp. 17	: **Shidou**	
Sp. 18	: **Tianxi**	
Sp. 19	: **Xiongxiang**	
Sp. 20	: **Zhourong**	
Sp. 21	: **Dabao**	- Second Luo-Connecting point. (Major Luo point.).

From Dabao (Sp. 21) the vital Yin energy flows on to Jiquan (H. 1.).

Note: The Spleen and the Stomach are related to the soft tissues and the four limbs. These two Organs are also connected to the lips and the mouth.

In summary—the Spleen Channel is used to treat,

(1) disorders along the Channel,

(2) digestive disorders,

(3) chronic infections and allergies,

(4) disorders of muscles, and other soft tissues, including oedema and ascites,

(5) disorders of the lips and the mouth cavity,

(6) genito-urinary disorders,

(7) General Tonification.

THE CIRCULATION OF ENERGY IN THE SPLEEN

The Spleen Channel of Foot-Taiyin has its deep connection originating from the superficial channel as it runs upwards in the anterior abdominal wall. In the abdominal cavity it connects with the Organ Spleen and its Coupled Organ the Stomach. From the Stomach it runs upwards internally along the oesophagus to enter the root of the tongue and spreads on its lower surface and the mouth cavity.

An internal branch from the stomach also communicates with the Organ Heart and via its channel with all the soft tissues.

SYNDROMES OF THE SPLEEN

A. **The Spleen Channel:** Eructation of gas from the Stomach (belching), nausea, vomiting, pain at the root of the tongue.

B. **The Organ Spleen:** Diseases of the Spleen are described under two main headings.

1) **Weakness of the qi (vital energy) of the Spleen.** This syndrome may be caused by irregular food intake or excessive mental strain. Poor appetite causes the qi of the Spleen to be weak. Anorexia and symptoms of malnutrition are seen. A pale tongue and a thready pulse are associated.

2) **Invasion of the Spleen by cold and damp factors.** This is caused by the overeating of raw chilled food. Poor appetite, loose stools with a white sticky tongue and thready pulse occurs.

■

HEART CHANNEL (H.)

"The Heart is the root of life; it is reflected in the blood vessels and its Qi communicates with the tongue."

— *Ling Shu*

— Polarity : Yin.

— Number of points : 9.

— Pertaining Organ : Heart.

— Related Channel : Small Intestine Channel (S.I.).

— Element : Fire.

— Energy flows : Centrifugal.

— Course :

The Heart Channel originates its superficial course in the centre to the axilla. It runs distally on the anterior and medial aspect of the arm to end near the lateral edge of the base of the nail of the little finger (It runs on the commonest pathway of referred cardiac pain).

Connections with the Small Intestine Channel:

Yuan – Source point: Shenmen (H. 7.).

Lou – Connecting point: Tongli (H. 5.).

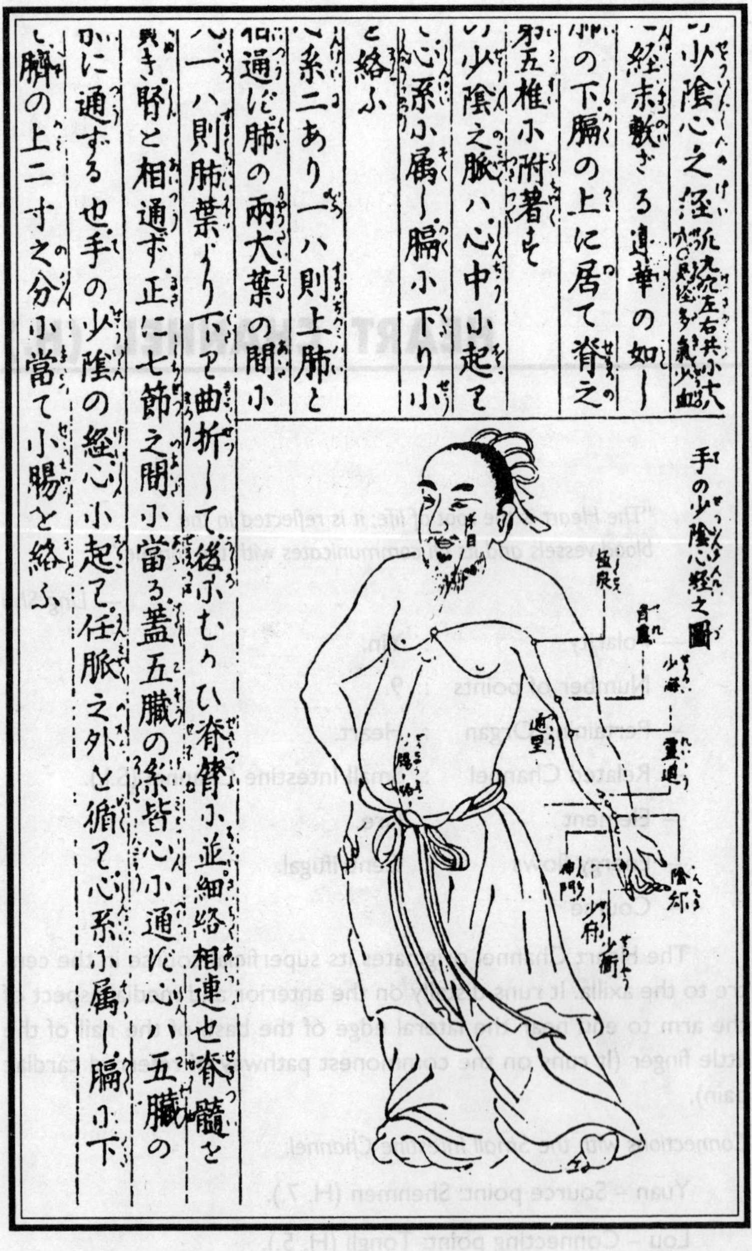

少陰心之経〈凡九穴左右共ニ十八穴 此経多気少血〉
経未敷ざる蓮華の如し
の下膈の上に居て脊之
五椎ニ附著せ
少陰之脈ハ心中ニ起て
心系ニ属し膈ニ下り小
と絡ふ
系二あり一ハ則上肺と
通じ肺の両大葉の間ニ
一ハ則肺葉より下て曲折して後ニむかい脊膂ニ並細絡相連せ脊髄を
き腎と相通ず正に七節之間ニ當る蓋五臓の系皆心ニ通じ心ハ五臓の
に通ずる也手の少陰の経心ニ起て任脈之外を循て心系ニ属し膈ニ下
臍の上二寸之分ニ當て小腸を絡ふ

Clinical uses:

1) Diseases along the Channel.
2) Heart diseases.
3) Mental disorders (Heart is related to the Brain). e.g., anxiety, hysteria, schizophrenia, insomnia, epilepsy.
4) Tremors, chorea-athetosis parkinsonism.
5) Speech disorders (Heart is connected to the tongue).
6) Autonomic disturbances, e.g. increased sweating.

Commonly used acupuncture points:

Elbow: H. 3,

Forearm: H. 5, H. 6, H. 7.

Hand: H. 8 H. 9.

Note: 1) The Organs Heart and Pericardium together with tneir Channels form one functional unit.

2) The Heart, Pericardium and the Brain functions are closely related.

Description of the commonly used points:

Shaohai (*H. 3.*). (*Shaohai*).

Location: Midway between the medial end of the elbow crease and medial epicondyle of the humerus when the elbow is *fully* flexed.

Note: Quchi (L.I. 11.). is located when the elbow is *semi*-flexed.

Indications: Disorders of the elbow and soft tissues around it, numbness of upper limb, angina pectoris, golfer's elbow, tremors of the forearm (e.g. chorea, athetosis, parkinsonism).

Puncture: 1.0 cun perpendicularly.

Tongli (*H. 5.*). (*Tungli*). Luo-Connecting point.

Location: 1 cun proximal to Shenmen (H. 7.), on the radial side of the tendon of the flexor carpi ulnaris.

THE HEART CHANNEL

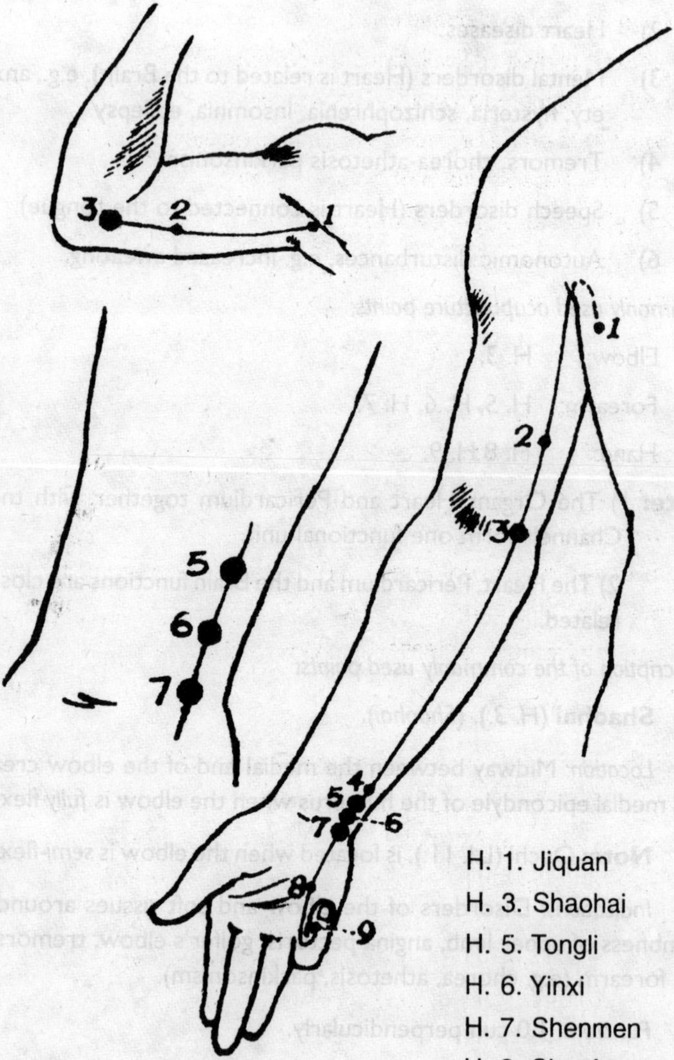

H. 1. Jiquan

H. 3. Shaohai

H. 5. Tongli

H. 6. Yinxi

H. 7. Shenmen

H. 8. Shaofu

H. 9. Shaochong

Indications: Aphasia dysphasis, hoarseness of voice, stammering.

Note: Heart is connected to the tongue.

Puncture: 0.5 cun perpendicularly.

Yinxi (*H. 6.*). (*Yinhsi*). Xi-Cleft point.

Location: 0.5 cun proximal to Shenmen (H. 7.).

Indications: Angina pectoris, palpitation, excessive sweating.

Puncture: 0.5 cun perpendicularly.

Note: This is the *Xi-Cleft point* and is therefore used in treating the symptoms of *acute Heart disease:* e.g., palpitation, angina pectoris, maniacal behaviour, severe depression.

Shenmen (*H. 7.*). (*Shenmen*). Yuan-Source point. An important tranquilizer point. Shenmen in Chinese means "God's door".

Location: On the radial side of the tendon of the flexor carpi ulnaris muscle, at the wrist crease.

Note: H. 5, H. 6 and H. 7 are all located on the radial border of the tendon of the flexor carpi ulnaris.

Indications: Palpitation, anxiety, hysteria, insomnia, mental disorders, rhythm disorders of the heart.

Puncture: 0.5 cun perpendicularly.

Note: According to traditional Chinese medicine, the functions of the heart and brain are closely allied. Disorders of the brain are, therefore, treated with points of the Heart and Pericardium Channels. The points commonly used in those disorders are: Shenmen (H. 7.) and Neiguan (P. 6.). The points Shenmen (H. 7.) and Baihui (Du 20.) are the important sedative and tranquilizer points of the body. The Ear Shenmen also has similar therapeutic effects.

Shaofu (*H. 8.*). (*Shaofu*).

Location: In the palmar surface of the hand, between the tips of the ring finger and little finger on lightly clenching the fist.

Indications: Disorders of the palm, rheumatoid arthritis of the carpal joints, Duputryen's contracture.

Puncture: 0.5 cun perpendicularly.

Note: This is a painful point. All points on the palms and soles of the feet are painful.

Shaochong (*H. 9.*). (*Shaochung*). Jing-Well point.

Location: 0.1 cun proximal to the radial corner of the nail of the little finger.

Indications: Pain in the chest, apoplexy, palpitation and other acute emergencies.

Puncture: 0.1 cun perpendicularly to cause bleeding or acupressure in emergencies, if a needle is not available.

List of all the acupuncture points of the Heart Channel:

H.	1	:	**Jiquan**	
H.	2	:	**Qingling**	
H.	3	:	**Shaohai**	- Water point.
H.	4	:	**Lingdao**	- Metal point.
H.	5	:	**Tongli**	- Luo-Connecting point.
H.	6	:	**Yinxi**	- Xi-Cleft point.
H.	7	:	**Shenmen**	- Yuan-Source point; Earth point.
H.	8	:	**Shaofu**	- Fire point.
H.	9	:	**Shaochong**	- Jing-Well point, Wood point.

THE CIRCULATION OF ENERGY IN THE HEART

The Heart Channel of Hand-Shaoyin originates form the Organs Heart and Pericardium. It has internal connections with the Organs Small Intestine and all other Zang-Fu Organs. A deep connection runs upwards along the oesophagus to connect with the tongue and the brain (via the eyes). The energy flows to the superficial channel from the Organ Heart at the mid-point of the axilla.

SYNDROMES OF THE HEART

A. **The Heart Channel:** Pain along the medial aspect of the upper limb, night sweating, dryness of the throat.

B. **The Organ Heart:** Diseases of the Heart are described under 5 main syndromes.

1) **Insufficient vital energy (qi) of the Heart.** This is usually caused by asthenia after a prolonged illness. The symptoms are palpitation, dyspnoea, profuse sweating, mental confusion and thready pulse.

2) **Deficiency of the Yin of the Heart.** This is usually a result of a prolonged febrile illness or mental worry. The symptoms are those of insomnia, poor memory and dream-disturbed sleep.

3) **Stagnation of the blood in the Heart.** Stagnation of qi and blood occurs when the heart is too weak to effectively circulate the blood. Symptoms are those of cardiac failure.

4) **Hyperactivity of the fire of the Heart.** This syndrome is due to anxiety. The symptoms may be insomnia, fever with a red tongue, bitter taste and a flushed face.

5) **Derangements of the mind.** This syndrome is due to a depression of the qi by high fevers, coma and delirium. Servere mental symptoms may result.

■

SMALL INTESTINE CHANNEL (S.I.)

"The Small Intestine is the official who recieves the abundance from *the Stomach and is concerned with the transforming of this matter."*

— *Su Wen*

— Polarity : Yang.

— Number of points : 19.

— Pertaining Organ : Small Intestine.

— Related Channel : Heart Channel (H.)

— Element : Fire.

— Energy flow : Centripetal.

— Course:

Originates its superficial course at the medial side of the base of the little finger. It runs on the posterior and medial aspect of the arm, zig-zags over the back of the shoulder, and runs over the side of the neck to the side of the face to end in front of the ear.

Connections with the Heart Channel:

Yuan-Source point: Hand-Wangu (S.I. 4.).

Luo-Connecting point: Zhizheng (S.I. 7.).

こゝに示す故に其交經授受支別に假すと云○靈道ハ掌後一寸五分にあり通里
腕後一寸陥なる中にあり。陰郄ハ掌後の脈中腕を去ヿ五分にあり。神門
掌後鋭骨之端。陥なる者の中にあり少府ハ手の小指本節の後陥なる中。
勞宮に同ヿ少衝ハ手の小指の内廉の端にあり。爪甲を去ヿ韭葉の如し
是動ずる則ハ病。嗌乾き
心痛渇して飲ん欲す。是
臂厥と云。是心を主る所
生病者目黄き。脇痛。臑臂
内の後廉痛厥掌中熱痛
す。盛なる者ハ寸口大な
ると人迎に再倍す。虚す
る者ハ寸口反て人迎よ
り小也

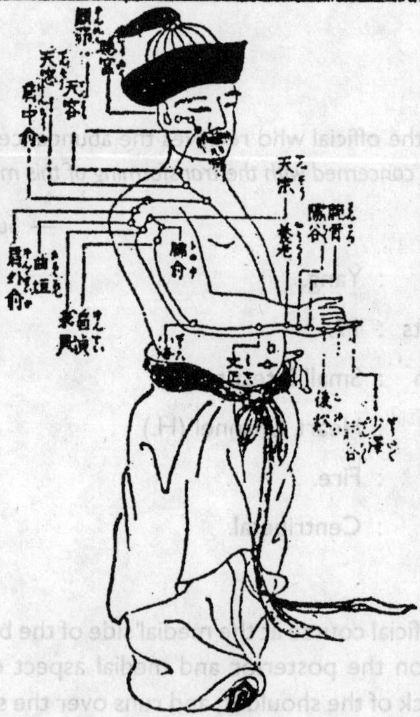

手の太陽小腸經之圖

Clinical uses:

1) Diseases along the course of the Channel e.g., deafness swelling of the cheek, stiff-neck, sore throat.

2) Disorders of the small intestine. (Generally in disorders of small intestine, the lower He-Sea point, Exajuxu (St. 39.) is the preferred point).

Commonly used acupuncture points:

Hand: S.I. 3.

Forearm: S.I. 6.

Shoulder: S.I. 9.

Neck: S.I. 17.

Face: S.I. 18, S.I. 19.

Description of the commonly used acupuncture points.

Houxi (*S.I. 3.*). (*Houhsi*), Confluent point of the Du Channel.

Location: At the medial end of the main transverse crease of the palm on clenching the fist.

Indications: Acute stiffness of the neck, acute low backache severe occipital headache.

Puncture: 0.5 cun perpendicularly, with strong manual stimulation of the needle.

Note: This is a very painful point and should be used only in very acute conditions.

Yanglao (*S.I. 6.*). (*Yanglao*). Xi-Cleft point.

Location:

a) In the depression on the lateral aspect of the styloid process of the ulna. (It is easier to locate this point with the hand pronated)

b) On the back of the wrist, in the depression proximal to the inferior radio-ulnar joint.

THE SMALL INTESTINE CHANNEL

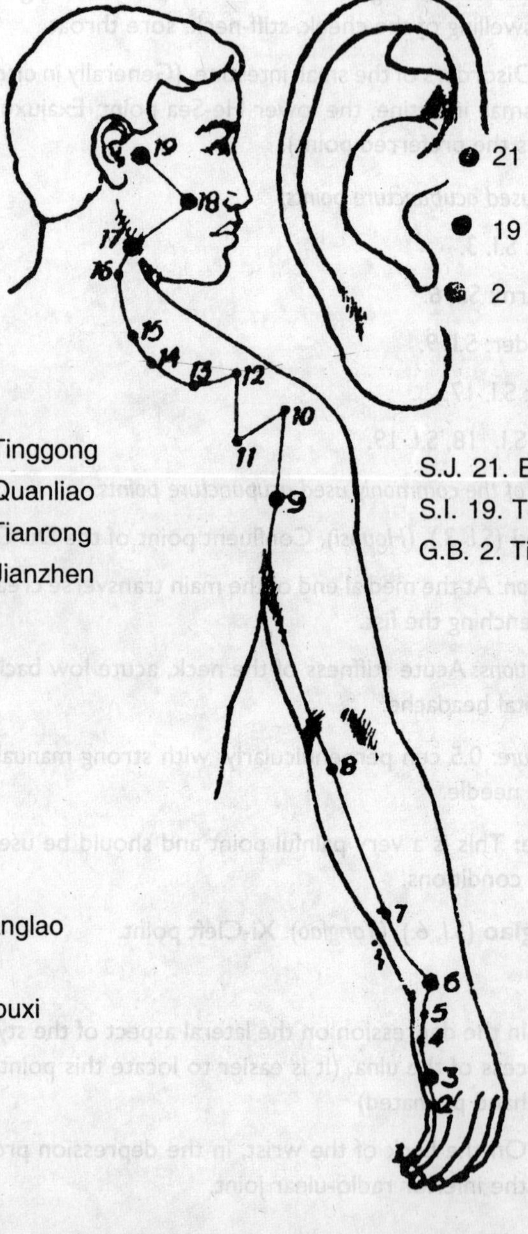

S.I. 19. Tinggong

S.I. 18. Quanliao

S.I. 17. Tianrong

S.I. 19. Jianzhen

S.J. 21. Erman

S.I. 19. Tinggong

G.B. 2. Tinghui

S.I. 6. Yanglao

S.I. 3. Houxi

Indications: Pain in wrist, stiff neck, cervical spondylosis. An acute stiff neck could be dramatically relieved by strong manual stimulation of this point. Failing vision in the elderly. (The energy at the end of this channel flows over the orbit to reach the next (U.B.) Channel).

Puncture: 1.0 cun obliquely towards Neiguan (P. 6.)

Jianzhen *(S.I. 9.)*. (*Chienchen*).

Locations: 1.0 cun superior to the highest point of the posterior axillary fold.

Indications: Frozen shoulder, sprains and strains of the shoulder muscles, paralysis of the upper limb.

Puncture: 1.0 – 1.5 cun perpendicularly.

Note: This point is often used in combination with two other local points, Jianyu (L.I, 15.) and Jianliao (SJ. 14.), and with Distal point Hegu (L.I. 4.) and Influential point Yanglingquan (G.B. 34.), for disorders of the shoulder joint. Ah-Shi points are also needled.

Tianrong (*S.I. 17.*). (*Teinjung*). Dangerous point.

Location: On the anterior border of the sterno-cleidomastoideus at the level of the angle of the jaw.

Indications: Tonsillitis, sore throat, aphasia.

Puncture: 1.0 cun perpendicularly.

Note: This point is a Dangerous point as it is situated near the great vessels of the neck. The needle should be directed towards the tonsils *not* backwards as it may affect the carotid body.

Quanliao (*S.I. 18.*). (*Chuanliao*). Regional analgesic point.

Location: In the depression below the prominence of the zygomatic bone on a vertical line drawn (downwards) from the outer canthus of the eye.

Indications: Toothache, trigeminal neuralgia, facial paralysis.

Puncture: 0.3 – 0.5 cun perpendicularly. (If inserted too far downwards, the needle may enter the mouth cavity and may cause bleeding inside the mouth).

THE SMALL INTESTINE CHANNEL

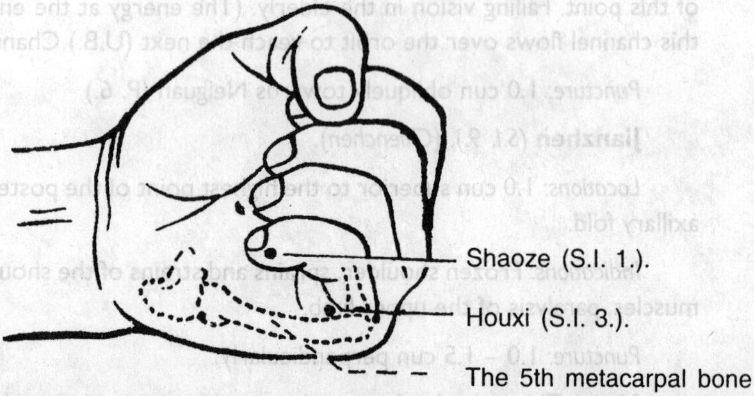

ACUPUNCTURE POINTS IN FRONT OF THE EAR

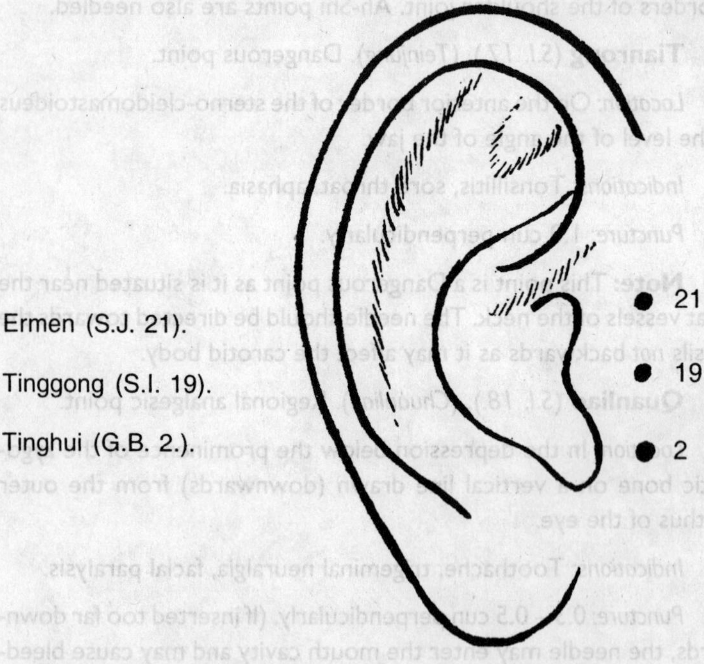

Note: This is the best regional analgesic point in the head and neck region. It is often used in tooth extractions, ear, nose, throat surgery and in brain surgery.

Tinggong (*S.I. 19.*). (*Tingkung*).

Location: In the depression felt between the tragus and the mandibular joint when the mouth is slightly open.

Indications: Ear disorders, e.g., deafness, tinnitus, vertigo, Meniere's disease, (chronic) ear infections.

Puncture: 0.5 cun perpendicularly. It is more usual, however, to puncture through the points Ermen (S.J. 21.), Tinggong (S.I. 19.) and Tinghui (G.B. 2.) horizontally downwards. This is known as the "puncturing-through technique".

Note: A case of rupture of the ear drum has been reported after a perpendicular puncture.

List of all the acupuncture points of the Small Intestine Channel:

S.I. 1 : **Shaoze** – Jing-Well point, Metal point.

S.I. 2 : **Qiangu** – Water point.

S.I. 3 : **Houxi** – Wood point, Confluent point.

S.I. 4 : **Hand-Wangu** – Yuan-Source point.

S.I. 5 : **Yanggu** – Fire point.

S.I. 6 : **Yanglao** – Xi-Cleft point.

S.I. 7 : **Zhizheng** – Luo-Connecting point.

S.I. 8 : **Xiaohai** – Earth point.

S.I. 9 : **Jianzhen**

S.I. 10 : **Naoshu**

S.I. 11 : **Tianzong**

S.I. 12 : **Bingfeng**

S.I. 13 : **Quyuan**

S.I. 14 : **Jianwaishu**

S.I. 15 : **Jianzhongshu**

S.I. 16 : **Tianchuang**

T.I. 17 : **Tianrong** – Dangerous point, if inserted backwards.[1]

S.I. 18 : **Quanliao** – The best regional analgesic point of the head and neck area.

S.I. 19 : **Tinggong**

From Tinggong (S.I. 19.) the vital Yang energy flows on to Jingming (U.B. 1.) across the eye. The point Yanglao (S.I. 6.). may, therefore, be used to treat failing vision particularly in elderly people.

Note: The Heart and the Small Intestine are related to the blood vessels. These two Organs are also connected to the tongue and mouth. The Heart and Pericardium together with the blood vessels are related to the Brain. The Brain is considered an Extraordinary Organ in traditional Chinese medicine.

Note: Treatment of Ear Disorders.

Local Points:

Ermen (S.J. 21.).

Tinggong (S.I. 19.). through and through insertion.

Tinghui (G.B. 2.).

Distal Points (select from):

Sanjiao Channel:

Zhongzhu (S.J. 3.).

Waiguan (S.J. 5.).

Small Intestine Channel:

Yanglao (S.I. 6.)

Gall Bladder Channel:

Foot-Linqi (G.B. 41.).

1 Pressure on the baro-receptors of the neck may cause fainting.

THE CIRCULATION OF ENERGY IN THE SMALL INTESTINE

The Small Intestine Channel of Hand-Taiyang as it traverses the scapular region communicates with the Du Channel at Dazhui (Du 14.). Then at the supraclavicular fossa a deep branch commences which connects with the Heart and then this branch descends along the oesophagus and passes through the diaphragm reaching the Stomach and it finally enters the Organ Small Intestine, its pertaining Organ.

Another branch arises from the Organ Small Intestine and connects to the Inferior He-Sea Point, Xiajaxu (St. 39.). This point is the preferred point in treating the disorders of the Organ Small Intestine.

SYMDROMES OF THE SMALL INTESTINE

A. **The Small Intestine Channel:** Pain along the channel, sorethroat, swelling of the cheek, deafness, lower abdominal pain.

B. **The Organ Small Intestine:** Symptoms of disorders are similar to those of Spleen disorders.

■

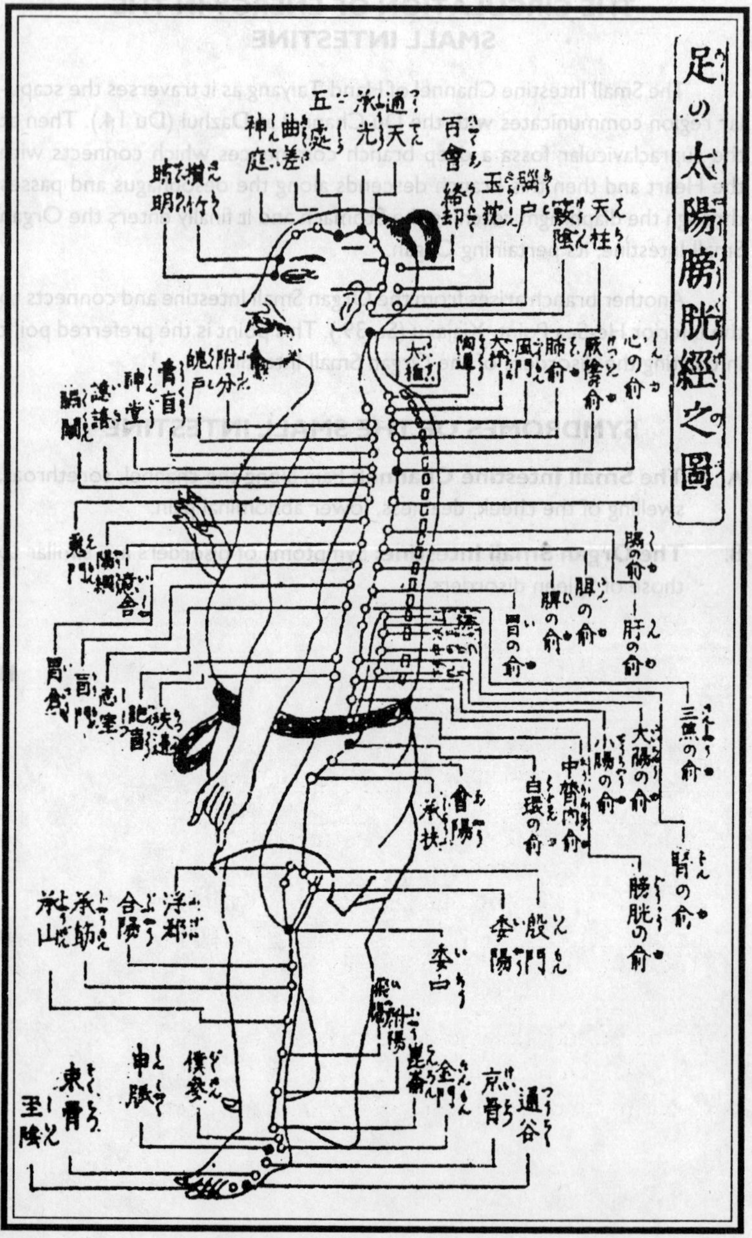
足の太陽膀胱經之圖
通天
承光
曲差
五處
神庭
百會
絡却
玉枕
天柱
攢竹
睛明
風門
肺の俞
厥陰の俞
心の俞
膏肓
神堂
譩譆
膈関
魄戸
附分
陽綱
意舎
胃倉
肓門
志室
胞肓
秩邊
膈の俞
肝の俞
膽の俞
脾の俞
胃の俞
三焦の俞
腎の俞
大腸の俞
小腸の俞
膀胱の俞
中膂内俞
白環の俞
會陽
承扶
殷門
委陽
浮郄
合陽
承筋
承山
附陽
金門
僕參
申脈
京骨
束骨
通谷
至陰

URINARY BLADDER CHANNEL (U.B.)

"The Kidneys unite at the Bladder, where the fluid is stored.
— Urine is the surplus of the fluid of the body".

— Chaoshi Bingyuan

- Polarity : Yang.
- Number of points : 67.
- Pertaining Organ : Urinary Bladder.
- Related Channel : Kidney Channel (K.)
- Element : Water.
- Energy flow : Centrifugal.
- Course:

This channel begins at the medial corner of the eye and runs over the top of the head, close to the midline. At the nape of the neck it divides into two branches. The branch (the one more often used in therapy) courses down the back of the trunk at a distance of 1.5 cun from the midline, till it reaches the level of the fourth posterior sacral foraman. Here it abruptly reverses direction and runs obliquely and medially to the first posterior sacral formen from where it descends vertically over all the other posterior sacral foramina. It then deviates obliquely to the midline and reaches the coccyx, thereafter it descends on the back of the leg. The lateral branch of the

Channel descends from the neck on a line parallel to the medial branch, but at a distance of 3 cun from the midline. It passes over the buttock and posterior aspect of the thigh to reach the midpoint of the popliteal fossa and then reuniting with the medial branch at this point, descends over the calf muscle and reaches the foot after passing behind the lateral malleolus. After traversing the lateral border of the foot it ends near the lateral corner of the little toe-nail.

Connections with the Kidney Channel:

Yuan-Source point: Jinggu (U.B. 64.)

Luo-Connecting point: Feiyang (U.B. 58.)

Clinical uses:

1) Points on the face are used mainly for eye disorders.

2) There are twelve pairs of points on the back of the trunk called Back-Shu points, which are related to each of the twelve internal Organs. These points become tender or may show other abnormal reaction when the corresponding internal Organ is diseased and are therefore also categorised as Alarm points.

3) Points on the lumbar region are used commonly for the treatment of low backache and genito-urinary disorders.

4) Points on the lower limb are used for pain, muscular cramps and other local disorders, while those below the knee also serve as Distal points for the treatment of diseases on the proximal course of the Channel.

Commonly used acupuncture points:

Face : U.B. 1, U.B.2.

Neck : U.B. 10.

Back of trunk: U.B. 11, U.B. 13, U.B. 14, U.B. 15, U.B. 17, U.B. 18, U.B. 19, U.B. 20, U.B. 21, U.B. 22, U.B. 23, U.B. 25, U.B. 27, U.B. 28, U.B. 32, U.B. 54.

Note: 1. U.B. 11 to U.B. 23 are Dangerous points.

II. The lateral branch of this Channel is numbered differently by some German authors.

Lower limb: U.B. 36, U.B. 37, U.B. 40, U.B. 57, U.B. 58, U.B. 60, U.B. 62, U.B. 67.

Description of the commonly used acupuncture points:

Jingming (*U.B. 1.*) (*Chingming*). Dangerous point.

Location: 0.1 cun medial and superior to the inner canthus of the eye, near the medial border of the orbit.

Indications: Diseases of the eye.

Location: As this is a Dangerous point, puncture superficially 0.2 cun, or insert slowly (without any attempt at manipulation), 0.5-1.0 cun along the medial wall of the orblit.

Zenzhu (*U.B.2.*). (*Tsanchu*).

Location: In the depression at the medial end of the eyebrow, directly above the inner canthus of the eye.

Indications: Diseases of the eye, sinusitis, frontal headache.

Puncture: 0.3-0.5 cun horizontally downwards, or laterally.

Tianzhu (*U.B. 10.*) (*Tienchu*).

Location: In the lower border of the occiput, between the transverse processes of the first and second cervical vertebrae, 1.3 cun lateral to the midline. (1.3 cun lateral to Yamen (Du 15.).

Indications: Stiff nedi, occipital headache, sore throat, cervical spondylosis. This point is rarely used.

Puncture: 0.5 cun perpendicularly.

Dashu (*U.B. 11.*). (*Tachu*), Influential point for bone and cartilage.

Location: 1.5 cun lateral to the lower border of the spinous process of the first thoracic vertebra.

Indications: Pain in the shoulder girdle area, arthritis of the joints. Used in all joint, bone, and cartilage disorders.

THE URINARY BLADDER CHANNEL

U.B. 1. Jingming — Dangerous point

U.B. 2. Zanzhu

U.B. 10. Tianzhu

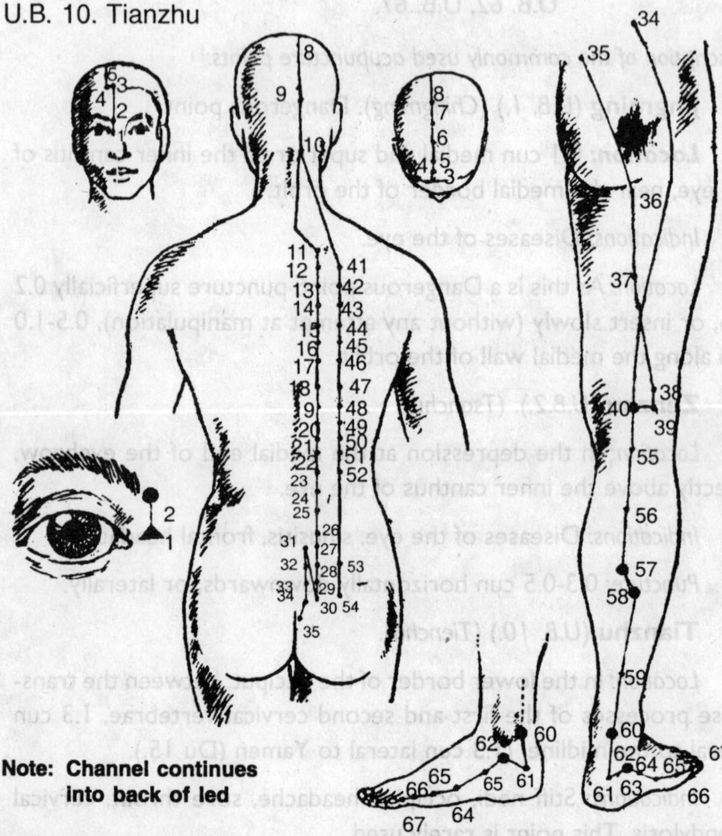

Note: Channel continues into back of led

Back-Shu Points:

U.B. 11.	U.B. 19.	U.B. 32. Ciliao
U.B. 13.	U.B. 20.	U.B. 54. Zhibian
U.B. 15.	U.B. 21.	U.B. 40. Weizhong
U.B. 16.	U.B. 23.	U.B. 57. Chengshan
U.B. 17.	U.B. 25.	U.B. 58. Feiyang
U.B. 18.	U.B. 28.	U.B. 60. Kuntun
	U.B. 29	U.B. 62. Shenmai

Puncture: 0.3 cun perpendicularly or obliquely downwards.

Feishu (*U.B. 13*). (*Feishu*). Back-Shu point of the Lung.

Location: 1.5 cun lateral to the lower border of the spinous process of the third thoracic vertebra.

Indications: Lung disease, nose disorders, disorders of the skin (Lung is connected to the skin), lesions of the soft tissue of the soft tissue of the dorsal spine area.

Puncture: 0.3 – 0.5 cun perpendicularly or obliquely downwards.

Jueyinshu (*U.B. 14.*). (*Chuehyinshu*) Back-Shu point of the Pericardium.

Location: 1.5 cun lateral to the lower border of the spinous process of the fourth thoracic vertebra.

Indications: Heart disease, brain disorders.

Puncture: 0.3-0.5 cun perpendicularly or obliquely downwards.

Xinshu (*U.B. 15.*). (*Hsinshu.*). Back-Shu point of the Heart.

Location: 1.5 cun lateral to the lower border of the spinous process of the fifth thoracic vertebra.

Indications: Heart disease, neurasthenia, hysteria, epilepsy, schizophrenia, insomnia, anxiety, addictions, behavioural disorders.

Puncture: 0.3 – 0.5 cun perpendicularly or obliquely.

Geshu (*U.B. 17.*). (*Keshu*). Influential point for Blood, Back-Shu point of the diaphragm.

Location: 1.5 cun lateral to the lower border of spinous process of the seventh thoracic vertebra (at the level of the lower border or the scapula).

Indications: Paralysis of diaphragm, hiccough, anorexia nervosa, anaemia, chronic hemorrhagic diseases, leukaemia.

Puncture: 0.3 – 0.5 cun perpendicularly or obliquely downwards.

Ganshu (*U.B. 18.*). (*Kanshu*). Back-Shu point of the Liver.

BACK - SHU POINTS

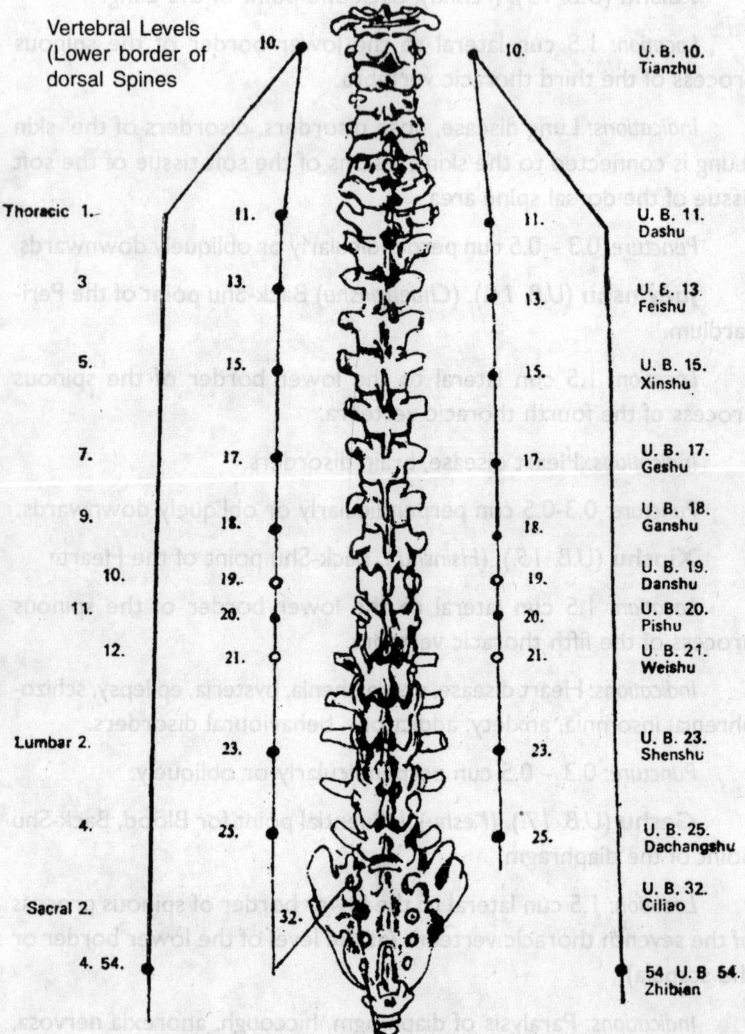

The level of sympathetic outflow from the sympathetic ganglia to the respective internal organs has a close parallelism to the levels of the Back-shu points. This is a meeting point of the anatomist, neurologist, chiropractor osteopath, neuro-surgeon, orthopaedist and the acupuncturist.

Location: 1.5 cun lateral to the lower border of the spinous process of the ninth thoracic vertebra.

Indications: Liver disease, eye disease, muscle and tendon disorders, local disorders of the spine.

Puncture: 0.3 – 0.5 cun perpendicularly or obliquely downwards.

Danshu (*U.B. 19.*). (*Tanshu*). Back-Shu point of the Gall bladder.

Location: 1.5 cun lateral to the lower border of the spinous process of the tenth thoracic vertebra.

Indications: Gall bladder diseases, local disorders of the spine.

Puncture: 0.3 – 0.5 cun perpendicularly or obliquely downwards.

Pishu (*U.B. 20.*). (*Pishu*). Back-Shu point of the Spleen.

Location: 1.5 cun lateral to the lower border of the spinous process of the eleventh thoracic vertebra.

Indications: Gastro-intestinal disorders, oedema, allergic disorders, soft tissue disorders.

Puncture: 0.3 – 0.5 cun perpendicularly or obliquely downwards.

Weishu (*U.B. 21.*). (*Weishu*). Back-Shu point of the Stomach.

Location: 1.5 cun lateral to the lower border of the spinous process of the twelfth thoracic vertebra.

Indications: Stomach disorders.

Puncture: 0.3 – 0.5 cun perpendicularly or obliquely downwards.

Sanjiaoshu (*U.B. 22.*). (*Sanchiaoshu*) Back-Shu point of the *Sanjiao* (the Three Body Cavities).

Location: 1.5 cun lateral to the lower border of the spinous process of the first lumbar vertebra.

Indications: Abdominal distension, flatulence, loss of appetite, incontinence of urine, local disorders of the spine.

Puncture: 0.5 – 1.0 perpendicularly.

THE URINARY BLADDER CHANNEL

U.B. 1. Jingming — Dangerous point

U.B. 2. Zanzhu

U.B. 10. Tianzhu

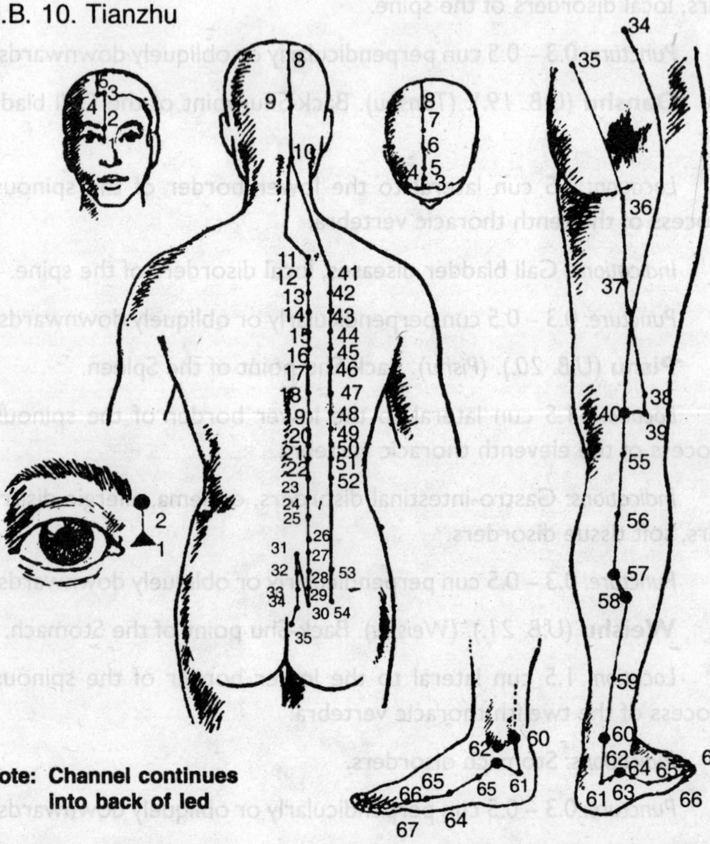

Note: Channel continues into back of led

Back-Shu Points:

U.B. 11.	U.B. 19.	U.B. 32. Ciliao
U.B. 13.	U.B. 20.	U.B. 54. Zhibian
U.B. 15.	U.B. 21.	U.B. 40. Weizhong
U.B. 16.	U.B. 23.	U.B. 57. Chengshan
U.B. 17.	U.B. 25.	U.B. 58. Feiyang
U.B. 18.	U.B. 28.	U.B. 60. Kuntun
	U.B. 29	U.B. 62. Shenmai

Shenshu (*U.B. 23.*). (*Shenshu*). Back-Shu point of the Kidney.

Location: 1.5 cun lateral to the lower border of the spinous process of the second lumbar vertebra (at the level of the lower border of the rib cage in the renal angle).

Indications: Genito-urinary disorders, ear disease, bone disorders, alopecia, local disorders of the spine.

Puncture: 1.0 cun perpendicularly or obliquely towards the vertebral column. See page 85 references K. Fukuda *et. al*).

Dachangshu (*U.B. 25.*). (*Tachangshu*). Back-Shu point of the Large Intestine.

Location: 1.5 cun lateral to the lower border of the spinous process of the fourth lumbar vertebra (at the level of the upper border of the iliac crest).

Indications: Diarrhoea, constipation, low backache, sciatica, paralysis of the lower extremities.

Puncture: 1.0 – 1.5 cun perpendicularly.

Xiaochangshu (*U.B. 27.*). (*Hsiaochangshu*). Back-Shu point of the Small Intestine.

Location: 1.5 cun lateral to the midline, level with the first posterior sacral foramen, in the depression over the sacro-iliac joint.

Indications: Low backache, enteritis, sacro-iliac diseases.

Puncture: 1.0-1.5 cun perpendicularly or 2 to 3 cun obliquely towards Dachangshu (U.B. 25.).

Pangguangshu (*U.B. 28.*). (*Pangkuangshu*). Back-Shu point of the Urinary Bladder.

Location: 1.5 cun lateral to the midline, level with the second posterior sacral foramen, in the depression just over the sacro-iliac joint.

Indications: Genito-urinary disorders, lumbo-sacral disorders.

Puncture: 0.5 – 1.0 cun perpendicularly.

THE URINARY BLADDER CHANNEL

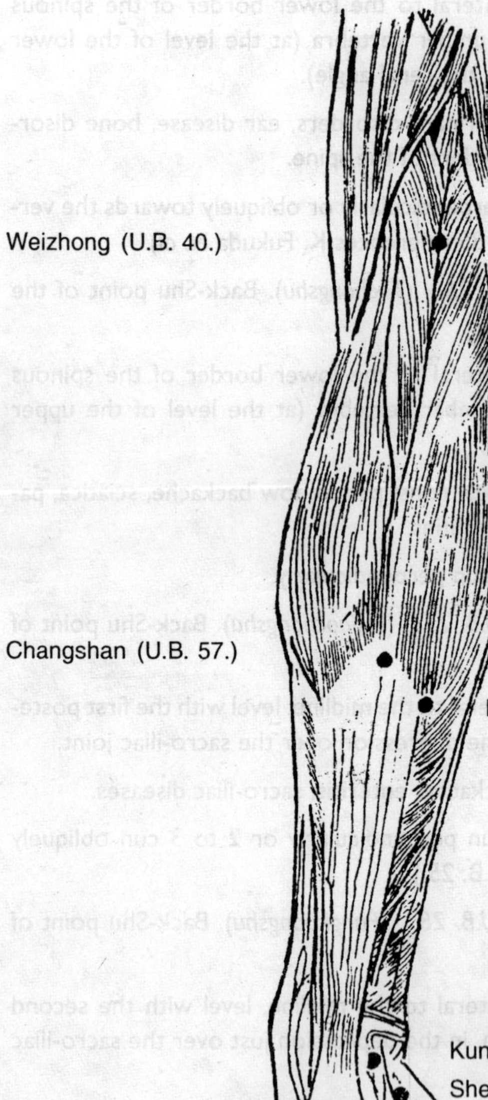

Ciliao (*U.B. 32.*). (*Tzuliao*).

Location: On the second sacral foramen.

Indications: Genito-urinary disorders, haemorrhoids, sciatica.

Puncture: 1.0 – 1.5 cun perpendicularly. Moxa on a needle is used in nocturnal eneuresis.

Chengfu (*U.B. 36.*). (*Chengfu*).

Location: In the middle of the gluted fold.

Indications: Sciatica, paralysis of the Lower Limb, Haemorrhoids.

Puncture: 1.5 - 2.0 cun perpenditularly

Yinmer (U.B. 37) Yinmer.

Location: Midpoint of a line joining Chengfu (U.B. 36.) and Weizhong (U.B. 40.), or 6 cun distal to Chengfu (U.B. 36.).

Indications: Sciatica, lumbo-sacral disorders paralysis of the lower limb.

Puncture: 1.0 – 2.0 cun perpendicularly.

Weizhong (*U.B. 40.*). (*Weichung*). One of the six important Distal points.

Location: At the midpoint of the popliteal transverse crease.

Indications: Sciatica, lumbago, paralysis of the lower limb, genito urinary disorders, disorders of the knee joint, skin disease.

Puncture: 0.5 – 1.0 perpendicularly; or prick to bleed with a three edged needle in skin disease.

Zhibian (*U.B. 54.*) (*Chihpien*).

Location: At the level of the fourth sacral foramen, 3.0 cun lateral to the midline.

Indications: Genito-urinary disorders, haemorrhoids, sciatica, hip disorders, paralysis of the lower limb.

Puncture: 1.5 – 2.0 cun perpendicularly.

Chengshan (*U.B. 57.*). (*Chengshan*).

Location: At the level where the two bellies of the gastrocnemius unite to form the tendo Achilles, 8 cun below Weizhong (U.B. 40), or half way between Weizhong (U.B. 40.) and the ankle joint.

Indications: Sciatica, cramps of the calf muscles,[1] pain in the sole of foot, paralysis of the lower limb, haemorrhoids.

Puncture: 1.0 – 1.5 cun perpendicularly.

Feiyang (*U.B. 58.*). (*Feiyang*). Luo-Connecting point.

Location: 7 cun directly above Kunlun (U.B. 60.), on the lateral aspect of the calf muscle. One cun inferior and lateral to Chengshan (U.B. 57.).

Indications: Ophthalmoplegia.

Puncture: 1.5 cun perpendicularly.

Kunlun *U.B. 60.* (*Kunlun*).

Location: Midway between the prominence of the latera malleolus and the lateral border of the tendo Achilles.

Indications: Painful disorders of the ankle region (arthritis, Achilles tendinitis), sciatica, lumbago, paralysis of the lower limb.

Puncture: 0.5 – 0.8 cun perpendicularly.

Shenmai (*U.B. 62.*). (*Shenmo*). Confluent point.

Location: 0.5 cun inferior to the tip (or lower border) of the lateral malleolus.

Indications: Convulsions, epilepsy, apoplexy, mental disorders, drug addictions, foot-drop.

Puncture: 0.3 – 0.5 cun perpendicularly.

Note: This is the most important sedative and tranquilizer point of the lower limb.

Zhiyin (*U.B. 67.*). (*Chihyin*). Jing-Well point.

---

1 Acupressure is very helpful in treating muscle cramps during pregnancy (Needles may cause abortion).

Location: 0.1 cun proximal to the lateral end of the proximal border of the little toe-nail.

Indications: Malposition of the foetus, difficult labour helps to reinforce uterine contractions and expedite delivery at full term. (Abortion may be caused in the earlier months of pregnancy.)

Puncture: 0.1 cun perpendicularly. Moxibustion on a needle.

List of all the acupuncture points of the Urinary Bladder Channel:

U.B. 1	:	**Jingming**	– Dangerous point.
U.B. 2	:	**Zanzhu**	
U.B. 3	:	**Meichong**	
U.B. 4	:	**Quchai**	
U.B. 5	:	**Wuchu**	
U.B. 6	:	**Chengguang**	
U.B. 7	:	**Tongtian**	
U.B. 8	:	**Luoque**	
U.B. 9	:	**Yuzhen**	
U.B.10	:	**Tianzhu**	
U.B.11	:	**Dashu**	- Influential point for bone and cartilage.
U.B.12	:	**Fengmen**	
U.B.13	:	**Feishu**	- Back-Shu (Lung) point.
U.B.14	:	**Jueyinshu**	- Back-Shu (Pericardium) point.
U.B.15	:	**Xinshu**	- Back-Shu (Heart) point.
U.B.16	:	**Dushu**	- (Specific point for pruritus).
U.B.17	:	**Geshu**	- Influential point for blood, Back-Shu point of the diaphragm.
U.B.18	:	**Ganshu**	- Back-Shu (Liver) point.
U.B.19	:	**Danshu**	- Back-Shu (Gall Bladder) point.
U.B.20	:	**Pishu**	- Back-Shu (Spleen) point.
U.B.21	:	**Weishu**	- Back-Shu (Stomach) point.

U.B.22 : **Sanjiaoshu** - Back-Shu (Sanjiao) point.
U.B.23 : **Shenshu** - Back-Shu (Kidney) point.
U.B.24 : **Qihaishu**
U.B.25 : **Dachangshu** - Back-Shu (Large Intestine) point.
U.B.26 : **Guanyuanshu**
U.B.27 : **Xiaochangshu** - Back-Shu (Small Intestine) point.
U.B.28 : **Pangguangshu** - Back-Shu (Urinary Bladder) point.
U.B.29 : **Zhonglushu**
U.B.30 : **Baihuanshu**
U.B.31 : **Shangliao**
U.B.32 : **Ciliao**
U.B.33 : **Zhongliao**
U.B.34 : **Xialiao**
U.B.35 : **Huiyang**
U.B.36 : **Chengfu**
U.B.37 : **Yinmen**
U.B.38 : **Fuxi**
U.B.39 : **Weiyang**
U.B.40 : **Weizhong** - One of the 6 important Distal points, Earth point.
U.B.41 : **Fufen**
U.B.42 : **Pohu**
U.B.43 : **Goahuang**
U.B.44 : **Shentang**
U.B.45 : **Yixi**
U.B.46 : **Geguan**
U.B.47 : **Hunmen**
U.B.48 : **Yanggang**
U.B.49 : **Yishe**

U.B.50 : **Weicang**

U.B.51 : **Huangmen**

U.B.52 : **Zhishi**

U.B.53 : **Baohuang**

U.B.54 : **Zhibian**

U.B.55 : **Heyang**

U.B.56 : **Chengjin**

U.B.57 : **Chengshan**

U.B.58 : **Feiyang** - Luo-Connecting point.

U.B.59 : **Fuyang**

U.B.60 : **Kunlun** - Fire point.

U.B.61 : **Pushen**

U.B.62 : **Shenmai** - Confluent point.

U.B.63 : **Jinmen**

U.B.64 : **Jinggu** - Yuan-Source point.

U.B.65 : **Shugu** - Wood point.

U.B.66 : **Tonggu** - Water point.

U.B.67 : **Zhiyin** - Jing-Well point, Metal point.

Note I: The Back-Shu points are used:

1) to treat disorders along the spine.

2) to treat disorders of the related Organ-they lie at the level of the sympathetic ganglia which supply these organs.

3) to treat disorders of the sense organs connected to the related Organs.

4) to treat disorders of the tissues connected to the related Organ.

5) for diagnosis and prognosis, as they are also Alarm points.

6) as Influential points in the case of Dashu (U.B. 11.) and Geshu (U.B. 17.).

7) in combination with Mu-Front points, as an effective method of treating Internal Organ disorders. (No Distal points need then be used).

8) frequently, for moxibustion.

9) also, we have reported a case of collapse of a lung after needling at Dushu (U.B. 16.). Great care must therefore be exercised when using these points.

Note II: The Back-Shu points coincide with the surface marking of the sympathetic ganglia. The order of the acupuncture points exactly correspond sequentially to the sympathetic outflow to the internal organs.

THE CIRCULATION OF ENERGY IN THE URINARY BLADDER

The Urinary Bladder Channel of Foot-Taiyang joins the Du Channel at the point Baihui (Du 20.) and there communicates directly with the brain. While coursing down along the paravertebral muscles it communicates with the Organs Urinary Bladder and the Kidney. At the Back-Shu points deep communications exist with all the other Internal Organs as well.

SYNDROMES OF THE URINARY BLADDER

A. **The Urinary Bladder Channel:** Lacrimation, when exposed to the wind, rhinitis, epistaxis, vertical and occipital headaches, backache and sciatica.

B. **The Organ Urinary Bladder:** Diseases of the Urinary Bladder are recognized under two main syndromes:

1) **Damp-heat in the Urinary Bladder:** Damp heat injures the Urinary Bladder causing frequency, urgency and pain on micturition. Blood clots may appear in the urine. Renal stones may be formed. The tongue is red with a black coating. The pulse may be rapid.

2) **Disturbance in the Urinary Bladder functions:** This is due to a kidney insufficiency. The symptoms are retention or dribbling. The tongue is pale and a deep thready pulse may be felt.

■

TABLE OF THE IMPORTANT URINARY BLADDER CHANNEL POINTS OF THE BACK OF THE TRUNK

		LOCATION	NAME	No.	Related Organ	DISORDERS
Cervical		1.3 cun lateral to the midpoint between C.1 and C.2	Tianzhu	U.B.10.	—	Stiff neck, occipital headache, cervical spondylosis
thoracic vertebrae	1	1.5 cun lateral to spinous process of T.1	Dashu	U.B.11.	Bone and cartilage	*Influential Point for bone and cartilage:* pain in the shoulder girdle area.
	3	1.5 cun lateral to Spinous precess of area. T.3	Feishu	U.B.13.	Lung (Lu.)	Lung disease, nose disorders, skin disorders, lesions of the soft tissue of the dorsal spine
		1.5 cun lateral to spinous process of T.4	Jueyinshu	U.B.14.	Pericardium (P.)	Heart disease, brain disorders, local disorders of the spine.
	5	1.5 cun lateral to spinous process of T. 5	xinshu	U.B.15.	Heart (H.)	Heart disease, brain disorders, speech disorders local disorders, of the spine.
	7	1.5 cun lateral to spinous process of T.7	Geshu	U.B.17.	Blood (Diaphgram)	*Influential point tor blood:* anaemia, chronic hemorrhagic diseases, paralysis of diaphgram, hiccough.
	9	1.5 cun lateral to spinous process or T.9	Ganshu	U.B.18.	Liver (Liv.)	Liver disease, eye disease, muscle and tendon disorders, local disorders of the spine.
		1.5 cun lateral to spinous process of T.10	Danshu	U.B.19.	Gall Biadder (G.B.)	Gall bladder disease, liver disease, local disorders of the spine.
	11	1.5 cun lateral to spinous process of T.11	Pishu	U.B.20.	Spleen (Sp.)	Gastro-Intestinal disorders, oedema, allergic disorders, soft tissue disorders
		1.5 cun lateral to Spinous process of T.12	Weishu	U.B.21.	Stomach (St.)	Gastric disorders.

Lumbar vertebrae		1.5 cun lateral to spinous process of L.1	Sanjiaoshu	U.B.22.	Sanjiao (S.J.)	Abdominal distension, flatulence, local disorders of the spine.
	2	1.5 cun lateral to spinous process of L.2	Shenshu	U.B.23.	Kidney (K.)	Genito-urinary disorders, ear disease, bone disorders, alopecia, local disorders of the spine.
	4	1.5 cun lateral to spinous process of L.4	Dachangshu	U.B.25.	Large intestine (L.I.)	Diarrhoea, constipation, low backache, sciatica paralysis of the lower extremities.
Sacral		1.5 cun lateral to the midline, level with S.1	Xiaochangshu	U.B.27	Small intestine (S.I.)	Low backache, enteritis, sacro-iliac disease genito-urinary disorders.
		1.5 cun lateral to the midline, level with S.2	Pangguangshu	U.B.28	Urinary Bladder (U.B.)	Genito-urinary disorders, lumbo-sacral disorders.
	2	On the second sacral foramen	Ciliao	U.B.32.		Genito-urinary disorders, haemorrhoids, sciatica.
	4	3.0 cun lateral to the midline, level with S.4	Zhibian	U.B.54.		Genito-urinary disorders, haemorrhoids, sciatica hip disorders, paralysis of the lower limb.

Note: The U.B. Channel points situated lateral to verterbrae from T.I. to L. 4. are located by reference to the lower border of each dorsal spine.

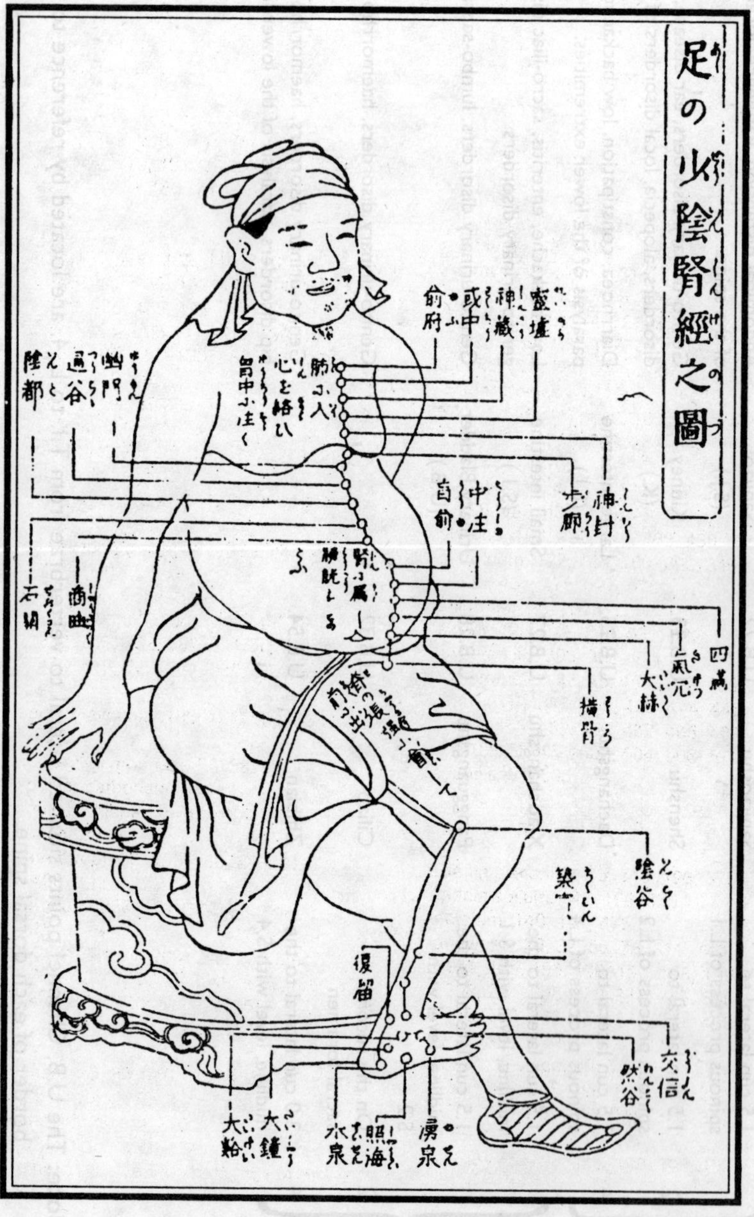

足の少陰腎經之圖
兪府
或中
神藏
靈墟
神封
歩廊
幽門
通谷
陰都
肺に入
心を絡い
胸中に注く
中注
肓兪
商曲
石関
腎に属
膀胱を絡ふ
四満
氣穴
大赫
横骨
陰谷
築賓
復溜
交信
然谷
大鐘
大谿
照海
水泉
湧泉

KIDNEY CHANNEL (K.)

"The Kidneys control water. The Kidney Qi penetrates to the ears."

— Ling Shu

- Polarity : Yin.
- Number of points : 27
- Pertaining Organ : Kidney.
- Related Channel : Urinary Bladder Channel (U.B.).
- Element : Water.
- Energy Flow : Centripetal.
- Course :

Commencing at the sole of the foot, it travels towards the medical side of the ankle where it makes a loop; thereafter it ascends along the medial side of the leg, passes along the medial side of the popliteal fossa, and travelling up the postero-medial aspect of the thigh, reaches the front of the abdomen close to the midline to end in the upper part of the chest.

Connections with the Urinary Bladder Channel:

Yuan-Source point: Taixi (K.3.).

Luo-Connecting point: Dazhong (K.4.).

THE KIDNEY CHANNEL

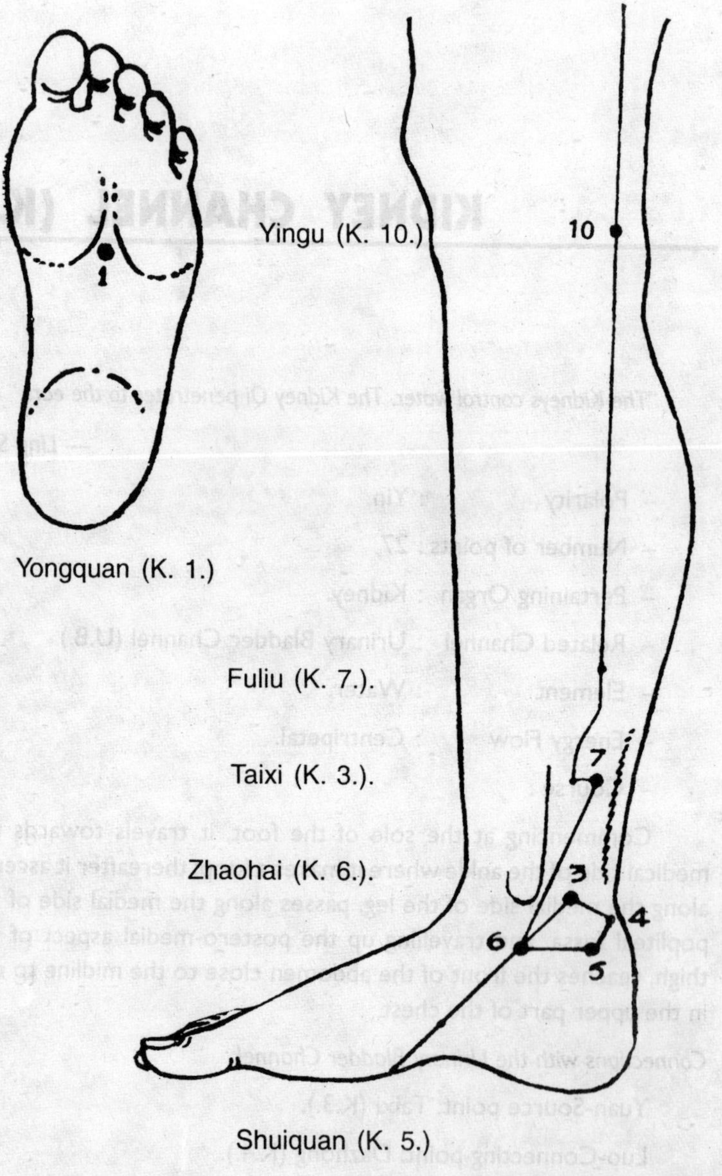

Clinical uses:

1) Genito-urinary disorders. (The Organ Kidney of traditional Chinese medicine represents both the urinary and genital functions; the concept of 'Kidney' also includes the adrenal glands, particularly the stress mechanisms.

2) Low back pain, pain and paralysis of the lower extremities.

3) Excess Lung disorders: Water (K.) is the son of Metal (Lu.).

4) Oedema, excessive sweating (disorders of the Element Water).

5) Convulsions and other acute emergencies (at Yongquan (K.1.)).

6) Bone cartilage and nail disorders, ear disorders, alopecia (the Kidney is connected to bone, cartilage, the head hair and the ears).

Commonly used acupuncture points:

K. 1, K. 3, K. 5, K. 6, K. 7.

Description of the commonly used acupuncture points:

Yongquan (*K.1.*). (*Yungchuan*). Jing-Well point.

Location: In the sole of the foot, on a line drawn posteriorly between the 2nd and 3rd toes, in the depression formed between the anterior one-third and posterior two-third parts of the sole when the toes are plantar flexed.

Indications: This is the most effective Jing-Well point for needling and is used in fainting, coma, shock, hysteria, epileptic attack infantile convulsions, cyclical vomiting, hyperemesis gravidarum and other acute emergency conditions. It is also indicated in plantar fascitis, plantar warts and excessive sweating of the sole of the foot.

Puncture: 0.5 cun perpendicularly.

Taixi (*K.3.*) (*Taihsi*). Yuan-Source point.

Location: Midway between the prominence or tip of the, medial malleolus and the medial border of the tendo-Achilles.

Indications: Genital and urinary disorders, impotence, low back ache, disorders of the ankle. In acute asthma or in cases of frequent asthmatic attacks, ("excess of Lung"), mild stimulation of this point or Fuliu (K.7.) may be usefully carried out.

Puncture: 1.0 cun perpendicularly, or towards Kunlun (U.B. 60.).

Shuiquan (*K.5.*). (*Shuichuan*). Xi-Cleft point.

Location: 1.0 cun below Taixi (K.3.), on the medial surface of the calcaneum.

Indications: Renal colic.

Puncture: 1.0 cun perpendicularly and employ very strong stimulation.

Zhaohai (*K.6.*). (*Chaohai*).

Locations: In the depression 1.0 cun directly below the prominence of the medial malleolus. (0.4 cun below the tip or lower border of the medial malleolus).

Indications: Genito-urinary disorders, oedema of the ankle.

Puncture: 0.5 cun perpendicularly.

Fuliu (*K.7.*). (*Fuliu*).

Location: 2 cun proximal to Taixi (K.3.), on the medial border of the tendo-calcaneus.

Indications: Excessive sweating, bronchial asthma.

Puncture: 1.0 cun perpendicularly.

Note: For excessive sweating, this point may be effectively combined with Hegu (L.I.4.) and Yinxi (H.6.) and the local points of the areas where there is excessive sweating:

Palm: Yuji (Lu. 10.); Laogong (P.8.); Shaofu (H.8.).

Axilla: Jiquan (H.1.).

Sole: Yongquan (K.1.).

The specific points used for oedema and ascites may also be added.

Yingu (*K.10.*). (*Yinku*).

Location: At the popliteal crease on the medial border of the semitendinosus.

Indication: Knee disorders, impotence, baldness.

Puncture: 1.0 cun perpendicularly.

List of all the acupuncture points of the Kidney Channel:

K. 1 : **Yongquan** - Jing-Well point, Wood point.
K. 2 : **Rangu** - Fire point.
K. 3 : **Taixi** - Yuan-Source point, Earth point.
K. 4 : **Dazhong** - Luo-Connecting point.
K. 5 : **Shuiguan** - Xi-Cleft point.
K. 6 : **Zhaohai**
K. 7 : **Fuliu** - Metal point.
K. 8 : **Jiaoxin**
K. 9 : **Zhubin**
K. 10 : **Yingu** - Water point.
K. 11 : **Henggu**
K. 12 : **Dahe**
K. 13 : **Qixue**
K. 14 : **Siman**
K. 15 : **Abdomen - Zhongzhu**
K. 16 : **Huangshu**
K. 17 : **Shangqu**
K. 18 : **Suiguan**
K. 19 : **Yindu**
K. 20 : **Abdomen - Tonggu**

K. 21 : **Youmen**

K. 22 : **Bulang**

K. 23 : **Shenfeng**

K. 24 : **Lingxu**

K. 25 : **Shencang**

K. 26 : **Yuzhong**

K. 27 : **Shufu**

From Shufu (K.27) the Yin vital energy flows on to Tianchi (P.1.)

Note: The Kidney and the Urinary Bladder are related to bone, cartilage and to head hair. The Kidney is also connected to the sense organs, the ears.

THE CIRCULATION OF ENERGY IN THE KIDNEY

The Kidney Channel of Foot-Shaoyin, as it travels upwards, branches to communicate, with Changqiang (Du 1.) and it then enters the Organ Kidney and thereafter communicates with the Organ Urinary Bladder. A branch ascends from the Organ Kidney to reach the pharynx and then terminates at the root of the tongue.

SYNDROMES OF THE KIDNEY

A. **The Kidney Channel:** Feverish sensation of the soles, weakness of the lower limbs, irregular menstruation, nocturnal emissions, sorethroat (Pharyngitis).

B. **The Organ Kidney:** Diseases of the Kidney are described under two main syndromes.

1) **Weakness of the qi (vital energy) of the Kidney:** This is due to asthenia after a long illness. Insufficiency of the Yin of the Kidney occurs. Urinary disorders, nocturnal eneuresis, infertility and asthmatic breathing may occur. A thready pulse may result. Alopecia often occurs.

2) **Insufficiency of the Yang of the Kidney:** This may be due to excessive sexual activity. The symptoms are low backache, joint disorders, impotence and oedema of the legs. Chronic pharyngitis, bone, cartilage and joint disorders may occur. Loss of hear-

ing, tinnitus, vertigo and chronic ear infections may also often occur. A pale tongue with a deep thready pulse may result.

Note: The Kidney Channel may be used in treating:

1) disorders of the Kidney (pertaining Organ).

2) other genito-urinary disorders (associated with the Organ).

3) Urinary Bladder disorders (coupled Organ).

4) disorders along the Urinary Bladder Channel, e.g., sciatica lowbackache (coupled Channel).

5) 'excess' disorders of the Lung. e.g., frequent asthmatic attacks (Water is son of Metal).

6) 'excess' disorders of the Heart and Brain, and Small Intestine disorders (Water destroys Fire).

7) disorders of the Liver and Gall Bladder and diseases along their Channels (Wood is the son of Water).

8) ear disorders (Kidney 'opens to' ear).

9) disorders affecting bone and head hair (related tissues).

This is an example of how one Channel has a multiplicity of functions. This wide spectrum of therapeutic latitude displayed by a single channel is a point to the fact that no two acupuncturists in the world may use the same combination of points to treat any one disorder. The best combination to choose, no doubt, depends on the experience of the individual acupuncturist and the response of the patient.

■

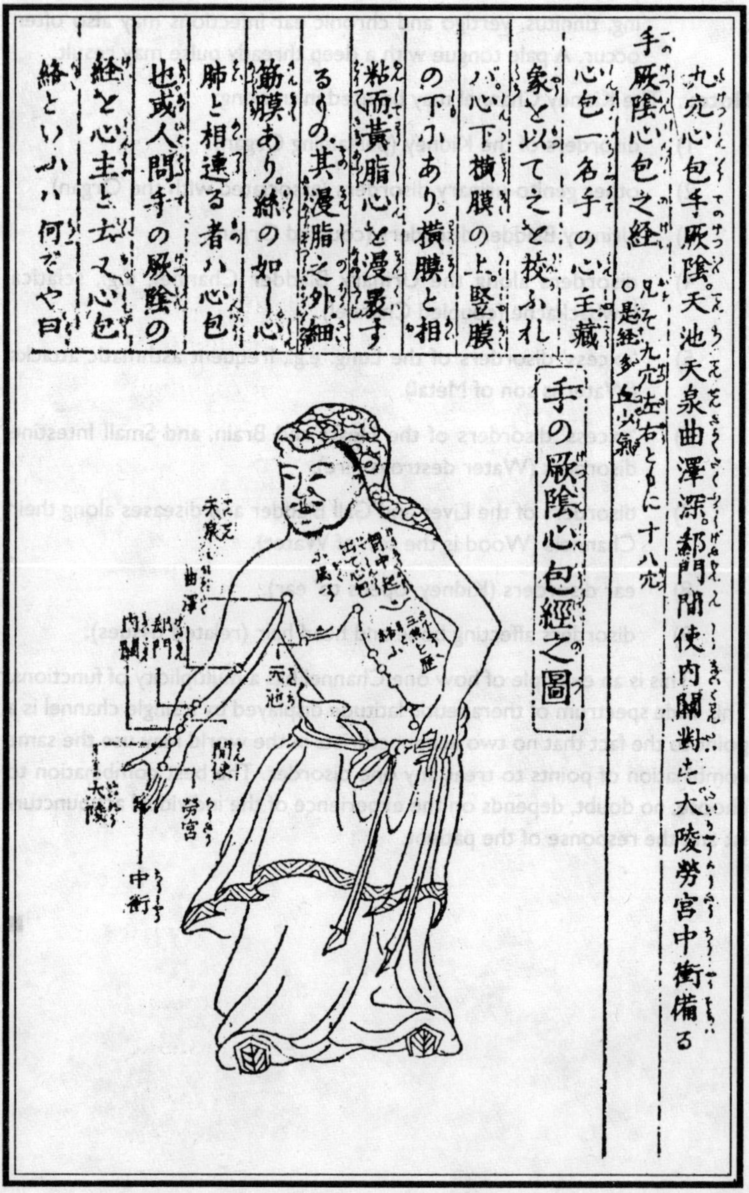

九穴心包手厥陰。天池天泉曲澤深。郄門間使内關對。大陵勞宮中衝備る
凡そ九穴左右ともに十八穴
○是經多血少氣
手の厥陰心包經之圖
手厥陰心包之経
心包一名手の心主藏
象を以てこれを挍ふれ
バ心下横膜の上竪膜
の下にあり。横膜と相
粘而黄脂心を漫裹す
るもの其漫脂之外細
筋膜あり。絲の如し心
肺と相連る者ハ心包
也或人問手の厥陰の
経と心主と云又心包
絡といふハ何ぞや曰
天池
天泉
曲澤
郄門
間使
内關
大陵
勞宮
中衝

PERICARDIUM CHANNEL (P.)

"The Pericardium is part of, and a protector of the Heart. They help the brain to function."

— *Ling Shu*

Called the *Xin Pao Luo Jing* in Chinese the name of this Channel is also translated as 'Circulation', 'Circulation Sex' and 'Heart Constrictor'.

- Polarity : Yin.
- Number of points : 9.
- Partaining Organ : Pericardium.
- Related Channel : Sanjiao (S.J.).
- Element : Fire.
- Energy flow : Centrifugal.
- Course :

Commencing 1 cun lateral to the nipple, it runs along the front of the upper limb between the Lung Channel and the Heart Channel and ends at the tip of the middle finger.

Connections with the Sanjiao Channel:

Yuan-Source point: Daling (P.7.).

Luo-Connecting point: Neiguan (P. 6.).

THE PERICARDIUM CHANNEL

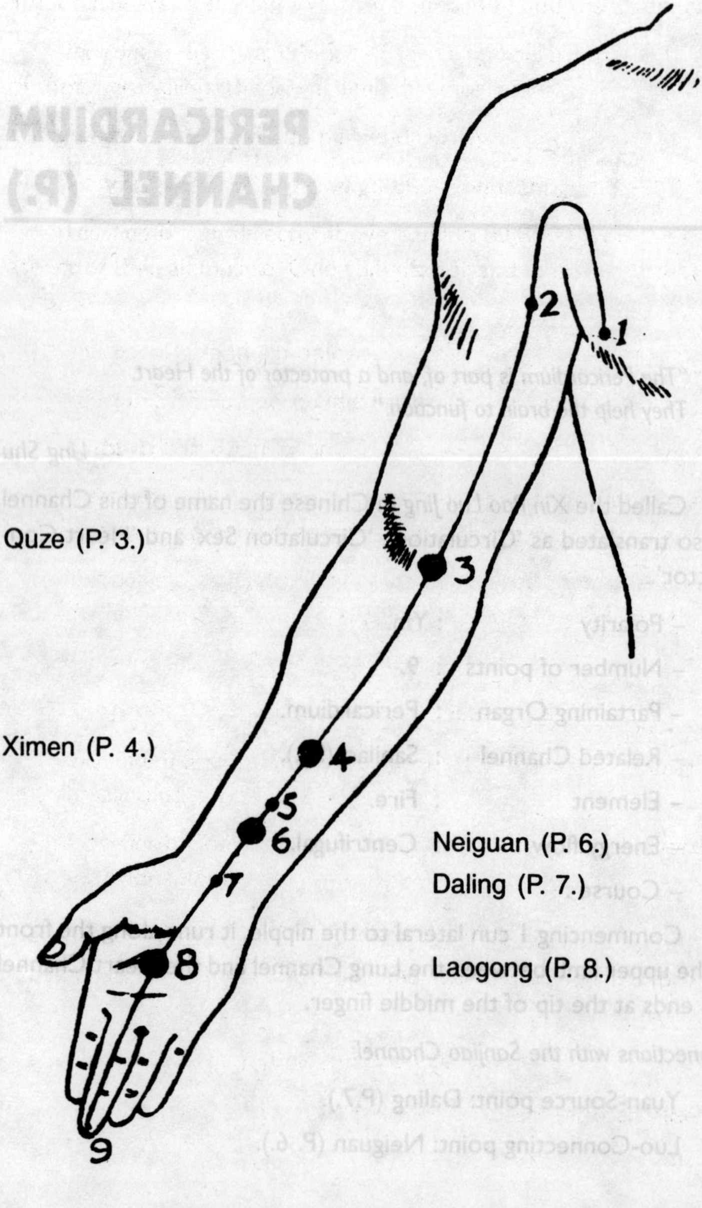

Clinical uses:

1) Heart diseases, especially angina pectoris, palpitation, disorders of rhythm.
2) Upper abdominal disorders such as gastritis, peptic ulcer, nausea, vomiting, morning sickness.
3) Mental disorders such as schizophrenia, nervous instability.
4) Diseases along the course of the Channel.

Note: In traditional Chinese medicine the Heart and the Pericardium are associated with the brain and its functions, although the brain is itself classified as an Extraordinary Organ. In the treatment of brain disorders therefore the main Channels to be selected are the Heart and Pericardium Channels. In appropriate cases however selection of points may also be made from the Du, Urinary Bladder, and Stomach channels, as they run on the scalp and over the brain. The following are the more common points used in disorders of the brain:

Shenmen (H. 7.).

Neiguan (P. 6.).

Baihui (Du 20.).

Shendao (Du 11.),

and the points on the three Yang Channels which run from the head to the foot:

Shenmai (U.B. 62.). Xinshu (U.B. 15.),

Yanglingquan (G.B. 34.),

Fenglong St. 40.).

Commonly used acupuncture points:

Elbow: P. 3.

Forearm: P. 4, P. 6, P. 7,

Hand: P. 8.

THE THREE YIN CHANNELS OF THE UPPER LIMB

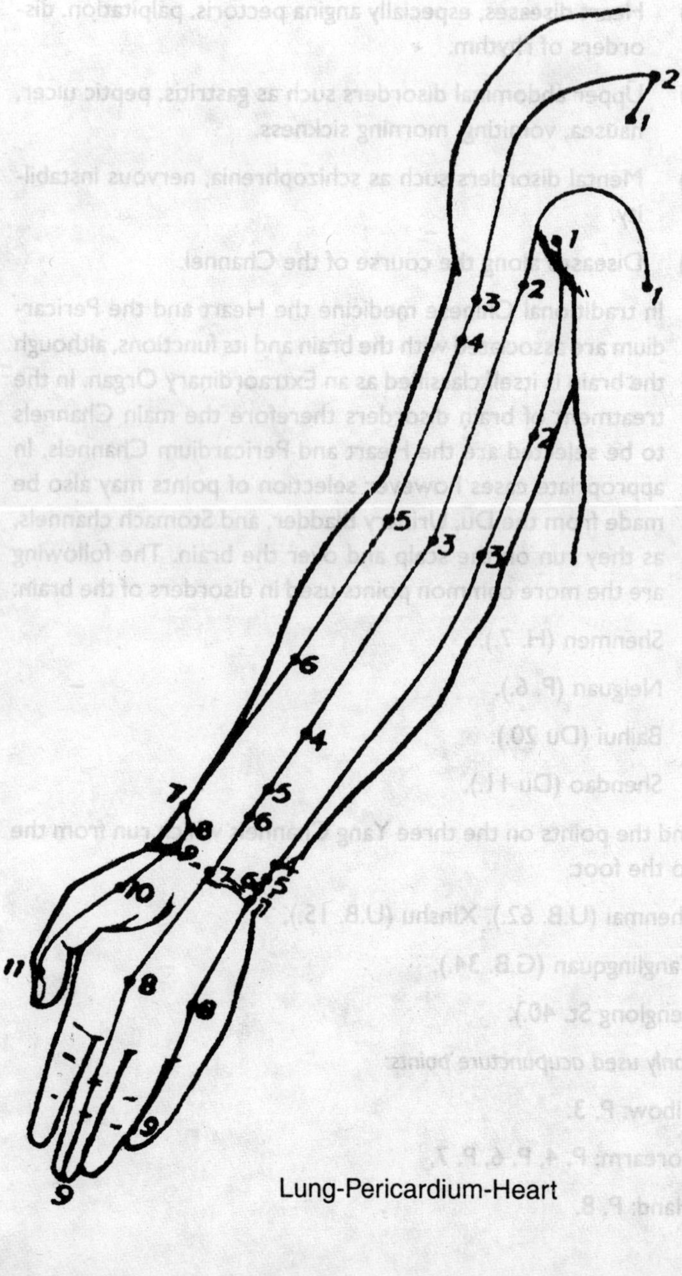

Lung-Pericardium-Heart

Description of the commonly used acupuncture points: **Quze** (*P. 3.*). (*Chutse*).

Location: In the ante-cubital crease, on the medial (ulnar) border of the biceps tendon.

Indications: Angina pectoris, palpitation, anxiety.

Puncture: 1.0 cun perpendicularly; in cases of fever or chronic yin diseases, prick to bleed with the three-edged needle.

Ximen (*P. 4.*). (*Hsimen*). Xi-Cleft point.

Location: 5 cun proximal to the midpoint of the wrist crease, between the tendons of the palmaris longus and flexor carpi radialis muscles.

Indications: As it is the Xi-Cleft point of the Pericardium Channel, it may be used to treat acute heart disease, e.g., angina pectoris, pericarditis tachycardia and other disorders of cardiac rhythm; acute depression and hysteria. This point is used for anaesthesia in cardiac surgery.

Puncture: 1.0 cun perpendicularly.

Neiguan (*P. 6.*). (*Neikuan*). One of the six important Distal points, Luo-Connecting point.

Location: 2 cun proximal to the midpoint of the wrist crease, between the tendons of the palmaris longus and flexor carpi radialis muscles.

Indications:

a) Heart disease: angina pectoris palpitation, carditis.

b) Brain disorders: mental disorders, epilepsy, hysteria, insomnia, anxiety.

c) Distal point for chest and upper abdominal disorders:

   i) Chest: pain in chest and costal region, hiccough;

   ii) Upper abdomen; nausea, vomiting, gastritis, peptic ul cer-, discomfort due to hiatus hernia.

d) Morning sickness, hyperemesis gravidarum.

e) Numbness of the forearm and hands.

f) For acupuncture anaesthesia in thyroidectomy and cardiac surgery.

Puncture: 1.0 cun perpendicularly or through to Waiguan (S.J. 5.).

Daling (*P. 7.*). (*Taling*). Yuan-source point.

Location: At the midpoint of the wrist crease between the tendons of the palmaris longus and flexor carpi radialis muscles.

Indications: Diseases of the wrist joint, early median carpal compression without positive objective neurological signs.

Puncture: 0.5 cun perpendicularly.

Note: In diseases of the wrist joint this point is usually combined with Shenmen (H. 7.). and Taiyuan (Lu. 9.). This illustrates the principle that when a Channel passes over a joint the acupuncture points in relation to that region are used to treat the joint disorder. (The principle that all points treat disorders of local and adjacent area).

Laogong (*P. 8.*). (*Laokung*).

Location: In the palmar surface, between the tips of the middle and ring fingers as these touch the central region of the palm on lightly clenching the fist.

Indication: Disorders of the palm, rheumatic arthritis of the carpal joints, Dupuytren's contracture, excessive sweating of the palm.

Puncture: 0.5 cun perpendicularly. This is a painful point.

List of all the acupuncture points of the Pericardium Channel:

P. 1 : **Tianchi**

P. 2 : **Tianquan**

P. 3 : **Quze** - Water point.

P. 4 : **Ximen** - Xi-Cleft point.

P. 5 : **Jianshi** - Metal point.

P. 6 : **Neiguan** - Luo-Connecting point.

P. 7 : **Daling** - Yuan-Source point, Earth point.

P. 8 : **Laogong** - Fire point.

P. 9 : **Zhongchong** - Jing-well point. Wood point.[1]

Note: The main sedative and tranquilizing points of the body are:

Baihui (Du 20.).
Sishencong (Ex. 6.).
Shenmen (H. 7.).
Neiguan (P. 6.).
Shenmai (U.B. 62.).
Xinshu (U.B. 15.)
Yanglingquan (G.B. 34.).
Fenglong (St 40.).
Shendao (Du 11.).
Anmain I (Ex. 8.).
Anmain II (Ex. 9.).
Yaoqi (Ex. 20.).

The point Hegu (L.I.4.) has also potent sedative and tranquilizing effects in addition to being the most important analgesic point.

THE ENERGY CIRCULATION IN THE PERICARDIUM

The Pericardium Channel of Hand-Jueyin originates from the Organ Pericardium, which is the protector of the Heart. It communicates with all the three body cavities. Its further connections are with the tongue and brain *via* the same internal pathways as the Heart.

SYNDROMES OF THE PERICARDIUM

These are the same as those of the Heart. (The Pericardium is the covering—the protector—of the heart).

1 According to some authorities this Jing-well point is located at the radial corner of the base of the nail of the middle finger.

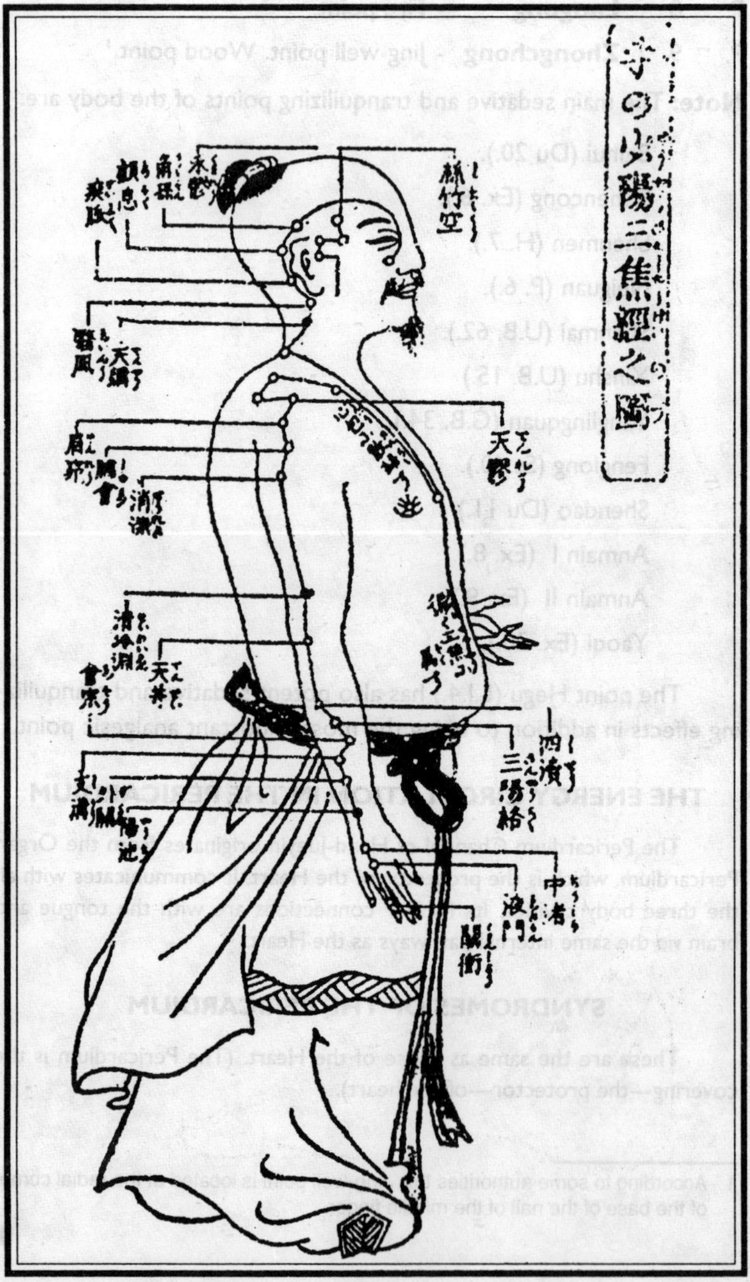
手の少陽三焦經之圖
絲竹空
角孫
顱息
瘈脈
翳風
天牖
天髎
肩髎
臑會
消濼
清冷淵
天井
會宗
四瀆
三陽絡
支溝
陽池
中渚
液門
關衝

SANJIAO CHANNEL (S.J.)

"The Sanjiao is the protector of the Zang and Fu."

— *Zangshi Leijing*

Sanjiao in Chinese means "Three Body Cavities"[1]. It is also translated as the "Triple Warmer" and the "Three Burning Spaces".

- Polarity : Yang.
- Number of points : 23.
- Partaining Organ : Sanjiao.
- Related Channel : Pericardium (P.).
- Element : Fire.
- Energy flow : Centripetal.
- Course:

Commencing in the ring finger, the Channel runs proximally on the back of the upper limb between the radius and the ulna, more or less parallel to and between the Large Intestine and Small Intestine Channels. From the tip of the shoulder it runs to the side of the

1 The Three Body Cavities are the thoracic cavity, the abdominal cavity and the pelvic cavity. It is the tissue enclosing the organs of these three areas that is considered as Sanjiao in traditional Chinese medicine. The Sanjiao is a conceptualization of the harmony that exists between the different internal organs.

THE SANJIAO CHANNEL

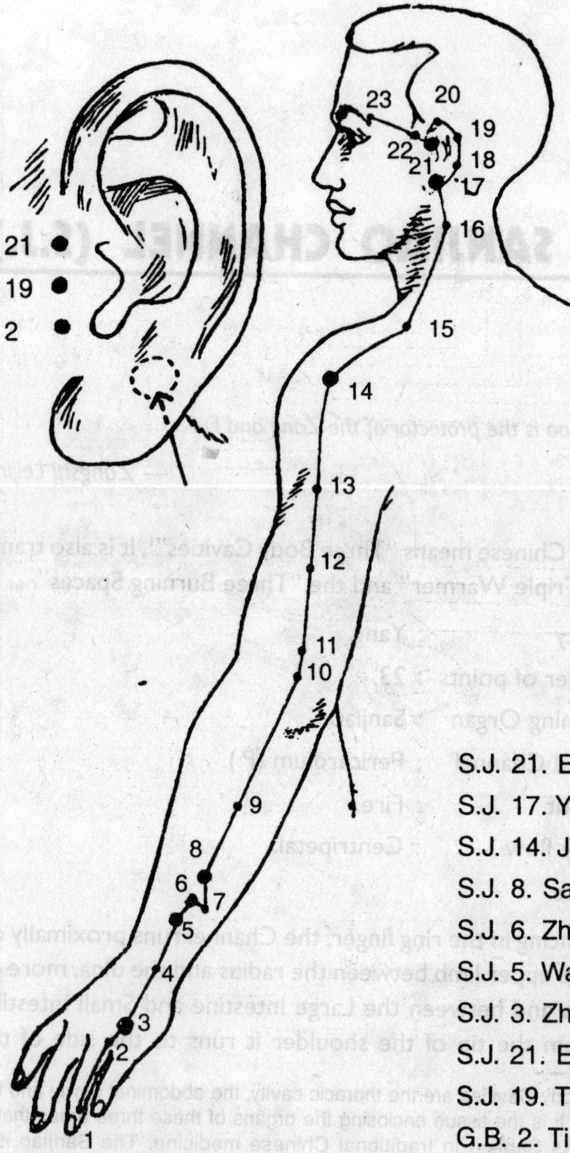

S.J. 21. Emen
S.J. 17. Yifeng
S.J. 14. Jianliao
S.J. 8. Sanyangluo
S.J. 6. Zhigou
S.J. 5. Waiguan
S.J. 3. Zhongzhu
S.J. 21. Ermen
S.J. 19. Tinggong
G.B. 2. Tinghui

neck, circles around the root of the external ear and terminates at the outer corner of the eyebrow.

Connections with the Pericardium Channel:

Luo-Connecting point: Waiguan (S.J. 5.)

Yuan-Source point: Yangchi (S.J. 4.).

Clinical uses:

1) Disorders of the ear.
2) Constipation (the commonest disorder of the abdominal cavity).
3) Paralysis, pain and polyneuropathy of the upper limb.
4) Pain in the shoulder and the back of the chest.
5) Eye diseases.

Commonly used acupuncture points:

Hand: S.J. 3.

Forearm: S.J. 5, S.J. 6, S.J. 8.

Shoulder: S.J. 14.

Ear: S.J. 17, S.J. 20, S.J. 21.

Eyebrow: S.J. 23.

Description of the commonly used acupuncture points:

Zhongzhu (*S.J. 3.*). (*Chungchu*).

Location: On the dorsum of the hand, in the depression between the heads of the 4th and 5th metacarpal bones. This point is best located by clenching the fist.

Indications: Ear disorders, paralysis of the upper extremities.

Puncture: 0.5 cun perpendicularly.

Waiguan (*S.J. 5.*). (*Waikuan*).

Location: 2 cun proximal to the midpoint of the dorsal transverse crease of the wrist, between the radius and the ulna.

Indications: Paralysis of the upper limb, temporal headache, ear disorders, stiff-neck.

THE SANJIAO CHANNEL

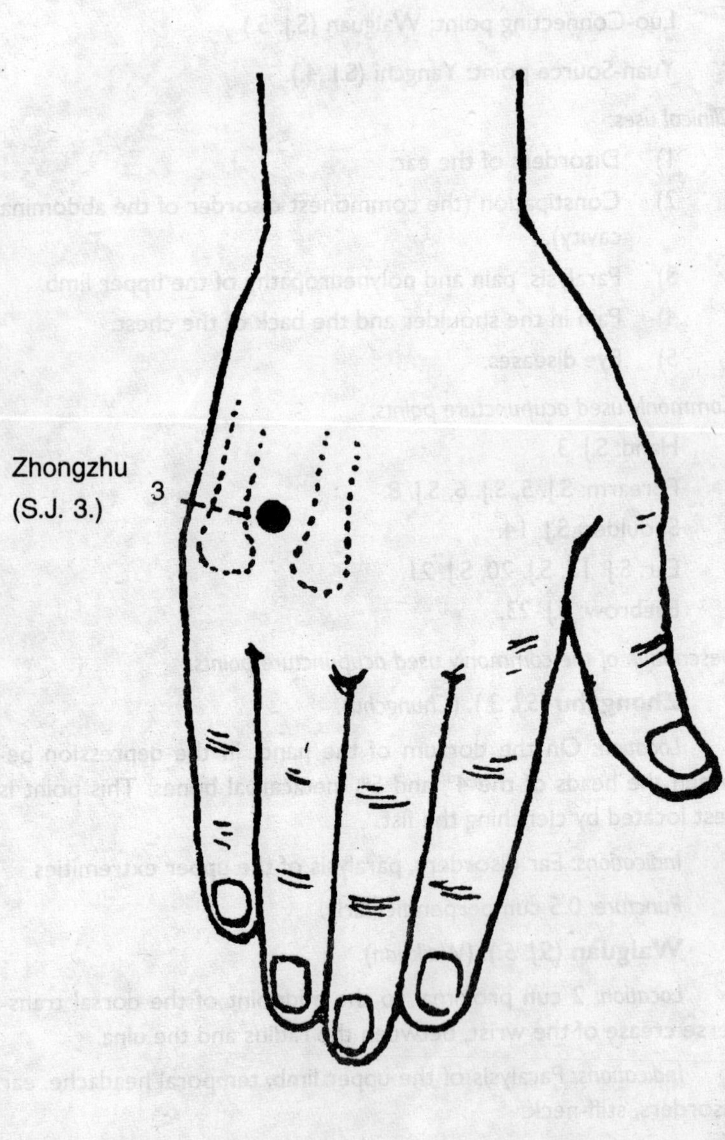

Puncture: 1.0 cun perpendicularly.

Zhigou (*S.J. 6.*) (*Chihkou*).

Location: 1.0 cun proximal to Waiguan (S.J. 5.).

Indications: Constipation.

Puncture: 1.0 cun perpendicularly.

Sanyangluo: (*S.J. 8.*). (*Sanyanglo*).

Location: 1.0 cun proximal to Zhigou (S.J. 6.).

Indications: Pain in the costal region (as in herpes zoster); acupuncture anaesthesia for thoracic surgery (e.g. lobectomy).

Puncture: 1.0 cun perpendicularly.

Jianliao: (*S.J. 14.*). (*Chienliao*).

Location:

a) With the arm abducted to a horizontal position, in the posterior depression of the origin of the deltoid muscle from the lateral border of the acromion.

b) With the arm by the side, between the acromion and the greater tuberosity of the humerus.

Indications: Frozen shoulder, pain in the arm, paralysis of the arm.

Puncture: 1.0 cun perpendicularly towards Jiquan (H.1.).

Yifeng (*S.J. 17.*) (*Yifeng*).

Location: In the highest point of the depression behind the ear lobe, between the angle of the mandible and the mastoid process.

Indications: Ear disorders, facial paralysis.

Puncture: 1.0 cun perpendicularly.

Jiasun (*S.J. 20.*). (*Jiasun*).

Location: On the scalp at the apex of the ear, when the ear is folded forwards. Endorcrine Point.

Indication: Endrocrine disorders, especially of pituitary origin e.g. dwarfism.

THE COMMONLY USED POINTS OF THE POSTERIOR ASPECT OF THE FOREARM AND THE HAND

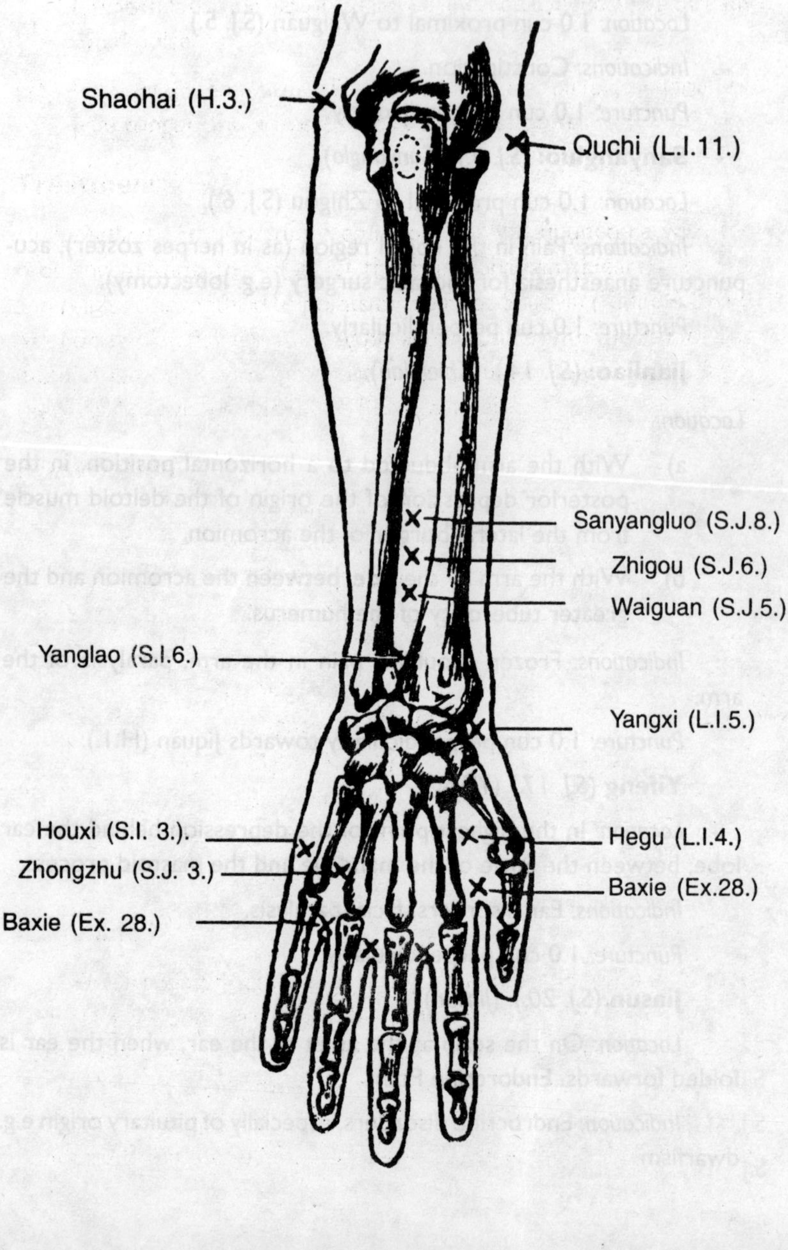

Puncture: 0.5 cun obliquely downwards.

Ermen (*S.J. 21.*). (*Erhmen*).

Location: In the depression in front of the supra-tragic notch. It is easier to locate this point when the mouth is slightly open.

Indication: Ear disorders.

Puncture: 0.5 cun perpendicularly, or more usually, horizontally downwards through Tinggong (S.I. 19.) to Tinghui (G.B. 2.) ("puncturing-through technique").

Sizhukong (*S.J. 23.*). (*Ssuchukung*). "The tip of the bamboo leaf".

Location: In the depression at the lateral end of the eyebrow.

Indication: Eye diseases, temporal headache, frontal sinusitis.

Puncture: 0.5 cun horizontally and posteriorly in the direction of Shuaigu (G.B. 8.). Sometimes a long needle is inserted connecting these two points, especially for temporal arthritis.

List of all the acupuncture points of the Sanjiao Channel.

S.J. 1	:	**Guanchong**	- Jing-Well point, Metal point.
S.J. 2	:	**Yemen**	- Water point.
S.J. 3	:	**Zhongzhu**	- Wood point.
S.J. 4	:	**Yangchi**	- Yuan-Source point.
S.J. 5	:	**Waiguan**	
S.J. 6	:	**Zhigou**	- Fire point.
S.J. 7	:	**Huizong**	- Xi-Cleft point.
S.J. 8	:	**Sanyangluo**	
S.J. 9	:	**Sidu**	
S.J. 10	:	**Tianjing**	- Earth point.
S.J. 11	:	**Qinglengyuan**	
S.J. 12	:	**Xiaoluo**	
S.J. 13	:	**Naohui**	
S.J. 14	:	**Jianliao**	

THE ACUPUNCTURE POINTS IN FRONT OF AND BEHIND THE EAR

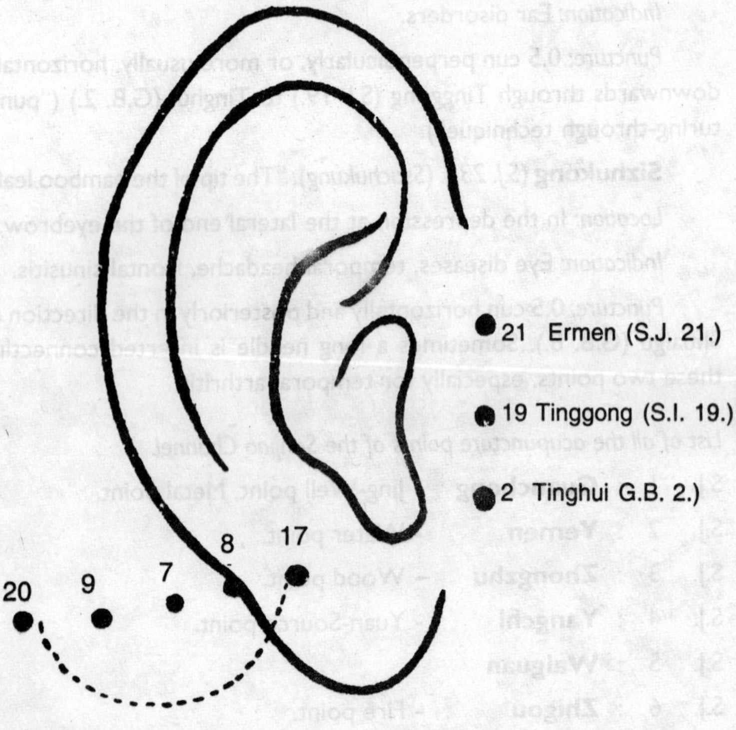

Dotted line outlines the mastoid process

Fengchi (G.B. 20.)

Anmian II (Ex. 9.)

Yiming (Ex. 7.)

Anmian I (Ex. 8.)

Yifeng (S.J. 17.)

S.J. 15 : **Tianliao**

S.J. 16 : **Tianyou**

S.J. 17 : **Yifeng**

S.J. 18 : **Qimai**

S.J. 19 : **Luxi**

S.J. 20 : **Jiaosun**

S.J. 21 : **Ermen**

S.J. 22 : **Ear-Heliao**

S.J. 23 : **Sizhukong**

From Sizhukong (S.J. 23.). the yang vital energy flows on to Tongziliao (G.B. 1.).

Note: Sanjiao Channel treats disorders of the 'Three Body Cavities' and disorders along the Channel.

1. Upper body cavity (chest cavity):

   i) Chest pain, intercostal neuralgia, pain following fracture of the ribs, herpes zoster of the chest area.

   ii) Chest surgery: pulmonary lobectomy can be carried out using the single point Sanyangluo (S.J. 8.).

2. Middle and lower body cavity (abdominal and pelvic cavity). Constipation.

3. Disorders along the Channel:

   Paralysis, numbness of the upper limb, shoulder disorders, stiff neck, ear and eye disorders.

Note: The Sanjiao is not intelligible on Western medical concepts of anatomy. According to some authorities, the Sanjiao is a conceptualization of the preservation of the homoeostasis of the Internal Organs. According to some authorities the 3 body-cavities represent (a) the cardio-respiratory, (b) digestive and (c) metabolic, excretory and reproductive functions respectively.

THE ENERGY CIRCULATION IN THE SANJIAO

The Sanjiao Channel of Hand-Shaoyang, as it runs over the supraclavicular fossa, branches internally to connect with the Organ Pericardium and then with all the three body cavities and their Internal Organs.

The three body cavities are also connected with a branch which traverses the thigh to communicate with the point. Weiyang (U.B. 39.), the lower He-Sea point of this Channel.

SYNDROMES OF THE SAN JIAO

A. **The Sanjiao Channel:** Pain along the channel, ear and eye disorders.

B. **The Organ Sanjiao:** This includes disorders, related to and imbalances of all the Zang-Fu Organs.

■

GALL BLADDER CHANNEL (G.B.)

"The Gall Bladder is appended to the Liver and they mutually assist one another to perform their functions".

—Zhangshi Leijing

- Polarity Yang.
- Number of points : 44.
- Pertaining Organ : Gall Bladder.
- Related Channel : Liver Channel (Liv.).
- Element : Wood.
- Energy flow : Centrifugal.
- Course:

The Channel runs from head to foot on the lateral aspect of the body. It commences at the outer corner of eye and runs to the front of the ear. It then zig-zags over the side of the head, and from the postero-lateral aspect of the neck it courses down the lateral aspect of the trunk and the lower limb to end in the foot near the lateral corner of the base of the 4th toe nail.

Note: The Channel lies in relation to the eye, the ear, the head, brain and neck, ribs, breast, liver, gall bladder and sciatic nerve areas. A number of important Distal points of the Channel treat proximal diseases in these regions.

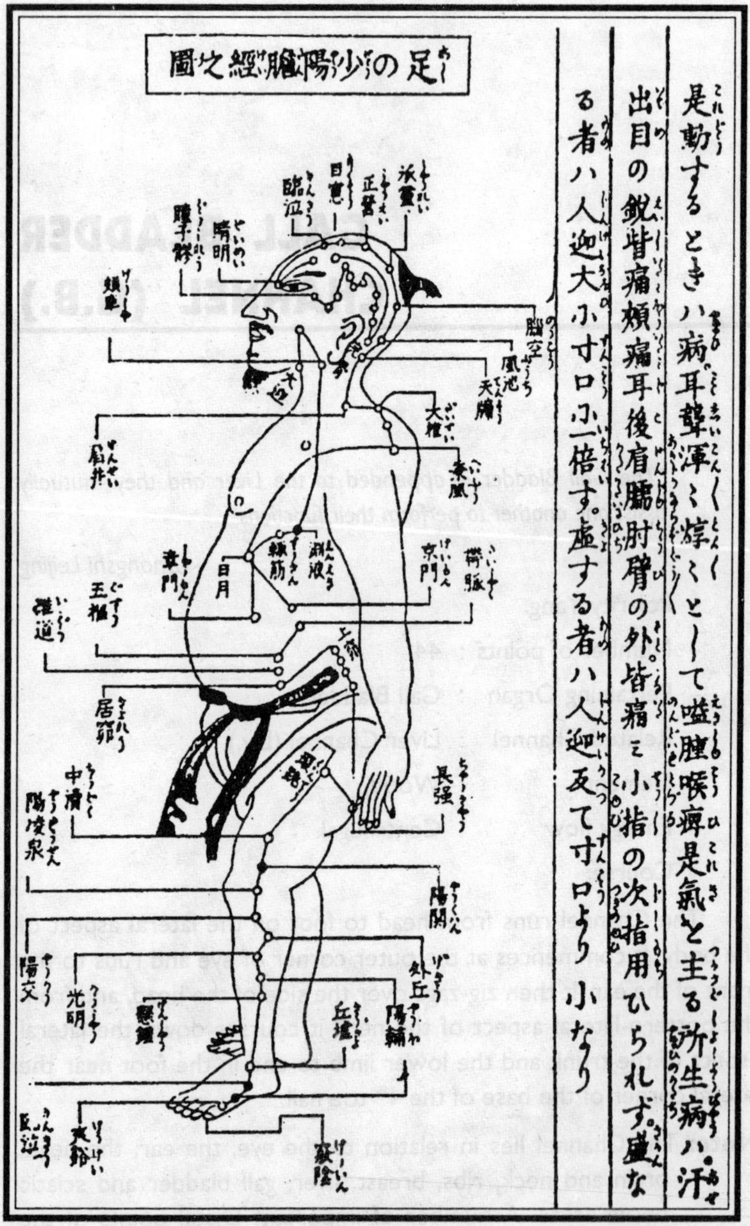
足の少陽膽經之圖
是動するときハ病耳聾渾々焞々として嗌腫喉痹是氣を主る所生病ハ汗
出目の鋭眥痛頰痛耳後肩臑肘臂の外。皆痛ミ小指の次指用ひられず。盛な
る者ハ人迎大ふ寸口ふ一倍す。虚する者ハ人迎反て寸口より小なり
承靈
正營
目窗
臨泣
睛明
瞳子髎
頰車
腦空
風池
天牖
大椎
肩井
秉風
帶脈
京門
淵液
輒筋
日月
章門
五樞
維道
居髎
中瀆
陽陵泉
長強
陽關
陽交
外丘
光明
懸鐘
陽輔
丘墟
臨泣
夾谿
竅陰

Connections with the liver Channel:

Yuan-Source point: Qiuxu (G.B. 40.).

Luo-Connecting point: Guangming (G.B. 37.).

Clinical uses:

Disorders along the course of the Channel such as diseases of the eye, ear, neck, mental disorders, lactation disorders, gall bladder and liver disorders pain in the gluteal region, low backache, sciatica, paralysis of the lower limbs.

Commonly used acupuncture points:

Eye area: G.B. 1, G.B. 14.

Ear area: G.B. 2.

Temporal area: G.B. 8.

Neck: G.B. 20.

Shoulder: G.B. 21.

Breast: G.B. 24.

Trunk:

Gall Bladder area: G.B. 25.

Loin: G.B. 26.

Hip:

Sciatic nerve area: G.B. 30.

Thigh: G.B. 31.

Leg: G.B. 34, G.B. 37, G.B. 39.

Ankle: G.B. 40.

Foot: G.B. 41.

Description of the commonly used acupuncture points:

Tongziliao (*G.B. 1.*). (*Tungtzuliao*).

Location: 0.5 cun lateral to the outer canthus of the eye.

Indications: Eye diseases, facial paralysis, headache, trigeminal neuralgia.

Puncture: 0.5 cun horizontally and posteriorly.

Tinghui (*G.B. 2.*). (*Tinghui*).

THE GALL BLADDER CHANNEL

G.B. 14. Yangbai
G.B. 8. Shuaigu
G.B. 1. Tongziliao
G.B. 2. Tinghui
G.B. 20. Fengchi

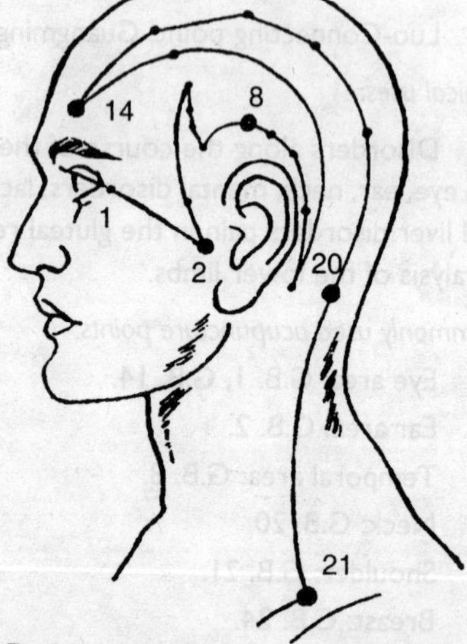

G.B. 21. Jianjing

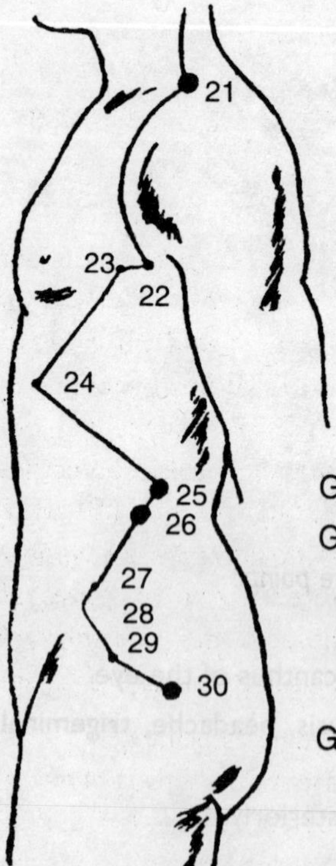

G.B. 25. Jingmen
G.B. 26. Daimai

G.B. 30. Huantiao

Location: In the depression immediately in front of the intertragic, notch, when the mouth is open.

Indications: Ear disorders, chronic infections of the auditory canal and the external ear, arthritis of the mandible, trismus, facial paralysis, trigeminal neuralgia.

Puncture: 1.0 cun perpendicularly, or use the puncturing through technique (see under Ermen S.J. 21.).

Shuaigu (*G.B. 8.*). (*Shuaiku*).

Location: Directly above the apex of the ear, 1.5 cun above the hairline. (The apex of the ear may be conveniently located by folding the ear over forwards, on itself).

indications: Migraine, ear diseases, dizziness, vertigo.

Puncture: 1.0 cun horizontally either anteriorly or posteriorly.

Yangbai (*G.B. 14.*) (*Yangpai*).

Location: 1.0 cun above the midpoint of the eyebrow.

Indications: Facial paralysis, frontal headache, frontal sinusitis, night blindness, glaucoma and other eye diseases.

Puncture: 0.5 cun horizontally and inferiorly through towards or through to Yuyao (Ex. 3.).

Fengchi: (*G.B. 20.*) (*Fengchih*).

Location: In the depression medial to the mastoid process between the origins of the trapezius and sterno-mastoid muscles.

Indications: Occipital headache, common cold, influenza, stiff neck, cervical spondylosis.

Puncture: 1.0 cun with the needle directed towards the inner canthus of the opposite eye. Strong stimulation of this point is said to relieve or abort an attack of the common cold.

Note: Too deep an insertion should be avoided.

Jianjing: (*G.B. 21.*). (*Chienching.*) Special Alarm point of the Gall bladder. Endocrine point.

THE COMMONLY USED ACUPUNCTURE POINTS OF THE FRONT OF THE CHEST WALL

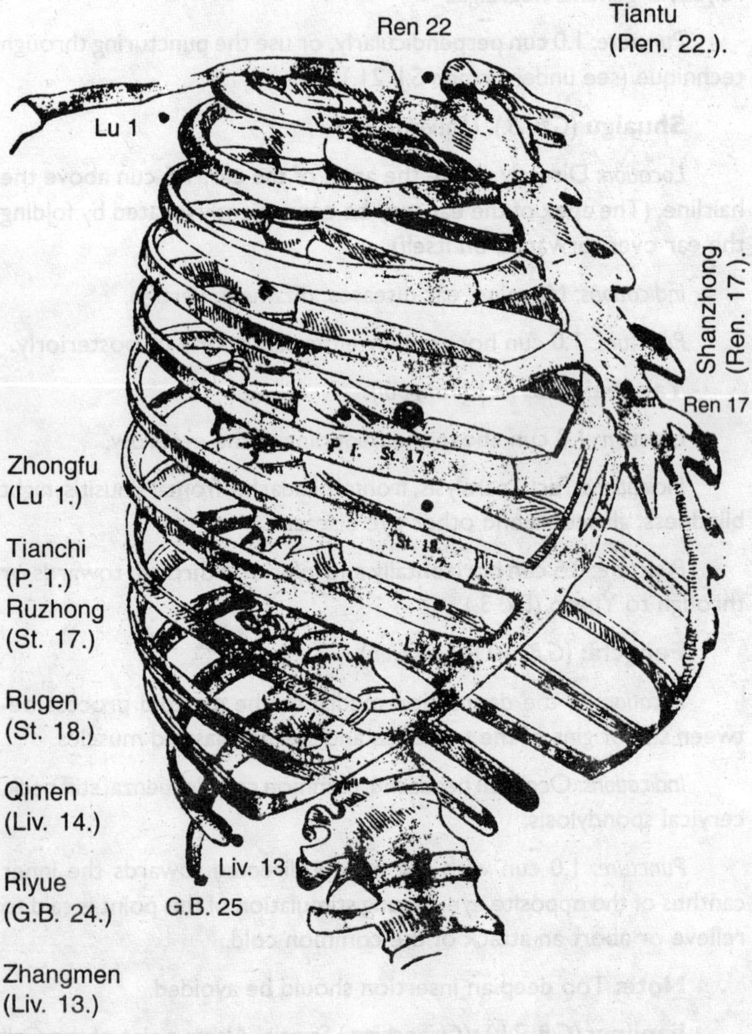

Location: Midway between Dazhui (Du 14.). and Jianyu (L.I. 15.). (Directly posterior to midpoint of clavicle, halfway between it and the superior border of the spine of the scapula).

Indications: Pain in the shoulder region, stiffness of the neck in conditions like cervical spondylosis and ankylosing spondylitis, hyperthyroidism, dysfunctional uterine bleeding.

Puncture: 1.0 cun perpendicularly.

Note: This point is used to treat endocrine disorders.

Riyue (*G.B. 24.*). (*Jihyueh*). Alarm point (Mu-Front) of the Gall bladder.

Location: On the nipple line in the 7th intercostal space (directly below Qimen (Liv. 14.) which lies in the 6th intercostal space.).

Indications: Cholecystitis, hepatitis, hiccough, gastritis.

Puncture: 0.5 cun obliquely.

Note: Insertion must be done obliquely as this is a Dangerous point.

Jingmen (*G.B. 25.*). (*Chingmen*). Alarm point (Mu-Front) of the Kidney.

Location: At the free end of the 12th rib.

Indication: Nephritis, costal pain, abdominal distension, flatulence.

Puncture: 0.5 cun perpendicularly.

Daimai (*G.B. 26.*). (*Taimai*).

Location: At the level of the umbilicus, on a vertical line drawn from the free end of the 11th rib.

Indications: Pelvic disorders, costal pain, back pain.

Puncture: 1.0 cun perpendicularly.

Huantiao (*G.B. 30.*) (*Huantiao*).

Location: Draw a straight line between the highest point of the greater trochanter and the sacral hiatus: the point is situated at the junction of the outer third with the medial two-thirds on this on this line.[1] It is located more easily in a lateral or prone position.

1 According to some Chinese authorities it is on the midpoint of this line.

THE FREQUENTLY USED POINTS IN THE LOW-BACK AREA

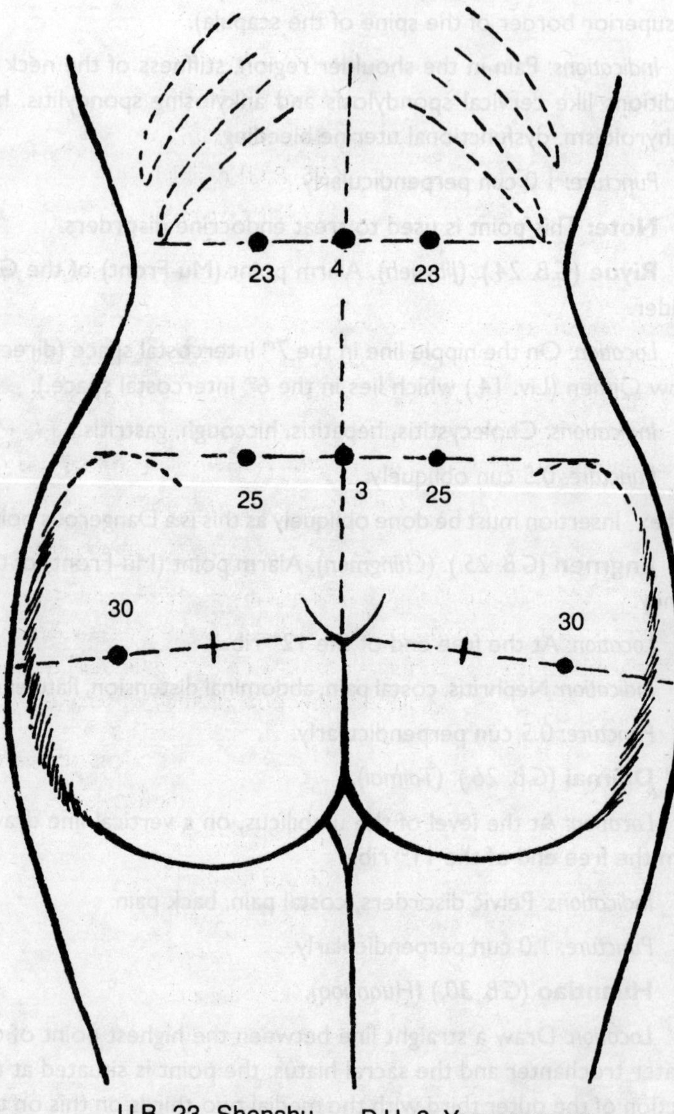

U.B. 23. Shenshu
U.B. 25. Dachangshu
G.B. 30. Huantiao
D.U. 3. Yaoyangguan
D.U. 4. Mingmen

Indication: Sciatica, prolapsed lumbar disc, paralysis of the lower extremities, disorders of the hipjoint.

Puncture: Perpendicular insertion with a long needle (about 5 cun in length). When the needle reaches the sciatic nerve, a sensation like an electric current will be felt travelling down the leg to the ankle region. When this sensation (*deqi*) is elicited, good therapeutic results may be expected.

Note: This is a very effective point for treating acute sciatica.

Fengshi (*G.B. 31.*). (*Fengshih*).

Location:

a) On the lateral aspect of the thigh, 7 cun proximal to the transverse popliteal crease, between the vastus lateralis and biceps femoris muscles: or

b) with the patient standing erect or lying supine, hand placed on the lateral side of the thigh, this point lies immediately distal to the tip of the middle finger.

Indications: Paralysis and pain of the lower extremities, paraesthesia in the distribution of the lateral cutaneous nerve of the thigh (*meralgia paraesthetica*).

Puncture: 1.5 cun perpendicularly.

Yanglingquan (*G.B. 34.*). (*Yanglinchuan*) Influential point for muscles and tendons.

Location:

a) In the depression anterior and inferior to the head of the fibula; or

b) at the meeting point of two straight lines, one drawn vertically on the anterior margin of the head of fibula, the other horizontally at the neck of the fibula.

Indication: Hemiplegia, pain in or paralysis of the leg, diseases of the gall bladder, muscle and tendon disorders, mental disorders, epilepsy headaches.

THE GALL BLADDER CHANNEL IN THE LOWER LIMB

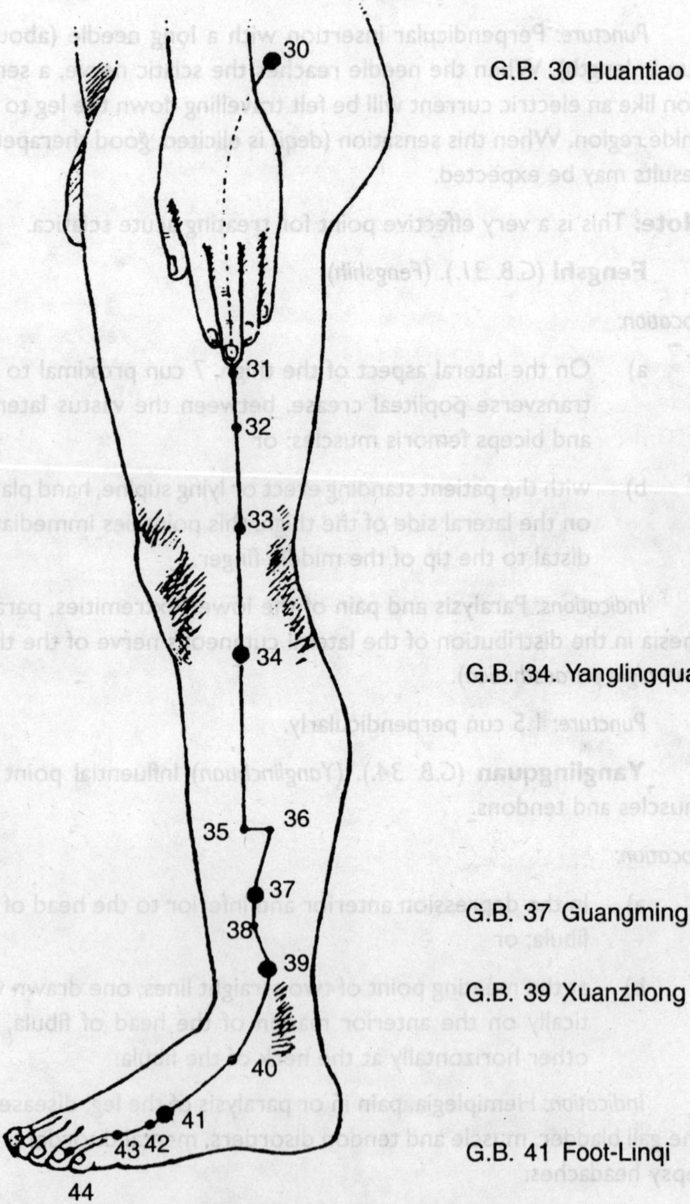

Puncture: 1.5 cun perpendicularly towards Yinlingquan (S.p. 9.), or obliquely downwards, forwards and medially.

Guangming (*G.B. 37.*) (*Kuangming*). Luo-Connecting point. "Guangming" in Chinese means "Bright Sight".

Location: 5 cun above the tip of the lateral malleolus, on the anterior border of the fibula, (According to some Chinese authorities it is located on the posterior border of the fibula.)

Indications: Eye disorders.

Puncture: 1.0 cun perpendicularly.

Xuanzhong (*G.B. 39.*). (*Hsuanchung*). Also called **Juegu.** Influential point for bone marrow.

Location: 3 cun above the tip of the lateral malleolus on the posterior border of the fibula.

Indications: paralysis of the lower limbs, stiffness of the neck, disorders of the marrow.

Puncture: 1.0 cun perpendicularly.

Qiuxu (*G.B. 40.*). (*Chiuhsu*). Yuan-Source point.

Location: At the meeting point of two lines, one drawn vertically on the anterior border of the lateral malleolus, the other horizontally on its inferior border.

Indications: Ankle disorders, pain in the chest wall.

Puncture: 0.5 cun perpendicularly.

Foot-Linqi (*G.B. 41.*). (*Tsulinchi*).

Location: In the depression immediately distal to the junction of the base of the 4th and 5th metatarsals.

Indications: Pain in the foot, breast disorders, ear disorders.

This is a supplementary point used in frozen shoulder.

Puncture: 0.5 cun perpendicularly.

List of all the acupuncture points of the Gall bladder Channel

G.B. 1 : **Tongziliao**

G.B. 2 : **Tinghui**

COMMONLY USED ACUPUNCTURE POINTS OF THE DORSUM OF THE FOOT

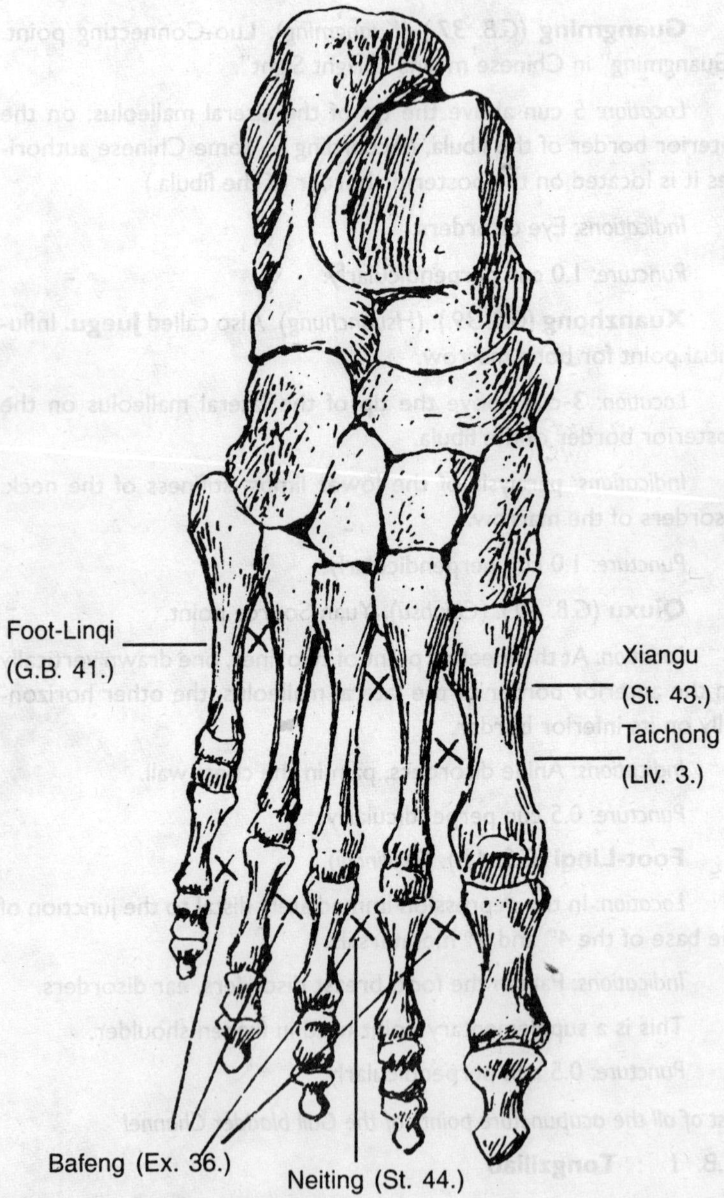

G.B. 3 : **Shangguan**

G.B. 4 : **Hanyan**

G.B. 5 : **Xuanlu**

G.B. 6 : **Xuanli**

G.B. 7 : **Qubin**

G.B. 8 : **Shuaigu**

G.B. 9 : **Tianchong**

G.B.10 : **Fubai**

G.B.11 : **Head-Qiaoyin**

G.B.12 : **Head-Wangu**

G.B.13 : **Benshen**

G.B.14 : **Yanghai**

G.B.15 : **Head-Linqi**

G.B.16 : **Muchuang**

G.B.17 : **Zhengying**

G.B.18 : **Chengling**

G.B.19 : **Naokong**

G.B.20 : **Fengchi**

G.B.21 : **Jianjina** – Special Alarm point of the Gall bladder.

G.B.22 : **Yuanye**

G.B.23 : **Zhejin**

G.B.24 : **Riyue** – Alarm point (Mu-Front) of the Gall bladder.

G.B.25 : **Jingmen** – Alarm point (Mu-Front) of the Kidney.

G.B.26 : **Daimai**

G.B.27 : **Wushu**

G.B.28 : **Weidao**

G.B.29 : **Femur-Juliao**

G.B.30 : **Huantiao**

G.B.31 : **Fengshi**

G.B.32 : **Femur-Zhongdu**

G.B.33 : **Xiyangguan**

G.B.34 : **Yanglingquan** - Influential point for muscle and tendon Earth point.

G.B.35 : **Yanjiao**

G.B.36 : **Waiqiu** - Xi-Cleft point.

G.B.37 : **Guangming** - Luo-Connecting point.

G.B.38 : **Yangfu** - Fire point.

G.B.39 : **Xuanzhong** - Influential point for marrow (**Juegu**).

G.B.40 : **Qiuxu** - Yuan-Source point.

G.B.41 : **Foot-Linqi**[2] - Wood point.

G.B.42 : **Diwuhui**

G.B.43 : **Xiaxi** - Water point.

G.B.44 : **Foot-Qiaoyin** - Metal point.

Note: The Gall bladder Channel has two Influential points (G.B. 34 and G.B. 39.).

This Channel has three Alarm points (G.B. 21, G.B. 24, and G.B. 25.).

Dannang (Extra), although an Extraordinary point, lies on the Gall bladder Channel and it is also an Alarm point of the Gall bladder. Thus the Gall bladder has altogether four Alarm points.

CIRCULATION OF ENERGY IN THE GALL BLADDER

The Superficial Gall Bladder Channel of Foot-Shaoyang arises at the outer canthus (Tongzillao G.B. 1.). A deep branch also arises here and traverses the deeper tissues of the face and neck, and enters the chest cavity through the supraclavicular fossa. Descending further it passes through the

2 Also spelt Lingqi

diaphragm to connect with the Organ Liver and then its own pertaining Organ, the Gall bladder. A further branch arising in the Gall bladder Organ descends through the abdomen to connect with the superficial channel at Huantio (G.B. 30.).

SYNDROMES OF THE GALL BLADDER

A. **The Gall bladdar Channel:** Eye disorders, parietal headache, bitter taste, pain along the pathway of the superficial channel.

B. **The Organ Gall bladder:** Diseases of the Organ Gall bladder are described under the syndromes which are closely related to Liver disorders e.g.:

Syndrome of Damp-heat in the Gall bladder and Liver:

This syndrome is usually due to prolonged indulgence in alcohol, rich and excessively spicy foods. This causes a depression of the functions of both the Liver and Gall bladder. The symptoms are pain in the hypochondrium, Jaundice, bitter taste, nauses and vomiting. The tongue coating is greenish-yellow and sticky.

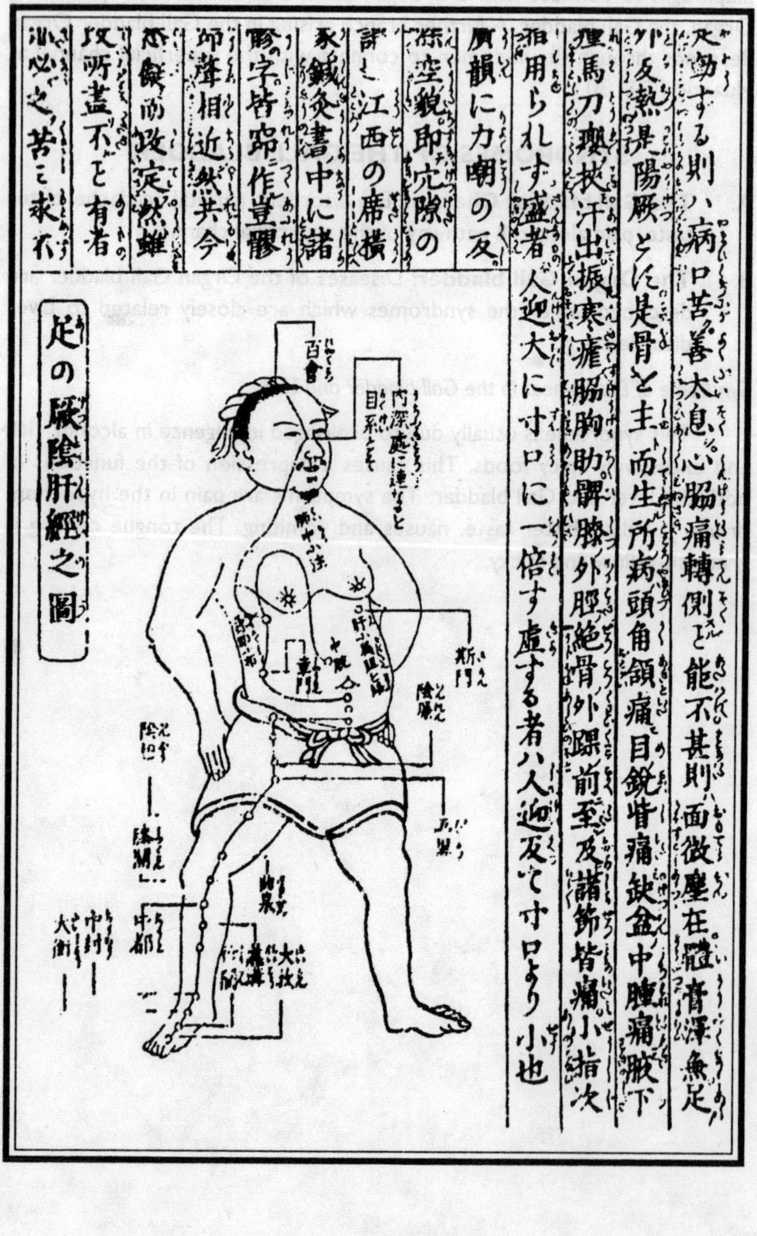

足動する則ハ病口苦ク善太息ス心脇痛轉側ヿ能不甚則ハ面微塵在體膏澤無足
外反熱是陽厥とに是骨と主而生所病頭角頷痛目鋭眥痛缺盆中腫痛腋下
腫馬刀瘻挾汗出振寒瘧胸脇肋髀膝外脛絶骨外踝前至及諸節皆痛小指次
指用られず盛者人迎大に寸口に一倍す虚する者ハ人迎反て寸口より小也
足の厥陰肝經之圖
百會
期門
章門
陰廉
陰包
膝關
曲泉
中都
中封
大衝

LIVER CHANNEL (LIV.)

"The Liver is the important organ which stores and transforms the blood."

— *Ling Shu*

- Polarity : Yin.
- Number of points : 14.
- Pertaining Organ : Liver.
- Related Channel : Gall bladder Channel (G.B.).
- Element : Wood.
- Energy flow : Centripetal.
- Course:

This Channel originates at the big toe and runs over the dorsum of the foot, along the medial aspect of the leg and the medial side of the knee; then ascending further along the medial aspect of the thigh it reaches the inguinal region; from here it courses to the tip of the 11th rib and runs anteriorly along the costal border to its last point between the 6th and 7th ribs on the nipple line.

Connections with the Gall Bladder Channel:

Yuan-Source point: Taichong (Liv. 3.).

Luo-Connecting point: Ligou (Liv. 5.).

THE LIVER CHANNEL

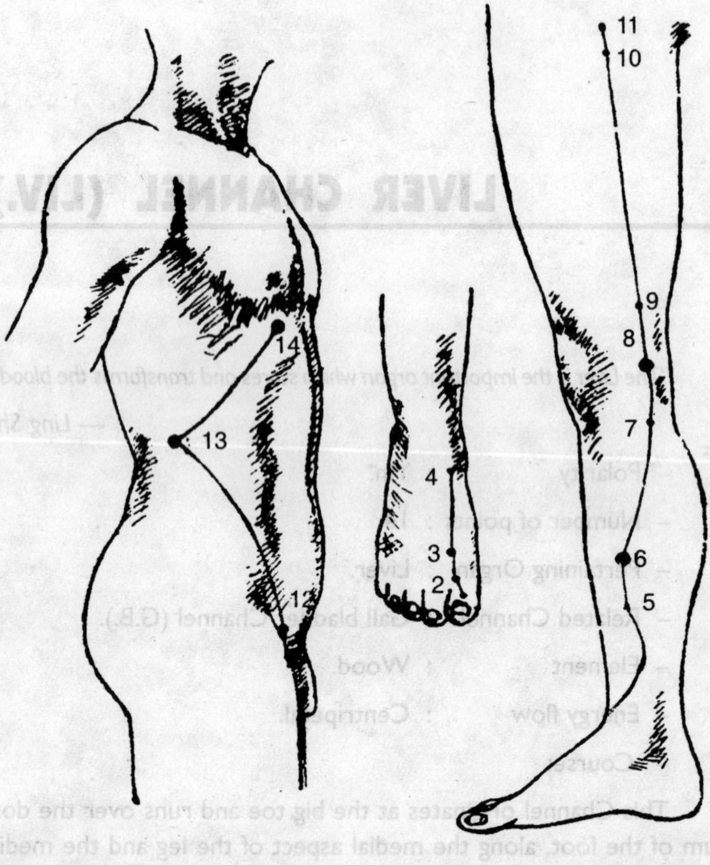

Liv. 3. Taichong
Liv. 6. Chongdu
Liv. 8. Ququan
Liv. 13. Zhangmen

Clinical uses:

1) The Distal points are used for

   i) disorders of the Liver (the pertaining Organ),

   ii) proximal disorders such as eye disorders (the eye is the connected sense organ).

2) The points on the leg are used for genito-urinary disorders and muscle and tendon disorders (diseases along the channel; muscle and tendon are connected tissues of the liver).

3) The points on the trunk are used for Liver and Gall bladder disorders, Spleen disorders (Liv. 13.) and pain in the flanks.

4) Headaches and mental disorders are treated using Taichong (Liv. 3.).

Commonly used acupuncture points:

Leg: Liv. 3, Liv. 6, Liv. 8.

Abdomen: Liv. 13, Liv. 14.

Description of the commonly used acupuncture points:

Taichong (*Liv. 3.*). (*Taichung*). Yuan-Source point.

Location: 2 cun proximal to the margin of the web of the 1st and 2nd toes.

Indication: Eye diseases, hypertension, headaches.

Puncture: 1.0 cun obliquely in a proximal direction.

Note: I) This is a good homeostatic point, being most effective in treating hypertension. However caution must be observed as it could cause a sudden fall of blood pressure. It is advisable therefore to have the patient supine when using this position. Acupuncture normally causes homeostasis; this is an exceptional instance when homeostasis can be overshot.

II) This point is located in the foot at a place which is the equivalent of the Hegu (L.I. 4) in the hand, and its properties are similar.

Zhongdu (*Liv. 6.*). (*Chungtu*). Xi-Cleft point. Special Alarm point of the liver.

Location: 7 cun superior to the tip of the medial malleolus on the medial border of the tibia.

Indications: Liver and gall bladder disorders.

Puncture: 1.5 cun perpendicularly.

Ququan (*Liv. 8.*).

Location: In the transverse crease of the knee joint, at the medial border of the semimembranous tendon.

Indications: Disorders of the knee joint. This point is specific for the treatment of impotence.

Puncture: 1 cun perpendicularly, or towards Yingu (K. 10.).

Zhangmen (*Liv. 13.*). (*Changmen*). Influential point for the Zang Organs. Alarm Point (Mu-Front) of the Spleen.

Location: At the free end of the 11th rib.

Indications: Liver disorders, disorders of the Spleen.

Puncture: 0.5 cun perpendicularly.

Qimen (*Liv. 14.*). (*Chimen*). Dangerous point, Alarm point (Mu-Front) of the Liver.

Location: Vertically bellow the nipple, in the intercostal space between the 6th and 7th ribs.

Indications: Hepatitis, chest pain.

Puncture: 0.5 cun horizontally and laterally along the skin.

List of all the acupuncture points of the Liver Channel:

Liv. 1 : **Dadun** - Jing-well point, wood point.
Liv. 2 : **Xingjian** - Fire point.
Liv. 3 : **Taichong** - Yuan-source point, Earth point.

Liv. 4 : **Zhongfeng** - Metal point.

Liv. 5 : **Ligou** - Luo-Connecting point.

Liv. 6 : **Zhongdu** - Xi-Cleft point.

Liv. 7 : **Xiguan**

Liv. 8 : **Ququan** - Water point

Liv. 9 : **Yinbao**

Liv. 10 : **Femour-Wuli**

Liv. 11 : **Yinlian**

Liv. 12 : **Jimai**

Liv. 13 : **Zhangmen** - Influential point Alarm point (mu-Front) of the Spleen.

Liv. 14 : **Qimen** - Alarm point (Mu-Front) of the Liver.

From Qimen (Liv. 14.), the Yin vital energy (Qi) flows on to Zhongfu (Lu. 1.) at about 3 a.m. thus re-establishing the cycle of the flow of vital energy.

Note:

Qi = Vital Energy

Jingqi = Vital Energy flowing along the Channels.

Sieqi = Disease factors. (Pathological Energy)

Deqi = Acupuncture sensations.

Taqi = Energy from the air.

Kuqi = Energy from the food.

THE CIRCULATION OF ENERGY IN THE LIVER

The deep branch arises from the Channel in the abdomen and than runs along the Stomach to enter the Organs Liver and Gall Bladder. From the Organ Liver a branch travels upwards to connect with the eyes. From the eyes this branch connects with the Du Channel at the vertex of the scalp, after traversing through the brain.

SYNDROMES OF THE LIVER

A. **The Liver Channel:** Pain along the Channel, fullness of the chest.

The Liver Channel, as it curves around the external genitalia, may be blocked by sieqi so that stagnation of Qi and blood may occur. This causes lower abdominal symptoms and pain in the genitalia. Frigidity or impotence may also result.

B. **The Organ Liver:** Disorders of the Organ Liver may be described under four main syndromes.

1) **Depression of the qi of Organ Liver.** This is due to mental disorders. Apart from cerebral symptoms, pain in the upper abdomen, vertical headaches, dysmenorrhoea (in women) may occur.

2) **Excess of fire of the Organ Liver.** This is due to excess consumption of alcohol. The clinical features are headaches, red eyes, bitter taste flushed face. A red tongue with a yellow coating is often seen. A rapid and wiry pulse may be felt. The excess of fire may injure the blood vessels causing epistaxis and haematemesis.

3) **Insufficiency of the blood of the Organ Liver.** This occurs due to anaemia following any chronic illness. The clinical features are dizziness, blurring of vision, pallor of the skin, scanty menstrual flow in women, impotence in men, weakness of muscles and tendons, and numbness of the extremities.

4) **Stirring of the wind in the Organ Liver by the Heart.** This is due to external heat stirring up the endogenous wind. The clinical features may be high fever, convulsions, coma and other signs of liver failure. A deep-red tongue with a rapid, wiry pulse may result.

Note: The Liver and Gall Bladder are invariably affected together in disorders of the Wood Element.

■

DU CHANNEL (DU)[1]

"The governing vessel unites the yang Qi of the whole body".

— Ling Shu

– Polarity : Yang.

– Number of points : 28.

– Related Channel : Ren Channel (Ren.)

– Course:

In the back midline, from the anus to the mouth.

Note: a) The Du Channel is one of the two unpaired channels, the other being the Ren Channel which runs in the front midline. These two midline channels are also classified with the Eight Extra Channels (as distinct from the Twelve paired (Regular or Organ) Channels. However, the modern practice is to classify them with the paired channels to make up the Fourteen Channels.

b) The Du Channel is not linked to any definite "Organ"; but it has a controlling or "governing" influence on all the other. Yang channels, and hence occupies a very important place in acupuncture, "Du" in Chinese means "the Governor".

1 Also called Governor Vessel."

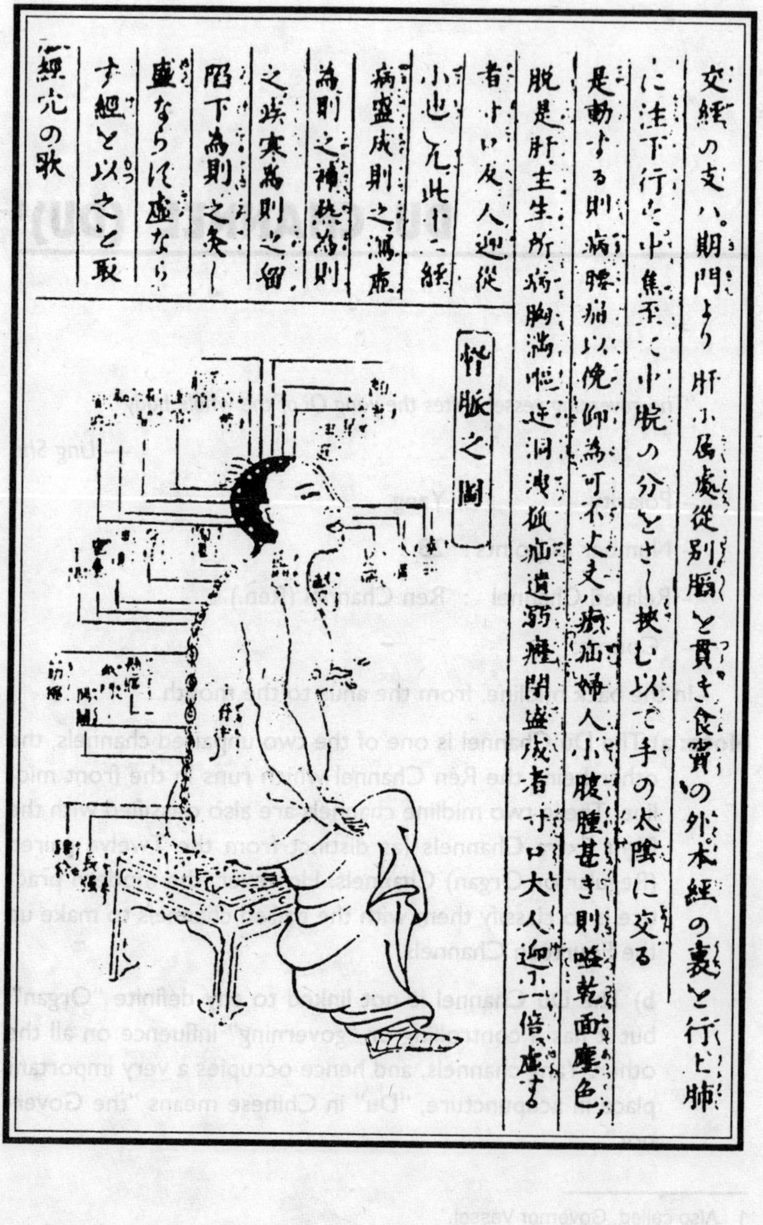
督脈之圖
交經の支ハ期門より肝に属處從別脳と貫き食竇の外本經の裏と行上肺
に注下行た中焦至こ中脘の分とさし挾む以て手の太陰に交る
是動する則病腰痛以俛仰為可不丈夫ハ㿗疝婦人小腹腫甚き則嗌乾面塵色
脱是肝主生所病胸滿嘔逆洞洩狐疝遺溺癃閉盛成者寸口大人迎一倍虚する
者寸口反人迎從
小也凡此十二經
病盛成則之瀉虚
為則之補熱為則
之疾寒為則之留
陷下為則之灸し
盛ならず虚なら
ず經を以之を取
經穴の歌

Connections with the Ren Channel:

Lue-Connecting point: Changqiang (Du 1.)

Clinical uses:

1) Ano-rectal disorders, low backache.
2) Immune disorders.
3) Infective disorders
4) Mental and neurological disorders, deaf-mutism.
5) Oral disorders.

Note: This channel runs over the spinal cored and the brain, and its functions are closely linked to those of the central nervous system.

Commonly used acupuncture points:

Back of trunk: Du 1, Du 3, Du 4, Du 6, Du 11, Du 14.

Neck: Du 15, Du 16.

Head: Du 20, Du 23, Du 25, Du 26, Du 28.

Description of the commonly used acupuncture points:

Changqiang (*Du 1.*). (*Changchiang*).

Location: Midway between the tip of the coccyx and the anus. The point is best located with the patient in the prone or lateral position.

Indications: Haemorrhoids, rectal prolapse, anal fissure, pruritus of anus.

Puncture: 0.5 cun perpendicularly.

Yaoyangguan (*Du. 3.*). (*Yaoyangkuan*).

Location: On the back midline, between the dorsal spines of the 4th and 5th lumbar vertebrae (at the level of the upper border of the iliac crest).

Indication: Low backache, genito-urinary disorders, impotence.

DU CHANNEL

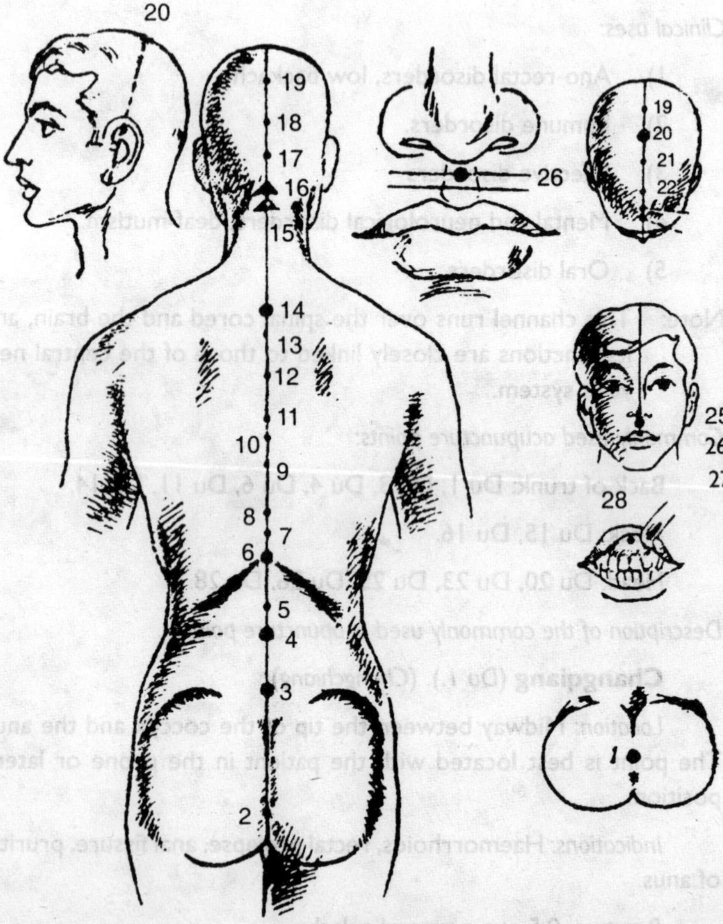

Du. 1. Changqiang	Du 15. Yamen } Dangerous Points
Du 3. Yaoyangguan	Du 16. Fengfu } Dangerous Points
Du 4. Mingmen	Du 20. Baihui
Du 6. Jizhong	Du 26. Renzhong-Jing-well point
Du 14. Dazhui	Du 28. Yinjiao

Puncture: 1.0 cun perpendicularly; the needle may be pointed slightly upwards. (Superiorly).

Mingmen (*Du 4.*) (*Mingmen*).

Location: On the back midline, between the dorsal spines of the 2nd and 3rd lumbar vertebrae (at the level of the lower border of the rib cage).

Indications: Low backache, genito-urinary disorders, impotence.

Puncture: 1.0 cun perpendicularly the needle may be tilted slightly upwards. (Superiorly).

Jizhong (*Du 6.*) (*Chichung*).

Location: On the back midline, between the dorsal spines of the 11th and 12th thoracic vertebrae.

Indications: Haemorrhoids, epilepsy. This point causes muscular relaxation in spastic states. It is also used during abdominal surgery with Yaoshu (Du 2.) or Yaogi (Ex. 20.) and electrically stimulated.

Puncture: 0.5 cun obliquely upwards.

Shendao (*Du 11.*). (*Shentao.*)

Location: On the back midline, between the dorsal spines of the 5th and 6th thoracic vertebrae.

Indications: Loss of memory.

Puncture: 0.5 cun obliquely upwards.

Dazhui (*Du 14.*). (*Tachui*).

Location: On the back midline, between the dorsal spines of the 7th cervical (vertebra prominens) and the 1st thoracic vertebra.

Indications:

a) Mental disorders, epilepsy, convulsions in children, headache, migraine.

b) Local disorders, e.g., stiff neck, cervical spondylosis, torticollis, sprain of cervical muscles, neck injuries, hypotonia of neck muscles.

THE FREQUENTLY USED POINTS IN THE LOW-BACK AREA

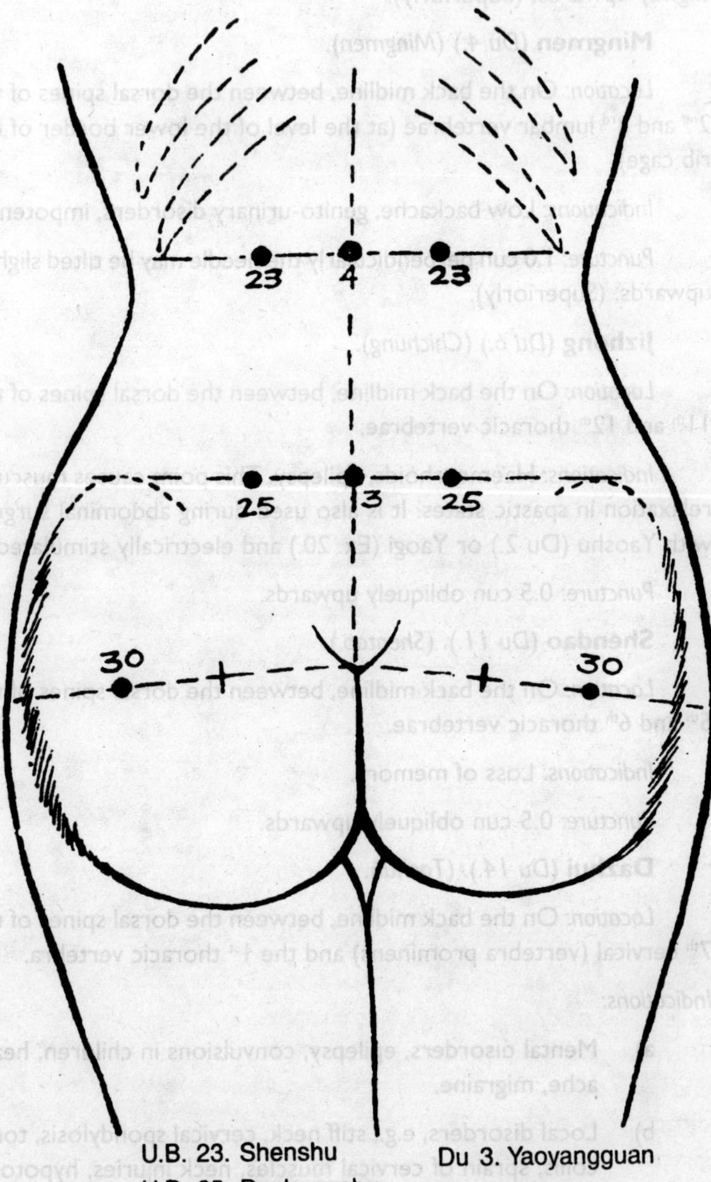

U.B. 23. Shenshu
U.B. 25. Dachangshu
G.B. 30. Huantiao
Du 3. Yaoyangguan
Du 4. Mingmen

c) Frozen shoulder with pain radiating to the back of the chest, paralysis of the upper limb.

d) Pain along the thoracic, (dorsal) spine ankylosing spondylitis.

e) Lung disorders, cough e.g., bronchial asthma, bronchitis, cough, whooping cough.

f) Eczema and other skin disorders.

g) Infective and immune disorders, e.g., cold influenza, fevers, malaria, infections.

Puncture: 1.0 cun perpendidularly or pointed upwards at a slight slant.

Note: This is one of the most potent immune enhancing acupuncture points. In very high fever, strong stimulation of the needle at this point tends to bring down the fever quickly, often in a matter of minutes. It is especially useful in children who are toxic and will not tolerate drugs.

Yamen (*Du 15.*). (*Yamen*). Dangerous point.

Location:

a) At the nape of the neck on the midline, between the dorsal spines of the 1st and 2nd cervical vertebrae.

b) On the midline 0.5 cun above the posterior hairline.

c) On the midline 3.5 cun above the spinous process of the 7th cervical vertebra when the head is erect.

Indications: Deaf-mutism, aphasia, aphonia, speech difficulties following paralytic strokes.

Puncture: This is a Dangerous point and improper needling can cause serious complications from damage to the medulla oblongata. The patient should be instructed to bend the neck slightly forwards, and the needle should be inserted perpendicularly and slowly in the direction of the point of the chin. *The depth of insertion should not generally exceed 1.0 cun and there should be no manipulation.* If any

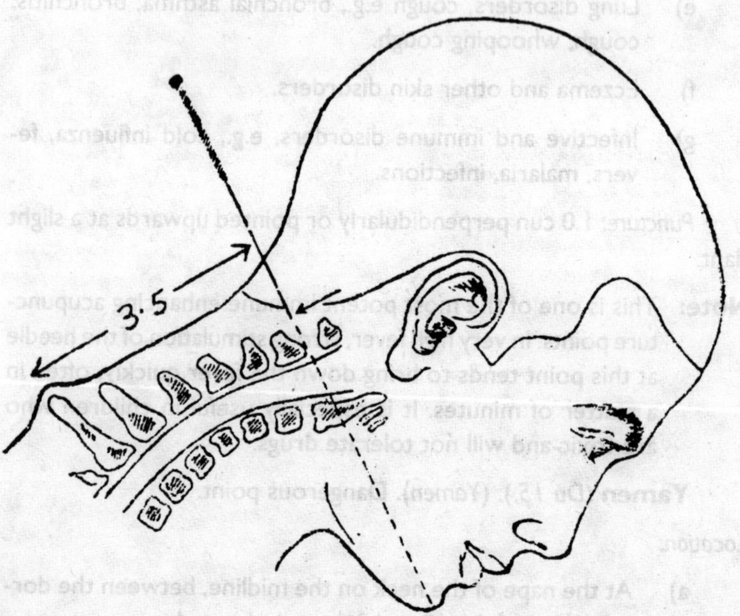

YAMEN (DU 15.)

Correct location, depth and direction.

Location: 0.5 cun above the posterior hairline in the back midline.

Depth: 1 cun.

Direction: With head semi-flexed towards the point of the chin. No stimulation.

discomfort is felt the needle should then be removed immediately. (Many clinicians believe it is best not to retain the needle here).

Fengfu (*Du 16.*). (*Fengfu*). Dangerous point.

Location:

a) At the nape of the neck, on the midline in the depression directly below the occipital protuberance.

b) On the midline 1.0 cun above the posterior hairline.

Indications: Mental disorders, common cold, headache.

Puncture: This is a very dangerous point. As in needling Yamen (Du 15.), care should be taken not to damage the medulla oblongata. It is perhaps the most vulnerable acupuncture point in the body and it is best that the novice treats this as a Prohibited point. Also, unlike Yamen (Du 15.), its usefulness is limited.

Baihui (*Du 20.*). (*Paihui*). ("Baihui" in Chinese means "meeting point of a hundred points". This point controls all other points and channels in the body).

Location:

a) Draw a straight line from the tip of the ear lobe to the apex of the auricle and extend this line upwards on the scalp till it intersects the midline: the point lies at this intersection.

b) On the vertex of the skull, 5 cun behind the anterior hairline and 7 cun above the posterior hairline, in the midline.

c) On the midline, 8 cun behind the glabella, Yintang (Ex. 1.).

d) On the midline, 7 cun above the posterior hairline.

e) On the midline, 10 cun above the vertebra prominens.

Indications:

a) This is the best tranquilizing and sedative point of the body. It treats all psychiatric and neurological disorders, e.g., schizophrenia, epilepsy, insomnia, parkinsonism, neuras-

THE DU CHANNEL

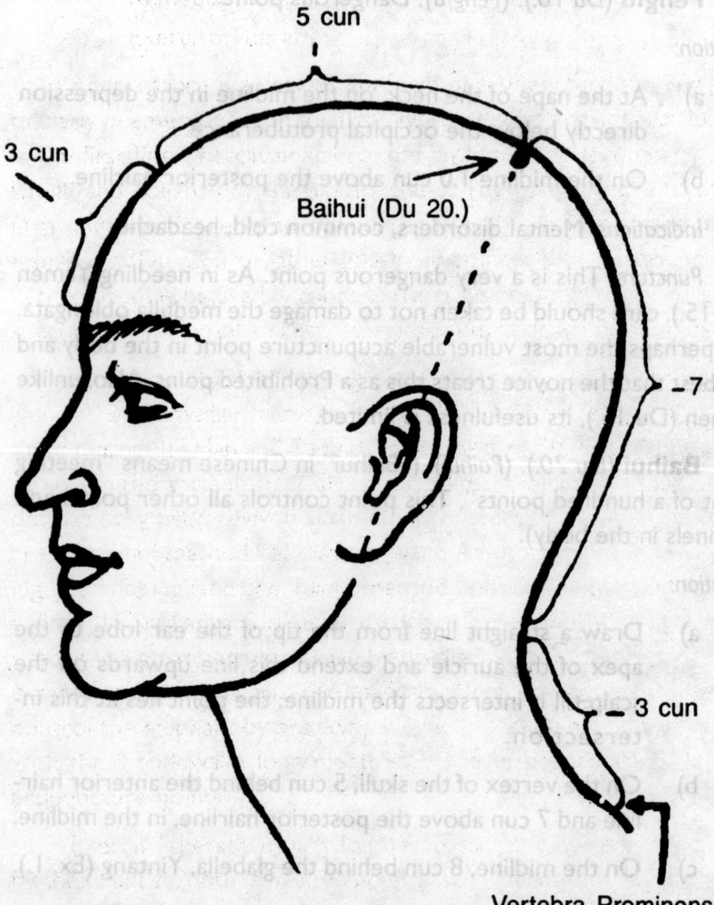

Baihui (Du. 20.)

There are six methods to locate this point

thenia, and all conditions where psychogenic factors may exist, such as bronchial asthma, impotence, skin disorders.

b) Headache (especially vertical headache).

c) Apoplexy and other cerebral vascular disorders (in the early stages).

d) Loss of memory.

e) Diseases of the anal region (as a Distal point).

f) Falling of head hair due to pathological causes (alopecia areata).

Puncture: 0.3-0.5 cun obliquely or horizontally, with the needle directed posteriorly.

Note:a)This is a powerful sedative and tranquilizing point. As psychogenic factors are present in almost all diseases, the use of this point on a general basis with other specific points is recommended for good therapeutic results.

b) This point also acts as "governor", having a coordinating effect when points are used on a number of different channels.

c) This is a good point to commence the first therapy as it is a relatively painless point and the patient cannot see the point of insertion of the needle.

Shangxing (*Du 23.*). (*Shanghsin*).

Location: 1.0 cun above the midpoint of the anterior hairline.

Indications: Nasal obstruction, epistaxis.

Puncture: 0.5 cun obliquely downwards.

Suliao (*Du 25.*). (*Suliao*).

Location: At the tip of the nose.

Indications: Nasal obstruction, epistaxis.

Puncture: 0.2 cun, perpendicularly.

THE DU CHANNEL

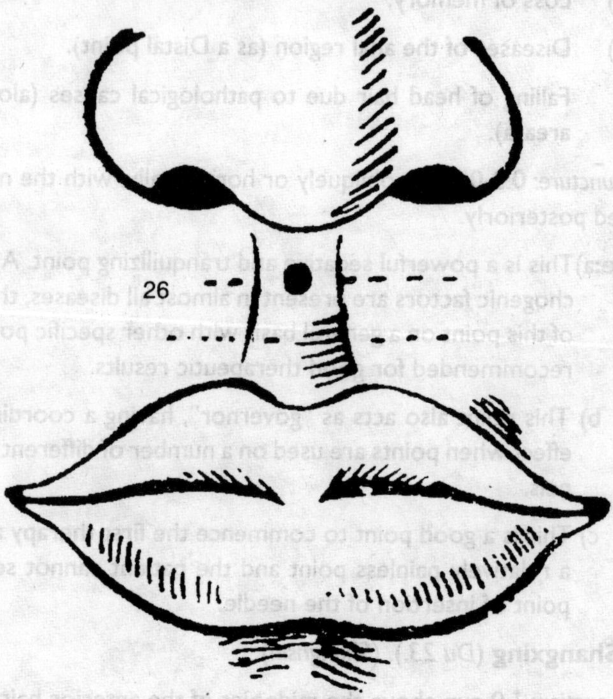

Renzhong (Du 26.)

Note: This point is also called Shigou in South China

Renzhong (*Du 26*). (*Jenchung*). Also called **Shigou** (*Shuikou*).

Location: At the junction of the upper third and lower two thirds of the philtrum of the upper lip, in the midline.

Indications:

a) Jing-Well point for use in acute emergencies, e.g., fainting, epileptic fits, convulsions, shock, heat stroke, hysterical attack.

b) Acute low-backache, as a Distal point.

c) Facial paralysis, painful disorders and swelling of the face.

Puncture: 0.3-0.5 cun obliquely backwards and upwards.

Note: a) In traditional Chinese medicine this point is known as "the point of re-animation" as it is used as emergency treatment for sudden fainting.

b) In the treatment of emergency conditions, the needle may be manipulated and removed as soon as pain is felt by the patient. It is not necessary to keep the needle longer.

c) Acupressure applied with the nail of the index finger (and applied obliquely backwards and upwards) is often found to be equally effective. Firm pressure should be maintained till the patient recovers.

d) This point is the meeting point of three yang channels.

Yinjiao (*Du 28.*). (*Yinchiao*).

Location: Between the gum and upper lip in the frenulum of the upper lip.

Indications:

a) Pain and swelling of the gums and other oral diseases.

b) Heamorrhoids, as a Distal point.

Puncture: 0.1-0.2 cun obliquely upwards, or prick to bleed with the three-edged needle.

DIAGRAM TO ILLUSTRATE THE FLOW OF ENERGY IN THE REN AND DU CHANNELS

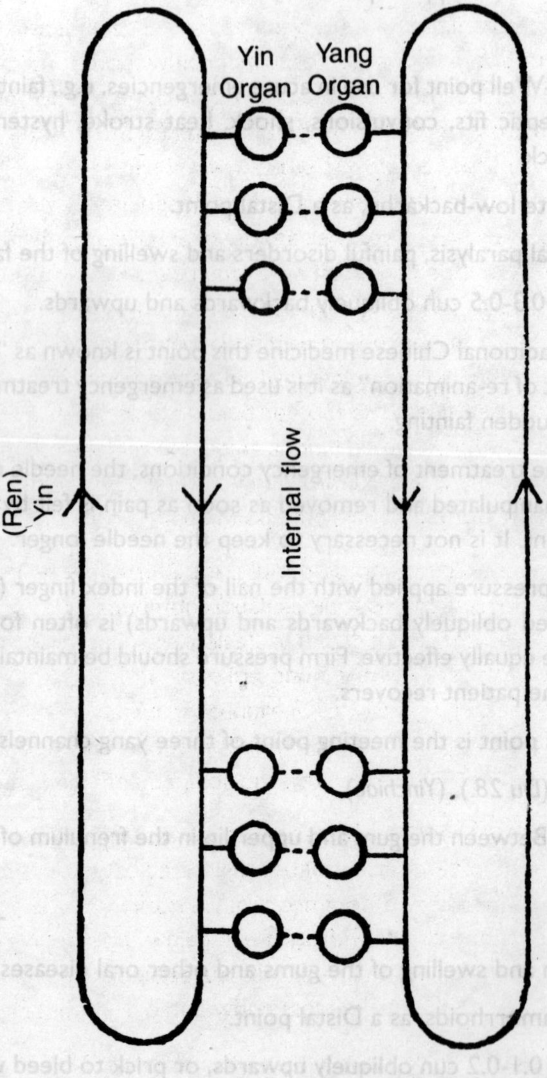

List of all the acupuncture points of the Du Channel:

Du 1 : **Changqiang** - Luo-connecting point.
Du 2 : **Yaoshu**
Du 3 : **Yaoyangguan**
Du 4 : **Mingmen**
Du 5 : **Xuanshu**
Du 6 : **Jizhong**
Du 7 : **Zhongshu**
Du 8 : **Jinsuo**
Du 9 : **Zhiyang**
Du 10 : **Lingtai**
Du 11 : **Shendao**
Du 12 : **Shenzhu**
Du 13 : **Taodao**
Du 14 : **Dazhui**
Du 15 : **Yamen**
Du 16 : **Fengfu**
Du 17 : **Naohu**
Du 18 : **Qiangjian**
Du 19 : **Houding**
Du 20 : **Baihui**
Du 21 : **Qianding**
Du 22 : **Xinhui**
Du 23 : **Shangxing**
Du 24 : **Shenting**
Du 25 : **Suliao**
Du 26 : **Renzhong**
Du 27 : **Duiduan**
Du 28 : **Yinjiao**

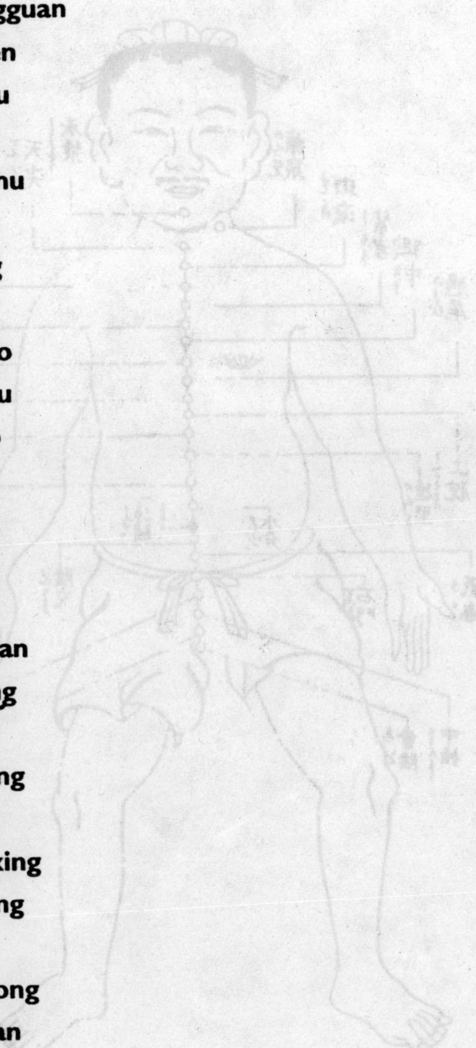

■

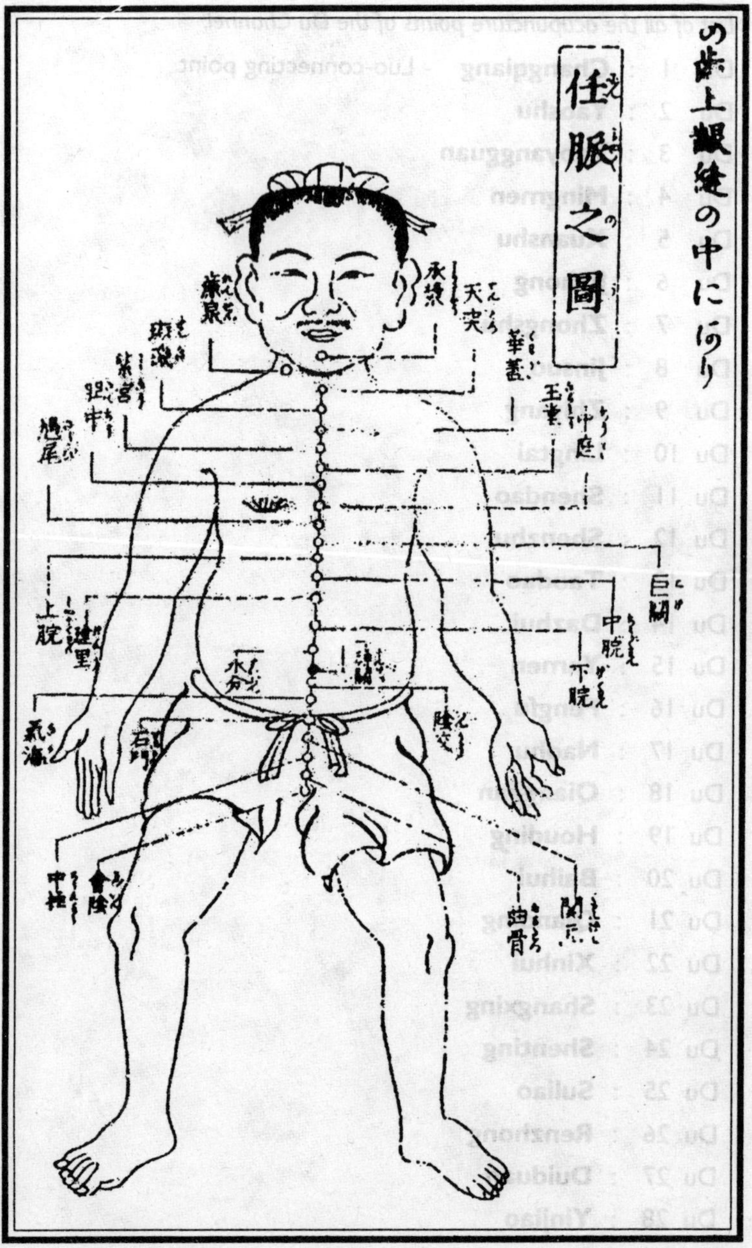

任脈之圖
廉泉
承漿
天突
璇璣
華蓋
紫宮
玉堂
膻中
中庭
鳩尾
巨闕
上脘
建里
中脘
下脘
水分
神闕
陰交
氣海
石門
中極
會陰
關元
曲骨

REN CHANNEL (REN.)[1]

"The vessal of conception connects the way so that the menses de scends at the right time. It is the root of conception and controls the nourishment of pregnancy".

— Ling Shu

- Polarity : Yin.
- Number of point : 24.
- Related Channel : Du Channel (Du).

In the front midline, from the front of the anus to below the mouth.

Note: 1) The Ren Channel, like the Du Channel, is not linked to any definite Internal Organ. It has however a controlling influence over all the Yin Channels and on the anteriorly situated Alarm points of certain Internal Organs.

2) It has an influence on the reproductive functions, on account of which it is also called the "Conception Vessel."

Connections with the Du Channel:

Luo-Connecting point: Jiuwei (Ren 15.).

Clinical uses:

Disorders along the pathway of the Channel, such as genitourinary and gastro-intestinal disorders, heart and lung disorders, aphasia, aphonia, dysarthria, facial, paralysis excessive salivation.

1 Also called "Conception Vessel".

Commonly used acupuncture points:

Perineum: Ren 1.

Lower abdominal area: Ren 2, Ren 3, Ren 4, Ren 5, Ren 6.

Upper abdominal area: Ren 9, Ren 12.

Chest: Ren 17.

Neck: Ren 22, Ren 23.

Face: Ren 24.

Description of the commonly used acupuncture points:

Huiyin (*Ren 1.*). (*Huiyin*).

Location: In the centre of the perineum.

Indications: Haemorrhoids.

Puncture: 1.0 cun perpendicularly.

Note: This point together with Changqiang (Du 1.), is very effective for early haemorrhoids.

Qugu (*Ren 2.*) (*Chuku.*).

Location: Immediately above the midpoint of the superior border of the pubic symphysis.

Indication:

Genito-urinary disorders, e.g.

a) incontinence and retention of urine, chronic inflammation, nocturnal enuresis in children;

b) impotence, spermatorrhoea, ejaculatio poraecox;

c) menstrual disorders.

Puncture: 1.5 cun perpendicularly.

Zhongji (*Ren 3.*). (*Chungchi*), Alarm point (Mu-Front) of the Urinary bladder.

Location: In the front midline, 4 cun below the umbilicus, 1 cun above Qugu (Ren 2.).

Indications: Same as for Qugu (Ren 2.).

Puncture: 1.5 cun perpendicularly.

Guanyuan *(Ren 4.).* (*Kuanyuan*). Alarm point (Mu-Front) of the Small Intestine.

Location: In the front midline, 3 cun below the umbilcus, 2 cun above Qugu (Ren 2.).

Indications: Same as for Qugu (Ren 2.); also diarrhoea.

Puncture: 1.0 cun perpendicularly.

Shimen (*Ren* 5.). (*Shihmen*). Alarm point (Mu-Front) of the Sanjiao.

Location: In the front midline, 2 cun below the umbilicus.

Indication: Oedema and ascites.

Puncture: 1.5 cun perpendicularly.

Note: A very effective combination of points for oedema and ascites is: Shimen (Ren 5.), Shuifen (Ren 9.), Yinlinquan (Sp. 9.), Pishu (U.B. 20.), There is also an oedema point in the ear.

Microfilarial swellings of the leg (elephantiasis), swelling of the arm following breast surgery, varicose veins and chronic oedema in dependent areas also respond well to these points.

Qihai (Ren 6.). (*Chihai*).

Location: In the front midline, 1.5 cun below the umbilicus.

Indications: Neurasthenia. This is a good Tonification point and used in conjunction with Zusanli (St. 36.) and Sanyinjiao (Sp. 6.) for chronic fatigue and hypotension.

Puncture: 1.5 cun perpendicularly.

Shenjue[2] (*Ren 8.*) (*Shenchueh*). *Forbidden point for acupuncture.*

Location: In the centre of the umbilicus.

Indications: While it is *forbidden* for acupuncture, it is an anatomical landmark to locate other points. Moxibustion point for chronic diarrhoea and other Yin disorders.

2 Also spelled Shenque.

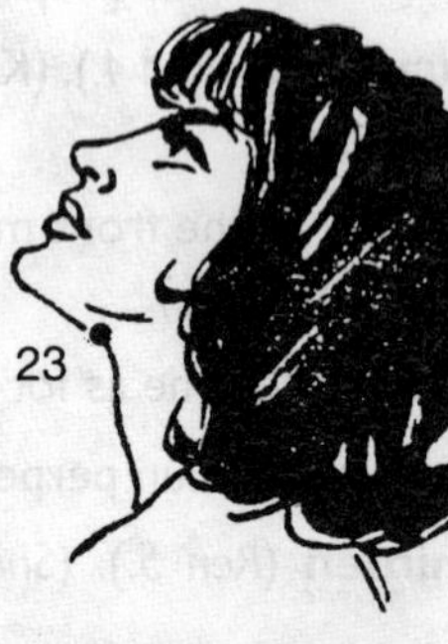

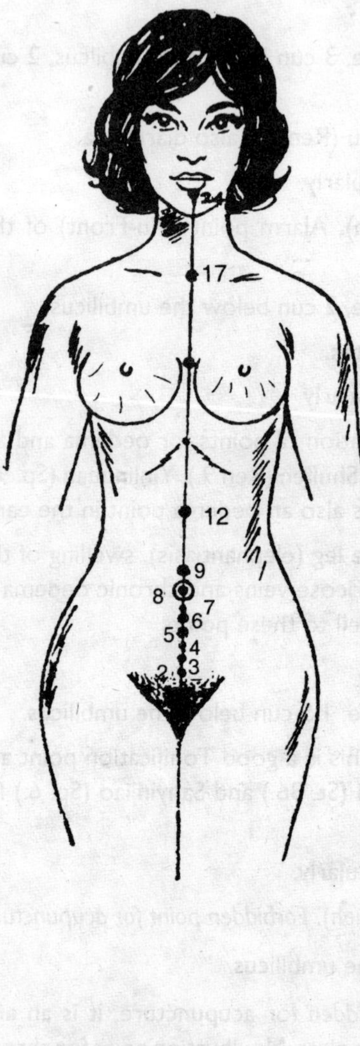

Ren 24. Chengjiang
Ren 23. Lianquan
Ren 22. Tiantu
Ren 17. Shanzhong
Ren 12. Zhongwan
Ren 9. Shuifen
Ren 8. Shenjue

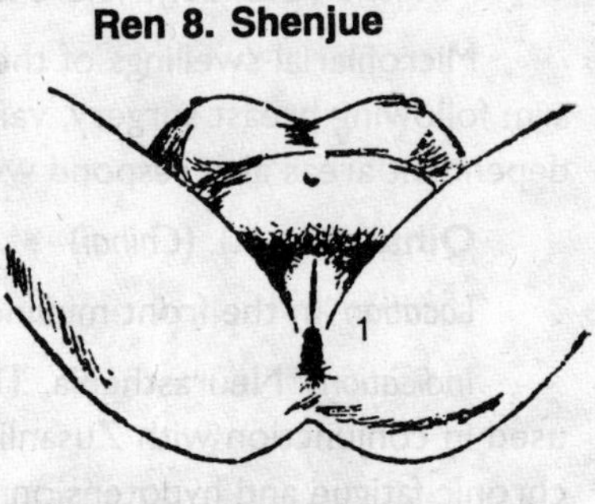

Ren 7. Abdomen - Yinjiao
Ren 6. Qihai
Ren 5. Shimen
Ren 4. Guanyuan
Ren 3. Zhongji
Ren 2. Qugu
Ren 1. Huiyin

Shuifen (*Ren 9I*). (*Shuifen*).

Location: In the front midline, I.0 cun above the umbilicus.

Indications: Specific point for oedema and ascites.

Puncture: I.5 cun perpendicularly.

Zhongwan (*Ren I2.*). (*Chungwan*). Alarm point (Mu-Front) of the Stomach. Influential point for Fu Organs.

Location: In the front midline, midway between the xyphoid process and the umbilicus (or 4 cun directly above the umbilicus).

Indications: Peptic, ulcer, abdominal distension, flatulence, dyspepsia, nausea and vomiting.

Puncture: I.5 cun perpendicularly.

Shanzhong (*Ren I7.*). (*Shanchung*). Influential point for the respiratory system, Alarm point (Mu-Front) of the Pericardium.

Location: On the sternum, midway between the two nipples (at the level of the 4th intercostal space).

Indications: Heart disease, bronchial asthma and other lung disorders, breast disorders.

Puncture: I.0 cun horizontally downwards; in breast disease the needle may be directed laterally, towards the diseased breast.

Tiantu (*Ren 22.*). (*Tientu*). Dangerous point.

Location: At the centre of the suprasternal fossa, 0.5 cun above the sternal notch.

Indications: Bronchial asthma, hiccough, dysphagia.

Puncture: As this is a Dangerous point, the following procedures should be observed in sequence:

a) Have the patient comfortably seated.

b) Locate the point.

c) Insert the needle about 0.3 cun perpendicularly.

d) Extend the patient's neck.

THE MU-FRONT ALARM POINTS

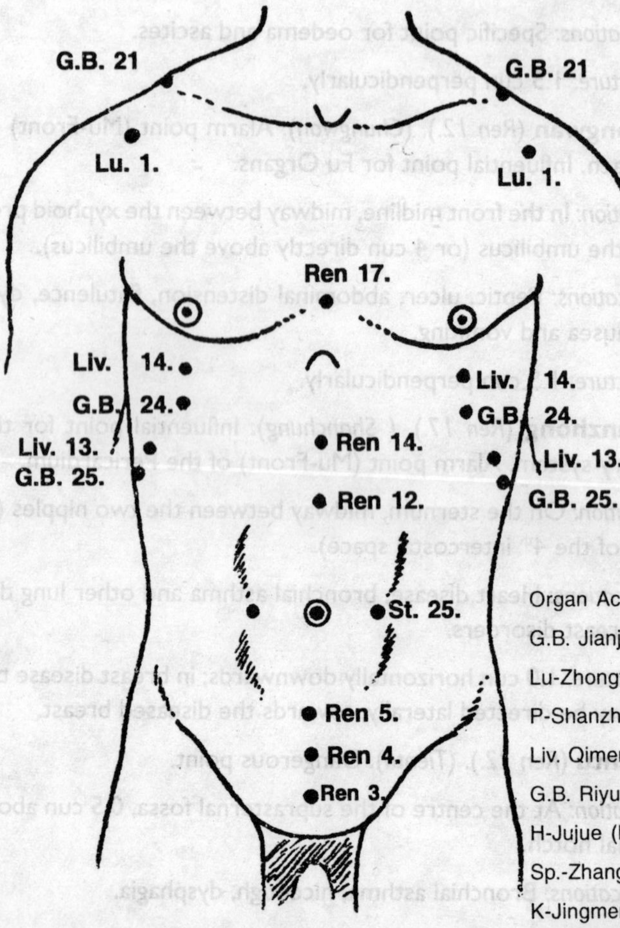

Organ Acupuncture Point

G.B. Jianjing (G.B. 21.)

Lu-Zhongfu (Lu. 1.)

P-Shanzhong (Ren 17.)

Liv. Qimen (Liv. 14.)

G.B. Riyue (G.B. 24.)

H-Jujue (Ren 14.)

Sp.-Zhangmen (Liv. 13.)

K-Jingmen (G.B. 25.)

St. Zhongwan (Ren 12.)

L.I. Tianshu (St. 25.)

S.J. Shimen (Ren. 5.)

S.I. Guznyuan (Ren. 4.)

U.B. Zhongji (Ren. 3.)

Note: The Special Alarm point of the Gall Bladder at the shoulder is also included.

e) Change the direction of the needle and then insert further 1.0-1.5 cun downwards along the posterior border of the sternum.

f) Ensure that the patient can swallow without pain and is otherwise comfortable.

All manoeuvers must be carried out gently and precisely.

Note: This is the best point for treating an acute attack of bronchial asthma or hiccough. This point should not however be used until proficiency has been gained under the guidance of a trained acupuncturist. Incorrect insertion may lead to serious complications as a result of damage to the great vessels and other structures in the mediastinum.

Lianquan (*Ren 23.*). (*Lienchuan*).

Location: On the midline of the neck, midway between the Adam's apple and the lower border of the mandible.

Indications: Aphasia, mutism, dysarthria, sudden loss of speech, dysphagia, speech difficulties following paralytic strokes, stammering, excessive salivation, pharyngitis laryingitis, pseudo-bulbar palsy, speech disorders due to parkinsonism.

Puncture: 1.0-1.5 cun obliquely towards the root of the tongue, or towards Baihui (Du 20.).

Note: Care should be taken to insert in the midline and in the correct direction.

Chengjiang (*Ren 24.*). (*Chengchiang*).

Location: In the middle of the mental labial groove, in the depression between the point of the chin and midpoint of the lower lip.

Indications: Facial paralysis, trigeminal neuralgia, toothache of the lower incissors, swelling of the gums, excessive salivation, anaesthetic point for tooth extraction.

Puncture: 0.3 cun perpendicularly or pointed downwards.

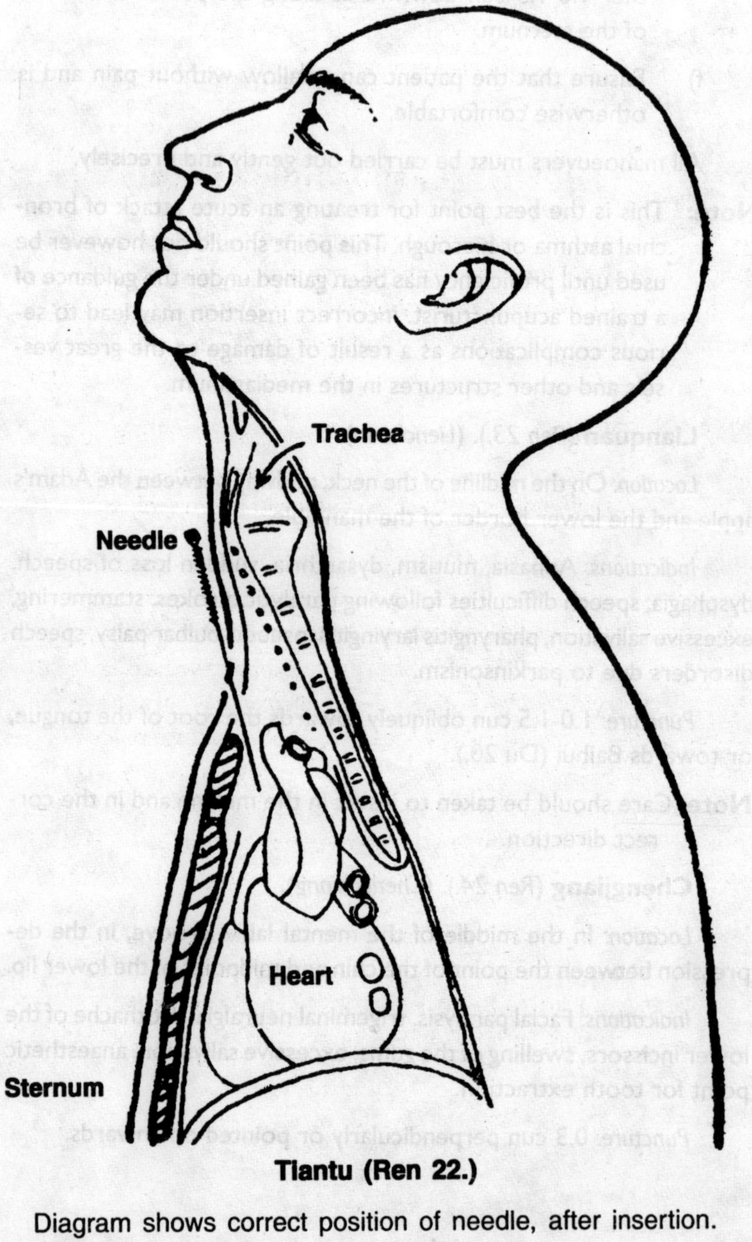

Diagram shows correct position of needle, after insertion.

List of all the acupuncture points of the Ren Channel:

Ren 1 : **Huiyin**

Ren 2 : **Qugu**

Ren 3 : **Zhongji** – Alarm point (Mu-Front) of the Urinary Bladder.

Ren 4 : **Guanyuan** – Alarm point (Mu-Front) of the Small Intestine.

Ren 5 : **Shimen** – Alarm point (Mu-Front) of Sanjiao.

Ren 6 : **Qihai**

Ren 7 : **Abdomen – Yinjiao**

Ren 8 : **Shenjue or Shenque**

Ren 9 : **Shuifen**

Ren 10 : **Xiawan**

Ren 11 : **Jianli**

Ren 12 : **Zhongwan** – Influential point for Fu Organs; Alarm point (Mu-Front) of the Stomach.

Ren 13 : **Shangwan**

Ren 14 : **Juque** – Alarm point (Mu-Front) of the Heart.

Ren 15 : **Jiuwei** – Luo-Connecting point.

Ren 16 : **Zhongting**

Ren 17 : **Shanzhong** – Influential point for the respiratory system; Alarm point (Mu-Front) of the Pericardium.

Ren 18 : **Yutang**

Ren 19 : **Chest-Zigong**

Ren 20 : **Huagai**

Ren 21 : **Xuanji**

Ren 22 : **Tiantu**

Ren 23 : **Lianquan**

Ren 24 : **Chengjiang**

THE ACUPUNCTURE POINTS OF THE REN CHANNEL ON THE HEAD AND NECK

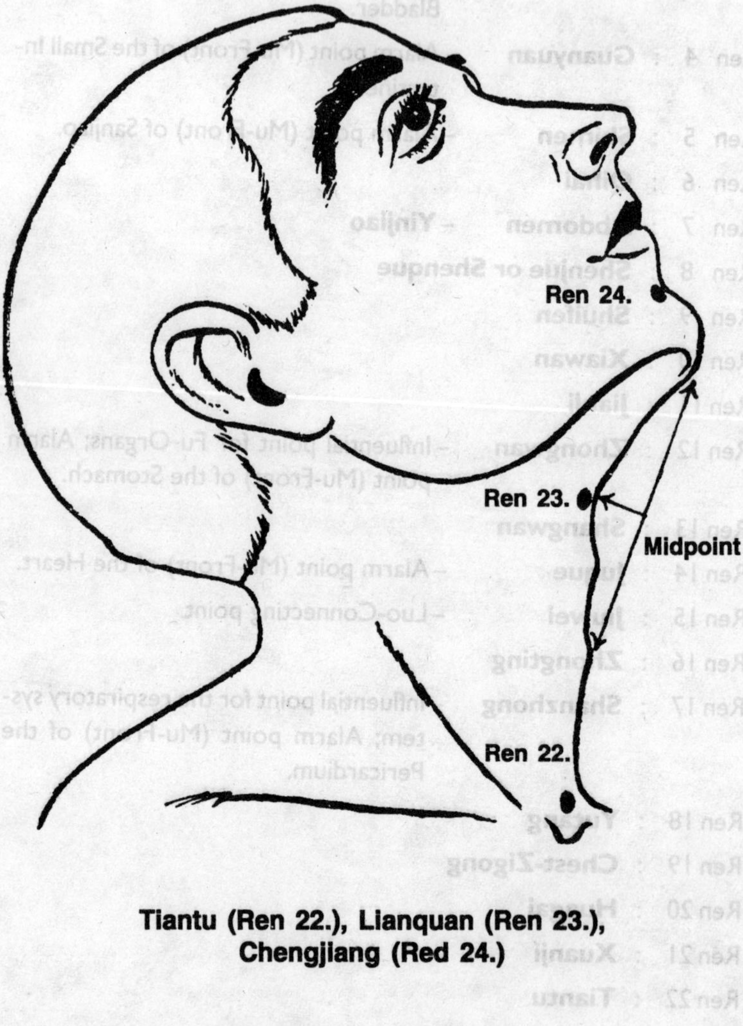

Tiantu (Ren 22.), Lianquan (Ren 23.), Chengjiang (Red 24.)

CIRCULATION OF ENERGY IN THE DU AND REN CHANNELS

The energy circulates in both superficial channels in the midline sof the body from below upwards. They enter the interior at the mouth and travel downwards along the gastro-intestinal tract as shown in diagram at page 270. In doing so they balance the energies of the six sets of Coupled Internal Organs. A complete cycle of circulation takes twenty four hours.

According to some authorities however the circulation takes the form of a figure of eight as follows: The Yin energy changes to Yang energy in the morning hours, and vice-versa at sunset. (This situation may be reversed in on night shift workers).

There is a Luo-connecting point in the Du as well as the Ren Channels. These two points are connected to each other via the internal Organs where the change of polarity of the energy may occur.

■

THE EXTRAORDINARY POINTS (EX.)

After the points had been numbered in ancient times and placed in their apopropriate Channels, many new points were discovered during the course of the succeeding centuries. These new points are termed "Extraordinary points". While the majority fall outside the Fourteen Channels, some are located on the course of a Channel, and a few even coincide with regular points of the Channels.

Commonly used Extraordinary points:

Head: Ex. 1 to Ex. 10.

Trunk: Ex. 17, Ex. 20, Ex. 21.

Upper limb: Ex. 28, Ex. 21.

Lower limb: Ex. 31, Ex. 32, Ex. 33, Ex. 35, Ex. 36.

Description of the commonly used Extra-ordinary points:

Yintang (*Ex. 1.*). (*Yinthang*). Modern acupuncturistis call this point Du 24.5.

Location: On the ridge of the nose, midway between the medial ends of the two eyebrows.

Indications: Rhinitis, headache, eye disease, endocrine disroders.

(Some workers believe that this point controls pituitary functions and improves extrasensory perception).

THE ACUPUNCTURE POINTS OF THE VERTEX OF THE SCALP

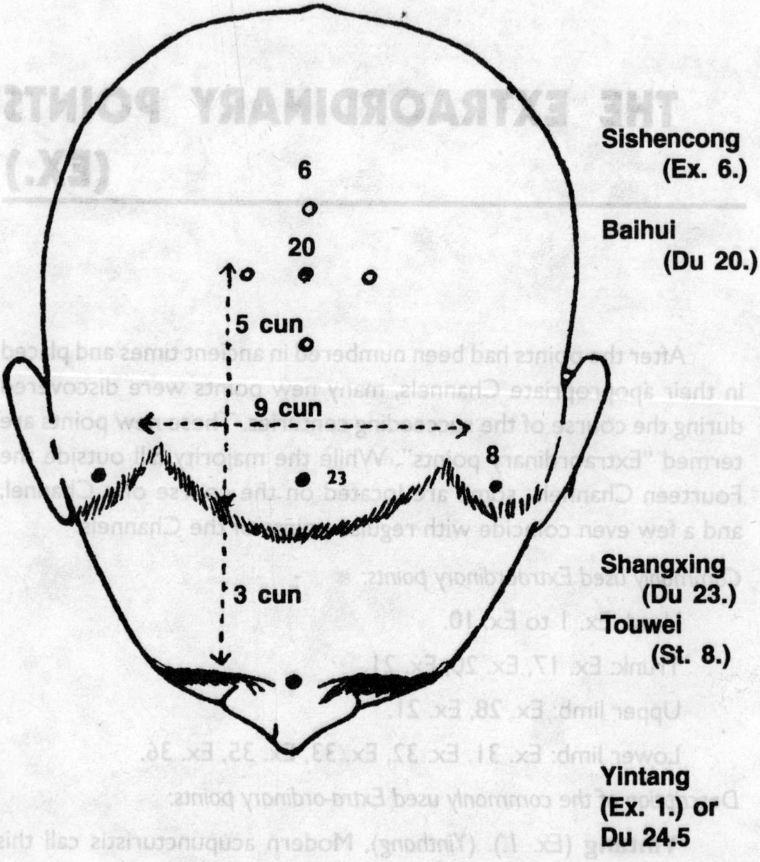

Puncture: 0.5 cun horizontally downwards.

Taiyang (*Ex.* 2). (*Taiyang*).

Location:

a) On the temple, in the depression 1.0 cun directly posterior to the midpoint of a line connecting the outer end of the eyebrow with the outer canthus of the eye.

b) Extend the curved lines of the eyebrow and the lower eyelid outwards: the point lies where these two lines cross.

Indications: Headache, migraine, eye diseases, facial paralysis, trigeminal neuralgia, toothache, sinusitis.

Puncture: 0.5 cun perpendicularly or obliquely:

i) perpendicular insertion for headache, migraine, facial paralysis, trigeminal neuralagia;

ii) oblique insertion towards the eye, for eye disorders;

iii) oblique insertion downwards for toothache, maxillary sinusitis.

Yuyao (Ex. 3.). *Yuyao).*

Location: At the midpoint of the eyebrow, vertically above the midpoint of the pupil.

Indications: Frontal sinusitis, eye disorders, facial paralysis.

Puncture: 0.5 cun horizontally along the skin:

i) directed medially for frontal sinusitis:

ii) directed downwards for eye disorders;

iii) directed laterally for facial paralysis.

Usually this point is punctured in a through and through insertion commencing at Yangbai (G.B. 14.).

Qiuhou (*Ex.* 4.). (*Chiuhou*). Dangerous point.

Location: At the junction of the lateral fourth and the medial three-fourths of the infra-orbital border.

SISHENCONG (Ex. 6.)
(THE FOUR MENTAL WISDOMS)

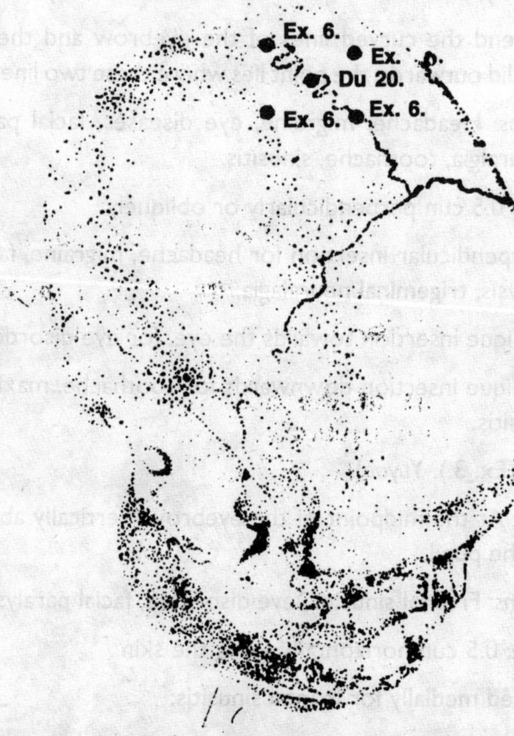

Indications: Myopia, optic nerve disorders, glaucoma and other eye disorders.

Puncture: 1.0 cun perpendicularly with the patient looking upwards. The needle should be directed along the floor of the orbit in the direction of the optic foramen (i.e. slightly medially and superiorly).

Note: This is a Dangerous point as it is located in the orbit. The beginner should not attempt insertion at this point without the supervision of a trained acupuncturist. Good sterilization of the needle must also be ensured when using this and the other points located in the orbit. viz., Chengqi (St. 1.) and Jingming (U.B. 1.).

Jiachengjiang (*Ex. 5.*). (*Chiachenchiang*).

Location: In the depression on the mental foramen, 1.0 cun lateral to Chengjiang (Ren 24.).

Indications: Facial paralysis, trigeminal neuralgia, lower toothache.

Puncture: 0.2 cun perpendicularly.

Sishencong (*Ex.6.*) (*Szushentsung*). ("Sishencong" in Chinese means "The Four intelligences").

Location: These are four points situated on the vertex 1.0 cun anterior, posterior and lateral to the point Baihui (Du 20.).

Indications: Headache, apoplexy, epilepsy.

Puncture: 0.5 cun horizontally towards Baihui (Du 20.).

Note: These four points are usually used together with Baihui (Du 20.). They may also be used as an alternative to Baihui (Du 20.) if the patient experiences undue pain at the latter point as sometimes happens.

Yiming (*Ex. 7.*). (*Yiming*).

Location: 1.0 cun posterior to Yifeng (S.L. 17.). This point lies on a straight line connecting Yifong (S.J.17.) and Fengchi (G.B.20.).

THE ACUPUNCTURE POINTS BEHIND THE EAR

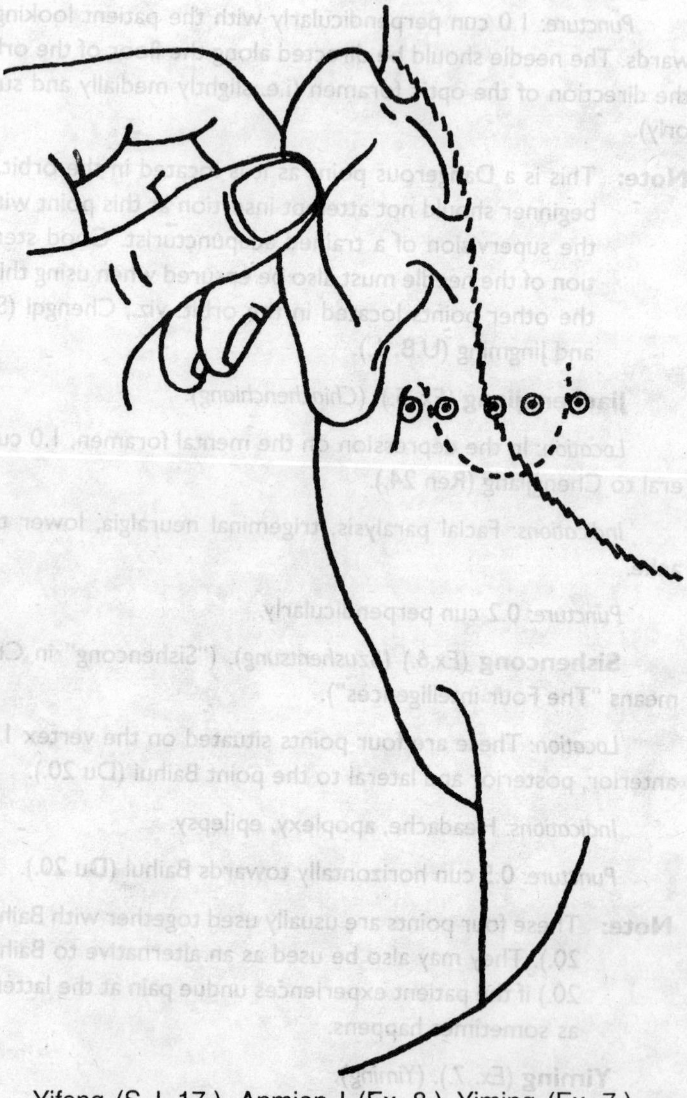

Yifeng (S.J. 17.). Anmian I (Ex. 8.). Yiming (Ex. 7.), Anmian II (Ex. 9.), Fengchi (G.B. 20.)

Note: The dotted curved line is the mastoid process

Indications: Ear and eye disorders.

Puncture: 0.5 cun perpendicularly.

Anmian I (*Ex.8.*). (*Anmian I*).

Location:

a) Between Yifeng (S.J. 17.) and Yiming (*Ex.* 7.).

b) 0.5 cun posterior to Yifeng (S.J.17.).

Indications: Insomnia.

Puncture: 0.1 cun perpendicularly.

Anmian II (*Ex.* 9) (*Anmian II*).

Location: Between Yiming (Ex. 7.) and Fengchi (G.B. 20.).

Indications: Insomnia.

Puncture: 0.1 cun perpendicularly.

Anmian I and Anmian II are generally used together.

Jinjin (*left*), **Yuye** (*right*). (*Ex.* 10). (*Chinchin, Yuye.*)

Location: On the sublingual veins on either side of the root of the tongue.

Indications: Swelling of the tongue, ulceration of the mucous membrane of the mouth, thrush, aphasia, nausea, vomiting, aphthous stomatitis.

Puncture: With the tongue rolled upwards, 0.5 cun perpendicularly, or prick to bleed with the three-edged needle.

Dingchuan (*Ex.* 17.). (*Tingchuan*). ("Dingchuan" in Chinese means "Soothing Asthma"). In South China this point is called Pingchuan.

Location: 0.5 cun lateral to Dazhui (Du 14.). (This is also one of the Huatuojiaji (Ex. 21.) points).

Indications: Bronchial asthma.

Puncture: 0.5 cun with the needle directed slightly medially.

THE EXTRAORDINARY POINTS

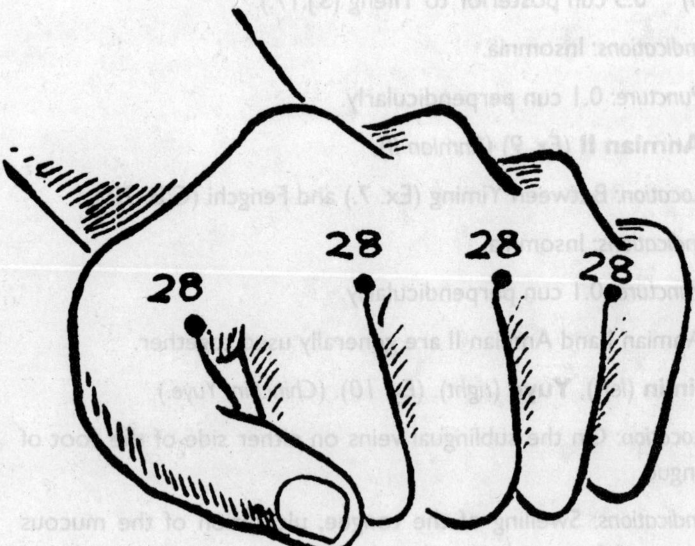

Baxie (Ex. 28.)

Yaoqi (*Ex. 20.*). (*Yaouqi*).

Location: 2 cun directly above the coccyx.

Indications: Epilepsy, muscular relaxation together with Jizhong (Du 6.). stimulated electrically.

Puncture: 1.0-2.0 cun upwards, horizontally along the skin.

Huatuojiaji (*Ex. 21.*) (*Huatuo chiachi*). Named after the famous *surgeon Hua Tuo* (circa 200 B.C.).

Location: These are a series of 28 pairs of points situated 0.5 cun lateral to the lower ends of the dorsal spines of the 1st cervical to the 4th sacral vertebrae.

Indications: Pain along the spine, pain along the segmental nerve, disorders of the Internal Organ at the corresponding level.

Puncture: 0.5 – 1.0 cun in the cervical and thoracic regions 1.0 – 1.5 cun in the lumbar and sacral regions. The needle should be directed slightly obliquely towards the median plane.

Baxie (*Ex. 28*). (*Pahsieh*). Eight points.

Location: On the dorsum of the hand, on the webs between the 5 fingers; 4 points in each hand, totalling 8 points. ("Ba" means eight in Chinese.) These points are best located having the patient form a fist.

Indications: Disorders of the fingers, rheumatoid arthritis, numbness of the fingers, polyneuropathy.

Puncture: 1.0 cun obliquely and proximally

Shixuan (*Ex. 30.*). (*Shixuan*). Ten points.

Location: On the tips of the ten fingers, about 0.1 cun posterior to the apex of the nail.

Indications: For emergencies such as shock, coma, heat strokes, apoplexy, fever.

Puncture: Prick with three-edged needle or filiform needle to cause bleeding.

THE EXTRAORDINARY POINTS

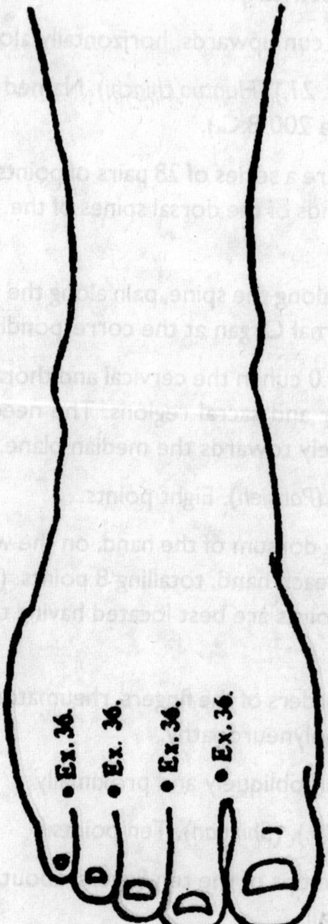

Bafeng (Ex. 36.)

Heding (*Ex. 31*). (*Heting*).

Location: On the midpoint of the upper border of the patella.

Indications: Disorders of the knee joint.

Puncture: 0.5 cun perpendicularly.

Xiyan (*Ex. 32.*). (*Hsiyen*).

Location: In the depression on the medial side of the ligamentum patellae.

Indication: Disorders of the knee-joint.

Puncture: 0.5 cun perpendicularly, or obliquely towards Lateral-Xiyan.

Note:a) The point on the lateral side of the ligamentum patellae coincides with Dubi (St. 35.) but it is also called "Lateral-Xiyan", and for this reason the point proper is sometimes referred to as Medial-Xiyan (Nei-Xiyan). "Xiyan" in Chinese means "Knee-Eye" and "Dubi" means "Nose of the Calf."

b) These two points together with Heding (Ex. 31.), are commonly used in treating disorders of the knee.

Lanwei (*Ex. 33*). (*Lanwei*). Alarm point of the vermiform appendix.

Location: 2 cun below Zusanli (St. 36.), on the Stomach Channel.

Indications: Appendicitis, post-operative pain after appendicectomy.

Puncture: 1.0 cun perpendicularly.

Note: "Lanwei" in Chinese means the "vermiform appendix". This point becomes tender in acute appendicitis and is therefore particularly useful in confirming the diagnosis.

Dannang (*Ex. 35.*) (*Tannang*). Distal Alarm point of the Gall Bladder Channel.

Location: 1.0 cun below (distal to) Yanglingquan (G.B. 34.), on the Gall Bladder Channel.

THE ACUPUNCTURE POINTS ON THE DORSUM OF THE FOOT

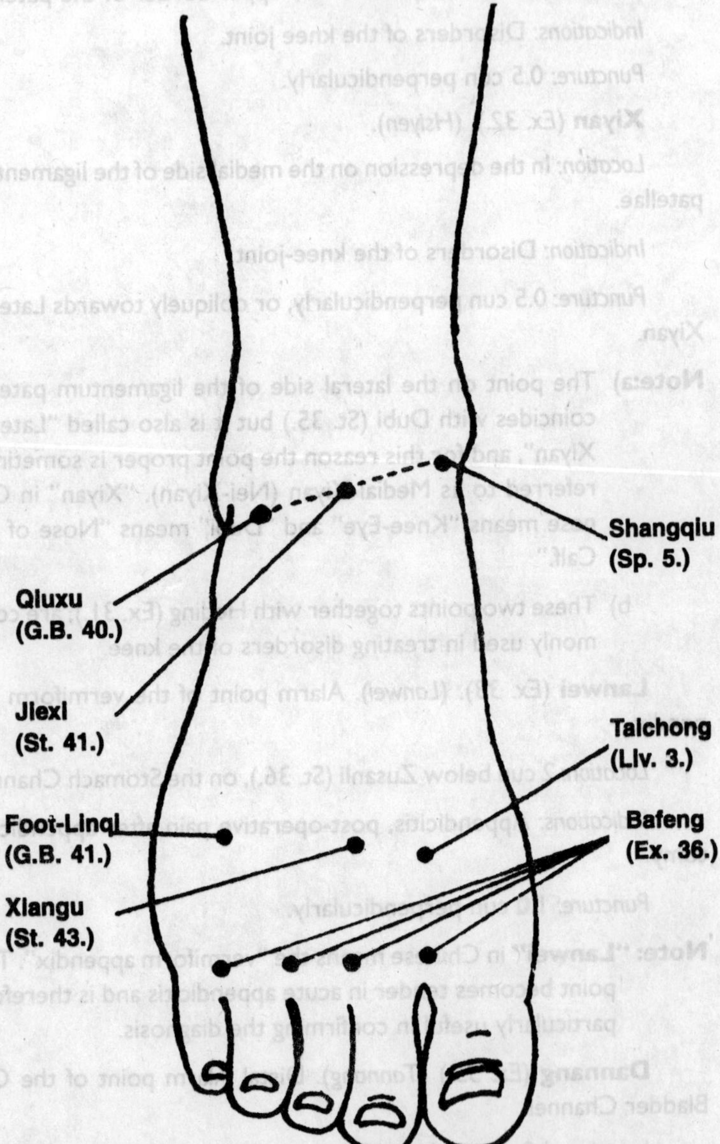

Note: Neiting (St. 44.) is one of the Bafeng (Ex. 36.) points

Indications: Diseases of the gall bladder and the liver.

Puncture: 1.0 cun perpendicularly.

Note: This is the Alarm point in the leg of the Gall Bladder.

Bafeng (*Ex. 36*). (*Pafeng*). Eight points.

Location: On the dorsum of the foot, 0.5 cun proximal to the borders of the webs between the 5 toes; 4 points on each foot, totalling 8 points.

Indications: Arthritis of the toes, numbness of the foot and the toes, polyneuropathy.

Puncture: 0.5 cun obliquely and proximally.

Note: Three of these points coincide with Xingjian (Liv.2.), Neiting (St. 44.) and Xiaxi (G.B. 43.).

There are no universal criteria, as yet, for the recognition of new acupuncture points. *Ronald Melzack* has pointed out that the tender points described by authorities such as Janet Travel correspond to such acupuncture points. Zhang Xiang-tong and co-workers believe that it is an area of aggregation of deep pressor receptors. The methods adopted by Becker and co-workers to detect points of lowered electrical resistance on the skin are also helpful.

Clinically the production of adequate *deqi* at the site and the cure of illness or relief of symptoms by using the point is, in the final analysis, the most important test for the recognition of new point.

In any event the recent odious practice of some egotistical acupuncturists who try to perpetuate their own names in new points must be deplored. It can only serve to further confuse both the student and the practitioner. The interest in the plethora of new points described in China during the Cultural Revolution seem to have all but evaporated

As there is a differing numbering system between Beijing (Peking) and other centres in China there is currently a move to do away with the numbers of the Extraordinary points.

THE UN-NUMBERED EXTRAORDINARY POINTS (U.EX.)

These are points which have been discovered in recent times, most of them by medical workers in the People's Republic of China, especially the points used in acupuncture anaesthesia. There is still no universal agreement among acupuncturists regarding the uses of these points; time must elapse and more experience gained before they could be more precisely categorised. Although there is a large collection of these points, only those in common use have been described. The total number described in international literature exceeds a staggering 1500. Small wonder these are also known as strange points!

Bientao (*also called Tungfeng and Bientaotih*).

Location:

a) At the level of the lower margin of the angle of the jaw, immediately anterior to the carotid artery.

b) 1.0 cun directly inferior to Jiache (St. 6.).

Indications: Acute tonsillitis, especially with trismus.

Puncture: 1.0-1.5 cun perpendicularly, avoiding the cartoid artery.

Note: This is a Dangerous point as it is close to the baro-receptors.

Posterior-Tinggong (*Houtingkung*).

Location: On the root of the ear, level with Tinggong (S.I. 19.).

Indications: Deafness, deaf-mutism, dizziness, vertigo, chronic ear infections, pain of middle ear disease.

Puncture: Insert needle along the junction of the external ear with the scalp so that the tip of the needle rests in the crus of the helix. Penetrate 0.5-1.0 cun forward and slightly upwards in the directions of the crus of the helix.

Xia-Yifeng (*Hsiayifeng*).

Location: 1.0 cun below Yifeng (S.J. 17.).

Indications: Tonsillitis, sore throat, aphasia.

Puncture: 0.5-1.0 cun perpendicularly.

Bipay

Location: At the upper end of the anterior crease of the axilla.

Indications: Heart disease, especially angina pectoris and rhythm disorders.

Puncture: 1.0 cun perpendicularly.

Note: We have found excellent results with this point combined with Neiguan (P.6.), in rhythm disorders of heart disease. This is a frequently used point.

Jianneiling (*Jianqian*).

Location: Midway between Bipay (U.Ex) and Jianyu (Li.15)

Indications: Tendinitis of the long head of biceps associated with frozen shoulder.

Puncture: 1.0 cun perpendicularly.

Jianquan (Chienchuan)

Location: Midway between Jianyu (L.I. 15.) and Jianliao (S.J. 14).

Indications: Supra-spinatus tendinitis.

Puncture: 1.0 cun horizontally through to Jianyu (L.I. 15.). or to Jianliao (S.J. 14).

Taner (*Thaner*) Motor point of the deltoid.

Location: Midpoint of the deltoid muscle. (on the S.J. Channel).

Indications: Paralysis of the deltoid muscle, stroke.

Puncture: 1.5 cun perpendicularly.

Tunzhong (*Tunchung*).

Location: Midpoint between Huantiao (G.B. 30.) and the anterior superior iliac spine.

Indications: Low backache, sciatica, paraplegia, urticaria, sacro-iliac disease.

Puncture: 2-3 cun perpendicularly.

Yaoyang (*Yaoyang*).

Location: In the depression over the sacra-iliac joint.

Indications: Low backache, sacro-iliac disease, pain of secondary carcinoma of the spine.

Puncture: 0.5 cun perpendicularly.

Dingchan (also called **Chienhsi**).

Location: 3 cun directly above (Proximal) to Heding (Ex.31.).

Indications: Arthritis of the knee, paralysis of the lower limb. Particularly useful for knee disorders with wasting of the quadriceps.

Puncture: 1.0-2.0 cun obliquely, directed proximally.

Neima. (*Neima*). In Chinese "Nei" means medial, and "Ma" means anaesthetic.

Location: On medial border of tibia, midway between the ankle joint and the knee joint. This point coincides with Zhongdu (Liv. 6.).

Indications: This is an anaesthetic point used in lower abdominal, pelvic and perineal surgery. It is also used to achieve childbirth together with the point Sanyinjiao (Sp. 6.).

Puncture: 1.0 cun perpendicularly.

Weima. (*Weima*). In Chinese "Wei" means lateral, and "Ma" means anaesthetic.

Location:

a) on the same level as Neima on the lateral side of the leg on the Stomach Channel.

b) 9 cun above the tip of the lateral malleolus on the Stomach Channel.

Indications: All abdominal and pelvic surgery.

Puncture: 1.0 cun perpendicularly.

See also Appendix page 898.

PHILOSOPHICAL CONCEPTS

"As in heaven, so on earth."

THE THEORY OF YIN AND YANG

The edifice of traditional Chinese medicine was built on the solid foundation of careful clinical observations, and it was presented within the framework of the all-embracing philosophical concepts of Yin and Yang.

According to the Yin-Yang theory, the Universe was originally in a state of primordial chaos without force, form or substance. It then resolved into the negative (Yin) and Positive (Yang) forces, and order was produced out of Tao. It is said, therefore, that a balance exists in the Universe in its normal state, because Yin and Yang relate to each other in harmony. Natural disasters such as earthquakes, floods, and volcanic eruptions are brought about by an imbalance of the Yin and Yang forces. However, these forces are constantly interacting with each other; this is why everything in the Universe is neither stable nor final. It is, in fact, the dynamic balancing of this duality which brings about both equilibrium and change. They are therefore, like the different but inseparable poles of a magnet, or the pulse and interval of an oscillation. As is written in the *Huang Di Nei Jing*, "The universe is in a state of oscillation of the forces of Yin and Yang and their changes."

This dyamic concept is the keystone of the entirety of Chinese philosophy and of Chinese medicine. Yin is conceptualized as being cold, dark and female. Yang is warm, light and male. Yin is passive and signifies that which is deep and hidden. Yang is active and signifies that which is above the surface. Since Yin and Yang are constantly changing their relationship to each other, one cannot exist, materially or conceptually, without the other. Thus there is no night without day, no inside without outside and no virtue without vice. As described by the philosopher Chuangtzu, "One Yin and one Yang is called the Tao. The passionate union of Yin and Yang is the eternal pattern of the Universe."

Yet nothing is absolutely Yin or absolutely Yang in every Yin there is always some Yang, and in every Yang there is some Yin. In other words, an excess of Yang is a deficiency of Yin, and an excess of Yin is a deficiency of Yang.

Health and Disease are also explained in terms of this universalistic Chinese philosophy. As man is made out of the same elements as the universe, he is subject to the same laws, the Universe being the macrocosm, Man the microcosm.

Even in terms of modern physiology we know that there are mechanisms to raise and lower the blood pressure, mechanisms to raise and lower the rate of respiration, and mechanisms to regulate the levels of blood sugar. Each individual cell is miniature chromosomic representation of the whole individual and a myriad of biochemical reactions unceasingly occur to preserve the dynamic state of life. For instance, if we consider the distribution of the two ions Na^+ and K^+, inside and outside the cell, we can clearly see how Yin-Yang type of reactions occur unceasingly in order to preserve the vitality and integrity of the living cell. The hormonal balance in a healthy individual is a perfect example of this Yin-Yang dynamism. In fact the concept of homeostasis in modern physiology is none other than the establishment of a Yin-Yang balance as applied to the known parameters of the biochemical physiology of the organism. The basic postulates of the Yin-Yang theory are therefore valid, even in the context of today's scientific *milieu,* if we can adjust our minds to these ancient semantics.

The Yin-Yang relationship of the body areas are described in the *Essentials of Chinese Acupuncture*, Beijing (1980), as follows :

"The tissue and organs of the human body may pertain either to *yin* or *yang* according to their relative locations and functions. Viewing the body as a whole, the trunk surface and the four extremities, being on the exterior, pertain to *yang*, while the *zang-fu* organs are inside the body and are *yin*. Viewing the body surface and the four extremities alone, the back pertains to *yang*, while the chest and abdomen pertain to *yin*, the portion above the waist pertains to *yang* and that below partains to *yin*, the lateral aspect to *yin*; the channels running along the lateral aspects of an extremity pertain to *yang*, while those along the medial aspect pertain to *yin*. When speaking of the *zang-fu* organs alone, the *fu* organs with their main function of transmitting and digesting food pertain to *yang*; while *zang* organs with their main function of storing vital essence and vital energy pertain to *yin*. Each of the *zang-fu* organs itself can again be divided into *yin* and the *yang* e.g., the *yin* and the *yang* of the kidney, the *yin* and the *yang* of the stomach, etc. In short, however complex the tissues and structures of the human body and their functional activities be, they can be generalized and explained by the relationships of *yin* and *yang*.

The interdependent relation of *yin* and *yang* means that each of the two aspects is the condition for the other's existence and neither of them can exist in isolation. For instance, without daytime there would be no night; without excitation there would be no inhibition. Hence, it can be seen that *yin* and *yang* are at once in opposition and in interdependence; they rely on each other for existence, coexistence in a single entity. The movements and changes of a thing are due not only to the opposition and conflict between *yin* and *yang* but also to their relationship of interdependence and mutual support.

There can be very little doubt that the philosophical use of the terms Yin and Yang began in the early 4th century B.C. and that the passages in older texts which mention these terms Yin-yang are most likely interpolations made later by copyists.

Etymologically, the characters are certainly connected with darkness and light respectively. The character Yin (shady side of a hill) involves an ideogram of a hill with shadows and clouds; the character Yang has slanting sunrays or a flag fluttering in the sunshine. It may also represent a person holding a perforated disc of jade which was the symbol of heaven, the source of all light, and which may have been originally the ideogram of the most ancient astronomical instrument. These ideas correspond with the way in which these terms were used in the *Shih Ching*, a collection of ancient folksongs. Yin evokes, to the Chinese mind, the idea of cold and damp, of rain, of femaleness of that which is inside and dark, such as the underground chambers in which ice was conserved during the summer for the affluent, in ancient China. Yang evokes the idea of sunshine and heat, of spring and summer months, of maleness, and may refer to the appearance of a male ritual dancer. In several ancient classics Yin meant the shady side of a mountain or a valley (north of the mountain and south of the valley), while yang, meant the sunny side (south of the mountain and north of the valley).

Historians who have examined the first appearance of the two words as philosophical terms, find the first definition in the fifth chapter of the fifth appendix of the book *I Ching where* the statement is made '*one Yin* and *one Yang*, that is the Tao!' (*I Yin I Yang chih wei Tao*). The general sense must be that there are only these two fundamental forces or operations in the universe, now one dominating now the other, in a wave-like succession. This appendix would date, at the earliest, from the late Warring states period (early 3rd century B. C.).

In the *I Ching* (Book of Changes), each hexagram is composed of six lines, whole or broken, corresponding to the Yang and the Yin respectively. Each of the hexagrams has primarily Yin or primarily Yang, and by a judicious arrangement it was possible to derive all sixty-four of them in such a way as to produce alternating Yin and Yang. It was only by the establishment and maintenance of a real balance between the two equal forces that happiness, health or good order could be achieved. The Chinese tendency was to find in all things an underlying harmony and unity rather than a struggle and chaos.

The famous symbolic representation of Yin and Yang is similar to the now infamous swastika[1] designs found on Chinese Neolithic pottery and also on Chou bronzes. There has been great divergence of opinion about the origins of the swastika, as seen in the ancient literature, but it is certainly Neolithic, almost certainly a dualistic fecundity symbol. Hence its connection with Yin and Yang. Perhaps it has a correlation with the S-spiral designs commonly seen on Yangshao pottery.

The *Li Wei Chi Ming Ching*[2] states:

"The changes of the seasons accord with the *Qi* of Heaven and the *Qi* of Earth. When the four seasons are in mutual accord, when the Yin and Yang complement each other, when the sun and moon give forth their light unimpeded by fogs or eclipses and when superiors and inferiors are in intimate harmony with one another, then all things, all persons and all animals, are in accord with their own natures and function harmoniously."

If the two aspects seemed to be closely connected, it was not by means of a cause and effect relationship, but rather "paired" like the obverse and the reverse of a coin, like echo and sound or shadow and light. The ancient thinkers attempted to lay foundations upon which the world of the natural sciences could have been built. Perhaps the most significant thing about them is that they show an unmistakable tendency towards dialectical rather than Aristotelian logic, expressing it in precise, subtle, paradox conscious of the contradictions when confronted with the grey areas of the realities of life.

Existence and non-existence mutually generate each other; they complement each other, the long and the short demonstrate each other, high and low explain each other, instrument and voice harmonise with each other. By the first century B.C. the Chinese were familiar with the south-pointing properties of pieces of magnetite made into short lengths and capable of turning about the axis on

1 Han dynasty

2 The Swastika of Adolf Hitlet was cycled in the opposite direction. It was therefore, symbolically an unlucky sign.

blancing. One is at liberty to assume whether it was a coincidence that in a world where everything was connected to everything else, according to definite correlation rules, it should have occurred to the Chinese-experimenters, as natural or possible, that a piece of carved lodestone of special design should partake of its cosmic directivity. In a way, the whole idea of Yin-Yang was the idea of a field of force. All things orientated themselves according to it, without having to be instructed to do so, and without the application of a mechanical compulsion. The same idea springs to one's mind, as will be clearly seen, in connection, with the hexagrams of the *I Ching;* Ying and Yang acting as the positive and negative poles respectively of a cosmic field of force. It is not therefore surprising, that it should have been in China that men stumbled upon what was indeed the field of magnetic force of their own planet.

TAO

The essence of the universalistic Chinese philosophy is the concept of *Tao* (pronounced "dow"). It is difficult to translate the exact meaning of this word. The "Way" is probably the closest equivalent. All the ideas of Chinese philosophy converge in Tao. Tao has been described as "formless, nameless, the motive force of all movements and actions, and the mother of all substances."

The celebrated Chinese philosopher Lao-Tse in a well-known poem in the *Tao-Teh-king* sang to Tao as follows:

Something there is, whose veiled creation was

Before the earth or sky began to be,

So silent, so aloof, and so alone,

It changes not, nor fails, but touches all.

Conceive it as the mother of the world.

I do not know its name,

A name for it is the "way"

Pressed for a definition

I call it the Greatest.

The concept of the Tao is not an abstract concept dissociated from everyday life. It is postulated in the *Nei Jing* that the Tao operates at three levels: in heaven above, on earth below and within man (as also in all other living things).

These three manifestations of Tao are called.

The Tao of Heaven (*Thien*).

The Tao of Earth (*Jen*), and

The Tao of man (*It*). By man here we may also include animal and vegetable life forms as well.

It is within the ordered harmony of this triology that the good life was attainable.

The Tao was the all-inclusive name for this order, an efficacious totality, a reactive natural medium; it was not a creator, for nothing is created in the world, even the world was not created! The sum of wisdom consisted in adding to the number of analogical correspondences in the repertory of worldly correlations. Chinese ideals involved neither God nor Law. The uncreated universal organism, whose every part, by a compulsion internal to itself and arising out of its own nature, willingly performed its functions in the cyclical recurrences of the whole, was mirrored in human society by a universal ideal of mutual good understanding, a flexible regime of interdependences and solidarities which could never be based on unconditional ordinances; in other words, it functioned according to natural laws.

The important preaching of the ancient Chinese was to "live according to the Tao". Living according to Tao means to integrate one's self with the rules of nature, which regulate both earthly and heavenly changes. It is a code of physical, mental and ethical conduct based on unchanging cosmic truths and not on the rules and regulations codified by man. Thus Tao means the way of shaping one's earthly conduct in accordance with the operation of the natural laws, in order to reach the goal of perfection (which is oneness with the Tao), both now and hereafter. Not only mental and moral discipline but also sound physical health and freedom from disease and infirmity were considered essential for this purpose. Acupuncture, moxibustion, proper diet, exercise, work, leisure, herbal therapy, as a preventive, are regarded as useful ancillary measures to help living in accordance with the Tao. The *Nei Jing* describes a number of sages who enjoyed eternal youth by virtue of their strict adherence to the Tao. "Those who follow Tao achieve the formula of perpetual youth and maintain a youthful appearance. Although they are old in years, they are yet able to produce offspring!" Tao is the goal; Tao is the absolute.

Taoism is the only system of mysticism which man has experienced which is not profoundly anti-scientific.

Toaism had two origins. First, there were the philosophers of the Warring States period who followed a Tao of Nature rather than a Tao of human society and therefore, instead of seeking employment at the courts of the feudal princes withdrew into the wildernesses, the forests and mountains, there to meditate upon the Order of Nature, and to observe its manifold manifestations. They attacked Confucian scholastic knowledge of the rank and observances of feudal society. They believed that the true knowledge was the study of the Tao of Nature.

The other root of Taoism was the body of ancient shamans[3] and magicians who entered Chinese culture several centuries before

3 Shamanism has been the native religion of the Ural-Altaic people from the Bering Straits to the borders of Scandinavia, including the Lapps and Eskimos. American-Indian medicine-men have often been called shamans by anthropologists, as their practices are analogous. The cult, which may still be observed in many tribes today, is one of polytheistic or polydemonistic nature-worship, sometimes involving a supreme god, but often not. The "priest", whose equipment consists characteristically of drums, spears and arrows, was primarily occupied with magical healings (the expulsion of evil spirits which have possessed the patient) and divination employing scapulimancy. Aided by abnormal trance-like states , the shaman, who is a mediator between the spirits and men, goes into

Christ from the northern and southern areas respectively and which later concentrated on the northeastern coastal regions, specially in the States of Chhi and Yen. Under the names of *wu* and *fang shih* they played an important part in ancient Chinese life as the adherents of a kind of mystical religion (Shammanistic and magic), closely connected with the rural masses of the people and opposed to the orthodox state religion encouraged by the elite Confucians.

It may at first sight be curious to understand how these two different elements of ancient Chinese society could have combined so completely to form the "Taoist religion" of later times. Science and magic are , in their earliest stages, indistinguishable. The Taoist philosophers, with their emphasis on Nature, were bound in due course to pass from the purely observational to the experimental method.

These beginnings from the history of alchemy, a purely Taoist proto science; and the beginnings of pharmacology and medicine were also very closely associated with Taoism. Indeed, the differentiation

---

autohypnotic *Contd....*

trances, during which he journeys to the abodes of gods and demons, afterwards announcing the results of his conversations with them. Dancing has always been a particularly important element in shamanic rites, but ventriloquy was also used, as well as juggling and tricks, whereby the shaman releases himself from bonds. Sha-men is the transliteration of the Sanskrit sramana, or samanera which meant in pre-Buddhistic times an ascetic, and later a trainee Buddhist monk. Shamans were Taoist magicians, celebrants or exorcists.

Certain traits are found which point to a wide culture throughout the northern latitudes below the Arctic Circle, i.e. Northern Asia and Northern America. This culture area may be called the Shamanism area. A typical implement common to all parts of this vast area is the rectangular or semilunar stones knife, quite unlike anything known in Europe or the Middle East, but found among Eskimos and American-Indians, as also among Chinese and in Siberia. Needham points out that such knives were common in the Shang dynasty, and continued to be made of iron down to recent times in China. Another characteristic of this northern culture is the use of pit-dwellings or earth-lodgas: the beehive shape of which may have descended to the peasants house of the Thang period which may be seen painted on the frescoes of Tunhuang. The sinew-backed or composite bow seems to have been an invention of this area. If America was peopled by migrations across the Bering Straits at the beginning of the Neolithic, we might have en explanation of some of those strange similarities which exist between Amerindian and East Asian civilisations. Joseph Needham, *Science and Civilization in China,* Vol. 2, Cambridge University Press (1956).

of science and magic did not occur before the birth of modern science and technology in the early 17th century A.D. Such considerations may help us to understand how Taoist philosophy combined with magic (*wu*) to form the popular pragmatic "Taoist religion". The *Tao Te Ching,* 4th Century B.C. (Canon of the Virtues of the Tao), Which may be regarded as the most profound and beautiful work in the Chinese language, was written by Lao Tzu. Lao Tzu was from a noble family. For the Taoists, the Tao or Way, was the manner in which the universe operated; in other words the *Order of nature.* The Tao as the Order of Nature brought all things into existence and governed all their actions.

Lao Tzu says.

> "The supreme "Tao, how it floods in every direction!
>
> This way and that, there is no place where it does not go.
>
> All things look to it for life, and it refuses none of them;
>
> Yet when its work is accomplished it possesses nothing
>
> Clothing and nourishing all things, it does not Lord over them.
>
> Since it asks for nothing from them
>
> It may be classed among things of low estate;
>
> It may be named supreme.
>
> But since all things obey it, without coercion,
>
> It does not arrogate greatness to itself
>
> And so it fulfils its Greatness."

We have, therefore, a naturalistic pantheism, which emphasizes the unity and spontaneity of the operations of Nature. The Taoist texts are full of explanations about Nature. The *Chuang Tzu*[4] is the next greatest book on Taoism. It was written shortly after the *Tao Te Ching.* The *Chuang Tzu* authored by Chuang Chou states:

4 4th century B.C. This work appeared shortly after the *Tao Te Ching.*

"How ceaselessly heaven revolves! How constantly earth abides at rest! Do the sun and the moon contend about their respective places? Is their someone presiding these things? Who binds and connects them together? Who causes and maintains them, without trouble or exertion? Or is there perhaps some secret mechanism, in consequence of which they cannot but be as they are? Is it that they move and turn without being able to stop by themselves? Then how does a cloud become rain, and does rain again re-form cloud? What diffuses them so abundantly? Is there someone, with noting to do, who urges them on to all these things for his enjoyment? Winds rise in the north, one blows to the west, another, to the east, while some rise upwards, each in their own direction. Who is sucking and blowing all this? Is there someone, with nothing to do, who thus rules the world for his amusement? I venture to ask about these causes."

"The Tao has reality and evidence of existence but no material and no form. It may be transmitted but cannot be received. It may be attained but cannot be seen. It exists by and through itself. It existed before Heaven and Earth, and indeed for all eternity. It causes the Gods to be divine and the world to be Natural. It is above the zenith, but it is not high. It is beneath the nadir but it is not low. Though prior to heaven and earth, it is not ancient. Though older than the most ancient, it is yet young."

If there was one idea which the Taoist philosophers stressed more than any other it was the unity of nature and the eternity and uncreatedness of the Almighty Tao. The Taoists were close to an appreciation of the problems of causality, though they never embodied it in formal logical propositions.

Chuang Tzu also emphasises:

"Life is the follower of death, and death is the predecessor of life; but who knows their cycles and the connections between them (i.e. the Tao)? Man's life is due to the conglomeration of the *Qi* and when they are dispersed death occurs. Since death and life thus complement each other, why should I account for either of them as evil? ... Life is accounted beautiful because it is spirit-like and wonderful. Death is accounted hateful because it is foetid and putrid. But the foetid and putrid, on returning, is transformed again into the spirit-like by metamorphoses and then the cycle of changes occurs once more. Therefore it is said that all through the universe there is one *Qi* and consequently the sages prized that unity both in life and in death."

One can see the tendency to incorporate an appreciation of and resignation to these changes, as part of an understanding of Nature which was the basis of Taoist ataraxy, or calmness of the mind. "The Tao is that which accompanies all other things and meets them, which is present when they are evolved and when they come to their perfection; it is the tranquility at the centre of all disturbances. It produces fullness and emptiness, but it is neither fullness nor emptiness; it produces fullness and emptiness, but it is neither fullness nor emptiness; it produces withering and killing, but it is neither withering nor killing; it produces root and branches, but it is neither root nor branch; it produces accumulation and dispersion but it is itself neither accumulated nor dispersed."

Chapter II of the *Tao Te Ching* further states.

"Thirty spokes combine to make a cart wheel,

When there was no private property carts were made for use.

Clay is formed to make vessels;

When there was no private property, vessels were made for use.

Windows and doors go to make a house;

When there was no private property, houses were made for use.

Thus having private property leads to profit for the feudal lords,

But not having it leads to use by the people."

There can be little doubt as to which political line was in accord with the ancient Taoistic teachings.

From the beginning Taoist thought was captivated by the idea that it was possible to achieve a material immortality (*Hsien*) by indulging in certain practices.

These practices fail into several categories:

1) respiratory techniques;

2) heliotherapeutic techniques;

3) gymnastic techniques e.g. *tai-chi-chuan;*

4) sexual techniques;

5) alchemical and pharmaceutical techniques;

6) dietary techniques;

7) meditation techniques.

All these techniques went under the collective name of "nourishing the *qi,* of the nature". The sexual techniques, owing to the Confucian and the Buddhist conservatism, have remained totally uninvestigated, yet they have considerable physiological interest. It was quite natural, in view of the general acceptance of the Yin-Yang theories, to think of human sexual relations against a cosmic background, and indeed as having intimate connections with the mechanism of the whole universe. The Taoists considered that sex, far from being an obstacle to the attainment of *hsien*-ship, could be made to aid it in important ways. Techniques practised in private were called "the method of nourishing life energy by enhancing the Yin and Yang" and their basic aim was to conserve as much as possible the seminal essence and the divine element, specially by "causing the semen to return". At the same time, the two great forces, as incarnated in two separate human individuals, were to act as indispensable spiritual nourishment for each other. This is in direct contradistinction to the Judeo-Christian attitude to sex. There are many detailed parallelisms between Taoism and Indian Tantrism. The practice of "making semen return" was done by force exerted on the male urethra by the female partner using perineal pressure at the moment of ejaculation. The seminal discharge was thereby forced into the bladder and later voided in the urine. It is believed, even by modern Hindus, that hormones from the seminal fluid are thereby reabsorbed. This sexual technique was described and practised by Taoists as well as the followers of Tantrism. Both civilizations practised respiratory exercises to reinforce this sexual technique, particularly by developing the perineal musclature. It was believed that the vital fluids from the semen thereby ascended to the thousand petalled lotus at the top of the head (the brain).

Owing to the prude values of present day Chinese society these important historical connections remain uninvestigated.

The recognition of the importance of the female in the scheme of things, the acceptance of equality of women with men, the conviction that the attainment of health and longevity needed the cooperation of the sexes, the exquiste admiration of certain feminine psychological characteristics, the incorporation of the physical phenomena of sex in therapeutic group catharsis, free alike from asceticism and class distinctions, reveal several aspects of ancient Taoism which had no counterpart in Confucianism or Buddhism. There is probably some connection between these practices and the matriarchal elements in primitive tribal collectivism, with much of the prominence given to the female symbol in ancient Taoist philosophy. It may be no coincidence that in ancient China the Taoists were the supreme representatives of social solidarity, of aggregation and unity, of all that was opposed to division and separation. Indeed, their thought and practice went so deep as to be universal love, the power of affinity and union of opposites in the universe, to achieve universal harmony.

The philosophy of Taoism, though containing the elements of political collectivism, religious mysticism and the training of the individual for an intellectual immortality, developed many of the most important features of the scientific attitude, and is therefore of cardinal importance in the history of science in China. Moreover, the Taoists acted on specific principles, and that is why we owe to them the beginnings of chemistry, mineralogy, botany, zoology and phamacology in East Asia. They show many parallels with the scientific pre-Socratic and Epicurean philosophers of Greece. However, they failed to reach any precise definition of the experimental method, or any systematisation of their observations as they realized Nature is in a state of dynamic flux.

The Taoists were profoundly conscious of the universality of change and transformation—this was one of their deepest scientific insights. Taoist patterns of thought and behaviour include all kinds of rebellion against conventions, the withdrawal of the individual from society, the love and study of Nature, the refusal to take office, and the living embodiment of the paradoxical non-possessiveness of the *Tao Te Ching:* production without possession, action without self-assertion development without domination. Many of the most attractive elements of the Chinese character derive from Taoism. China without Taoism would be a dwarfed plant where its tap root has perished.

The main motivation of the Taoist philosophers in observating Nature was that they were attempting to gain that peace of mind which comes from having formulated a rational hypothesis to allay the terrifying manifestations of the natural world surrounding and penetrating the frail structure of human society. Whether the phenomena be those of inclement weather, earthquakes, eruptions, storms or floods, or of the varied forms of disease; man at the beginning of the path of science felt stronger and more confident when once he had differentiated and classified them, and especially named them, after formulating naturalistic theories about their origins, development and likely future incidence. This distinctive peace of mind the Chinese called *ching hsin.* The Chinese scientific correlative thinking always involved the two fundamental principles or forces in the universe, the Yin and the Yang, negative and positive projections of man own sexual experience and the Five Elements of which all known universal phenomena were composed. The five elements were aligned and associated, in symbolic correlation, with everything in the universe which could be got into a fivefold order and much ingenuity was shown in fitting the classification to include diverse phenomena.

The keywords in Chinese philosophical thought are *Order* and above all *Pattern*. The symbolic correlations or correspondences all formed part of one colossal pattern. Events behaved in particular ways, not necessarily because of prior actions or impulsions of other things, but because their position in the ever-moving cyclical universe was such that they were endowed with intrinsic natures which made that behaviour for them. If they did not behave in those particular ways they would lose their relational positions in the whole (which made them what they were), and change into something other than themselves. They were thus parts in existential dependence upon the whole world-organism and they reacted upon one another not so much by mechanical impulsion or causation as by a kind of metaphysical resonance.

Events influence each other by a kind of abstract pattern of inductance. A myriad of patterns are subsumed in the Great Pattern Tao. Harmony was regarded as the basic principle of a world-order "spontaneous and organic". With this is mind, we can see in a new light the poetical philosophy of Hsun Tzu[5], who went so far as to exalt *li* (good customs and traditional observances sanctioned by generally accepted morality) to the level of a universal cosmological principle. Not only in human society, but also throughout the world of Nature, there was a give and take, a kind of mutual courtesy rather than strife among inanimate powers and processes, a finding of solutions by compromise. Chinese though developed their organic aspect, visualising the universe as a hierarchy of parts and wholes, suffused by a harmony of wills. Chinese correlative thinking was *not* primitive thinking in the sense that it was an alogical or pre-logical chaos in which anything could be the cause of anything else, and where men's ideas were guided by the pure fancies of one other medicine-man; it was a picture of a sophisticated and precisely ordered universe, in which things "fitted" exactly. It was a universe in which this organisation came about, not because of fiats issued by a supreme creatorlawgiver which things must obey subject to sanctions imposed by attendant spirits, nor because of the physical clash

5 An ancient Toaist humanist who attacked all kinds of superstition by preaching a rationalist doctrine.

of innumerable billiard-balls in which the motion of the one was the physical cause of the impulsion of the other. It was an ordered harmony of wills without an ordainer; it was like the spontaneous yet ordered and exquistely patterned movements of a group of dancers none of whom are bound by law to do what they do, nor yet pushed by others coming behind, but cooperate in a voluntary harmony. "No one was ever seen to command the four seasons", yet they never swerve from their course. However absurd may have been the conviction that dreaded evils would follow his failure, the ritual of the Emperor was the supreme manifestation of this belief in the oneness of the universal pattern. In the proper pavilion of the Ming Thang or Bright House, also in his dwelling-place and in the Temple of Heaven, the Emperor, clad in the robes of the colour appropriate to the season, faced the proper direction, caused the musical notes appropriate to the musical notes appropriate to the time to be sounded, and carried out all the other ritual acts which signified that the unity of heaven and earth is in tune with the cosmic pattern.

If the moon stood in the mansion of a certain equatorial constellation at a certain time, it did so not because anyone had ever ordered it do so, nor because it was obeying some mathematically expressible regularity depending upon such and such unique formula—it did so because it was part of the pattern of the universal organism that it should do so, and for no other reason whatsoever. Horoscopy and astrology also derived their inspiration from these changes and patterns of the cosmos.

The idea of corraspondence has great significance and replaces the idea of causality, that things are *connected* rather than caused. The universe itself is a vast organism, with now one and now another component taking the lead—spontaneous and uncreated it is, with all the parts of it cooperating in a mutual service. Apart from this vision of the Taoists, there runs throughout Chinese history a current of rational naturalism and of enlightened scepticism, often much stronger than what was found at corresponding periods in Europe, where modern science and technology grew up.

In the realm of philosophical theory and practice, early Taoism owed much both to the Indian Upanishad literature for its theory

THE RELATIONSHIPS OF THE FIVE ELEMENTS AND THE ZANG FU ORGANS

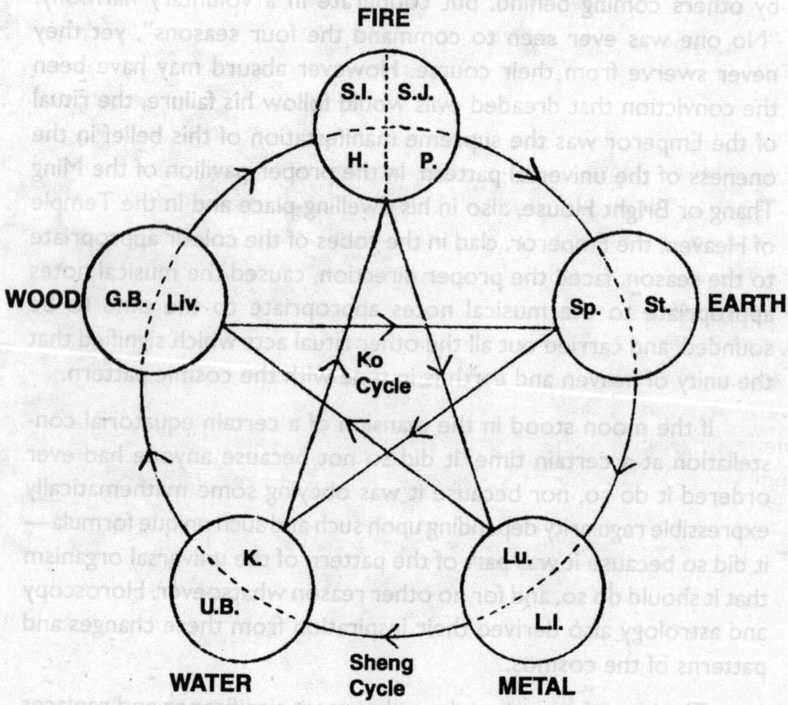

Sheng = Generative
Ko = Destructive

and to Indian yogism for some of its practices. Further, Chinese Buddhism was also an importation from India. The Upanishads are metaphysical commentaries on the Vedas, and date from the 8th to the 4th centuries B.C., so that they are little earlier than the first period of elaboration of the Taoist doctrine. The Vedas strongly marked metaphysical idealism, which is the concept of the unity of the *brahman* and the *atman,* the absolute and the self, and greatly emphasised the unity of nature, and the incorporation of the individual within it. The influence of Yoga practices, especially the breathing exercises from ancient India, upon early Taoism is considerable. Some Taoist schools practised self-hypnosis by concentrating on the inhaling and exhaling processes, but this was not universal. In any case the aims of this *samadhi or* dhyana among the Taoists were different from those of the Indian *rishis.* Both wished to master organic life and to attain supernatural powers, but while the Rishis sought for an ascetic virtue which would enable them to dominate the Gods themselves, the Taoists sought a material immortality in a universe in which there were no Gods to overcome, and asceticism was only one of the methods which were often used to attain their ends. Besides contemplation of the universe during quiet self-hypnosis, they were also interested in the techniques of sexual intercouse by which they thought that life might be prolonged, and above all in the preparation of drugs which would render the taker immortal. Admittedly, both the latter elements have parallels in ancient Indian thought. Sex has been outstandingly significant in all Hindu myth and religion, particularly in the theme of the *Saktis,* the ancient intoxicating sacred Indian drink called *soma,* which was regarded as an aphrodisiac and an elixir of immortality.

VITAL ENERGY (Qi)

"Life is like flame of a lamp,

Soon extinguished when the fuel (Qi) is exhausted."

— *Huan Than, 40 B.C.*

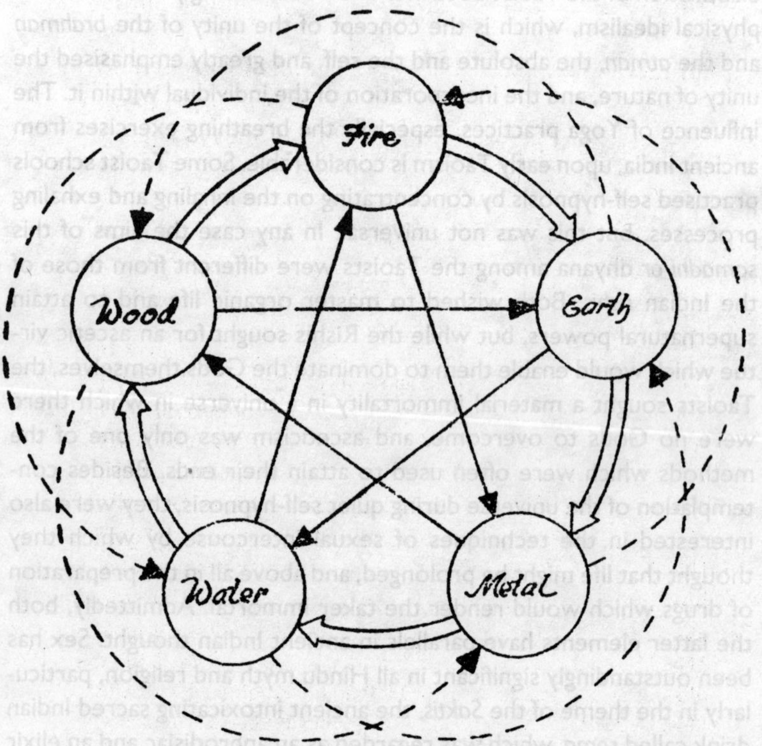

⟹ Inter-promoting relationship (Sheng)
⟶ Inter-acting and over-acting relationship (Ko)
– – → Counter-acting relationship

From the Essentials of Chinese Acupuncture, Beijing (1984)

The interaction of Yin and Yang produces "*Qi*", the bipolar flow of energy which pervades the entire Universe. It is bipolar because it is as every thing else in them universe subject to the fluctuations of Yin and Yang. Qi is the prime energy which motivates the Tao.

There are many forms of Qi. Heat, light and sound, for example, are various forms of Qi. The Qi that can be manipulated with acupuncture needling is called "*Jing Qi*" of the vital energy circulating in the Channels. It regulates the circulation of blood, the processes of digestions of food, the autoprotection of the organism and all other vital activities. The body carries a certain amount of Qi at birth. This is depleted by the daily activities of living; it is augmented by the intake of food and air. This depletion or reinforement, if balanced, maintains growth and health. Imbalance of Qi—its excess or deficiency within the organism—is the cause of ill health. Its absence is death. The purpose of acupuncture is to restore the imbalance of body Qi by puncturing the correct combination of points.

Qi is an abstract philosophical concept which is not adequately translatable from the Chinese medical lexicon to other languages. Qi infuses life with all its protein manifestations. It is an imponderable entity. However it has a multiplicity of materials manifestations as well, such as the circulation of blood and the essences of the body causing growth of the organism. "The spirit" being responsible for the state of consciousness and mental activities, and the secretion of "fluids" such as tears, saliva, sweat, bile and urine, which co-ordinates the smooth functioning of the various organs and tissues.

THE THEORY OF THE FIVE ELEMENTS

In the words of the *Huang Di Nei Jing, Su Wen* "There are Five Elements in heaven, as also on earth." The Chinese classified all phenomena of the Universe into the Five Elements.

The five Elements are: *Wood, Fire, Earth, Metal and Water.* They are related in two cyclic sequences which are termed the generative and the destructive cycles.

In the generative cycle (called the "*Sheng*" cycle) Fire is fed by Wood; the ashes which form become the Earth; Metal is formed in the Earth; Water springs from Metal (fluidity arises from the solid state); and Water nourishes trees which become Wood, thus completing the cycle.

In the destructive cycle (called the "*Ko*" cycle) Fire melts Metal; Metal cuts Wood; Wood covers the Earth; and the Earth dams Water.

The Five Elements are therefore not independent entities but exist in an intimate relation to each Element which governs and is governed by another Element.

As Professor Joseph Needham points out[6], it is quite likely that the Five Elements may refer not to five material substance but to five characteristics namely :

Wood - solidity and ease of workability;
Fire - Combustion and development of heat;
Earth - fertility;
Metal - fusibility; and
Water - fluidity.

Yet there is nothing which is wholly one Element and free from all the others; every entity possesses all Five Elements but one Element predominates, and it is that Element which confers its name to the entity concerned. The relationship of the Elements of each other is essentially a conceptual relationship.

According to *The Essentials of Chinese Acupuncture,* Beljing (1980):-

The theory of the five elements holds that wood, fire earth, metal and water are basic materials constituting the material world. There exists among them an interdependence and inter-restraint which determines their state of constant motion and change."

"The theory of the five elements basically explains the interpromoting, inter-acting, over-acting and counter-acting relationships among them. Its application to traditional Chinese medicine is in classifying into different categories, natural phenomena plus the tissues and organs of the human body and the human emotions and interpreting the relationship between the physiology and pathology

6 "Science and Civilization in China" Cambridge University Press (1954).

of the human body and the natural environment with the laws of the inter-promoting, over-acting and counter-acting of the five elements. This theory is used as a guide in medical practice."

The theories of *yin-yang* and the five elements are two outlooks on nature in ancient China, both encompassing rudimentary concepts of materialism and dialectics and to some extent reflecting the objective law of things. They are of practical significance in explaining physiological activities and explaining pathological changes in guiding medical practice. In clinical application the two are usually related with and supplement each other and cannot be entirely separated. As for shortcomings in the two theories, by adhering to the scientific attitude of dialectical and historical materialism, we can continue making progress in our medical practice and promote the further development of traditional Chinese medicine in the light of constantly summing up our experience."

The classification into Five Elements of the main phenomena of the Universe (as also applicable in traditional medicine) is as follows:

Five Elements	Five Cardinal Points	Five Seasens	Five Perverse Climates	Five Colours	Five Stages of Development
WOOD	East	Spring	Wind	Green	Birth
FIRE	South	Summer	Heat	Red	Growth
EARTH	Center	Late Summer	Humidity	Yellow	Transformation
METAL	West	Autumn	Dryness	White	Harvest
Water	North	Winter	Cold	Black	Storage

Traditional Chinese medicine was well aware that external factors in the environment influence the body in health and disease. The five seasons and the five perverse climates are ready examples. (These are among the exogenous factors that cause disease).

Since 350 A.D. the Five Element Theory had been discussed often, especially in the eastern seaboard states of Chhi and Yen, in the works of the famous Tsou Yen. His sayings were vast and profound and not in accord with the accepted beliefs of the classics. First he examined small objects, and from these he drew conclusions about large ones, until he reached what was without limit[7]. First he spoke about modern times, and from this went back to the time of Huang Di. The followers of Tsou Yen's teachings and methods were known as the Naturalists. These ideas crystallised, in the late 3rd century B.C. in a short treatise known as the *Wu Ti Te* (The Virtues by which the Five Emperors Ruled). There is much evidence which connects the Naturalists with the beginnings of alchemy. The Historical classic *Shu Shing*[8] describes the Five Elements as follows:

"Of the elements, the first is called Water, the second Fire, the third Wood, the fourth Metal, and the fifth Earth. Water is that quality in Nature which we describe as soaking and descending. Fire is that quality in nature which we describe as blazing and uprising. Wood is that quality in nature which permits of curved surfaces or straight edges. Metal is that quality in Nature which can follow the form of a mould and then become hard. Earth is that quality in Nature which permits of sowing, and reaping."

That which soaks, drips and descends causes saltiness. That which rises up generates bitterness. That which permits of curved surfaces or straight edges gives sourness. That which can follow the form of a mould and then become hard, produces acidity. That which permits of sowing, growth and reaping, gives rise to sweetness."

The conception of Five Elements suggests five types of fundamental biophysical processes as follows:

WOOD	accepting form by submitting to cutting and carving instruments	solidity involving workability	sourness
FIRE	heating, burning, ascending	heat, combusting	bitterness
EARTH	producing edible vegetation	nutritivity	sweetness
METAL	accepting form by moulding when in the liquid state, and the capacity of changing this form by re-melting and re-moulding	solidity involving congelation and re-congelation (mouldability)	acidity
WATER	soakig, dripping, descending, dissolving	liquidity, fluidity, solution	saltiness

7 Similar to the Newtonian-Cartesian paradigm of modern science.
8 3rd Century B.C.

The Five Elements are five powerful natural forces in everflowing cyclical motion, and not passive motionless, fundamental, material substances.

Tung Chung-Shu writing "On the Five Elements", in 135 B.C. states:

"Heaven has Five Elements first Wood, second Fire, third Earth, fourth Metal, and fifth Water. Wood comes first in the cycle of the Five Elements and water comes last, earth being in the middle. This is the order which Heaven has made. Wood produces fire, produces earth (i.e. as ashes), earth produces metal (i.e. as ores), metal produces water, and water produces wood (for woody plants require water). This is their "father-and-son" relationship. Wood dwells on the left, metal on the right, fire in front and water behind, with earth in the centre This, too, is their father-and-son order, each receiving from the other in its turn. Thus it is that wood receives from water, fire from wood, and so on. As transmitters they are fathers, as receivers they are sons. There is an unvarying dependence of the sons on the fathers, and the direction is always from the father to the son. Such is the Tao of Heaven."

"This being so, wood, having produced fire, nourishes it; while metal having melted, is stored up in water. Fire delights in wood, and through the operation of the Yang is nourished by it. Water, having conquered metal, through the operation of the Yin buries it. Earth, in its service to Heaven, "uses all its loyalty" Thus it is that the Five Elements correspond to the actions of filial sons and loyal ministers. Putting the Five Elements into words like this, they really seem to be five kinds of actions, do they not?"

The idea of successive mutual conquests as phenomena succeed one another in the eternal round of Nature, was well known to the Chinese since 400 B.C. in many writings. The classic *Wen Tzu* further clearly states: "Metal may overcome wood, but with one axe a man cannot cut down a whole forest. Earth may overcome water, but with a single handful, one cannot dam up a river. Water may overcome fire, but with no more than a bucket-full one cannot put out a large conflagration." This is the counteracting property of the Five Elements.

The Five Elements gradually came to be associated with every conceivable category of phenomena in the universe which it was possible to classify in fives. Such correspondences were the common modes of thought from the Chhin dynasty onwards. The Five Elements Theory fashioned Chinese thinkings a great deal down the ages up to the present time.

Joseph Needham in *Celestial Lancets* states:

"Different environments gave rise to different incidences of endemic disease, hence the invention of different therapeutic methods. Thus moxibustion came mainly from the North, materia and pharmacy from the west, and gymnastics, remedial exercises and massage from the Centre. But acupuncture originated in the East, where people suffered greatly from boils and carbuncles; while its elaborations (in the form of the nine needles) came from the South. As for apotropaics (exorcisms, magical spells, and sacrifices to the gods and ancestors) this, it was considered, had been fairly universal from the earliest times. In part, it may be, this ancient proto-historical presentation was following the system of symbolic correlations, five types of medical treatment, being analogised with the 5 Elements classification and especially the five directions of space, but there may be rather more to it than that. For we know that ancient Chinese society was built upon, or greatly influenced by a number of 'local cultures', environing societies which brought various distinguishable traits into the eventual common Sinic stock. In this case, acupuncture would have been associated with the south-eastern quasi-Indonesian aquatic element, while moxa would have come down to join it from the northern quasi-Tungusic nomadic element, and the pharmaceutical influence would have come from the western Szechuanese and quasi-Tibetan element."

THE THEORY OF ZANG-FU

The concepts of Yin and Ying, Qi, and the Five Elements also apply to Man, the microcosm. In this manner, Man fits into the totality of the Universe and becomes a part of it.

According to the ***Huang Dinei Jing*** the different Internal Organs are described as having the division of labour exhibited by a properly run state. This is known as the *state analogy:*

The Organ	Official Function
The Heart	"The supreme Controller or the Emperor"
The Small Intestine	"The separator of the pure and impure"
The Pericardium	"The protector of the Emperor"
The Sanjiao	"The controller of temperature (internal environment"
The Liver	"The official for judgement and planning"
The Gall Bladder	"The official for decision making"
The Lung	"The Receivar of Qi from the heavens"
The Large Intestine	"The official for the drainage of the dregs"
The Stomach	"The official for rotting and ripening"
The spleen	"The official for transport and distribution"
The Kidney	"The controller of the storage of vital energy"
The Urinary Bladder	"The controller of water"

Another analogy is the *universe analogy:* the upper half of man, including the heart and brain, represents heaven; the lower half, including the stomach and genitalia, represents the earth. Man is the son of heaven and earth.

The ancient Chinese related the body functions into twelve Organ systems, which were classified according to their characteristics into Zang (Yin) and Fu (Yang), and into the Five Elements.

The Zang Organs have the function of storing and are known as the "Solid Organs". They are Yin in character. The Fu Organs have the function of digesting and absorbing food and excreting wastes, and are known as the "Hollow Organs". They are Yang in character. Although the different Organs have separate functions, they work in close co-ordination with each other to preserve the unity of the organism and to carry out its vital functions.

The classification of the Twelve Organs into Yin and Yang and into the Five Elements is correlated as follows:

a) Each Yin Organ is coupled to a Yang Organ and they are both identified with one of the Five Elements.

b) Each pair of these coupled Organs relate to the other such pairs of coupled Organs in the generative (Sheng) cycle and in the destructive (Ko) cycle that govern the relationship of the Five Elements.

Each of the Zang and Fu Organs relates to a vital function of the body. These relationships are illustrated in the following table:

TABLE ILLUSTRATING THE ZANG-FU THEORY

5 ZANG ORGANS[9]	**6 FU ORGANS**
Lung Respiration	**Large Intestine** Excretion of wastes
Heart (Pericardium) Circulation of blood. Mental activity	**Small Intestine** Separation of the essence from food and transport of waste to the Large Intestine.
Sanjiao	Maintaining homeostasis of the body.

9 In this functional classification the number of Zang Organs are reduced to Five because the heart and pericardium form one functional unit.

Spleen Digestion. Water metabolism. Circulation of blood. Immunity.	**Stomach** Ingestion, digestion, and transport of food and water.
Liver Bile secretion and transport. Regulation, storage and transport of blood. Control of tendons. Control of endocrines.	**Gall Bladder** Storage of bile. Mental acitivity.
Kidney Regulation of blood pressure Growth of bone, cartilage, teeth, nails and head hair, Promotion of "new life" as an extention of genital functions.	**Urinary Bladder** Water balance. Genital functions.

The ancient Chinese also discovered that the Zang and Fu Organs were connected to certain areas of the body in such a manner that pathological changes in a Zang or Fu Organ also brought about corresponding changes in related areas or tissues. Some of these changes could be related to the Five Colour. This made it easy to ascertain which set of Zang and Fu Organs needed treatment. These relationships are tabulated as follows:

YIN (ZANG) ORGAN	YANG (FU) ORGAN	Connected Tissues	Connected sense Organ	Connected structures for colour reference	The five Colour Changes
Lung	Large Intestine	Skin, Body hair	Nose	Skin	White
Heart Pericardium	Small Intestine Sanjiao	Brain, Blood vessels	Tongue	Mouth	Red
Spleen	Stomach	Soft tissue, Four extremities (limbs)	Mouth	Lip	Yellow
Liver	Gall Bladder	Muscle, Tendon	Eyes	Nail	Green
Kidney	Urinary Bladder	Bone, Cartilage, Nails Teeth, Head hair	Ears	Inside of forearm	Black

In the same way that pathological changes in the internal Organs could be caused by external (exogenous) factors, changes, could also be brought about by internal factors, these being mainly emotional causes (called endogenous factors). The relationship of the five human emotions to the Zang-Fu and their connections, in turn, to several areas of reaction were also of help to the traditional physician in his diagnosis. This set of relationships are shown below:-

ZANG ORGAN	**FU ORGAN**	**The Five Emotions**	**The Five Sounds**	**The Five Fluids**
Lung	Large Intestine	Sadness	Sobbing	Mucus
Heart (Pericardium)	Small Intestine Sanjiao	Joy	Laughing	Sweat
Spleen	Stomach	Anxiety	Singing	Lymph
Liver	Gall Bladder	Anger	Shouting	Tears
Kidney	Urinary Bladder	Fear	Groaning	Saliva

Joseph Needham[10] discussing ancient correlations states:

"Some of these correlations were a natural and benign outcome of the basic hypothesis itself. The association of the elements with the seasons was obvious enough, and it had been on their association with the cardinal points that the various sequences had been built up. What could have been more unavoidable than to link fire with summer and the south? This must have been of the highest antiquity, since we find fire (i.e. heat, and the grain ripened by it) in the autumn harvest character and its existence in the character for the south as well. Then the tastes (and probably also the smells, though the relation is not so clear) strongly suggest primitive chemistry. The colours invite much speculation. Since the cradle of Chinese civilisation was the land of the yellow soil in the upper *Yellow River basin* (modern Shansi and shensi), it is quite plausible to suppose that, for the centre, that colour imposed itself. Then white in the west would stand for the perpetual snows of the Tibetan massif, with green (or blue) in the east for the fertile plains or the seemingly infinite ocean. Finally, red in the south may have taken its origin from the red soil for Szechuan, the region which, lies just south of Shensi and Shansi; there are, moreover, large areas also of red soil in Yunnan and towards Vietnam."

"The *Huang Di Nei Jing. Su Wen* was responsbile for the physiological correlations of the Five Elements. There are associations between the elements and the viscera, the parts of the body, the sense-organs, and the affective states of the mind. No names of personalities connected with this medical group have come down to us. Thus was established the far-reaching system of symbolic correlations."

---

10 Joseph Needham, *Science and Civilization in China,* Cambridge University Press (1956).

THE THEORY OF JING-LUO

In traditional Chinese medicine, diagnosis and the treatment are based on the dynamic theory of energy flow, which postulates that Qi or vital energy flows continuously in the body in a definite time sequence and in definite pathways.

The Qi (vital-energy) in the body has three main levels of manifestation : superficial, deep and intermediate. Anything affecting Qi at one level may also affect it at the other levels. The ancient Chinese discovered that it was possible to cause changes in the body by skilfully influencing the Qi at the surface level-and this is, in fact, the object of all acupuncture therapy.

At the deep level, Qi travels along certain pathways which interconnect the Zang and Fu Organs in the Sheng (generative) and ko (destructive) cycles.

At the superficial level Qi flows along a system of conduits or channels called "Jing". These Jing-Channels may be classified into two groups : the regular Channels (known as the Twelve Paired Channels) and the extra Channels (known as the Eight Extraordinary Channels).

There are also several short collateral channels called "Luo" or Connecting Channels which maintain the cyclical flow of Qi in the body.

All these channels and collaterals are collectively referred to as the "Jing-Luo". They form the interlacing network which traverses the entire body carrying vital energy to every part of the body.

The main pathological manifestations of the Twelve Regular (Paired) Channels and the Eight Extraordinary Channels are described as follows in the ***Essentials of Chinese Acupuncture,*** Foreign Languages Press, Beijing (1980):

1. Pathological manifestations of the 12 regular channels

(1) The Lung Channel of Hand-Taiyin. Cough, asthma haemoptysis, congested and sore throat, sensation of fullness in the chest, pain in the supraclavicular fossa, shoulder, back and the lateral border of the anterior aspect of the arm.

(2) The Large Intestine Channel of Hand-Yangming. Epistaxis, watery nasal discharge, toothache, congested and sore throat, pain in the neck, anterior part of the shoulder and anterior border of the extensor aspect of the upper limb, borborygmus, abdominal pains, diarrhoea, dysentery.

(3) The Stomach Channel of Foot-Yangming. Borborygmus, abdominal distension, oedema, epigastric pain, vomiting, feeling of hunger, epistaxis, deviation of eyes and mouth, congested and sore throat, pain in the chest, abdomen and lateral aspect of the lower limbs, fever, mental disturbances.

(4) The Spleen Channel of Foot-Taiyin. Belching, vomiting, epigastric pain, abdominal distention, loose stools, jaundice, sluggishness and general malaise, stiffness and pain at the root of the tongue and mouth, swelling and coldness in the medial aspect of the thigh and knee.

(5) The Heart Channel of Hand-Shaoyin. Cardialgia, palpitation, hypochondric pain, insomnia, night sweating, dryness of the throat, thirst, pain in the medial aspect of the upper arm, feverishness in the palms.

(6) The Small Intestine Channel of Hand-Taiyang. Deafness, yellow sclera, sore throat, swelling of the cheek, distension and pain in the lower abdomen, frequent urination, pain along the posterior border of the lateral aspect of the shoulder and arm.

(7) The Urinary Bladder Channel of Foot-Taiyang Retention of urine, enuresis, mental disturbances, malaria, ophthalmodynia, lacrimation when exposed to wind, nasal obstruction, rhinitis, epistaxis, headache, pain in the nape, upper and lower back, buttocks and posterior aspect of the lower limbs.

(8) The Kidney Channel of Foot-Shaoying. Enuresis, frequent urination, nocturnal emission, impotence, irregular menstruation, asthma, hemoptysis, dryness of the tongue, congested and sore throat, oedema, lumbago, pain along the spinal column and the medial aspect of the thigh, weakness of the lower limbs, feverish sensation in the soles.

(9) The Pericardium Channel of Hand-Jueyin. Cardialgia, palpitation, mental restlessness, stifling feeling in the chest, flushed face, swelling in the axilla, mental disturbances, spasm of the upper limbs, feverishness in the palms.

(10) The Sanjiao Channel of Hand-Shaoyang. Abdominal distention, oedema, enuresis, tinnitus, pain in the outer canthus, swelling of the cheeks, congested and sore throat, pain in the retroauricular region, shoulder, and lateral aspect of, the arm and elbow.

(11) The Gall Bladder Channel of Foot-Shaoyang. Headache, pain in the outer canthus, pain in the jaw, blurring of vision, bitter taste in the mouth, swelling and in the axilla, pain along the lateral aspect of the chest, hypochondrium, thigh and lower limbs.

(12) The Liver Channel of Foot-Jueyin. Low back pain, fullness in the chest, pain in the lower abdomen, hernia, vertical headache, dryness of the throat, hiccup, enuresis, dysuria, mental disturbances.

2. Pathological manifestations of the eight extraordinary channels

(1) The Du Channel. Stiffness and pain along the spinal column, opisthotonus, headache.

(2) The Ren Channel. Leucorrhea, irregular menstruation, hernia, enuresis, retention of urine, pain in the epigastric region and the lower abdomen.

(3) The Chong Channel. Colic and pain in the abdomen.

(4) The Dai Channel. Abdominal pain, weakness and pain to the lumbar region, leucorrhea.

(5) The Yangqiao Channel. Epilepsy, insomnia.

(6) The Yinquiao Channel. Hypersomnia.

(7) The Yangwei channel. Chills and fever.

(8) The Yinwei Channel. Cardialgia.

The Channels described above are those at the superficial levels, by needling which, the acupuncturist is able to influence in order to readjust imbalances. The complete channel system however, by which is meant all the pathways of energy between the surface of the body and the Internal Organs, muscles and other parts of the body, are not and cannot be fully charted as they are so numerous and complex. The fact that the ear, nose, hand and foot are each used as self-contained systems of acupuncture, or that the tongue, the iris and other specific areas are used for diagnosis in respect of the entire body presupposes the existence of a very fine harmonious interconnecting network of channels. It must be remembered that the traditional Chinese physician was unaware of the nervous system as we know it today, and their postulation of the channel system must be regarded as a brilliant attempt to systematize the clinical interrelationship of the known functions of the body.

The main channels of energy which are of clinical importance to the acupuncturist are as follows:

a) The 12 Paired (Regular) Channels.

b) The 8 Extraordinary Channels.

c) The 12 Luo-Connecting Channels which join each Yin-Yang pair of the 12 paired Channels in the wrist or the ankle. The connection is achieved by the joining of the Luo-Connecting point of a Channel with the Yuan-Source point of its paired Channel and *vice versa.*

d) The 15 Luo Channels which also join the Paired Channels at the Luo-Connecting point. From these points they interconnect various parts of the body thus expanding the influence of the Paired Channels, e.g., the Luo Channel of the Spleen commences at the point Gongsun (Sp. 4.) and travels up the leg to the intestines and stomach. It is for this reason that the stimulation of this point is indicated in acute diarrhoea.

e) The 12 Divergent Channels which branch off from each of the Twelve Paired Channels (not necessarily always at the acupuncture points), travel through certain important tissues and eventually connect with the internal Organ related to the Channel from which it commences and with its Coupled Organ.

f) The 12 Muscle-Tendon Channels which originate from the Jing-Well points of the Paired Channels. They carry mainly Yang energy the influence of which explains the effect of the Jing-Well points to mobilise this Yang energy when needled in acute emergencies. They form a complex capilliary network.

THE FOUR TRADITIONAL LAWS OF ACUPUNCTURE

The Four Traditional Laws of Acupuncture may be used to select acupuncture points for therapy. They are known descriptively as:

1) the Mother-Son Law;

2) the Noon-Midnight Law (or Midday-Midnight Law);

3) the Husband-Wife Law; and

4) the Theory of the Five Elements (this has been discussed earlier).

These Laws are now briefly discussed:

1) Mother-Son Law:

This Law is a consequence of the cyclical flow of Qi (vital energy) along the Channels and the Organs. If the flow is blocked or hindered from circulating freely as the result of a disease factor then an abnormal surplus or deficiency of vital energy may occur. This affects not only that Channel or Organ but also the channel or Organs which precede and succeed it; disharmony of the entire organism is caused, and a condition of disease in manifest.

In the Mother-Son Law therefore, the recognition of the direction of the flow of vital energy is important. It flows from Channel or Organ just as "the mother nourishes her infant"

If a Channel or Organ shows an insufficiency of activity then it can be strengthened by so stimulating it so that it draws more vital energy from its mother.

The Mother-Son relationship of the Twelve Channels is in the sequence of the normal flow of vital energy of the Organ Clock in the Twelve Channels. The Mother-son relationship of the internal Organs is in the sequence of the generative cycle of the Five Elements (Sheng cycle).

THE ORGAN CLOCK

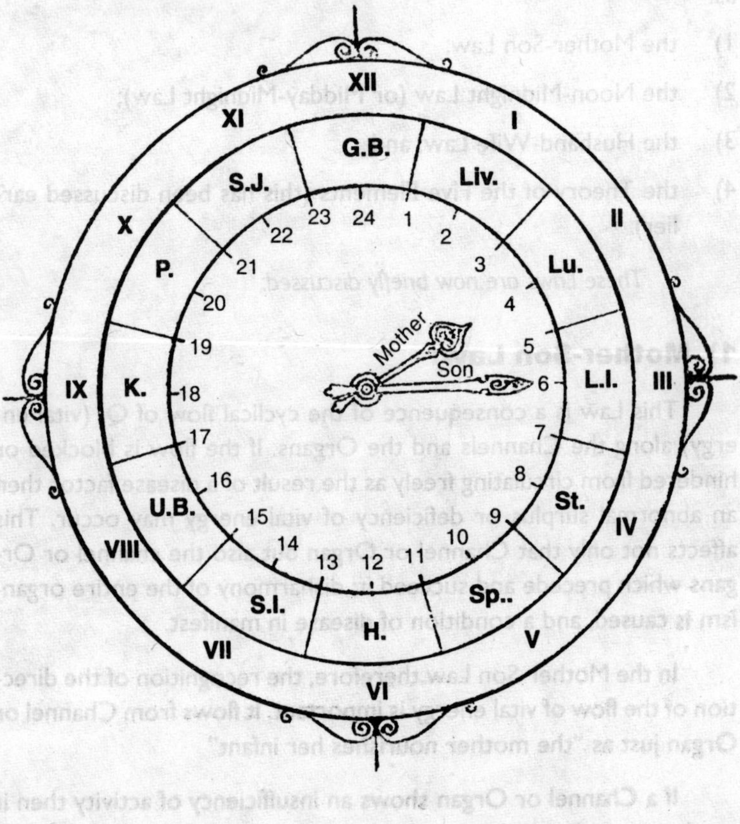

2) The Noon-Midnight Law or Midday-Midnight Law (tsu wu):

According to this Law, vital energy flows through the Twelve Channels in 24 hour cycles. Since the flow is through the Twelve Channels, it takes two hours for the surge of energy to pass through each Channel.

The ancient Chinese physicians found that, by utilizing this phenomenon, better results were obtained therapeutically.

The energy tide enters the Lung-Channel at 3.00 a.m. and leaves it to enter the succeeding Large Intestine Channel at 5.00 a.m. The vital energy flows in this manner successively through the twelve channels till it leaves the Liver Channel to re-enter the Lung Channel at 3 a.m. of the following day. This flow of energy in this time sequence is known as the **"Organ Clock".**

The times of the peak energy flow is as follows:

The Organ Clock

Channel	***Time***
Lung	3.00 a.m. — 5.00 a.m.
Large Intestine	5.00 a.m. — 7.00 a.m.
Stomach	7.00 a.m. — 9.00 a.m.
Spleen	9.00 a.m. — 11.00 a.m.
Heart	11.00 a.m. — 1.00 p.m.
Small Intestine	1.00 p.m. — 3.00 p.m.
Urinary Bladder	3.00 p.m. — 5.00 p.m.
Kidney	5.00 p.m. — 7.00 p.m.
Pericardium	7.00 p.m. 9.00 p.m.
Sanjiao	9.00 p.m. — 11.00 p.m.
Gall Bladder	11.00 p.m. — 1.00 p.m.
Liver	1.00 a.m. — 3.00 p.m.

THE ORGAN CLOCK

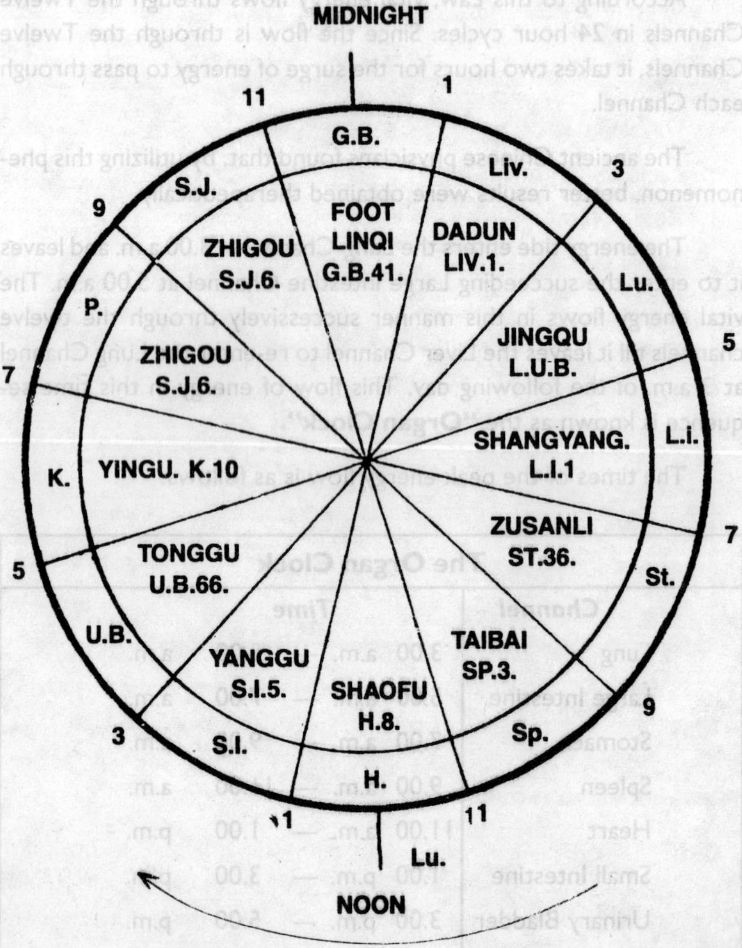

Diagram Illustrating the Horary Points

It has been stated, since ancient times, that there is a specific point in each Channel which is most effective, if used according to the relevant time of the Organ Clock. These points are known as the Horary points. The twelve Horary points are listed below:

Horary point	**Channel**
Jingqu (Lu.8).	Lung
Shangyang (L.I. 1.).	Large Intestine
Zusanli (St.36.).	Stomach
Taibai (Sp.3.).	Spleen
Shaofu (H.8.).	Heart
Yanqu (S.I.5.)	Small intestine
Tonggu (U.B.66.).	Urinary Bladder
Yingu (K.10.).	Kidney
Laogong (P.8.).	Pericardium
Zhigou (S.J.6.).	Sanjiao
Foot-Linqi (G.B.41.).	Gall Bladder
Dadun (Liv.1.).	Liver

These are not random points. A Horary point is a point on a Channel which corresponds to the same Element as the Element of that Channel e.g. Jiggqu (Lu.8). is the Metal point of the Lung. These points are in fact included among the sixty Command Points.

The Horary points are used during the appropriate period of the Organ Clock, when the vital energy is at a peak in a particular Channel. Thus when treating a disorder related to the Lung, the Horary point Jingqu (Lu.8.) may be used during the period 3.00 a.m. to 5.00 a.m. If the energy imbalance stems from a *deficiency* of energy in the Lung, this point may be punctured in the early part of this period (to take advantage of the surge of energy entering the Channel using the technique to tonification (the "*bu*" or re-enforcing method). If the imbalance is due to an *excess* in the Lung, then the point Jingqu (Lu.8.) is stimulated during the latter part of this period using the technique of sedation (the "*xu*" or reducing method).

The treatment according to the Organ Clock also corrects imbalances of vital energy involving the Organ or Channel diametrically opposite to it in the Organ Clock, e.g., treating the Urinary Bladder Channel at 3.00 p.m. at the point Tonggu (U.B. 66.) will have the opposite therapeutic influence on the Lung, into which the peak wave of energy enters at 3.00 a.m.

Even when using points other than the Horary points, particularly when a balancing of energy is carried out, timing the puncturing according to the Organ Clock may bring about more effective therapautic results.

Joseph Needham discussing the Chinese conceps of biorhythms in ***Celestial Lancets*** states:

"Some of the observations which form the stimuli for these questions are as old as the pre-Socratic and the Warring States, but so far all the resources of modern science have not sufficed to solve the basic problem, and two contrasting views have crystalised. The 'exogenous' view is that rhythmic geophysical forces provide living organism with informational inputs which regulate the timing of their recurrent processes. The 'endogenous' view is that organisms possess internal autonomous biological clocks, not immediately dependent on the external world, and constituting a self-sufficient timing mechanism. One can see that the insistence of the ancient Chinese physicians on the rhythmic character of physiological and pathological phenomena, both diurnal, monthly and annual, brought them clearly into the main line of human knowledge of this strange microcosm-macrocosm relationship. The natural ovulation and menstruation rhythm would always have given an incontestable paradigm."

Another idea was that the affairs of health and sickness proceeded according to a number of subtle rhythms, which, for effective intervention had to be caught at the right times and moments. Then again there was the conviction that man was not isolated from Nature, indeed mirrored in himself the whole, so that cylic astronomical, meteorological climatic and epidemiological factors mattered enormously for physiological and pathological processes; and there were conclusions to be drawn, and medical prognostications to be made from situations when the weather proved inappropriate for the season.

Just how right the Old Chinese bio-medical observers were in visualising regular cyclic change in the function and composition of living bodies especially those of human beings, can best be appreciated by those who are familiar with the researches of the last couple of decades on biological time keeping. A whole new department of the life sciences has opened. It has been established beyond doubt that there are a great number of inbuilt rhythms in organisms of all the phyla of the animal kingdom, and beyond that, in many plant forms also; biological clocks, as it were, which govern motion, rest and sleep, feeding and excretion, the chemical composition and the internal relations of tissue fluids, glands and other organs. The long known phenomena of plant photoperiodism may be a manifestation of such inbuilt rhythms. These may be of almost any length of time, but among the commenest are those which repeat every twenty four hours, and these are called diurnal or circadian rhythms (See page 932).

3) The Husband-Wife Law

Excess or depletion of vital energy may be accurately determined by pulse diagnosis by those who are familiar with this diagnostic method. There are twelve pulse positions on the two wrists, each wrist having three superficial and three deep pulses. Each of these position corresponds to a Channel and its related Organ. The deep pulses relate to the Zang (Ying) Organs and the superficial pulses relate to the Fu (Yang) organs.. The relative positions of these pulses are in accordance with the Theory of Zang-Fu and the Theory of the Five Elements.

The Husband-Wife Law describes the relationship between the left and right pulse positons and this has been found to be very useful in therapy. In traditional Chinese medicine the left side of the body is considered to be dominant over the right side. Hence all Organs represented as pulse positions on the left wrist are regarded as being dominant or "husband" in relation to the Organs represented on the **right** wrist, which are regarded as submissive or "wife" Organs. (women are always in the **right**!).

Pulse diagnosis is a great subjective art which takes decades to master. This is also the area of the greatest controversy in traditional Chinese Medicines. Different ancient authors describe different pulse positions. Although many attempts have been made to quantify or measure the different pulses using modern instrumentation, no satisfactory measure is yet available, as the parameters involved are very elusive.

Although most of traditional Chinese medicine bewilders the modern scientist, nevertheless scientific explanations as the *Gate control Theory* and the endorphin mechanisms are attempts to offer some degree of logical explanation. The mechanism of pulse diagnosis (or the ancient theory of angiology and splanchnology) however, seems to defy any explanation in terms of present day anatomy or physiology. A detailed discussion of pulse diagnosis is carried out in Chapter V).

I CHING

A significant work of Chinese scientific philosophy is the classic of the Book of Changes (*I Ching*). Originating from what was probably a collection of peasant omen texts; and accumulating a mass of material used in the practices of divination, it ended up as an elaborate system of symbols and their explanations, having no close counterpart in the texts of any other civilisation. Those symbols were believed to mirror, in some abstract way, all the processes of Nature. The sixty-four symbols in the system provided a set of abstract conceptions capable of explaining a large number of the events and processes of the phenomena of the natural world.

The *I Ching* is indeed a very complex book. The symbols are all made up of sets of lines (*hsiao*), some full or unbroken (*pang* lines), others broken, i.e. in two pieces with a space between (*Yin* lines). These may have been connected respectively with the long and short sticks of ancient divination procedures. By using all the possible permutations and combinations eight trigrams are formed and sixtyfour hexagrams, all known as *kua*. The *kua* are arranged in the book according to a definite order. Each *kua* is followed by a single paragraph of explanation; this is known as the *thuan* and attributed traditionally to King Wen of the early Chou dynasty (1050 B.C.). A commentary follows, usually in six sentences; this is known as the Appended Judgments (*hsi tzhu* or *hsiao tzhu*), and was traditionally attributed to Chou Kung (the Duke of Chou), another celebrated figure of the early Chou dynasty (1020 B.C.).

The canonical text originated from omen compilation which might be as old as the 7th or 8th century B.C. but did not reach its present form before the end of the Chou dynasty. With it one could know the most important 'dominant factors' or 'root causes' of events, and feel able to affirm with unshakable faith that though there was manifold complexity in the universe, there was no confusion.

Underlying these hexagrams, there is a recognition of the truth that all events are groups of relations. The diagrams themselves are clearly ideal constructions, expressing real facts, and built up from the real elements of experience, though conceptual. The diagrams are basically abstract types, substituting an ideal process for what is observed in Nature. They are formulas in which multifarious phenomena are stripped of their variety, and reduced to unity and harmony. Causation is represented as imminent change; as the constant interaction of the bipolar power of Nature, (which is never at rest, balanced or free) but is rather the mutually sustaining opposition of two forces which are essentially one energy, in the activity of which divergence and direction are inherent. The *I Ching* is a kind of translation of all natural phenomena into a mathematical language by means of a set of graphic symbols. The *I Ching* text was routinely consulted in ancient times before any therapy was administered.

Nothing could better illustrate the dialectical character of Chinese correlative thinking than the Book of Changes. No state of affairs is permanent, every vanquished entity will rise again, and every prosperous force carries within itself the seeds of its own destruction!

Superstitious practices flourished in China just as strongly as in all other ancient cultures. Divination of the future, astrology, geomancy, physiognomy, the choice of lucky and unlucky days, and the lore of spirits and demons were part of the common background of all Chinese thinkers, both ancient and medieval. The historian of science cannot simply dismiss these theories and practices, for they throw much light on ancient conceptions of the universe. Some of these magical practices led intensibly to important discoveries in the practical investigation of natural phenomena. Since magical practices and science both involve positive manual operations, the empirical element was always present in Chinese 'proto-science'. On the other hand, scepticism was an essential part of that critical spirit which was the second requirement for the development of scientific thinking, and it is worthy of remark that this sceptical element was never lacking the traditions of Chinese thought. The third element which would have been necessary for the unfolding of modern science in the purely Chinese *milieu* was the formation of mature hypothesis, couched in mathematical terms and experimentally verifiable.

It is now interesting to examine some of the metaphysics relating to the thinking of the Chinese philosophers. The disinclination of the ancient Chinese thinkers to draw any sharp distinction between spirit and matter was at one with their deeply organic philosophy, and their medical philosophy also developed on similar lines of thought.

CHINESE METAPHYSICS

Chinese thinkers did not at any time, believe in a single deity directing the cosmos, but rather thought in terms of an impersonal force (*Thien*) meaning "heaven" or "the heavens", or even better translated as "the cosmic order". Similarly, the *Tao* (or *Thin Tao*) was the "order of nature" Thus, in the traditional Chinese worldview, man was not regarded as the Lord of a Universe which was created for his use and enjoyment by God the Creator. From early times there was the conception of a *scale naturae* in which man was thought of as the highest form of life, but nevertheless without any authorisation to do what he liked with the rest of the universe. The universe did not exist specifically to satisfy man. His role in the universe was "to assist in the transforming and nourishing process of heaven and earth". And this was why, it was so often said that man formed a triad with heaven and earth (*Thien, It Jen*). It was not for man to question the way of Heaven or compete with it, but rather to harmonize his actions with it, while satisfying his own basic necessities. There are three levels, each with its own organisation expressed as : "Heaven has its seasons, man his government and the earth its natural wealth."

The keystone of Chinese philosophy is always *harmony*. The ancient Chinese sought for order and harmony throughout all natural phenomena and took this to be the ideal in all human relationships. Early Chinese thinkers were highly impressed by the recurrences and cyclical movements which they observed in Nature—the four seasons, the phases of the moon, the path of the planets, the return of the comets, the cycle of birth, maturity, decay and ultimate death in all living things. All dead matter is recycled to form new living things.

The Aristotelian doctrine of the ladder of souls in which plants were regarded as possessing a vegetative soul, and animals a vegetative and a rational soul was the thinking in the west. A very similar doctrine was taught by Hsun Tzu (Hsun Chhing) from 298 to 238. B.C. This idea is an obvious reflection on the *scala naturae*, a foreshadowing in fact, of the evolution-concept (of Charles Darwin) which ensues as soon as such a ladder is realised to exist.

According to Taoism there are three levels of life depending on their energy components, which are classified as follows:

Man : Living Qi+Sensitive Qi + Rational Qi

Animals : Living Qi+Sensitive Qi

Plants : Living Qi only.

Non-living matter possesses only material Qi.

Some later writers have, mistakenly, interpolated in man the concept of a soul needing salvation. This was not part of the rationalist Taoist philosoophy.

Thien or Heaven, was seen as an impersonal force generating the patterns of the world of Nature; phenomena were thought of as parts of a hierachy of wholes forming a cosmic pattern in which everything acted on everything else, not by mechanical impulsions, but by co-operation in accord with the spontaneous motivations of its own inner nature. Thus for the ancient Chinese, the natural world was not something hostile or evil which had to be perpetually subdued by willpower or brute force, but something akin to the greatest of all living organisms, the governing principles of which had to be understood by man, so that life could be lived in harmony with it. Organic naturalism has been, therefore, the basic attitude of Chinese culture through the ages. Man is central, but he is not the centre of the universe. Nevertheless, he has a definite function in it; a role to fulfil in the assistance of Nature, to act in conjunction with, not in disregard of, the spontaneous inter-related processes of the natural world.

There was, throughout Chinese history, a recognition that man is part of an organism far greater than himself. By corollary, he developed a great sensitivity to the possible depletion or pollution of the natural resources in the environment. For the Confucian and Taoist thinkers, morality, therefore arose out of the highest instincts of human beings themselves, not imposed by the decree of some imponderable, elusive, supernatural deity.

For the Chinese the greatest perfection has always consisted of the most perfect balance of the Yin and Yang, the female and male forces in the universe. These great opposites were always seen as relational, not contradictory; complementary, not antagonistic. This was far different from the Persian (Zoroastrian) dualism of antagonistic forces with which the Yin-Yang doctrine has often been confused.

In today's scientific *milieu* it is difficult to compare this ancient philosophy with the logic of controlled experimentation, mathematical hypothesis and their testing by statistical methods, which is the *sine qua non* of the modern scientific method.

According to modern scientific thinking, events occur in a linear fashion; that is A causes B, which with C causes D. Classical Chinese thought moves in an entirely different dimension, one in which various phenomena are interrelated as part of a pattern, According to the mythology surrounding the birth of the Chinese language, the legendary sage-ruler Fu Xi (also credited with discovering the triagrams of the *Book of Changes*) discerned the patterns in heaven and earth, and from them fashioned the characters of the Chinese language. The idea that phenomena are intertwined patterns has important ramifications. There is an overwhelming sense of context: events or objects by themselves have no meaning. Meaning is derived from participation in the patterns. From this grows the conviction that all things and events are closely interrelated.

In medical practice, these applications of philosophy appear in many ways. While the primary mode of thought in Western medicine is analytical, the causal links of Chinese medicine are exactly the opposite. Signs and symptoms are carefully analysed, integrated and synthesized, until a picture of the whole person appears.

Scientific thought has tended to place different qualities in discrete, non-interchangeable compartments. For example, mainstream Western thought posits a Mind-Body dichotomy. In this way of thinking, the Mind and Body are separate entities which sometimes interact with each other. Traditional Chinese thought on the other hand, tends to view all phenomena as existing along a transitional axis with two poles. Thus, there are differences of shades but not of kind. According to this model the Chinese realise a continuum between the two poles "Mind" and "Body", placing various aspects of human life along the line; one aspect may tend more to the "Mind-side" than another, and yet more to the "Body-side" when compared to still others. In traditional Chinese medicine, mental, emotional and physical illnesses are closely related, not absolutely different in kind. Traditional medicine takes the entire person into account, both in diagnosis and treatment. A traditional diagnosis is not a specific definition in a water-tight compartment, but rather a recognition of a shade of colour in an ever-changing dynamic spectrum of life, both in health and disease.

Another aspect of this perspective is that vital substances in the body are integrated forms of "matter" and "energy". Certain concepts such as Qi, Blood, Spirit, Essence, Fluids have attributes of both. If one realizes that some of these tend more to the energy scale of the continuum, and others more to matter, their meaning is easier to grasp.

The goals of modern science emphasize competition and confrontation. This view of the universe was very strong during the formative years of modern medicine, and has influenced it greatly. Disease is primarily due to causes that can be exterminated, extirpated or contained. When this is impossible treatment is usually unsuccessful. This is still the predominant paradigm of Western scientific medicine.

In social and personal relationships the Chinese traditionally prized harmony above all. A positive, harmonious feeling of "wellness" is the Chinese ideal of health. Disease is viewed as a disorder in the body, and treatment is directed towards properly "harmonizing" the organism. Disease and treatment are conceptualized in terms of the body. This perspective has given Chinese medicine a logical basis to manage many chronic debilitating conditions.

Modern medicine places a great deal of emphasis on a correct understanding of anatomy and how it changes during the course of a disease. Physiology and pathology are linked with structure; function is a by product of structure. Whenever possible, a disease is described by pathological changes in the biochemistry. Chinese medicine places its emphasis almost totally in function. What happens is considered more important than what a structure has come to look like. For example, the exact physical substrata of the organs were rarely subjected to intensive investigation in traditional medicine. In Chinese medicine the organs *are* the functions, and no mechanism, explicable on a structural or morphological level is necessary to prove a diagnosis.[11]

Traditional Chinese thinking made extensive use of a long chain of correspondences to rationalize the cosmos. This type of thinking was also prominent in medieval and renaissance Europe, but is no longer a part of modern western scientific thought. The correspondences, which in medicine linked aspects of the microcosm of man with the macrocosm of the cosmos, were one manifestation of the Chinese feeling for patterns and interrelationship. In some cases, however, these correspondences were based on superficial appearances and hindered the search for the truth. In other cases they were empirical lists whose underlying philosophical unity was based on metaphysical similarities. In modern science, precision of measurement and statistical analysis is the ideal. Traditional Chinese thought however, has an affinity for the abstract and metaphysical. This is due to an appreciation that in nature things are rarely black and white but instead are rather grey. This is also true of traditional medicine. The definitions, diagnostic entities, and therapeutic guidelines as presented in traditional medicine texts will, therefore, often seem imprecise to the Western scientist.

After the upsurge of modern chemistry and physics, there is the common belief that all phenomena of life and mind can be explained without hesitation by the properties of atoms, molecules and ultimately the subatomic particles themselves. Science is not the only valid form of human experience, and scientific objectivity is not the only authentic source of truth. Truth is a multidimensional experience. The confict between these two points of view has today given rise to what is popularly described as the "anti-science movement".

11 A diagnosis is a conceptual dynamic pattern of the imbalance of the vital forcas.

According to Joseph Needham of Cambridge University the whole of the anti-science movement has arisen because of the antagonism to two characteristics of Western civilisation; on the one hand the conviction that the scientific method is the only valid way of understanding and apprehending the universe, and on the other the belief that it is quite proper for the results of science to be applied in rapacious technology, often at the service of private gain ("capitalist profit").

A similar line of thought has been pursued by Frit of Capra, a nuclear physicist, in his celebrated book "*The Tao of Physics*"[12]. Essentially his argument is that: "Modern sub-atomic physics has made it quite clear that reality completely transcends all language, and that this was seen intuitively by the Taoist and Buddhist thinkers of ancient China and India. In the sub-atomic world the concepts of space and time, the idea of separable material objects, and the popular understanding of cause and effect have all lost their meaning. Mass and energy are interconvertible, radiation is not exactly waves and not exactly particles, time does not uniformly flow, changes always include the observer in an essential way, "measuring spoils the measurement", and no precise prediction is possible. Polar opposites are complementary rather than antagonistic, particles are both destructible and indestructible, matter is both continuous and discontinuous, and objects are rational events rather than substances; they are spontaneous dynamic patterns in a perpetual dance. Reality is beyond existence and non-existence. It is hardly surprising, therefore, that many minds, especially in the younger generation, are attracted to the thoughts of Lao Tzu and Chuang Chou, the strange systematisation of the *I Ching* (Book of Changes) and the insights of Tantrism and Zen Buddhism." The only unanswered question is, how it came about that the ancient and medieval thinkers of the Orient came to conclusions so close to those we have now arrived at with a great deal of effort, building gigantic cyclotrons, bubble-chambers, linear accelerators and the like, and following laboriously the traces of hadrons, electrons, photons, mesons and such particles. Even more enigmatic

12 *The Tao of Physics*, Frit of Capra, Berkley Shambhala (1975).

is, how the ancient physicians came to discover specific body points which have therapeutic effects for restoring the energy imbalances of disease. The greatest (Chinese) puzzle of them all is for us to understand today how they worked out an effective therapeutic modality such as acupuncture with so little understanding of either the anatomy or physiology of the human body.

LANGUAGE AND SEMANTIC PROBLEMS

In attempting to comprehend traditional Chinese medicine there are several difficulties.

It is not easy for even a Chinese to understand the whole of traditional Chinese medicine, less so for a foreigner whose knowledge of Chinese is only elementary. The *Huang Di Nei Jing* text (The Yellow Emperor's Classic of Internal Medicine) dated *circa* B.C. 200 is tremendous in volume and content. It consists of over forty thousand ideography amounting to a lifetime study. Several translations have been attempted by Western scholars like Ilza Veith, but there are many difficulties. Initially the translations are complicated because the manuscripts have gone through the hands of numerous copyists. These copyists were often mere scribes, rather than physicians of scholars, and consequently they have inadvertently introduced errors, inserted inappropriate characters, omitted characters, entire sentences and even paragraphs.

The classical Chinese language presents another great difficulty as there are no punctuation marks. One has to depend on the rhythm of the sentences to supply the commas and fullstops. Thus, it is difficult to search for scientific exactness in classical writings. Another difficulty is that the same Chinese character may have multiple meanings, in which case the proper interpretation depends on the context. The greatest difficulty in understanding comes from the fact that, the classical Chinese writer took great care in writing the most complicated thoughts as tersely as possible. Chinese medical and philosophical thoughts are difficult to comprehend on account of their symbolic and abstract conceptual content. During the course of its long history, the *Nei Jing* has been re-arranged, re-written, annotated, corrected, and supplemented several times. Therefore its present form must vary considerably from the traditional Chinese medicine practised in classical times. Other less important works present the same difficulties. At different periods of Chinese history acupuncture was banned; the last to do so were the Kuomindang. Books were burned and acupuncturists were banished; some like Hua Tuo (190 A.D.; even lost their lives. Much knowledge has thereby been progressively lost. Consequently, it is somewhat difficult to construct a coherent picture of traditional Chinese medicine right through history. On the other hand, an insuperable barrier to the understanding of Chinese, the oldest living language, is the use of an ideographic as opposed to an alphabetical script. Chinese is the only language which has remained faithful to ideographic, as opposed to alphabetic writing, for more than three thousand years. This may be because the language was strictly monosyllabic, and because it was non-agglutinative. There was no transition such as in Egyptian from hieroglyphic through hieratic to demotic, from which a syllabic alphabet arose. The most primitive elements of Chinese were generally *pictographs,* which were drawings reduced to essentials, conventionalised, and in time highly stylised. Naturally, concrete objects such as the heavenly bodies, animals and plants, tools and implements lent themselves most easily to such drawings. The scope of writing was latter extended to include *indirect symbols* formed by various kinds of substitutions, such as by taking parts for wholes, attributes for things, effects for causes, instruments for activities, gestures for actions, and so on, in a metaphorical way. For example, the word *fu,* meaning full or hollow, is derived from an ancient picture of an empty jar.

A third class of characters is composed of significant combinations of two or more pictographs, forming what might be called *associative compounds.* Thus *fu,* wife consists of one signs for woman, hand and broom; *fu* father consiss of the ancient signs for a hand and

13 Tantil is the next oldest

a stick; *hao* to love, or the adjective good, is a combination of the signs for a woman and a child. A particularly striking example is the word for male or man, *nan,* which shows the radicals for plough and for field, and implies 'that which employs its strength in the fields'.[14] In Chinese the sound of a pronounced word has no relation to the way in which it is written. This is true in the sense that the meaning of the written character is fixed and can be understood by speakers of different dialects, who may pronounce it in mutually incomprehensible ways. Whether a poem being read was written in the time of Christ, a thousand years later or yesterday; it is just as comprehensible and enjoyable in any case. In other cultures, where the written language has followed the spoken, a practically new literary language has evolved in the course of a few centuries. An Englishman of today can hardly go further back than three or four hundred years in his own literature; the earliest periods he can only appreciate after special philological study. To the Chinese, the literature of a millennia is open; and his unrivalled love for and knowledge of the ancient culture of his country is largely due to the peculiar genius of his literary heritage.

It is true that this old language, in spite of its ambiguity, has a concentrated, laconic, lapidary quality, making an impression of austere elegance, force and virility, unequalled by any other invented instrument of human communication. There are four tones, which increase the number of available sounds in Chinese. There is, therefore an average of some four meanings to every sound.

The invention of paper in the 2nd century was a great misfortune for China. Although the Chinese were ahead of the West in printing technology, this did not begin until the 9th century, leaving a gap of 700 years during which all manuscripts were written on perishable material instead of the durable parchment used in the West. China has often been called a 'bamboo' civilisation; there is evidence that the appreciation of the manifold uses of bamboo was already present in the Shang Dynasty. Its application was in the making of

---

14 Chaos is represented by two women under the same roof.

books of tablets, for which wood was also employed. These were probably similar to the books of the early Han which are still preserved; the lines of characters written on slips of wood or bamboo, and the slips held together with two strands of cord.

Traditional Chinese medical knowledge has many gaps, due to its chequered history and much knowledge has been lost on the way. Even among the highest respected authorities in China there is no unanimity or unitary concept of all traditional medical practices. There is, therefore, much diversity of practice of traditional Chinese medicine at the present time. The validity of this modality of therapy becomes all the more questionable in the eyes of the Western medicine practitioner.

The last chapter of Tao Te Ching aptly ends with the final conclusion:

True words are not beautiful;

Beautiful words are not true.

A good man does not argue;

He who argues is not a good man.

A wise man with no extensive knowledge is not a wise man.

The sage does not accumulate for himself.

The more he uses for others, the more he has himself.

The more he gives to others, the more he possesses of his own.

The way of Heaven is to benefit others and not to injure.

The way of the sage is to act but not to compete.

■

TRADITIONAL CHINESE DIAGNOSIS

"Nothing surpasses the examination of the pulse, for with it no errors can be committed."

— *Su Wen, Bk. 2 : 5*

With the modernisation of acupuncture in China, traditional methods of diagnosis are not in frequent use now. However, the modern practising acupuncturist must be familiar with the methodology of the traditional diagnostic procedures of Chinese medicine, at least as a historical background to his or her practice.

In several important features, the diagnostic procedures of traditional Chinese medicine are similar to those of modern Western medicine, but in certain other aspects there are many essential and remarkable differences.

To the traditional Chinese physician as well as to the Western trained physician, the patient presents his problems as a litany of symptoms. After examining the patient, it is the physician's duty to diagnose the disorder and administer the specific therapy. If this can be done without the introduction of unpleasant side-effects, the better it is for the reputation of the doctor, no less for the health of the

SCHEME OF MANAGEMENT OF DISEASE

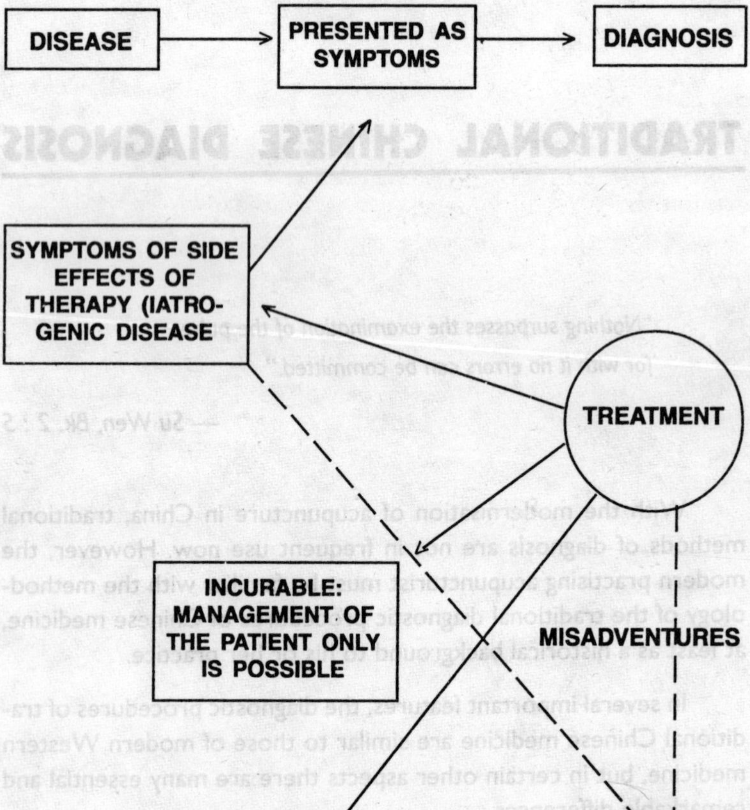

About 35% of patient get better or have amelioration of symptoms, whatever the therapy administered. This known as the PLACEBO EFFECT

patient. Side-effects are indeed undesirable. They usually set up a vicious circle complicating the clinical picture that leads to errors of diagnosis and therefore in treatment. Although the physician's aim is to cure the patient, he should do so in such a manner that side effects are minimized, if not altogether avoided.

There are many methods of therapy: for example, drug treatment; herbal therapy, acupuncture, moxibustion, chiropractic, massage, naturopathy, manipulation, surgery and so on.[1] Although all these have their sphere and range of usefulness, there is hardly any doubt that acupuncture is the modality which, considered from the effectiveness standpoint, is the least damaging to the human body. Logically this is why acupuncture should be the first line of treatment in most disorders. The use of acupuncture does not, of course, mutually exclude other modalities being combined with it, wherever or whenever such indications exist. As far as the patient is concerned, it must be realized, that he is generally not interested in the rationale of the therapy. His only objective in seeking the help of the physician is to get well. It is an error to suppose that the modern Western trained doctor obtains his success entirely through the rational applications of his scientific and technical knowledge. The doctor succeeds because he himself is a therapeutic agent. The patient sees him as a healer and the physician, consciously or unconsciously, assumes the role the patient has cast for him. The healer is the best drug. The healer is the most potent factor in the "therapy". This irrational part of medicine, whether the healer is the Western physician, the acupuncturist or any other, is an indispensable element in the healer/patient relationship, with great therapeutic potential. "It is not the needle but the man behind the needle" that initiates the cure.

In Western medicine the diagnosis is made by putting the patient through a grid of investigations; the logical order of which is as follows:

(1) The history.

1 Homoeopathy was not practised in China.

(2) Clinical examination, the steps of which in serial order are:-

(a) Inspection.

(b) Palpation.

(c) Percussion.

(d) Auscultation.

(e) Local examination of the affected part.

(f) General examination of the patient.

(3) Simple laboratory tests on urine, blood and stools are carried out as indicated.

(4) When the diagnosis is still not clear, more complicated tests such as X-rays, scanning, electromyography, cardiac catheterisation, tomography, etc., as indicated by the symptoms, are carried out.

(5) If the diagnosis is still elusive, more aggressive procedures such as biopsy, laparotomy and surgical exploration are carried out.

(6) Finally, in the event of death occurring without a diagnosis being made, the autopsy table is the last court of appeal. A diagnosis can still be made, even though the patient is dead!

In traditional Chinese medicine, there are some important differences from Western medicine, regarding the order in which diagnostic methods are carried out. Although it might appear logical to take a complete history of the case before embarking on the examination of the patient, Chinese medicine specifically prohibits elucidating the history of the illness as the first step in the procedure. The reasons are threefold:

(a) As soon as the patient reaches the consulting room, he is already anxious about his illness, and in the unfamiliar surroundings, is unable to communicate coherently the complete story of his problem, immediately.

(b) Deferment of the history taking gives time for the patient to get used to his new clinical surroundings, and enables the physician and the patient to discuss other subjects of mutual interest like the patient's family, the weather, or the latest news or gossip or some subject of mutual interest in order that they can establish a rapport and empathy with each. other, which is the *sine qua non* of good Medicine.

(c) Most of all, it gives the physician time to observe the patient as a whole, instead of directing his attention narrowly to that part of the body to which the patient assigns his symptoms.

Thus a general inspection is the first procedure, and by this means the physician obtains an unbiased picture of the total person, instead of a biased opinion diverted narrowly to the areas indicated by the symptoms only.

Even before first greeting the patient, the physician is advised to solicit the empathy of the patient by a friendly gesture of smile.

The scheme of the diagnostic steps in traditional Chinese medicine is as follows:

The Traditional Chinese Diagnostic Methods:

(1) Inspection.

(2) Auscultation[2]:

(a) Listening (The Chinese character is identical for
(b) Smelling for both these procedures.)

(3) History I (from the patient).

(4) Local Inspection.

(5) Percussion.

2 Auscultation was probably often carried out by placing the physician's ear directly on the patient's chest: this probably aided simultaneous smelling of the patient.

(6) Palpation :

(a) General Palpation (for pathological swellings and 'Alarm Points').

(b) Palpation and inspection of the affected areas, e.g., for '*Ah-Shi* Points' (Tender Points).

(c) The pulse – This is considered to be the most important step of the traditional diagnostic exercise. In modern China, the pulse diagnosis is not frequently practised. There is much debate today throughout the world on the importance and relevance of pulse diagnosis. This is the most controversial part of traditional Chinese medicine that has baffled modern scientists, who have critically investigated acupuncture.

(7) Special Tests : Naked eye examination of stools, urine, sputum and other excrescences of the patient.

(8) Special Examinations:-

(a) Eyes (conjunctiva, sclera, iris[3]).

(b) Tongue—The different areas of the tongue indicate the pathological state of the different Internal Organs.

(c) Lips.

(d) Skin.

(e) Hair (body hair, head hair).

(f) Formation of bones, teeth and nails.

(9) Ear-Inspection in a good light, palpation with the reverse end of an acupuncture needle or a matchstick.

(10) Interpretation of the dreams of the patient.

(11) History II (from a relative or a close friend). This confirms (or contradicts) the history as given by the patient. Also, it helps to ferret out information that the patient may be reluctant to

3 Iridodiagnosis — diagnosis by observing the iris changes.

convey readily such as traumatic experiences, alcoholism, indulgence in other vices, promiscuity, social diseases, family problems, financial worries, etc.

(A) Inspection, (B) auscultation and olfaction, (C) inquiring, and (D) palpation are known as "the four diagnostic methods" of traditional Chinese medicine.[4]

All the information needed by a Chinese physician in diagnosing disease and determining treatment is encompassed by these four areas of inquiry. The formulation of the diagnosis itself points to the strategy for treatment. In fact, without a proper understanding of the four methods of diagnosis, the optimal use of the Chinese therapeutic techniques, including acupuncture, is not possible.

In any form of medicine, diagnostics act as a bridge between recognition of the disease and treatment. Both diagnosis and treatment in Chinese medicine are very different from Western medicine. In traditional Chinese medicine the patterns emerge from observing the interplay of the causes of disease with the functional changes.

Several of the diagnostic techniques of Chinese medicine, such as palpation of certain groups of acupuncture points or diagnosis by tenderness at points on the ear are totally unknown to orthodox Western medicine. In Western medicine, most definitive diagnosis are made from the inside out through the use of various diagnostic tests, to examine parts of the body that are usually inaccessible by other means. The results of these tests are then reconciled with the clinical presentation of the signs and symptoms of the patient.

A. Inspection (Looking)

The first thing a physician carries out when a patient, consults him is to "look the spirit over". Spirit here means the combination

4 Pulse, Tongue and Ear diagnosis form the important clinical tripod (the 3 legs of the diagnostic stool).

of the patient's facial expression, muscle tone, posture, mode of speech and general appearance. If the disease is not serious he will be spirited, have a good complexion, clear eyes and speech, normal posture, and be quick in replying to any questions. When many diseases reach a certain point of seriousness, the patient's face becomes dark, he shows little interest in what goes on around, looses normal posture, talks slowly with frequent pauses and very often becomes dispirited. Sometimes one fact (e.g., speech or posture) of a dispirited patient will suddenly seem to change for the better, with no corresponding improvement in the other features. This is a sign that the disease has entered a very critical phase, because it represents a major imbalance in the body. It is particularly grave, if a seriously ill patient becomes euphoric.

Certain physical types are prone to certain disorders. Obese people are likely to suffer from diseases having Phlegm and Dampness as their source, while thin people suffer more easily from Deficient Yin.

Changes in skin, colour, especially of the face, are important. Frequently the appearance of colour indicates some problem with the Organ to which that colour corresponds. A pale complexion reflects a Deficient of Cold condition. If the face is dusty and swollen this signifies deficient Qi. If the face is pale and lustreless there is insufficient blood.

Red signifies the Heart. If it appears as a light tinge that shows primarily in the cheeks in the afternoons, it is a Deficient Heart. If the face is flushed and the eyes red, it is Excessive Heat. A Yellow colour comes from Dampness and Deficiency. In Chinese medicine, there are two kinds of jaundice: Yang jaundice caused by Damp Heat, where the skin is a bright orange-yellow and Yin jaundice caused by Damp Heat, where the skin is yellow Black, which is most commonly observed under the eyes, signifies Deficient Kidneys and Congealed blood.

One useful method employed in carrying out a diagnosis in infants and small children is to examine the veins on the radial side of the index finger to determine the nature and gravity of an illness. In normal children this vein turns faintly red when rubbed. Bright red signifies that the child has contracted a Hot disease. If it is purple, the Heat is very strong. If it is greenish-blue there is wind in the body. The first segment of the finger is called the Wind segment, the second the Qi segment, and the tip is called the Life segment. when the vein is only visible in the Wind segment, the disease is mild. When it reaches the Qi segment it is more severe. When the vein is visible in the Life segment, the disease is in a severe terminal stage. This technique is useful because it gives information about the condition of a patient in common childhood diseases, at an age when it is most difficult to palpate the pulses or obtain a personal history.

Inspection of the tongue occupies a prominent place in traditional Chinese diagnosis. The tongue is closely connected (through the internal channels) with the Heart and Spleen, and therefore reflects the condition of the blood. For diagnostic purposes, the body of the tongue is divided into areas representing various Organs, as shown in the illustration (page 410).

Localization of pathological change in a specific area of the tongue usually signifies a disorder of the corresponding Organ.

In diagnosis, changes in the shape, coating and body of the tongue are all important. The significance of these changes is expressed in terms of the Six Excesses and Eight Diagnostic Methods. When the tongue is examined, it must be done in as close to natural light as possible. Otherwise, there may be an incorrect observation of the colour of the body or coating. It is also necessary to ascertain whether the patient has eaten or drunk anything (e.g., beetroot, tea, coffee), that would affect the colour of the coating.

The healthy tongue is pinkish red, neither too obese nor too pointed, slightly moist with no fur or a thin white coating and usually without crevices. If a person has a tongue of this description it signifies that any disease, which he may have contracted, is mild.

The shape and the physical alterations of the tongue are the first things to look for. An obese tongue, with indentations of teeth along the edges, indicates either Deficient Qi or a surfeit of Dampness in the body. Differentiation depends on the coating. A white, moist coating reflects Deficient Qi, a greasy coating indicates Dampness. A tongue that is thin and narrow indicates either insufficiency of Yin fluids, or both deficient Qi and Yin. If the body of the tongue is red, then the disorder is that of Deficient Yin alone. If it is pale, both the Qi and Yin are weak.

Red eruptions on the tip or the edges of the tongue indicate intense Heat. Red or purplish eruptions on the sides of the tongue (in the Liver area) indicate Congealed Blood, pain, or tension, due to disturbances of the spreading functions of the Liver. They are often observed in menstrual disorders of women.

Cleavages in the tongue, either superficial or deep, indicate the presence of Heat or dryness in the body. In a small minority of cases it is congenital and is, therefore, not significant.

The colour of the tongue changes, depending upon the degree of Heat in the body and upon the condition of the Qi and Blood. A normal tongue is lighter; it is called pale; if darker it is called red, and if still darker it is called deep-red. Sometimes the tongue contains areas that are dark-blue or purple.

A pale tongue signifies Deficient Blood and Qi. If it is very pale, it may be a symptom of Interior Cold. A red tongue indicates the presence of Interior, Deficient Heat. In conditions of Excessive Heat the entire tongue is red, whereas with Deficient Heat only the tip is coloured. If the tongue is dark red, the Heat is located relatively deeply in the body. A deep-red tongue with ulcers is symptomatic of Fire in the Heart. When the tongue manifests purple or dark blue patches, there is an impediment to the flow of Qi and Blood. If these patches are localized, then the disorder is limited to that Organ of correspondence in the body.

Healthy people have a thin coating on the tongue. Changes in the appearance and colour of this coating are helpful in diagnosis. A normal tongue has a slightly moist coating. If there is too much moisture, such that there is a semi-transparent film over the tongue, the coating is called wet. This indicates the presence of Dampness in the body. Excessive dryness of the coating indicates on insufficiency of fluids (this is one of the first symptoms of this condition). If one can see the tongue through the coating, the coating is called thin. This signifies that the Excess indicated by the coating (usually Dampness, Heat or Cold) is mild. If the coating is very thick and appears to have a greasy layer upon it, it is called a greasy tongue. This characteristic indicates severe Dampness, or indigestion. If the Yin liquids are seriously depleted or the Stomach Qi is weak, the tongue will have no coating at all. This is called a bare tongue.

The colour of the coating is one of the most important indicators in determining the nature of a disease in the body. The coating is usually thin and white in a healthy person. If a patient has this type coating, the disease is not serious, or is still at the Exterior stage. A white, wet coating indicates Cold. A white, dry coating indicates that the Cold Excess is in the process of transforming into Heat. A thick, greasy, white coating indicates the presence of Phlegm and Dampness. A yellow coating signifies Heat.

In arriving at a diagnosis, many other parts of the body come under scrutiny. The hair[5] reflects the health of the Kidneys and the Blood. Thus, thinning, dry hair indicates Deficient Kidney Qi or weak Blood. The differences in colour and moisture of the lips are similar to those of the body of the tongue. If the corners of the lips do not close firmly and the groove between the nose and the upper lip is shrunken, then the Qi is close to exhaustion and the disease is probably terminal. Drooling saliva is due to either a Deficient Spleen or Heat in the Stomach. Red, swollen, or bleeding gums are caused by Stomach Fire. Pale swollen gums and loose teeth can be traced to Deficient Kidneys.

Inspection of the skin changes in the ears, is also useful in diagnosis.

5 Head hair.

B. Auscultation and Olfaction (Listening and Smelling)

A physician should note the patient's breathing, manner of speech and cough, as these are important indicators of the patient's health. In Deficient diseases, the breathing is shallow and soft; rough, heavy breathing occurs in diseases of Excess. Asthmatic wheezing is divided into two categories. Wheezing is characterized by rales and rhonchi during breathing, with the exhalations being particularly forceful. In cases of Deficient wheezing (the Kidneys not retaining the Qi is the main problem) the sound is low and there is more difficulty inhaling. Speech and coughs are differentiated as Excessive or deficient in the same manner. A cough that produces gurgling sounds in the throat is due to Phlegm or Dampness. A dry, hacking cough is caused by Dry Heat in the Lungs.

The nose is also an important diagnostic tool. In Excessive Hot diseases the various secretions and excretions of the body have a very foul odour; while in Excessive Cold diseases they may smell like putrified fish. Congestion of food in the gastro-intestinal tract may cause the patient to have a offensive breath.

The odours which correspond to the Organs through the 5 elements have two principal diagnostic functions. First, the physician may smell them[6] and distinguish which Organs are affected. Second, patients themselves may smell them[7] serially and be able to state if the particular Organ in question is recovering or otherwise.

C. Inquiring, Asking (Interrogation of the patient)

Asking the patient about his or her past medical history, present condition and life-style provides information which serves as important clues for the diagnosis. It must, however be combined with other methods of diagnosis, in order to correct the patient's subjective bias, and to elucidate information the patient does not readily di-

6 Smell emanating from the patient.

7 Testing the smell of the patient on selected natural substances.

vulge. Traditionally, there are several areas on which the Chinese physicians concentrate when interviewing patients. The important areas of inquiry are:

1) *Chills and Fever:* Chills and fever appearing simultaneously indicate exterior conditions. If the chills are stronger, it is a Wind-Cold disease; if the opposite, it is Wind-Hot condition. Alternating chills and fever is the primary symptom of half exterior disorders. Continuing fever without chills indicates that the disease has moved inwards. When the Heat has entered the Stomach and Intestines, there is a continual fever that rises in the evenings. Generally the fever increases during the night the disorder is grave. A patient with severely deficient Yin condition develops a low grade daily, or a feeling of heat in the soles and palms in the afternoons or evenings, which subsides late at night after the patient sweats heavily. Irregular periods of low fever accompanied by lassitude indicates Deficient Qi. Chills and coldness in the limbs are symptoms of Deficient Yang of the Kidneys.

2) *Perspiration:* If, during Exterior disorders perspiration is absent, this indicates that the excess has confined the Protective Qi, preventing the body from expelling the Excess. If there is sweating but no corresponding lowering of the fever, this indicates that the Protective Qi is too weak to expel the disease. If there is an excess of perspiration during the day, this is called spontaneous sweating and indicates Deficient Qi. Heavy sweating at night signifies Yin. Continuous sweating throughout the day producing a cold and clammy skin is a very bad prognostic sign.

3) *Head, Special Sense Organs and other parts of the Body:* Acute headaches are usually caused by exogenous Excesses, while chronic, recurring headaches are due to internal factors. Violent headaches indicate Excessive conditions, and dull headaches Deficient conditions. Headaches that increase in intensity after encountering cold are caused by Wind and Cold. Those which exacerbate in hot environments are usually caused by hyperactive Liver-Yang. When the head feels encased in a vice, the

cause is Dampness. Frontal headaches are associated with yang Brightness (Stomach and Large Intestine), and those concentrated behind the hairline with Greater Yang (Small Intestine and Bladder). These names refer to the channels which traverse that particular area of the head. Headaches at the vertex of the scalp are usually caused by Liver dysfunction. Often eye symptoms also occur in Liver dysfunctions.

In Chinese Medicine there are three kinds of vertigo. The first, related to hyperactive Liver Yang, feels as if one is walking unsteadily on a ship. In the second, associated with Wind and Phlegm, all objects seem to be spinning around. The third type, is caused by insufficient Blood and Qi, and it is characterized by dizziness, blurring of vision, and a ringing in the ears (tinnitus).

It is most important to ask the patient to identify any parts of the body that feel uncomfortable or painful. These points can be significant in themselves as identifying a local disorder, or they can reflect disease elsewhere in the channel along which they are located. Pain that moves around is due to Wind or Stagnant Qi. Pain which remains in one place is caused by Cold, Dampness or Coagulated Blood. Pain which lessens upon pressure or massage is Deficient. Conversely, pain which intensifies upon pressure is Excessive. Insufficiency of Blood and Qi can cause soreness in the muscles and tendons. Dampness may cause the body to feel heavy, swollen and lethargic.

4) *Urine and Stools:* An excess of urine especially at night is due to Deficient Kidney Yang which, if severe, can lead to incontinence. Spares urine can be caused by Heat drying up the liquids in the body or by Qi of the Bladder being too weak to pass urine Deficiency of the Kidney can result in dribbling of urine, impotence and amenorrhoea.

When Heat enters the body from outside and then penetrates the Stomach and Intestines, the abdomen feels distended painful and constipation results. In Deficient Yin conditions where there is an absence of fluids, constipation occurs without a feeling of distension. In old age. the body loses the energy to expel stools; this is called Cold constipation. Faecoliths may result, which may have to be mechanically removed.

Massive and sudden diarrhea is a condition of Excess. A Chronic diarrhea results from a Deficient Spleen. Frequent diarrhea with small stools each time and a feeling immediately afterwards that one has to evacuate again as in dysentery (tenesmus), is caused by Damp Heat in the Intestine. If diarrhea is accompained by pain in the abdomen which diminishes after the diarrhoea, the cause is usually congestion of food. This arises from a disorder affecting the Spleen-Stomach functions of transformation and transportation of food. If pain occurs under any kind of emotional stress and is not relieved by diarrhea, the cause is probably an imbalance between the Spleen and the Liver. Diarrhea every morning at dawn (called five o'clock or cock-crow diarrhoea) is caused by a deficient Spleen and Kidney Qi. It is most common among the elderly.

5) *Diet and Appetite:* Different types of thirst indicate disorders related to different Excesses. Not being thirsty or desiring warm drinks, indicates cold. A strong desire for cold drinks indicates Heat. The absence of thirst, or only a slight thirst, or spitting out immediately after drinking indicates Dampness. This occurs in patients who have a weak digestion.

Usually a good appetite shows that a disease is not too serious. Lack of appetite with a distended feeling after meals in caused by either a weak Spleen or a Damp Heat in the Sanjiao. Heat in the Stomach may cause a patient to overeat and be constantly hungry, and have borborygmy. The presence of certain tastes in the mouth has diagnostic significance (as determined by the correspondences of the Five Phases). Bitterness is associated with Heat; sweetness or blandness with Dampness or a week spleen; insipid tastes accompany congestion of food; sour tastes are associated with dysfunction of the Liver.

6) *Chest and Abdomen:* The basic principles governing pain in these areas are the same as those previously described for the head area. A feeling of compression in the chest accompanied by shortness of breath is due to Deficient Qi. A swollen and painful chest and sides indicate the dysfunction of the Liver or Gall Bladder. A feeling of distension in the abdomen that is relieved by belching or passing in the abdomen that is relieved by belching or passing gas is caused by the stagnation of either Qi or food.

7) *Eyes and Ears:* The eyes are the sensory organs associated with the Liver. Red, inflammed eyes are caused by a hyperactive Liver Yang. Loss of vision accompanied by dry, dull eyes is usually symptomatic of Deficient Liver and Kidney Yin. The ears are the sense organs of the Kidneys. A progressive loss of hearing or tinnitus is usually caused by a weakness of the Kidneys. The paths of the Lesser Yang channels (those associated with Sanjiao and Gall Bladder) travel around and into the ears. Hot diseases of exogenus origin often enter the body along these pathways and may cause a loss of hearing, which is sometimes permanent.

8) *Sleep:* Insufficiency of Blood in the Heart, or disturbances of the Spirit may result in insufficient sleep, much dreaming and palpitations of the Heart. If the Heart Yin is deficient, the person is irritable and finds it very difficult to fall asleep. Excessive sleepiness may be caused by heat in the Pericardium phlegm obstructing the opening of the energy pathways into the Heart, or a general Deficient Yang.

9) *Medical History:* By careful inquiry into the patient's past history a physician can place the results of the examination in proper perspective. The physician should pay careful attention to minor symptoms from the history that give certain clues as to the cause of the present illness. A detailed description of the progress of the disease and all medication taken prior to the time of the examination should be elucidated. Previous treatment should be noted carefully.

10) *Lifestyle and Habits:* These aspects should be ascertained in detail since they may prove an invaluable aid in diagnosing an illness. The whole person must be taken into account when making a diagnosis.

D. Palpation

Palpation in Chinese Medicine takes three principal forms. One is the palpation of local areas on the body that are painful, inflammed, swollen, or hot, in order to determine the nature of a local disorder. A swelling which is hot and painful belongs to the Yang type and is caused by Heat. That which is cold to the touch is usually a product of dampness and is therefore classified as Yin. Hard swellings or nodules are congealed Blood, while those with the sensation of elasticity whose borders are ill-defined are related to stagnant Qi. In fevers, when the palm is hotter than the back of the hand there is Deficient Yin; if the back of the hand is hotter, there is overactive Yang or excessive Heat.

The second form of palpation used in diagnosis is at specific acupuncture points on the front and back of the trunk. Usually, a point where the physician senses a "collapsed" feeling or which is tender to the touch is most likely to indicate disease in the related Internal Organ (Mu and Shu points).

The last category of diagnosis by palpation in Chinese Medicine is palpation of the pulse. There are many places on the body to palpate the pulse (each Organ has at least one) but traditionally it is the pulse on the Lung channel radial pulse on the wrist which is the principal site for diagnosis. This pulse, although specifically related to the Lungs and controlled by the Heart (as are all pulses), nonetheless reflects the condition of the Organs. Diagnosis by pulse is a subtle art and, even more than other diagnostic procedures, requires an enormous amount of concentration and experience in order to acquire the sensitivity necessary to obtain the correct results. While Chinese physicians agree that the pulse is best used in conjunction with the other diagnostic methods, physicians well-skilled in pulse diagnosis may discover an enormous amount of information about their patients by this method alone. A student should take as many pulses as possible because actually palpating the pulses is the only way to be proficient in pulse diagnosis.

Autopsy and dissection were prohibited in traditional Chinese Medicine, as the human body was considered sacred. Surgery, therefore, was not considered an important aspect of medicine. Surgery was mainly used for producing eunuchs for the imperial court and for treating war injuries, Surgery was the ultimate method used in treating an illness, when all other therapeutic methods had failed.

CAUSES OF DISEASE

The causes of disease are divided into four categories: (A) those originating from outside the body; (B) those arising inside the body; (C) miscellaneous causes, whose origins are neither outside nor inside the body; (D) Phlegm.

(Ancient treatises also described parasitic infestations, for example with intestinal worms, as a common cause of disease. Ancient physicians were also very familiar with trauma as a cause of disease particularly because, then as now, war and strife were frequent occurrences. Many ancient classics also describe quite accurately malnutrition and many food deficiency disorders. Boils, carbuncles, abscesses, new growths and enlargements of organs, particularly the malarial and bilharzial splenomegalies were well known to the physicians of ancient China).

When the different vital forces of the body are in a harmonious balance, there is positive health. When this balance, is disturbed, there is disease. The development of disease depends on two factors: the immunity level of the body, and the virulence of the disease causing agents. If the body is in positive health there is no way for disease to gain a foothold. Disorders may also arise from internal disharmonies without being caused by exogenous influences. In Chinese medicine much emphasis is placed on the prevention of disease by the promotion of general health and the early treatment of internal disharmonies.

In Chinese medical terminology, the physiological activities of the Organs, the Qi, and the Blood, all of which have the power to resist disease, are called the Normal Qi. The course of a disease is seen as a battle between the Normal Qi and the disease causing factors. Treatment of the disease, at any point in time, depends on the dynamic interaction between these two forces. Disorders which are primarily caused by internal disharmony require appropriate treatment so as to properly re-establish normal functioning of the affected Internal Organs.

A. The Six Excesses

The Six Excesses are the extrinsic causes of disease.

The Six Excesses are (1) Wind, (2) Cold, (3) Heat, (4) Dampness, (5) Dryness and (6) Summer Heat. They conform to the Five element correspondences (both Heat and Summer Heat correspond to Fire). The term Excess means "Abnormality, Evil, or Pernicious Influence". When normal environmental forces become excessive (e.g. a particularly cold spell in winter), or occur unseasonably (e.g., a warm spell in the middle of the winter, they may cause disease. However, because of individual physical make up and a latency period in some disease, different people may have different diseases at the same time or the same disease at different times. Clinical differentiation of the Excesses is made on the basis of symptoms, not tests aimed at discovering a precisely defined disease-causing agent. That is to say, the disease is described in terms of the body's response, rather than in terms of an autonomous disease entity. Two people may suffer from the same "disease" (in the Western medical sense) at the same, time, yet, because of differences in their environment and constitution they may exhibit completely different symptoms.

Sometimes an imbalance among the Internal Organs will lead to symptoms similar to those of an externally caused illness. It is usually possible to differentiate between symptoms caused by external Excess with those caused by an imbalance within the body itself from the history of onset of the disorder.

The Excesses. (with the exception of Heat) are each related to a particular season and associated with either Yin (which injures Yang forces) or Yang (which injures Yin). The symptomatic manifestations of each Excess resemble the characteristics of their seasonal counterparts in nature. (The original relationships between the Excesses and the seasons were based on the weather patterns in ancient China, and do not necessarily hold true for other parts of the world. In the Nei Jing it was recommended for each physician to familiarise himself with the seasonal epidemiology of different illnesses in his area.)

1) *Wind (Spring Yang):* Diseases caused by Wind arise suddenly and change their symptoms quickly. They may be accompanied by symptoms of muscle spasm, vertigo, pruritus or a pain, which often changes location. Wind diseases of an exogenous origin usually affect the skin, head, pharynx and lungs first. Wind is the Excess which carries others Excesses into the interior of the body.

   Internally, when the Liver (Wood -Wind) Yang is hyperactive, dizziness and convulsions occur; similar symptoms accompany high fevers. Both are caused by exterior Wind travelling to the interior of the Body.

2) *Cold (Winter Yin):* The principal symptom of this Excess is that the whole body or a part of it feels cold. Cold causes fluids to congeal in the body; this causes pain. Pain is caused by the obstruction in the flow of Qi or Blood. Cold causes material substances to coagulate in the channels; this causes cramps and spasms. When Cold diseases are present, the body excretions (mucus, tears, phlegm, urine, stools) are white or clear and watery.

   When the Yang Qi is weak, symptoms similar to those caused by Cold may occur.

3) *Heat (Yang):* The main characteristic of Heat is that the body or

a part feels hot. Heat easily injures the body fluids. Thus, the tongue and stools become dry and the patient is thirsty. Heat can cause the Blood to travel outside the channels, leading to haemorrhages or rashes. In the presence of Heat-caused diseases, body excretions are dark or yellow, sticky and foul smelling. Sometimes, the act of expulsion causes Heat in that area of the body. Often, diseases caused by one or the other Excesses, transform into Heat within the body. Heat is also a synonym for Fire.

4) *Dampness (Long Summer Yin)*: This Excess often appears during damp weather or when a person comes into contact with moisture for a prolonged period of lime. Dampness is sluggish and stagnating. Diseases caused by this Excess take a long time to be cured. When Dampness is on the external parts of the body the patient feels anxious, the limbs heavy, and the head feels swollen. When Dampness invades the muscles and joints, all movements become painful and oedema of the affected parts occur. Dampness tends to attack the Spleen. When the spleen's transforming and transporting functions are weak. Interior Dampness may result. (Damp diseases occurring during the Winter are liable to be very serious disorders).

5) *Dryness (Autumn Yang):* Dryness attacks the fluids of the body and may result in dry skin, chapped lips, hacking cough, constipation. When the body's Yin substances are seriously depleted (as in the later stages of a long febrile disease) similar symptoms may appear.

6) *Summer Heat (Summer Yang):* The primary characteristic of Summer Heat is fever with pronounced sweating. This injures the Yin and the Qi. Dampness almost always accompanies this Excess.

B. The Seven Emotions

The seven Emotions are excessive happiness, anger, worry, pensiveness, sadness, fear, and anxiety. They are linked with the Five

Elements system of correspondences, (both worry and sadness correspond to Metal; both fear and anxiety correspond to Water). Apart from the Seven Emotions, frustration upsets the free-flowing nature of the liver and, not surprisingly, often leads to anger. These are normal emotions which can lead to illness if sustained for a long period of time. These emotions either adversely affect those Organs associated with the same Element or upset the Yin-Yang balance in the body. Emotion related diseases, which might be labelled psychosomatic in Western medicine, are in Chinese medicine internal imbalances.

C. Causes Which Are Neither Outside Nor Inside (Miscellaneous Causes)

These refer to syndromes due to aetiologies that are neither Excesses nor Emotions. Inconsistency in the quantity, quality or time of eating causes indigestion and related diseases. Quality here refers both to the hygienic level of food and to the traditional classification of foodstuffs as either Cold or Hot. Each Organ is associated with a corresponding taste in the Five Element system. Too much of one taste will injure the corresponding Organs.

Sexual activity and the reproductive functions are linked with the Kidneys in men, and with the Kidneys and liver in women. When excessive sexual activity occurs, the Yin and Yang of these Organs may be damaged. If a woman gives birth too frequently, the Ren channel may be injured, resulting in menstrual problems. The same is true of manual labour; when performed in moderate amounts it benefits the body; when carried out in excess, the body is injured.

D. Phlegm

In traditional Chinese medicine the word Phlegm does not refer exclusively to the secretions that are coughed up from the Lungs, but also to stagnant fluids in the body. Traditionally, its formation is due to dysfunction in the water metabolism, especially in the transforming-transporting functions of the Spleen. Therefore, the Sp!een is the source of Phlegm. When the water in the body becomes stagnant, it transforms into Phlegm. There are many possible reasons for this stagnation, but the most common causes are Deficient Qi and Excess, Heat. Phlegm is both the result of dysfunction and the cause of further disease. When Phlegm collects in the lungs there is coughing and wheezing with profuse expectoration. When it enters the Stomach there is nausea and vomiting. When it invades the channels local swellings occur. When it surrounds the Heart delirium ensues.

(The concept of Phlegm caused disorders includes what is described in modern scientific medicine as endocrine disorders, metabolic disorders, enzymatic and other biochemical disorders).

In practice the various causes of disease often overlap and occur together. Diagnosis is directed towards determining the relationships which exist at a particular time between the different disease causing factors and their effects on the Organs, Channels and Tissues.

The Eight Principles of Chinese Diagnosis *(Ba Kang).*

After the examination of the patient, the physician classifies the illness according to the following scheme which embodies the "Eight Principles of Diagnosis" called "Be Kang" in Chinese.

Xu	I. YIN	3. Interior	5. Cold	7. Deficiency
Shi	2. YANG	4. Exterior	6. Hot	8. Excess

(This is a clinical classification).

The diagnosis in traditional Chinese medicine gives a conceptual picture of the basic dysfunctions of the body and suggests a basis for rational treatment. The first stage in the screening process utilizes the Eight Diagnostic Methods. There are four pairs of broad polarities that provide a preliminary understanding of the nature and intensity of the disease. The Eight Diagnostic Methods (also known as the Eight Principles) are Exterior/interior (depth of disease), Hot/Cold (nature of disease), Excessive/Deficient (strength of disease versus the resistance) and Yin/Ying (overall quality of the disorder). These parameters enable the physician to establish in general terms the location, quality and intensity of a disease. After this is done, other diagnostic methods are applied to identify the disease and select the appropriate treatment. It must be remembered that diseases are complex and ever changing. Sometimes two different or even contradictory parameters, will appear simultaneously. As the disease progresses, it may move from one parameter to another. It is, therefore important to monitor the changes and tailor specific treatment to fit the particular patient at that particular time. Consequently, Chinese physicians continuously adjust and modify their treatment as the disease evolves.

I/II Exterior – Interior

These features delineate the location of disease. The disease process evolves primarily in one of two ways. In the first, the body's balance between Yin and Yang is upset. These are always Interior diseases. In the second, an Excess enters the body from outside and the body reacts to it. Such diseases usually being Exterior disorders, may progress to become Interior. These two processes are not mutually exclusive. In fact, if there is no weakness in the body's Exterior defences, no Excess can penetrate, Here the skin, flesh, and channels are defined as Exterior, while the Internal Organs are defined as Interior.

Exterior symptoms include chills, fever, headaches, sore limbs, running nose, coughing, sore throat and a floating pulse. Ordinarily, Excesses first encroach upon the body through the skin or nose, which are both related to the Lungs. If the Excess succeeds in penetrating these outer defences there must be a weakness in the Protective Qi. Chills may result, which is the definitive symptoms of Exterior disorders. Sweating is an important indicator of the strength of the Protective Qi. If the Excess is in the outer and cephalic parts of the channels, headaches and soreness result. This is also reflected in a floating pulse. Some of the common clinical presentations are now discussed.

Exterior Cold: The chills are more pronounced than the fever; the coating on the tongue is white and moist; head and body pains are severe; mucus is clear or white, the throat may be inflammed and the voice raspy, the pulse is floating and tight.

Exterior Hot: The fever is high, the coating on the tongue is dry and yellow, the throat is vary painful and inflammed, mucus from the nose or lungs in yellow and congealed. The pulse is floating and rapid.

Exterior Excess: There is no perspiration. This usually occurs in a Wind-Cold disease when the Cold Excess is usually so strong that the sweat glands are obstructed.

***Exterior Deficiency*:** There is perspiration without the usual corresponding reduction of the fever. This is due to a weakness in the Protective Qi, which is not able to regulate the skin temperature.

Interior symptoms, as distinct from Exterior symptoms, are those involving the Organs and deeper tissues of the body. They may arise from Excesses located in the Exterior portions of the body which penetrate the external defences and enter the Organs, or from Excesses which directly attack the Organs themselves. Other frequent causes include emotional imbalance, improper living habits, alcoholism and addiction to drugs. All these disturb the harmony of the Organs.

There are some symptoms that commonly indicate the presence of Interior diseases rather than Exterior disorders. These include fever without chills, a feeling of coldness in the body, irritability, pain in the trunk, vomiting and changes in the tongue proper. The appearance of the stools and urine, and the presence of severe thirst (usually normal in Exterior conditions) are important signs in determining the nature of an Interior disease. A comparison between Interior Cold and Interior Hot diseases will serve to give a general idea how these symptoms are actually used in a differential diagnosis.

***Interior Cold*:** Typical symptoms include a pale complexion, sensitivity to cold at the extremities, no thirst or a desire to drink hot liquids, pain in the abdomen which diminishes upon the application of heat, copious and clear urine, watery stools, pale tongue with a white coating and a deep, slow pulse.

Interior Hot: Common symptoms include a flushed complexion, fever, irritability, thirst cold beverages, sweating, scanty dark urine, constipation or diarrhea containing pus or blood, a dark red tongue with a yellow coating and a quick pulse.

In the incubation period of an interior disorder and in diseases due to external factors, there is a period when symptoms are partially Interior. This occurs when there are alternating chills and fever, a fullness in the loins and chest, irritability and restlessness, nausea, lack of appetite, a bitter taste in the mouth, a dry parched mouth, vertigo and a wiry pulse. A carefully selected plan of treatment, focussing upon the channels which traverse the middle of the extremities, is required. Treating these channels (Liver, Gall Bladder, Sanjiao, Pericardium) allays at the symptoms of the half Exterior-half Interior level of the body.

If an Excess attacks both the Exterior and Interior portions of the body simultaneously, or if an Exterior disease complicates a pre-existing Interior condition, these two cases come into effect at the same time. In such instances the selection of points will depend on careful evaluation of the circumstances, with a decision as to the relative importance of each group of symptoms.

III/IV Hot-Cold

When the body is attacked by a Yang Excess, or when the Yin substances are depleted, then Hot symptoms develop. When the body is attacked by a Yin Excess or the Yang activities are weak, Cold symptoms develop.

***Hot*:** A flushed face, red eyes, heat in any part of the body, fever, irritability, thirst for cold liquids, constipation, scanty dark urine, dark red tongue, rapid pulse, dark putrid or thick secretions may occur.

Cold: A pale complexion, a quiet patient, tendency to curl up. feeling of cold, in many parts of the body, or a genera! feeling of cold lack of thirst or desire for hot liquids, severe localized pain, diarrhoea, copious clear urine, slow pulse and a clear or white phlegm are the common symptoms.

When different parts of the body are in different states, of disease the Hot and Cold symptoms may appear simultaneously. When either Hot or Cold is severe, 'false' symptoms may appear. In a Hot disease this usually takes the form of cold in the limbs because the Yang energy is blocked inside the trunk and cannot circulate in the limbs. In Cold diseases a flushed face, sore throat and irritability may appear due to the rising of the weak Yang. In such cases of disease the majority of the symptoms, particulary the appearance of the tongue and thirst factors, will accurately reflect the state of the illness.

V/VI Excessive – Deficient

These states describe the degree of the body's resistance (Normal Qi) in response to the virulence of the disease. If the disease occurs because of a weakness in the body defences rather than because of the strength of the Excess, the disease is called an Excessive disease. If the condition of the body is very weak and that of the disease process not necessarily strong or if the disease is caused primarily by internal disharmony or weakness, it is called Deficient. Generally speaking, acute disorders tend to be Excessive and chronic disorders are Deficient.

Excessive: Symptoms of Excess vary widely depending on the type and location of the disease. However, when compared to Deficient diseases, the following symptoms are important, the voice is normal or louder than normal, breathing is heavy, if Ah-Shi points exist in the chest or abdomen they are felt as hard or elastic lumps, which react painfully to pressure, the coating on the tongue is thick and the pulse has great force.

Note: An excess does not invariably lead to an Excessive condition, nor are all Excessive conditions caused by excesses. An excess refers to certain disease-causing factors. Excessive or a symptom of Excess, refers to the degree of the body resistance in relation to the intensity of the disease process.

Deficient: Deficient symptoms vary depending on whether it is the Qi, Blood, Yin or Yang of a particular Organ that is affected. However, when contrasted with symptoms of Excess, symptoms of Deficiency may be summarized as follows: the patient is quiet and withdrawn, the voice is soft and low, the complexion varies from sickly yellow to ghastly pale, breathing is light, pain diminished upon massage or pressure, swellings are soft, there is a scanty coating on the tongue and the pulse is weak and imperceptible.

As a disease progresses, changes occur with respect to these two signs and if conditions are appropriate, they can both appear simultaneously. In such cases an accurate diagnosis is essential to carry out the proper treatment of the patient.

VIII/VIII Yin-Yang

Yin and Yang are the larger clinical features within which the others are subsumed. Exterior, Hot, and Excessive symptoms are Yang; interior, Cold, and Deficient symptoms are Yin. The classic Yang symptoms correspond to Excessive and Hot conditions, while the classic Yin symptoms correspond to Deficient and Cold condition. Of course, all diseases include both Yin and Yang imbalances in their aetiology.

In traditional Chinese medicine diseases are broadly divided into **Shi** (diseases characterized by hyperactivity) and ***Xu*** (diseases characterized by hypoactivity) and the table of correspondences given above shows the essential points of difference. In diseases of a Shi nature, there is preponderance of the Yang element, manifestation of external warmth such as flushed face or fever, and general hyperactivity. This is usually seen in acute conditions where the patient's general condition is stable. In diseases of a *Xu* nature the reverse is true; there is preponderance of the Yin element the patient is pale and cold, and he feels listless and apathetic owing to general hypo-function. This is usually the case in chronic disorders. In Western medicine too, we clinically classify a patient as acute or chronic, hyperactive or hypoactive, extrovert or introvert, hypertrophic or atrophic, hypertensive or hypotensive, etc.

The other principles of diagnosis Commonly used are:

a) Differentiation of the syndrome according to the Theory of Zang - Fu.

b) Differentiation of the syndrome according to the Theory of Jing - Luo.

The method of therapy used, whether acupuncture, moxibustion or herbal therapy, is then decided on the basis of the disease classification according to the Eight Principles of Diagnosis described above. If acupuncture is the therapy of choice in a particular patient, then the disease classification serves as a pointer to the technique of needle insertion and manipulation. For example, if the disperse is Shi (hyperactive) in nature, the Xie (reducing) method of needle insertion is used. If it is Xu (hypoactive) in nature, the Bu (reinforcing) method is used. This is known as **The Great law of Flu-Xie.**

The therapy is first discussed with the patient and with the guardians before treatment is commenced, in order to obtain the co-operation of everyone concerned and thereby ensuring a better psychological framework for the cure.

The principles of diagnosis used in traditional Chinese medicine are the result of clinical observations; made on billions of patients over a millennia of clinical practice. As in the procedures of Western medicine (e.g. electro-cardiography, electro-encephalography, auscultation of the heart, etc.) these traditional diagnostic methods were not always the products of rationalization about disease, but grew out of empirical observations on the relations between various diseases and their protean manifestions. Some of these observations were recorded in symbolic language in accordance with the custom prevailing at the time, but to regard them as unscientific merely for this reason, would be about as scientific as rejecting the data of electrocardiography because they are expressed in alphabetical symbols. Some of these ancient observations ranged over a wide field of study and show much evidence of penetrative insight. Several thousands of years before Freud, the importance of examining the content of dreams was evident to Chinese physicians. That dreams were outlets for symbolic wish fulfilment, and therefore a guide to motivational factors, is clear from several passages in the *Nei Jing*. This is only an isolated example of the diagnostic ingenuity of the traditional practitioner, which can be appreciated from a modern clinical standpoint.

THE PULSE DIAGNOSIS

In traditional Chinese medicine, examination of the patient's pulse is the keystone in the diagnostic procedure. Twelve main pulses are recognized at the wrists of which; three are superficial and three are deep, at each wrist. The superficial pulses are felt by using only light pressure of the examining finger, while the deep pulses are felt by exerting stronger pressure.[8]

The best time to take the pulse is in the early morning, physiologically the least active time of the day. As far as possible, it is very important that both the patient and the physician be relaxed while the pulse is being taken. This means that the patient should wait at least ten minutes after arrival before examining. The physician must refrain from carrying out a hurried pulse examination and making a snap diagnosis. If this precaution is not observed, the resulting pulse readings will be inaccurate.

The patient should sit face to face with the physician during the pulse diagnosis. The hands should never be above the heart level. When taking the pulse three fingers should be used, the middle,

---

8 Superficial pulses are felt at the level of the systolic pressure of the deep pulses at slightly above the diastolic pressure.

index, and ring, with the index finger placed closest to the wrist crease.

At first, the three positions are palpated simultaneously, initially, lightly, then with medium pressure, and finally more strongly. After this, each position is checked separately.

Different systems are used whereby the pulse at each position is identified with certain Organs. The correlations most commonly used now in China are:

- left hand proximal position corresponds to *Kidney yin*.
- left hand middle position corresponds to *Liver*.
- left hand distal position corresponds to *Heart*.
- right hand proximal position corresponds to *Kidney Yang* (The Sanjiao is linked to this pulse)
- right hand middle position corresponds to *Spleen*
- right hand distal position corresponds to *Lungs*.

Because pulse taking is an art, it is not surprising that there is no single orthodox set of correspondences. Rather, there are many ways to integrate the same patterns.

When the pulse is taken, attention is given to the frequency, amplitude and quality of the pulse. A normal pulse is distinct, discernible to the fingertip upon medium pressure, and can still be palpated with the application of heavy pressure. It has what is traditionally known as Stomach Qi, Spirit, and Root. The more these qualities are present in the pulses of a patient, the less serious is the discernible.

'Stomach Qi' is the quality of moderation. The pulse is neither too fast nor too slow. It is unhurried and moderately strong. Because the Stomach is the entrepot for nutrition of the body, a patient with Stomach Qi can recover from a disease, whereas a patient without it cannot. 'Spirit' is similarly a quality of moderation, but it is moderation in the shape of the strength of the pulse. A weak pulse with Spirit has a core of strength. A strong pulse with, Spirit has a feeling of elasticity. 'Root' refers to the proximal half of the pulse of Kidney positions. Because the Kidneys are associated with the basal energy of the body, if their pulses have enough strength the body has defensive energy (Wei Qi.).

In a healthy person the distal position tends to be floating, while the proximal half of the pulse position is usually submerged. Frequency of the pulse is about four beats to each, respiration (72 beats per minute). Some variation is normal, Athletes often have a slow pulse. Young children have quick pulses. Fat people have deep pulses, while thin people have pulses with a tendency to be exaggerated than normal. Women's pulses are usually softer and slightly quicker than men's. Also, women's right pulses are usually stronger than their left, while the converse is true of men. Some use these sexual differences in the pulses to predict the sex of the foetus. If the mother's pulse is stronger on the right, the child will be a girl. If it is stronger on the left, it will be a boy.

There are many pathological pulses. Different schools name seventeen, twenty-eight, even thirty-two different pulse types. Some of these types are very rare and appear only in the late stages of terminal disease. Others vary only slightly from each other, and require considerable experience to differentiate. Generally, the pulses can be grouped together in categories which correspond to the steps in the procedure of taking the pulse. It must be borne in mind that, nearly always, a person's pulse, healthy or otherwise, will be a combination of the pulse, types discussed below.

Pulse Characteristics

DEPTH:

The first quality which the physician searches for is depth. There are two principal abnormal pulses in this category.

Floating. This pulse is distinct when lightly palpates, but fades under greater pressure. This pulse is usually associated with exterior conditions (chills, fever, running nose). Since these conditions primarily affect the Lungs, it is ordinarily most pronounced in the Lung, pulse. In a very weak person with a cold this pulse may disappear. In chronic diseases where the Qi and Blood have been seriously depleted (so that the body's Yang Qi is weak and floating, and lacks sufficient Yin) this pulse will fall even in the absence of the Exterior symptoms.

Submerged. This pulse is only distinct upon application of considerable pressure. The presence of this pulse signifies that the disorder has advanced to the Interior of the body. Specific symptoms accompanying this pulse depend on the nature of the disease.

RHYTHM:

The next characteristic of the pulse is rhythm. The normal pulse should pulsate about four beats to each breath of the patient. Athletes may have a slower pulse and children a faster one. Usually, however, there are two principal types of pulses which are distinguished by their characteristic rhythms:

Slow. The pulse rate is three or less heart beats per respiration. This signifies Cold or Deficient Yang. Symptoms include pronounced sensitivity to cold, poor circulation, loose bowels, white coating on the tongue and general lassitude.

Quick. The pulse rate is six or more beats per respiration. This signifies Heat caused either by the Heat Excess or Deficient Yang: Symptoms include fever, rash and pronounced thirst.

DURATION:

The length of the pulse is another important characteristic.

Long. This pulse can be felt even above the proximal position and beyond the distal position. When a person is ill, this pulse indicates that the disease (usually related to Heat and Blood) is well advanced. The symptoms include fever and irritability. In a healthy person, however, it represents a robust constitution.

Short. The short pulse can only be discerned in the middle position. It signifies insufficiency of Blood and Qi. Symptoms include a pale complexion, lack of energy, and the tendency to excessive sleep (hypersomnia).

FORCE:

There are two main pulse types in this group.

Weak. This pulse feels weak and hardly impresses the physician's fingers. Its presence signifies Deficiency, either general (Qi and/or Blood) or in the Organ corresponding to the specific pulse location.

Strong. This pulse responds strongly to the touch. It signifies the presence of an Excess in an ill person, but among the healthy it signified positive health.

QUALITY:

The last and most difficult aspect to ascertain in a pulse is its quality. This characteristic includes the texture, smoothness, and regularity of the pulse wave. Such differentiation is often crucial to the accuracy of the diagnosis.

Slippery. This pulse can definitely be discerned, but the boundaries are indistinct, as if feeling a ball through a layer of highly viscous liquid. A slippery pulse usually signifies the presence of Dampness or Phlegm in the body. Symptoms include mucus, sluggish digestion, difficulty in mobilising the joints and a heavy coating on the tongue. If a healthy woman exhibits this pulse at all positions, it usually indicates that she is pregnant.

Rough. The pulse feels choppy as if the waves of the pulse are irregular (in form, not in rhythm). This pulse signifies Congealed Blood (hard, painful nodules in the abdomen, menstrual irregularities), stagnant Qi (inflammed stomach, headaches, abdominal pains) or Deficient Blood.

Wiry. The feeling of this long and taut pulse is like that of a violin or guitar string. It is a strong pulse that pushes back. A wiry pulse appears in Liver diseases accompanied by pain.

Taut. This pulse feels like a taut clothesline (fuller than wiry), and as if it were fast, but in fact is not. The waves are short and follow each other closely. A taut pulse, when accompanied by a floating pulse, is characteristic of Excessive Cold disorders, in particular. Symptoms include severe chills, fever, pain in the joints, clear vomit and a white coating on the tongue.

Huge. This pulse can be felt at all levels and is slightly stronger at the proximal pulses and at the beginning of the pulse waves. It almost always signifies Excessive Heat conditions and is accompanied by high fever, great thirst, and pronounced sweating. However, if it appears suddenly in a long, debilitating disease, it reflects the exhaustion of Qi and is a very bad prognostic sign.

Fine. This pulse is small and thin like a fine thread, It signifies insufficiency of the Blood and Yin. Symptoms include thirst, irritability, low grade fever and a tongue with a red tip.

Irregular. There are three types of irregular pulses, all of which signify disorders of the Heat Qi; (1) Hasty is fast with irregular pauses, and shows Excessive Heat Yang or congested Qi in the Upper Burner. (2) Knotted is slow with irregular pauses, and signifies obstruction to Blood in the Heart, with Yin in excess or Phlegm in the Pericardium. (3) Intermittent is systematic but pauses abnormally. It signifies an exhausted condition in the Organs. All three pulses are very dangerous signs when they appear in an ill person, but may also occur in otherwise healthy people during periods of mental or emotional distress.

The main object of pulse diagnosis is to ascertain whether there is any imbalance of vital energy that requires correction. Imbalance of energy is shown by either excess or deficiency in one or more pulses in the respective positions assigned to each of the patient's wrists. Pulses are connected by internal Channels to the Internal Organs. It is important to note that these are not purely anatomical concepts, if the rationale behind pulse diagnosis is to be understood. In traditional Chinese medicine, the term " Organ " —does not refer only to the anatomical structure, which goes by that name. It also includes the whole complex of physiological functions and pathological variations arising in that organ, all local and remote effects of its activities, and all subjective sensations, which can be related to that Organ on the basis of clinical observations. For instance the Gall Bladder Organ is not merely an anatomical projection of that viscous, but relates to many other functional involvements such as the site of headache in bilious attacks, the site of the referred pain to the shoulder in gall bladder disease, and certain points on the leg which have been found effective in the treatment of such conditions. Similarly, the Gall Bladder pulse is not merely a measure of the emptiness or fullness of that viscera, but expresses the state of depletion or excess of the vital functions associated with the Gall Bladder as a whole.

Pulse diagnosis is a consuming and extremely, difficult art to time master but perhaps it is well worth the effort. Many obscure ailments are due to some kind of imbalance in the body energy which are difficult to detect by the usual methods of Oriental or Western diagnosis, and pulse diagnosis may be very helpful in the diagnosis of such obscure and complicated disorders.

Diagnosis of disease by pulse examination has been practised from ancient times in both the Eastern and Western systems of medicine. In traditional Chinese acupuncture, it is regarded as the diagnostic method *par excellence*. According to the *Nei Jing* (Yellow Emperor's Classic of Internal Medicine) written *circa* 300 B.C. "Nothing surpasses the examination of the pulse; for with it errors cannot be committed" (Bk. 2:5). Similarly, in the traditional acupuncture of Sri Lanka, its importance has been repeatedly emphasised as, for example, in the following verse:

"Be mindful of what the pulse reveals
Before thou doest apply
The needle science of Iswara:
Revealed in the days gone by.
(From an ancient Sinhala ola manuscript, 300 B.C.)

"*Nadi Sastra*" or the science of pulse diagnosis has, been time immemorial, been the cornerstone of the traditional systems of medicines as practised in Sri Lanka and the rest of the Orient.

In Western medicine too, pulse examination has long been recognised as a procedure of the highest diagnositc value. The Western trained physician is familiar with pulses such as the dicrotic pulse, pulses alternans, pulses bisferiens, pulses paradoxus and so on. Recognition of these pulses are considered important today, for diagnosis as well as for prognosis.

Nevertheless, when it comes to Chinese pulse diagnosis, the western trained practitioner is prone to become hypercritical and to dismiss the subject as rather nonsensical. From a superficial standpoint there may be some justification for this. When it is said that the sensation felt on palpating the pulse is "like a piece of wood floating on water" or "like a stone thrown into a pond" or "like a pearl rolling inside a basin" or "like a lute string" or "like a rope that is twisted and pulled tight at both ends" or "like an onion stalk which is hollow inside", or better still "like a weak wind that puffs up the feathers on the back of a bird, flustering and humming", it is natural for a Western physician to feel that the whole subject is in the realm of fantasy and therefore inaccessible to the kind of objective investigation which his scientific training demands. Again, the postulation of as many as 6 pulses (3 superficial and 3 deep) in the radial position serially arranged at each wrist, is totally alien to his way of thinking, as taught in Western medicine.

To add to his other difficulties the novice realizes that "pulse diagnosis may only be learnt from experience at the bedside, under the tutelage of an experienced traditional practitioner, after many long years" and that, "the distinction between the deep and superficial pulses requires a discriminating sense of touch and the ability to vary in a controlled manner the pressure exerted by the examining finger". Little wonder then, that many Western physicians after a few trials, or no experience at all, have dismissed Chinese pulse diagnosis as an impracticable art, based on highly subjective impressions, derived wholly from the amount of pressure exerted by the examining finger and therefore not worth bothering about.

Regarding this kind of objection it is pertinent to quote here the opinion of the eminent cardiologist, the late Paul Wood regarding the matter of varying the finger pressure when examining the Occidental pulse. Wood says, "the quality of the brachial pulse (which is the most convenient and revealing pulse to examine) can only be learned by experience. What is felt is a pressure wave, and to appreciate it fully, it is necessary to vary the pressure that thumb exerts on the artery until the maximum movement is detected. This implies exerting a force equal to the diastolic arterial pressure" (Paul Wood: Diseases of the *Heart and Circulation*. Eyre & Spottiswoode, London, 1968). Unless one is prepared to use double standards in judging a scientific issue, it is difficult to see how the Chinese method of varying the finger pressure differs in anyway from Wood's method of varying the thumb pressure in modern cardiology. The importance of experience too is stressed in both systems. When the picturesque imagery which is used in describing the objective event failed, the language of poetry was used by the Chinese. "The symphony of the pulses must be in harmony in a healthy person" states the *Nei Jing*.

Does pulse diagnosis work? Evidently yes, because for several thousands of years Oriental physicians have used it as a most important method for diagnosing diseases, selecting acupuncture points and for herbal therapy. The use of pulse diagnosis was mandatory throughout the ages, all other methods being regarded, at best, as mainly of supplementary value.

In recent years it is true that pulse diagnosis has receded somewhat into the background, even in the People's Republic of China, after the development of the neurophysiological theory of acupuncture, anaesthesia and the focusing of attention on ancillary methods like Ear Acupuncture and Head Needle Therapy. Pulse diagnosis does not receive even a passing mention in certain publications from China e.g., *"Outline of Chinese Acupuncture"* (1976).[9] Whether this is a reflec-

9 At the First National Symposium on Acupuncture, Moxibustion and Acupuncture Anaesthesia held in Beijing, People's Republic of China in June 1979 not a single paper on pulse diagnosis or other traditional diagnostic methods was presented. More than 100 research papers on Endorphins were presented.

tion of the general disbelief among modern acupuncturists in China, or whether it is a concession to Western beginners for the purpose of simplifying the subject is difficult to say, at the present. However, the older generation of practioners, nevertheless, continues to use this art.

In his latest book *"Scientific Aspects of Acupuncture"* (William Heinemann Medical Books, London, 1977), Felix Mann, the well-known British acupuncturist, throws doubt ,on the objective existence of acupuncture points and channels and says that the laws of Acupuncture are "largely mythical"; but nowhere does he question Chinese pulse diagnosis. Mann who has practised pulse diagnosis for several decades (and written several books on this subject) seems to have retained his confidence about this procedure, despite his critical re-examination of other basic ideas in the field of acupuncture. The majority of western physicians who have experimented with pulse diagnosis are inclined to think that *"there is something in it"* and that *"it seems to work, no doubt"*. Starting from these tentative conclusions, it is wise to accept quite candidly that if "it works" it may be curing patients, i.e. for reasons other than those traditionally postulated in Chinese Medicine. In other words, with pulse diagnosis we may be doing the right things for the wrong reasons. If so it should obviously be our aim to find out what the real scientific reasons are.

In the meantime we shall discuss briefly what pulse diagnosis is, what its objectives are, and the many pitfalls it is subject to, in clinical use. We shall confine our observations here to the radial pulse, which is this most commonly used. (Some traditional physicians in Japan and Korea use more proximal pulses in the forearm and even the brachial pulse, when carrying out a pulse diagnosis).

There are three pulse positions at each wrist, each having a superficial and a deep component, thus making a total of twelve pulses in both wrists. There is, therefore, one pulse pertaining to each Internal Organ. The consensus of opinion today in the West is that the pulse positions are as follows:

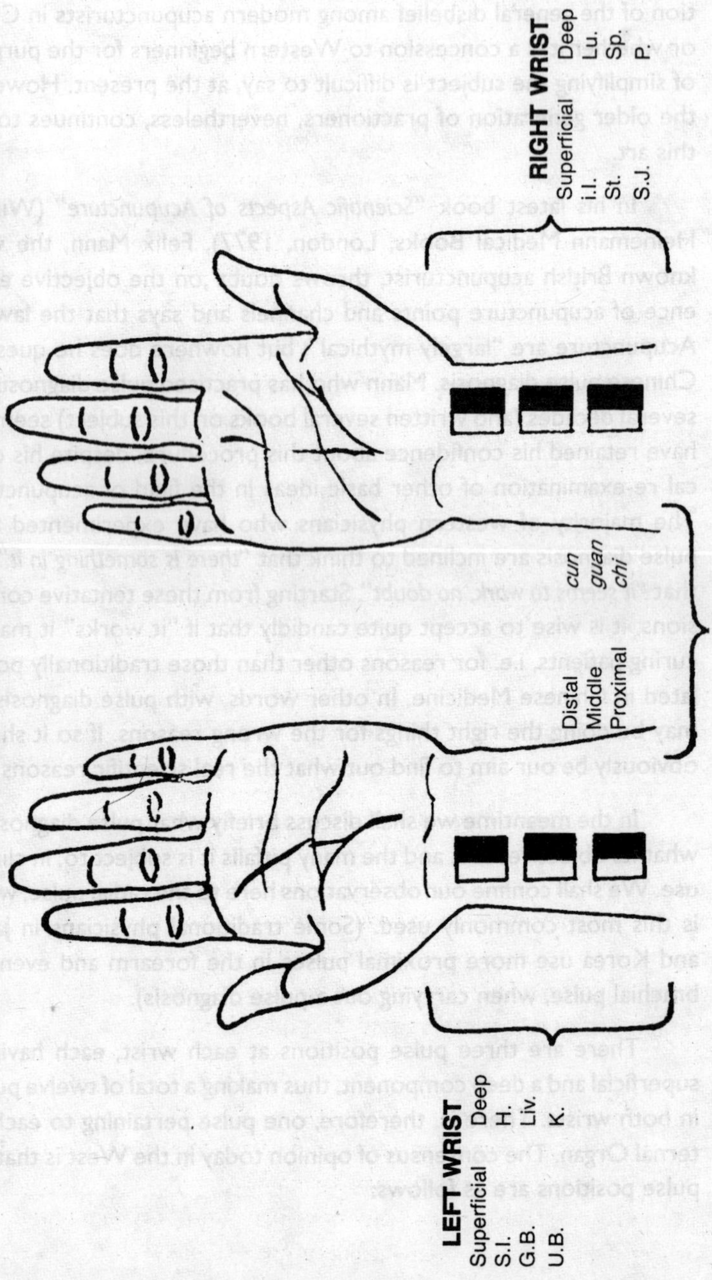

THE PULSE POSITIONS AS ADOPTED BY MOST WESTERN ACUPUNCTURISTS

THE PULSE POSITIONS

AS ADOPTED BY MOST WESTERN ACUPUNCTURISTS

LEFT WRIST				RIGHT WRIST	
Superficial	**Deep**			**Superficial**	**Deep**
S.I.	H.	Distal	*cun*	L.I.	Lu.
G.B.	Liv.	Middle	*guan*	St.	Sp,
U.B.	K.	Proximal	*chi*	S.J.	P.

In "*Essentials of Chinese Acupuncture*", Beijing, (1980) the following pulse positions are described:

LEFT WRIST				RIGHT WRIST	
Superficial	**Deep**			**Superficial**	**Deep**
S.I.	H. (P.)	Distal	*cun*	L.I.	Lu.
G.B.	Liv.	Middle	*guan*	St.	Sp.
U.B.	K. (Yin)	Proximal	*chi*	U.B. (S.J.)	K..(Yang)

(Different ancient authors describe varying pulse positions. Even the Nei Jing describes a different pulse arrangement to the above).

Twenty-eight pathological variants of each pulse form are described in traditional Chinese Medicine and, despite the overlay of poetic imagery, there is a descriptive core which, in many instances, may be compromised with western medical observations. The "halting pulse" for example, described as being "rapid, and giving the impression of undue haste, with intermittent, erratic stoppages," are referred to as the compensatory pauses, which follow the extrasystoles that occur in certain rhythm disorders. Confronted with such descriptions it has to be conceded that observations of a very astute nature have been made by the ancient physicians of China.

THE RADIAL PULSES

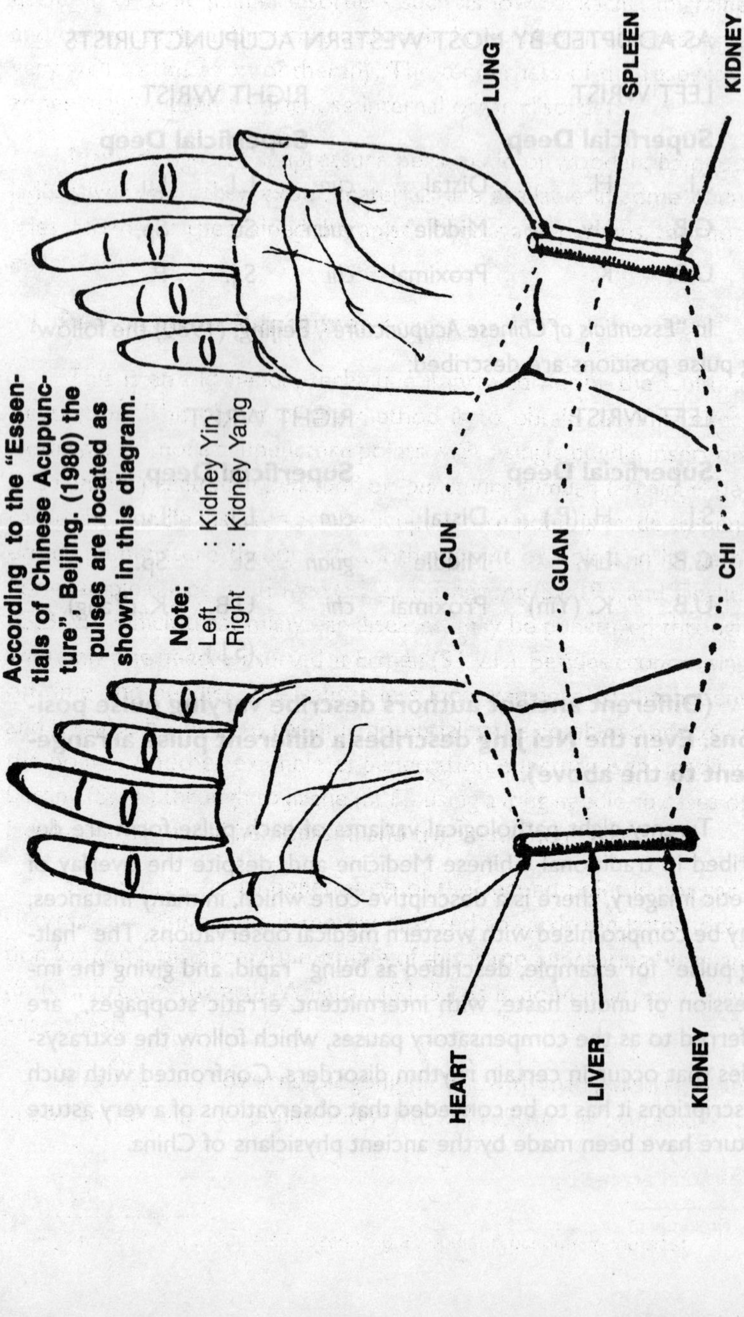

Some evidence which might be corroborative evidence of the Chinese pulse positions comes from the Ayurvedic medicine of India and Sri Lanka. In the Ayurvedic systems, there are 3 pulse positions at each wrist. They are called Va (windy or fiery) Pith (bilious) and Sem (phlegmatic or watery) situated from distal to proximal. For example, if we examine the left wrist, it is clearly seen that those positions correspond closely with the distal Heart and Small Intestine (fiery), the middle Liver and Gall Bladder (wood, bilious) and proximal Kidney and Urinary Bladder (watery) positions of the Chinese system. As there is no evidence whatever to suggest that Ayurveda was directly derived from Chinese Medicine or *vice versa,* the similarity of the pulse positions may have arisen from parallel observations made, independently, by physicians of the two schools. (Some scholars, however, believe that acupuncture probably evolved in prehistoric times out of the modifications of the principles of Ayurveda near the snowy bleaks of the Himalayas, where no herbs were available).

Apart from the recognition of the 28 pathological pulse modalities which require a degree of competence, which not many acupuncturists can easily attain, the principal object of Chinese pulse diagnosis is to ascertain by the 12 pulses whether there is an imbalance of energy as indicated, that requires correction. Imbalance of energy is shown by an excess or deficiency denoted by the pulse being full or empty at one or more of the pulse positions. The objects of acupuncture, according to traditional theory, is to correct such energy imbalances by needling the appropriate acupuncture points.

The following is a description of the more important pulses (*Essentials of Chinese Acupuncture,* Foreign Languages Press, Beijing, (1980):

Feeling the pulse

The location for feeling the pulse is above[10] the wrist, where the radial artery throbs. It is divided into three regions: ***cun, guan***

10 Proximal to

and ***chi.*** The region opposite the styloid process of the radius is known as *guan,* that distal to *guan* (i.e., between *guan* and the wrist joint) is *cun* and that proximal to *guan* is *chi.* The three regions of *cun, guan* and *chi* of the left hand reflect respectively the conditions of the Heart, Liver and Kidney, and those of the right hand reflect conditions of the Organs Lung, Spleen and Kidney.

In feeling the pulse, let the patient place the hand relaxed on a cushion, palm up. First locate the *guan* region with the middle finger, then put the index and ring fingers naturally on the *cun* and *chi* regions. Finger force is exerted first tightly, then moderately and finally heavily to get a general idea of the depth, frequency, rhythm, strength and form of the pulse. Any abnormal changes in any region of the pulse should be detected exerting an even force thereafter by feeling the three regions separately and making comparisons, in order to have a correct impression of the pulse as a whole.

A normal pulse is of medium frequency, i.e., 4-5 beats per breath, and regular rhythm. It is even and forceful.

Abnormal pulse readings and their clinical significance are as follows:

1) *Superficial pulse.* The pulse responds to the finger when pressed lightly and becomes weak on heavy pressure. This often occurs in the early stage of an exogenous disease, i.e., an exterior syndrome. It may also occur in patients suffering from prolonged illness and who are in a state of general weakness. In this situation, however, it is more often superficial and forceless.

2) *Deep pulse.* Superficial palpation reveals no clear pulse, which is felt only upon heavy pressure. This often occurs in interior syndromes.

3) *Slow pulse.* The rate is slow, with less than 4 beats per breath. This often occurs in cold syndromes.

4) *Rapid pulse.* The rate is quick, with more than 5 beats per breath, situation that often occurs in heat syndromes.

5) *Pulse of the xu type.* The pulse is weak and forceless and disappears on heavy pressure. It often occurs in syndromes of the *xu* type.

6) *Pulse of the shi type.* The pulse is forceful and is felt even on deep pressure. This often occurs in syndromes of the *shi* type.

7) *Wiry pulse.* The pulse feels taut and forceful, as though pressing on the string of a drawn bow. It often occurs where there is insufficiency of the *yin* and hyperactivity of the *yang* of the Liver.

8) *Rolling pulse.* The pulse feels smooth, flowing and forceful, and often occurs when there is excessive phlegm or retention of food. Rolling pulse may be observed in healthy people with ample *qi* and blood, and during pregnancy.

9) *Thready pulse.* The pulse is fine, as its name implies. It often occurs in the syndrome of *xu* (deficiency) of both *qi* and blood.

10) *Short pulse.* The movement is uneven and of short duration, with irregular missed beats. Short pulse of the *shi* type indicates hyperactivity of heat, excessive phlegm, stagnation of *qi* and blood and retention of food. Short pulse of the *xu* type is a sign of collapsing.

11) *Knotted pulse.* The pulse is slow and gradual with irregular missed beats, indicating endogenous cold or retention of cold phlegm and stagnant blood in the interior.

12) *Intermittent pulse.* The pulse is slow and gradual with missed beats at regular intervals. It often occurs in patients with impairment of qi and blood and declining *yang qi*.

Short pulse, knotted pulse may vary according to such factors as body build, activity, and general constitution of the patient, and weather. This should be taken into consideration in making a diagnosis.

Long clinical experience is required for correctly identifying the various kinds of pulses.[11] When two or more kinds of pulses are felt

11 A quarter century or more.

in one patient, e.g., a combination of thready and rapid, deep and thready, or thready and wiry, it is important to make a comprehensive analysis of the clinical significance of the combinations, at the same time, taking into consideration the general condition of the patient.

Recognition of the pitfalls of pulse diagnosis is absolutely essential to carry out an accurate pulse diagnosis. The practitioner who fails to heed them cannot expect to obtain anything except indifferent if not, inaccurate results. There are several common pitfalls of pulse diagnosis, which are now briefly discussed.

1. **Norms:** First, one has to establish a clinical norm. Norms, whether in pulse diagnosis or any other activity, vary from individual to individual. Even if a person looks normal there may be inner physical or mental distress, or there may be some latent or subclinical disease-process at work behind the facade of apparent normality. One can never be sure of an absolute norm in clinical medicine.

   Ideally, a healthy person's pulse should have neither deficiency nor excess at any of the pulse positions. All pulses should be equal. However, this is hardly ever the case. Constitutional types and temperamental differences (e.g. whether a person is ectomorphic, endomorphic or mesomorphic) may result in excess or deficiency in the pulses related to such types (e.g. the Fire Element Pulses H., P., S.I. and S. J. in ectomorphs, and the Water Element Pulses K. and U.B. in endomorphs). It is only by contincous observations and the maintaining of serial records that norms may be established in respect of any individual. Allowance also needs to be made for the emotional state of the patient at the time of the examination. The physical state, for example if a person is tired, profoundly affects the pulses.

   In ancient times, the physician was encouraged to stay healthy so that his own pulse could be taken as the norm.

2. **Technique:** Correct technique of the examination and much experience are essential. The surroundings must be peaceful

and a good rapport, between the examiner and patient, needs to be first established. It is best that the patient be rested for at least half an hour, especially if he has walked or travelled a long distance. At least 15 minutes should be spent in examining and evaluating the pulses.[12] Anyone who is observed to do in less time is either a maestro or a quack-more probably the latter, because even highly experienced adepts usually take half an hour more for its performance. There is no such thing as a "snap diagnosis" with the traditional Chinese pulses.

3. **Time of the day:** Early morning is the best time to carry out a pulse diagnosis. In the words of the Nei Jing "this is the time when the breath of Yin has not yet begun to diffuse, when food and drink have not yet been taken, when the Twelve Channels are not yet abundant, and when vigour and energy are not yet begun. Having established the imbalance, it is important, to check on the pulse at the time of the peak activity of the affected Organs as well, as depicted on the Chinese Organ Clock.

4. **The State of the Viscera :** In hollow " Fu " organs such as the Stomach, the Gall Bladder, the Large Intestine and the Urinary Bladder, it frequently happens that an excess or deficiency may appear on the pulse according to the state of fullness or emptiness of the viscus concerned. For example:-

Stomach Full (large meal).

Stomach Empty (hungry patient).

Gall Bladder Empty (fatty meal).

Large Intestine Full (constipation).

Urinary Bladder Full (distended bladder).

In all such cases the treatment is not acupuncture but to empty the bladder, give the patient a meal, or to postpone the pulse examination until the overloaded or empty viscus has regained its "normal" resting state.

12 In chronic, complicated cases the pulse must be examined several times, a day. The sleeping pulse is also important.

5. **Imbalance in a Single Organ:** Usually an imbalance is found in at least two Organs—excess in one and a deficiency in another. This is because the law of energy conservation holds good with regard to energy exchanges between the Organs and Channels. The Organs and Channels comprise a closed energy system and excess or deficiency in one is always accompanied by a corresponding deficiency or excess in another.

   Sometimes however an excess or deficiency is discovered only in one Organ or Channel. In such cases the situation must be considered as abnormal and it is mandatory to investigate further. A re-check of the pulse diagnosis may reveal a hitherto undetected excess or deficiency. However, if after repeated examination, it is not possible to locate a corresponding imbalance, there is no alternative but to assume a latent excess or deficiency as the case may be, on:

   a) the related Coupled Organ or Channel.

   b) the Mother Organ or Channel.

   c) the Son Organ or Channel.

   d) the Destructor Organ or Channel.[13]

   e) the Counteracting Organ or Channel.

Remedial action should be taken at the Luo-Connecting point in the case of (a) above, and at the appropriate Five Element (Five Shu) point in the case of (b) to (e).

6. **Operation of the Husband-Wife Law:** The Husband-Wife Law can effect the pulse reading in one of two ways:

   a) According to this Law, the pulses at the left wrist are usually stronger than the corresponding pulses at the right wrist. This is more so in a male patient. Hence, certain imbalances (e.g. Small Intestine in excess and Large Intestine deficient) may simply be manifestations of the Hus-

13 In the Ko cycle.

band-Wife Law, in which case no corrective action is indicated.

b) Tonification of an Organ on the left wrist has a dispersive action on the Organ belonging to the corresponding pulse position on the right wrist, and vice versa.

Therefore, at all stages-before, during and after treatment, it is necessary to be vigilant for the effects on the pulses created by the operation of the Husband-Wife Law.

7. **Emotions:** The emotional state of the patient, no doubt, has a direct bearing on all the 12 pulses. Such an erratic overall pulse pattern is also diagnostic of brain (mental disorders or heart disorders).

8. **Jet-Lag:** The rapid changes of longitude experienced today when travelling in modern aircraft causes many pulse changes in keeping with the concept of the Organ Clock. This is known as the phenomenon of bio-rhythms.[14]

9. **Occupation:** Night workers usually show a reversal of the diurnal rhythm. Those in stressful employments such as soldiers in combat, offshore oil-well workers, politicians on the campaign trail and the like, olympic athletes, may show many bizarre variations of the pulses.

10. **Anatomical and Pathological Irregularities:** An aberrant radial artery or pathological changes, such as arteriosclerosis, needs to be taken into consideration when carrying out a pulse diagnosis.

    Pathological changes such as localized atheromatous plaques may introduce serious errors when carrying out pulse diagnosis, particularly in the elderly. Vascular disorders such as Raynaud's disease may make the pulse imperceptible.

---

14 Space travel poses further problems and is now the domain of Space Medicine.

11. **Meditation:** Religious meditation, transcendental meditation and other similar forms of mental exercise may cause many variations of the pulse.[15]

12. **Drugs:** The intake of drugs or alcohol may profoundly alter the pulses.

13. **Smoking:** Smokers have many pulse variations.

It has been our unfortunate observation that many so-called "traditional acupuncturists", especially in Western countries perform pulse examination without paying any heed to these pitfalls. The result is improper diagnosis and poor results. If effective results are to be obtained with treatment based on pulse diagnosis, it is imperative that the pitfalls enumerated above be recognized and avoided. Inaccurate treatment, following incorrect diagnosis, can certainly make a patient worse (iatrogenic disease of acupuncture).

Instrumentation such as "pulsograms" and isochronous recordings of the pulses by electronic methods like those devised by Morita of Japan, Niboyet, of France, Beck of Korea and Yoo of West Germany, would certainly be useful in elucidating pulse diagnosis on a scientific basis. Meridian balancing by electrical methods such as Ryodoraku is another development which could potentially be useful in pulse research. There is indeed adequate scope in this field for studies monitored by modern electronic equipment. The problem arises in interpreting those pulse patterns. However, it would be premature to regard those developments as a substitute for the classical methods of pulse diagnosis as described in the Nei Jing and other ancient texts. Irrespective of what method is used, the basic prerequisite for meaningful research is that the classical methods be studied in their pristine purity, mindful of the pitfalls which await the unwary practitioner.

The mystery of pulse diagnosis is an art which cannot be learned by studying textbooks, inasmuch as one cannot become a cardiologist by learning to read electro-cardiograms or text books on the

15 Hypnosis and bio-feedback also change the pulses.

subject. The distinction between the qualities of the deep and superficial pulses, for instance, requires a discriminative sense of touch and the ability to vary in a controlled manner the pressure exerted by the examining finger. This is a knowledge which may only be gained from experience at the bedside with the help of an experienced acupuncturist.

Taking the pulse is like listening to a jazz band. Some players are in harmony with the rest, while others may go off at a tangent and strike a discordant note. It is the task of the physician to 'listen to these sounds and 'hear' what they convey. Even an experienced acupuncturist may take an hour or more to arrive at a correct assessment in a difficult case and in these days of commercialized assembly-line medicine, snap diagnosis and broad-specturm remedies, this might be considered a waste of time. Nevertheless it is a fact, that treatment based on a pulse diagnosis has often proved very effective in cases where 'shotgun acupuncture' (use of a few symptomatic and Ah-Shi points) has failed. It is still being used with 'confidence by many traditional practitioners, and all those who call themselves acupuncturists should endeavour to study this art seriously.

This description of the pulse diagnosis has been ,deliberately kept brief because pulse diagnosis is a great subjective art that must be learned at the bedside and no from any textbook. Readers who are interested in learning this practical diagnostic art should visit a clinic and spend a long time with the patients under the guidance of a competent practitioner. The pulse diagnosis must be supplemented with the symptomatology presented by the patient in order that the diagnosis becomes meaningful. "Any physician who teaches pulse diagnosis in a few lunar months may be spotlighted as a breeder of quackery"—The Classic of the Pulse. (200 B.C.).

THE EAR DIAGNOSIS

The details of the examination of the ear for diagnostic purposes is described in texts on Auriculotherapy.

TONGUE DIAGNOSIS

The different areas of the tongue reflect the state of the different Internal Organs as shown in the annexed diagram. The different colours of the tongue are also related to different Internal Organ disorders.

Colour	Internal Organ disorder
Red	Heart (P.) or Small Intestine (S.I.)
White	Lungs or Large Intestine
Green	Liver or Gall Bladder
Yellow	Spleen or Stomach
Black	Kidneys or Urinary Bladder

When examining the tongue the Yin or Yang nature of the disease may also be elucidated as follows:

Yin	Yang
Weak protrusion	Strong protrusion
Light coloured	Red or dark pink
Tooth marks at edges.	No tooth marks

The recent publication from China, *Essentials of Chinese, Acupuncture*, Foreign languages Press, Beijing, (1980) describes the pathological changes on the tongue as follows:

"Observation of the tongue:

Observation of the tongue, is including the tongue proper and its coating, an important procedure in diagnosis by inspection. There is a close connection between the tongue and the *zang-fu* organs, channels, collaterals, qi, blood and body fluid. Any disorder of these may result in a corresponding manifestation on the tongue. Indications of the nature of the disease can be learned by observing the colour, form and condition of both the tongue proper and its coating, and the motility of the tongue.

A normal tongue is of proper size, light red in colour, free in motion and with a thin layer of white coating over the surface which is neither dry nor too moist.

Below is described the main manifestations of abnormal (tongue) proper and of its coating, and their clinical significance:

1) Tongue proper

a. *Pale tongue*. A less than normally red tongue indicates syndromes of the *xu* or cold type caused by weakness of yang qi and insufficiency of qi and blood or due to the invasion by exogenous pathogenic cold.

b. *Red tongue*. An abnormally bright red tongue indicates various heat syndromes of the shi type due to invasion by pathogenic heat and various heat syndromes of the *xu* type resulting from consumption of *yin* fluid.

c. *Deep red tongue*. A deep red colour of the tongue occurs in the severe stage of a febrile disease in which pathogenic heat has been transmitted from the exterior to the interior of the body. It can also be seen in those patients suffering from a prolonged illness in which *yin* fluid has been exhausted and endogenous fire, which is of the *xu* type, is hyperactive.

d. *Purplish tongue*. A tongue purplish in colour, or with purple spots indicates stagnation of *qi* and blood. It also indicates preponderance of endogenous cold due to *xu* (deficiency) of *yang*.

e. *Flabby tongue*. A tongue larger than normal, flabby, and whitish in colour, sometimes with teeth prints on the border, indicates, *xu* (deficiency) of both *qi* and *yang* and retention of phlegm-damp in the interior. Flabby tongue deep red in colour indicates preponderance of pathogenic heat in the interior and hyperactivity of the fire of the heart.

THE AREAS OF THE TONGUE CORRESPONDING TO THE INTERNAL ORGANS

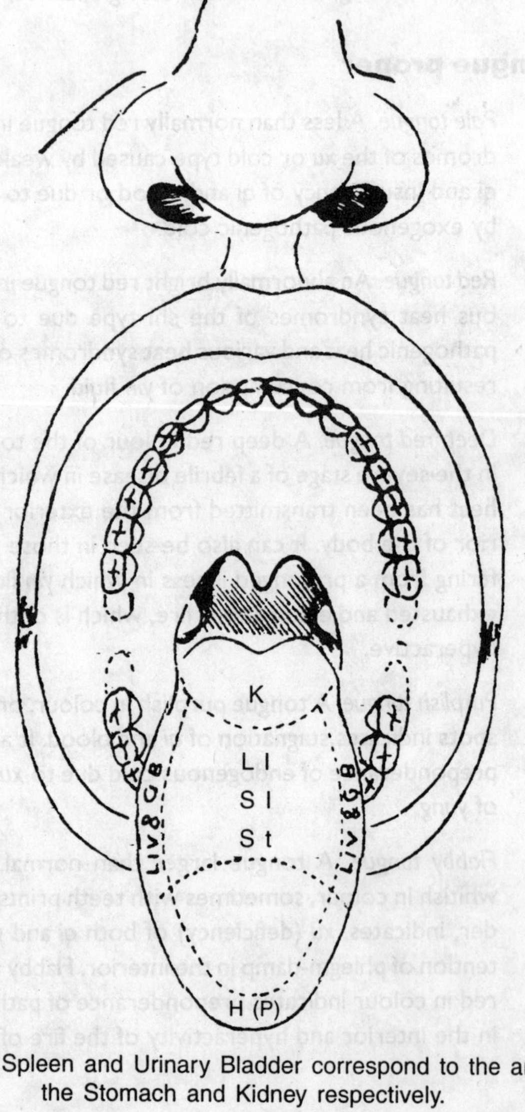

Note: The Spleen and Urinary Bladder correspond to the areas of the Stomach and Kidney respectively.

f. *Cracked tongue.* Irregular streaks or cracks on the tongue indicate consumption of body fluid by excessive heat, loss of the essence of the kidney and hyperactivity of fire due to *xu* (deficiency) or *yin.*

Congenital cracked tongue or a cracked tongue, without any morbid signs, are considered normal.

g. *Thorny tongue.* The papillary buds over the surface of the tongue swelling up like thorns, and usually red in colour, indicate hyperactivity of pathogenic heat.

h. *Rigid and tremulous tongue.* A tongue that is rigid and difficult to protrude, retract or roll, leads to stuttering and indicates invasion of exogenous heat and disturbance of the mind by phlegm-heat. It also indicates damage of the *yin* of the liver by strong heat which stirs up the wind, or obstruction of collaterals by wind-phlegm. The tremulous tongue seen in protracted illness often indicates *xu* (deficiency) of both *qi* and *yin.*

i. *Deviated tongue.* This indicates obstruction of the collaterals by wind-phlegm.

2. Tongue coating

a. *White coating.* The tongue's whitish coating may be thin or thick, sticky or dry. A thin white coating is normal, but when it is seen in an exogenous disease, it usually indicates invasion of the lung by wind-cold.

Thick white coating usually indicates retention of food. While sticky coating usually indicates invasion by the exogenous cold-damp or retention of phlegm-damp in the interior. Dry white coating usually indicates invasion by the pestilential factor.[16]

16 Epidemic factor.

b. *Yellow coating.* A yellow coating on the tongue may be thin or, thick, sticky or dry. A thin yellow coating usually indicates invasion of the lung by wind-heat, while a thick yellow coating usually indicates persistent accumulation of food in the stomach and intestines. Yellow sticky coating usually denotes accumulation of damp-heat in the interior or blockage of the Lung by phlegm-heat. Dry yellow coating usually indicates accumulation of heat in the Stomach and Intestines which results in damage to the *yin*.

c. *Greyish black coating.* A greyish black coating on the tongue may be moist or dry. Greyish black moist coating usually denotes retention of cold-damp in the interior or too much endogenous cold due to *xu* (deficiency) of yang. Greyish-black, dry coating usually indicates consumption of body fluid by excessive heat or hyperactivity of fire due to *xu* (deficiency) of yin.

d. *Peeled coating.* The tongue with its coating peeling off is known as a *"geographic tongue"*. If the entire coating peels off leaving the surface mirror smooth, the condition is known as glossy tongue. Both manifestations indicate the crisis in a long illness in which the antipathogenic factor is severely damaged and the yin is grossly deficient.

The abnormal changes of the tongue proper and coating suggest the nature and changes of disease from different aspects. Generally speaking, observations of the changes in the tongue proper is mainly to differentiate whether the condition of the *zang-fu* organs, *qi*, blood and body fluid is in a *xu* or *shi* state; while observation of the tongue coating is for judging the condition of pathogenic factors. Comprehensive analysis of the changes in both the tongue proper and its coating is therefore necessary when a diagnosis is made by observations of the tongue.

Attention should be paid to the exclusion of false phenomena, such as the tongue proper becoming redder and the coating thinner after eating or drinking hot beverages. Some food and drugs colour the tongue coating, e.g., olive, mulberry or plum may give it a greyish black hue; liquat, orange. coptis or riboflavin may make it yellow. Those who smoke or drink alcohol or tea often have a thick yellow or greyish yellow tongue coating. As observation of the colour, of both the tongue proper and its coating, is an important procedure in diagnosis; it is desirable that it be done in daylight."

Modern medicine also recognises many important pathological changes of the tongue as an aid to diagnosis:

1. An unduly enlarged tongue occurs in acromegaly, myxoedema, cretinism and mongolism. Amyloid disease of the tongue also causes enlargement of the tongue Myelomatosis is a common cause of amyloid disease of the tongue.
2. A fissured tongue occurs in mental defectives, mongols and in vitamin B complex deficiencies.
3. Angiomas of the lips or tongue may point to similar lesions in the central nervous system or the gastro-intestinal tract.
4. Frenal ulcers are due to whooping cough.
5. Thrush (*Candida albicans*) occurs commonly in infants. It may also occur in adults during antibiotic therapy (particularly with tetracycline).
6. Smoking, spirits, betel-chewing, spice or syphilis (tertiary) may give rise to leukoplakia of the tongue.
7. Dark brownish or black patches of the tongue are due to fungal infection following oral antibiotic therapy.
8. Vesicles of the tongue occur in varicella,
9. Branches of three different cranial nerves innervate the tongue. The tongue may be involved in disorders of any of these nerves.
10. In disorders such as uraemia, diabetes, bronchiectasis or the administration of certain drugs give rise to certain characteristic smells emanating from the patient's mouth and nose.
11. A furred dry tongue occurs in fevers, toxaemias and in acute abdominal disorders.

12. In diabetic coma a raw beefy tongue may be seen.
13. Atrophy of the villae on the tongue is seen in anaemias.

Pulse diagnosis, ear diagnosis and tongue diagnosis are the trinity of important diagnostic methods of traditional Chinese medicine. A mastery of the finer points of these clinical procedures is extremely difficult. However, acupuncture works equally effectively, if combined with Western methods of diagnosis. The Western diagnosis must then be so structured that the principles of the selection of points can be applied to modern scientific diagnosis. This approach is being used in many parts of the world today to combine the technology of scientific progress with the overwhelming effectiveness of acupuncture therapy in order to produce a more pragmatic medicine. At the Academy of Traditional Chinese Medicine, Peking a similar line of teaching is now being carried out.

In the final evaluation of acupuncture it must be borne in mind that this is not a system of medicine from which modern medical science has evolved, although it has been in existence in one form or another in many parts of the world for over four thousand years. On the other hand. the rationale for the many forms of therapy in modern medical treatment is still a matter of conjecture and are based of theories which have not been adequately substantiated by twentieth century criteria. However, they quite evidently continue to be used. A recent publication in an eminent medical journal by a famous lay statistician ridicules the statistical criteria used by Western medical writers to prove their theories, and it is quite likely that the future will see many of these theories or postulates discarded.

To the clinician, however, his primary consideration is the relief of pain and the alleviation of human suffering, and acupuncture has been shown positively to give relief in many illnesses. It would no doubt be rational to determine statistically whether acupuncture is beneficial or not. Having been found to be beneficial, there is no reason why it should not be used as a mode of therapy, accepting the theories and concepts and philosophies put forward by its originators, until such time definite and conclusive explanations for its mode of action are discovered.

THE CIRCULATION OF VITAL ENERGY (QI)

"Qi permeates all activities of the Universe. If a tree is planted, Heaven helps it to grow: if it is cut down, Heaven helps it to rot."

— Shih Tshu Lai Chi, 1005 A.D.

The circulation of energy is the central thesis of the universalistic Chinese philosophy, on which acupuncture is based. According to this philosopy the universe is in a state of cosmic energy flux. Energy exists in every material and living organism. Energy is transformable form one state to another and may exist even in the non-material state as well (e.g. Tao). These ancient metaphysical concepts, in many respects, show remarkable similarities to the present day Laws of Thermodynamics, and in certain features even anticipated the relativity theories of Einstein. Whereas Einstein hypothesised regarding the energy changes in the external world, the Chinese philosophers concentrated on the internal energy balances of the body, in order to understand disease and the life processes.

The basic difference between the orientation of scientific Western medicine and traditional Oriental medical philosophy is that the former is orientated to the biochemical changes in the body, whereas, the latter deals essentially with the energy imbalances in the body. While the therapeutics of Western scientific medicine are concerned mainly with altering the disease state by chemical means, acupuncture seeks to normalise the pathology by correcting the energy imbalances.

TYPES OF QI

In the living organism the principal energy responsible for the life process, according to traditional Chinese medicine, is called *Qi* or vital energy. The circulation of blood and vital energy, according to the *Huang Di Nei Jing*, is responsible for the vital functions in man and animals. There are many facets or subdivisions of the vital energy. The main subdivisions of the vital energy are described in the classical texts as follows:

1) Ku Qi : Physiological energy derived from the essences of food.
2) Zong Qi (Essential Qi) : Lung energy derived from the Ta Qi (the external energy from the inspired air).
3) Qin Qi (Clean Qi) : Nourishing energy originating in the Lungs from Ku Qi and Ta Qi. Qin Qi circulates in the Internal Organs.
4) Jeng Qi : Energy from Qin Qi, stored in the Kidneys.
5) Jing Qi : Energy circulation in the Channels, the Collaterals and muscular Channels.
6) Xian Tian Qi : Inherited ancestral energy.
7) Yuan Qi (Source Qi) : The active part of the Xian Tian Qi.
8) Ying Qi (Nutrient Qi) : This is formed from essential substances in the vessels and supplies the viscera.
9) Wei Qi (Defensive Qi) : This is also formed from food and circulates mainly in the soft tissues such

as skin, subcutaneous tissues and muscles. It defends the body against the exogenous aetiological factors of disease.

The three levels of Qi:

There are two main levels of circulating vital energy in a living organism:

(a) the superficial energy circulating in the channels.

(b) the deep energy circulating in the Internal Organs.

(c) there is also a third energy stratum permeating the muscular meridians diffusely like a capillary network, nourishing the soft tissues and the supporting structures like bone and cartilage.

The superficial energy circulates mainly in the 12 Channels in a cyclical manner(a 24 hours circadian cycle, biorhythm). The peak of the flow takes 24 hours to complete the full cycle through the Twelve Channels—(the Organ-Clock). The flow of energy in both the Du and Ren Channels is in an upward direction. Internally the energy descends in both Channels from mouth to anus. According to some authorities, the energy flow in the Du and Ren Channels occurs in the manner of a figure of eight, and takes 24 hours to complete one cycle. The Internal Organ energy circulates in the sequence of the Five Elements through the Internal Organs and it also exhibits a 24 hour cycle (the phenomenon of circadian rhythm).

The three levels of body energy closely communicate with each other. In a healthy person the total amount of energy in the superficial circulation is constant, while the quantum of Internal Organ energy is also constant (The Law of Conservation of Energy). These may be represented as follows:

SE of the 12 = C1

DE of 5 Zang + 6 Fu Organs = C2

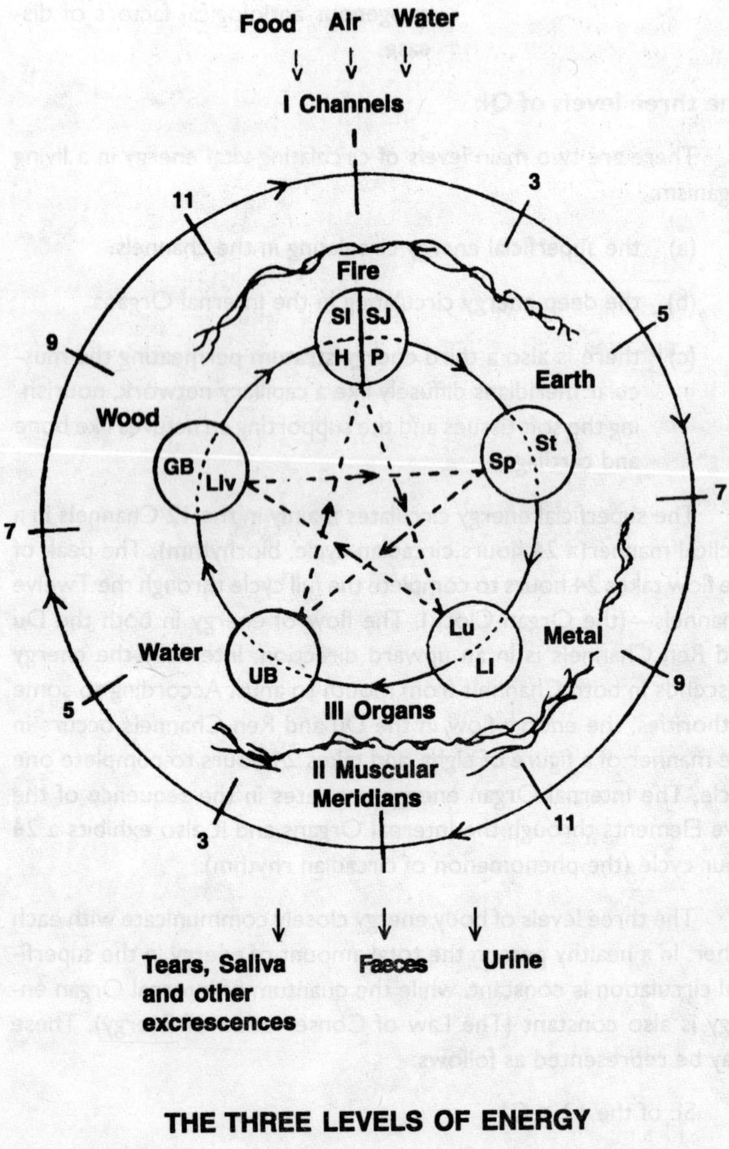

THE THREE LEVELS OF ENERGY

I. Channels. II. Muscular Meridians. III. Internal Organs.

Where SE = Superficial energy.

DE = Deep energy.

The muscular meridians are also a reservoir (C3) of a large amount of energy (ME).

SE + DE + ME = Total amount of vital energy or Qi in the body.

Yin and Yang are in equal quantities in the healthy state.

Therefore;

$$\frac{C1 + C2 + C3}{2} = \text{Yin} = \text{Yang, in a healthy individual (at rest).}$$

Although in a healthy individual it is said that the Yin and Yang are in equal quantities; this is not precisely true. There is a preponderance of Yin during the early hours of the morning and late at night; while Yang is in excess around midday. A diurnal rhythm thus exists. The Yin and Yang are, therefore, in a state of dynamic balance.

$$\frac{C1 + C2 + C3}{2} = \text{nearly equals Yin - nearly equals Yang.}$$

(occurs throughout the day).

There is a preponderance of Yin by midnight and a preponderance of Yang by midday in the Internal Organs of a healthy person. In the Channels the variations of the levels of Yin and Yang energy through the day are as follows:

3 a.m. – 5 a.m.	The Lung Channel of Hand-Taiyi (most strong of Yin).
5 a.m. – 7 a.m.	The Large Intestine Channel of Hand-Yangming (most strong of Yang).
7 a.m. – 9 a.m.	The Stomach Channel of Food-Yangming (most strong of Yang).
9 a.m. – 11 a.m.	The Spleen Channel of Foot-Taiyin (most strong of Yin).
11 a.m. – 1 p.m.	The Heart Channel of Hand-Shaoyin (less of Yin).

1 p.m. – 3 p.m.	The Small Intestine Channel of Hand-Taiyang (intermediate of Yang).
3 p.m. – 5 p.m.	The Urinary Bladder Channel of Foot-Taiyang (intermediate of Yang).
5 p.m. – 7 p.m.	The Kidney Channels of Foot-Shaoyir (less of Yin).
7 p.m. – 9 p.m.	The Pericardium Channel of Hand-Jueyin (intermediate of Yin).
9 p.m. – 11 p.m.	The Sanjiao Channel of Hand-Shao Yang (less of Yang).
11 p.m.—1 a.m.	The gall bladder Channel of Foot - Shao-Yang (less of Yang).
1 a.m. – 3 a.m.	The Liver Channel of Foot-Jueyin (intermediate of Yin).

Imbalances of body energy may occur either in (a) health or (b) in disease. For example, during violent muscular exercise there is a diversion of energy to the muscular channels (meridians) both from the superficial and the deep levels. The total amount of Qi may also need to increase when sustained exercise is carried out. This increase is brought about by supplementing the Qi with the body's reserves of (Jeng Qi and Ku Qi). These reserves can only be mobilized by an increase of the intake of Ta Qi (Air, Oxygen). Not only during muscular exercise but also during any emergency, acute disease or states of stress, a similar process may occur to shunt the energy to the required level of activity. These imbalances of energy so produced in the healthy state may be considered as purely temporary (i.e., physiological imbalances).

On the other hand, imbalance produced by disease state are of a serious nature. Pathological imbalances are caused by *sieqi* (disease factors). These concepts may be exemplified by the following equations:

In health:

Yin Energy (E Yin) = Yang Energy (E Yang).

In disease:

(E Yin) / (E Yang).

In deficiency disorders:

(E Yin) > (E Yang).

In an excess disorders:

(E Yang) > (E Yin).

In an absolute excess of Yang:

C1 + C2 + C3 > C1 + C2 + C3.

of disease. In the resting state of health.

In (cellular) death:

(E Yang) = 0,

and (E Yin) = infinity.

In the book *Yu Li Tzu* author Liu Chi (1365 A.D.)[1] describes death as the pouring back of a cup of water into the sea; the Qi returns to the universal mass of Qi.

In pregnancy the total amount of energy gradually increases till the time of delivery.

1 Liu Chi (1311 to 1375 A.D.) was an astronomer, mathematician and also a famous astrologer (like Kepler later).

DIAGRAM TO SHOW THE PATHWAYS OF THE ENERGY (5 ELEMENTS) CIRCULATION THROUGH THE INTERNAL ORGANS

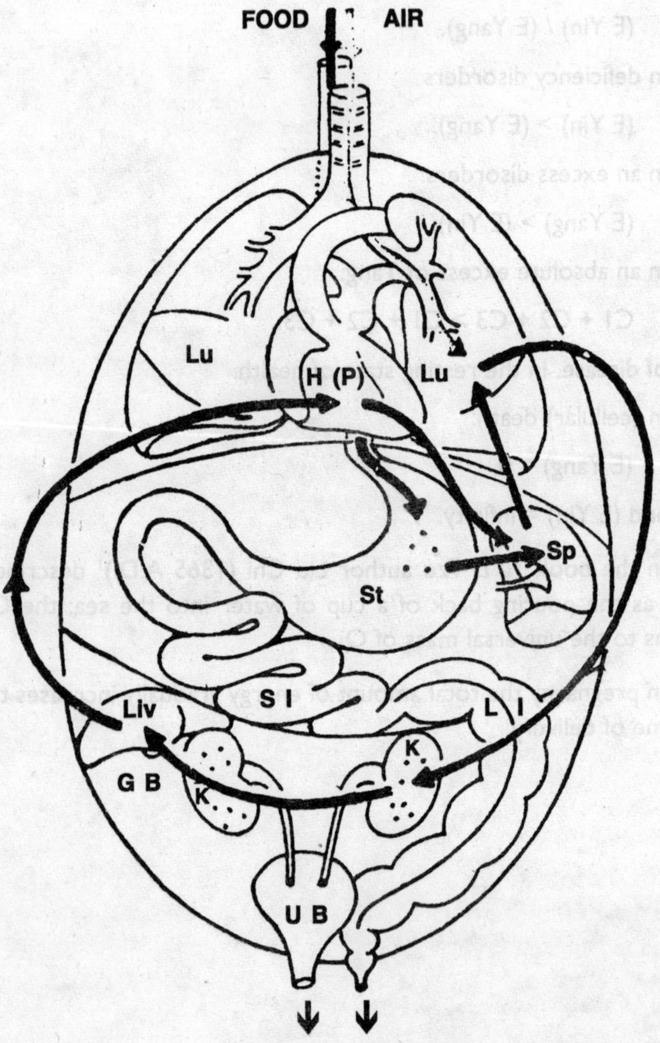

External energy enters the body mainly as food and air. Energy is lost as urine, faeces, heat, muscular activity, sweat, etc.

THE ENERGY CIRCULATION

Although the circulation of energy in the Channels and Internal Organs is considered as "within a closed system", this is not strictly so, as there are constant energy exchanges with the exterior (with the rest of the universe) as follows:

1) Energy is added on continually to the body by such processes as breathing (Ta Qi), food (Ku Qi), radiation from the external world (mainly *via* the acupuncture points).

2) Energy is continually lost by processes such as sweating, defaecation, urination, other excrescences and by radiation to the exterior.

The food enters the Stomach. The digestion occurs by the activity of the Spleen (the Spleen-Pancreatic complex). The metabolic energy of the food, the Ku Qi, enters the Five Element circulation *via* the Spleen and reaches the Lung. There it combines with the inspired energy, the Ta Qi, and forms the intrinsic Lung energy known as Zong Qi. From the Lung energy originates the energy known as Qin Qi, which circulates in the 5 sets of internal organs. The Qin Qi circulates from Lung—> Kidney—> Liver—> Heart—> Spleen and back to the Lung (A parallel circulation also occurs in the same sequence through the corresponding Yang Organs). As it circulates, a part of this energy is stored as a reserve energy (Jeng Qi) in the Kidney to be mobilized in states of stress. According to several ancient classics, the circulation of energy obtains its propulsive force from the respiratory movements of the lungs.

As the Internal Organs communicate with the Channels, a part of this Jeng Qi is shunted by each Internal Organ to circulate in the related Channel as Jing Qi the circulating energy of the channels.

SIEQI

Sieqi is a perverse form of energy which causes the disease factors to bring about imbalances in the organism and thereby gives

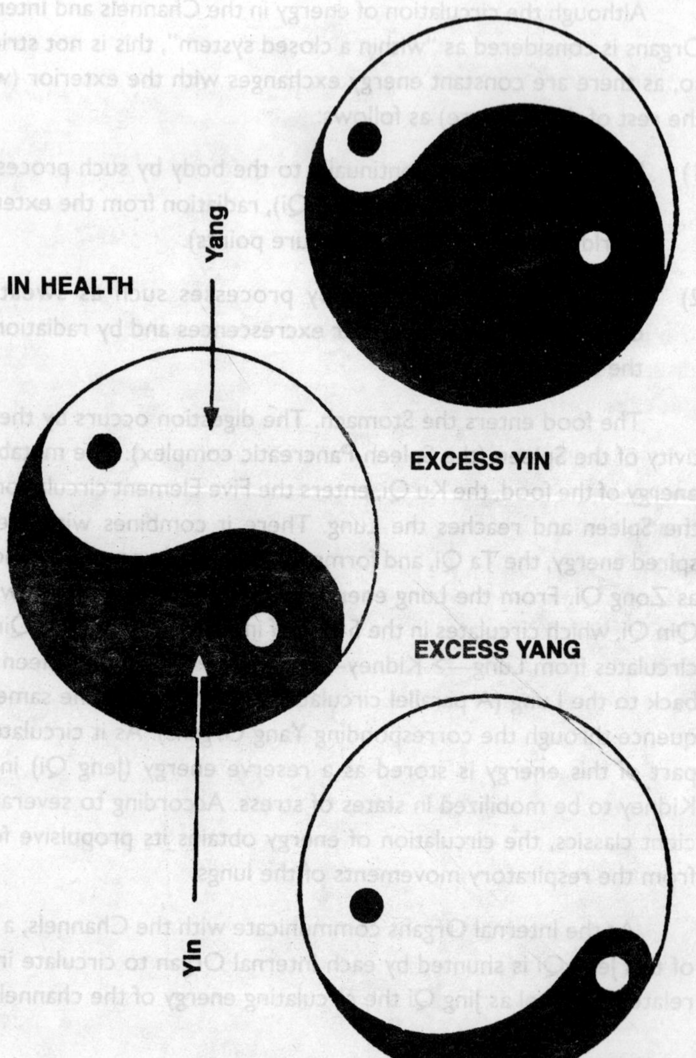

An excess may be either physiological or pathological.

rise to disorders. Pathogenic disease factors are divided into four groups:

A. Six exogenous factors.

B. Seven emotional factors.

C. Four miscellaneous factors.

D. Phlegm.

These factors have been discussed earlier.

The extrinisic factors cause disease mainly in the Channels; while the intrinsic factors cause disease in the Internal Organs. External diseases may, however, get interiorised; and internal diseases may, get exteriorized, if inadequately treated.

Diseases originate with the these aetiological factors by causing an imbalance of the Yin-Yang mechanism. In the state of positive health Yin-Yang are in dynamic balance. In disease there exists either an excess or a deficiency of Yang. The former are known as excess disorders (Yang diseases) with the latter are known as deficiency disorders (Yin diseases). The excess or deficiency may be an absolute, or only a relative excess or deficiency. In the former instance, the patient is acutely ill and emergency treatment and aggressive life saving measures are necessary.

A patient in a state of severe shock is one in which there is an absolute deficiency of vital energy. A patient, who is in the throes of an acute myocardial infarction, is in state of absolute excess of Yang. Both patients are, undoubtedly, seriously ill and need quick, intensive therapy. A severe excess of Yang may lead to a Yin deficiency disorder. The converse is also true.

Clinical death is a lack of Yang. When cellular death occurs it becomes an absolute lack of Yin and Yang.

In the symptomatology exhibited during an illness, there is a close relationship as follows:

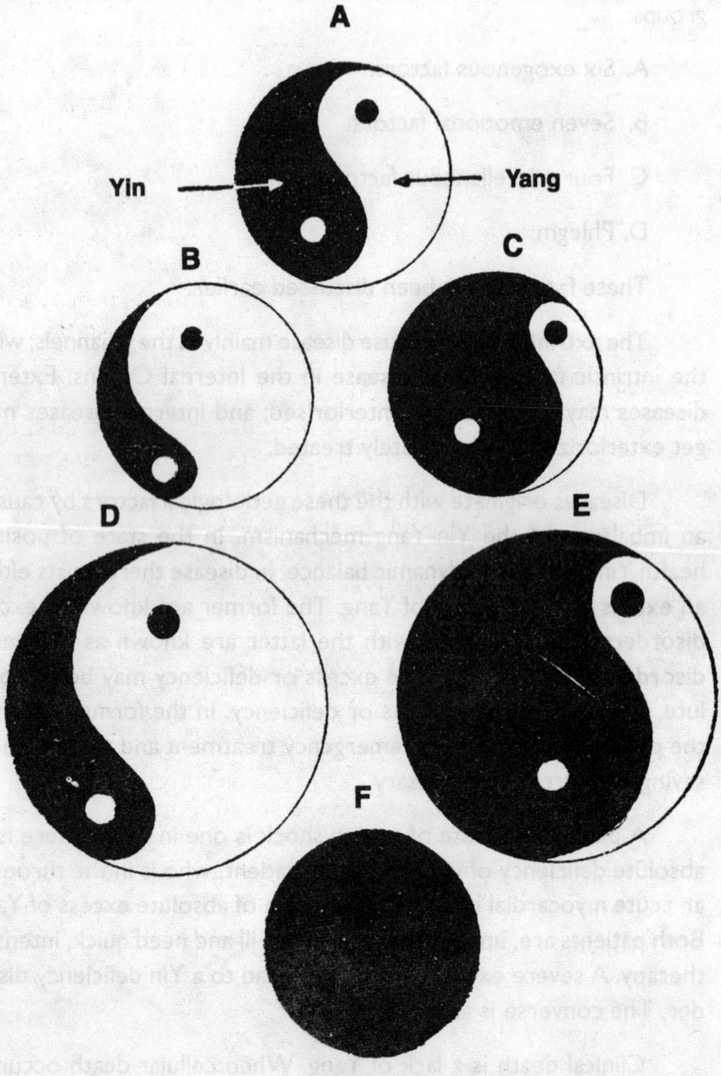

A Health
B Excess Yang C Excess Yin
D Absolute Excess of Yang
E Absolute Excess of Yin
F Death

Channel <—> Organ <—> Special Sense Organ <—> Connected Tissues. Often disease manifestations become interchangeable at these various energy levels, as for example bronchial asthma commonly becomes a skin disorder, a rhinitis, or a pharyngitis. The many Luo connections with various other Internal Organs and structures are also important. The pathology in these areas are also affected by any imbalance of the vital energy along the chain. Perverse energies may also be easily short-circuited along the Extraordinary Channels, with the Confluent point as the focus of activity, e.g., a pharyngitis (upper respiratory disorder) may lead to a Kidney disorder and the pharynx (e.g., streptococcal sorethroat leading to acute nephritis of Western medicine). Since the Urinary Bladder Channel has Internal connections with all the Internal Organs, it is the best Channel used for therapy when there are multiple imbalances involving many organs and tissue systems.

THE RECOGNITION OF ENERGY IMBALANCES

The energy imbalances may be diagnosed clinically by:

1) The history of the onset of the illness:

   e.g. exposure to cold denotes a disease of the energy imbalance in the channels of the exposed area—a facial paralysis, stiff-neck, polyneuropathy.

2) The symptoms exhibited: it is easy in most cases to determine whether the symptoms exhibited are a disorder of—

   a) the Channels, e.g., trigeminal neuralgia (Yang), facial paralysis (Yin).

   b) The Muscular Channels (meridians) e.g. muscular rheumatism, stroke, sprain, osteoarthritis.

   (c) the Internal Organs, e.g., nausea, vomiting due to gastritis, bronchial asthma, cirrhosis of the liver, angina pectoris.

3) The Alarm Points: The tenderness exhibited at the Alarm points is indicative of Internal Organ disorders.

4) The Ear: Auricular diagnosis is quite accurate in determining—

   a) Internal Organ disorders.

   b) Regional disorders of the muscular Channels, e.g., frozen shoulder, prolapsed intervertebral disc, stroke.

5) The Tongue: The tongue is called "the mirror of the heart" in Chinese medicine.

6) The Pulse: This is the final arbiter in determining the energy excess or deficiency in the Zang-Fu complex.

In the view of many authorities, it is likely that acupuncture points actually exist to carry out energy exchanges with the external environment of the body, so that man can exist in an equivocal state of cosmic energy balance with the universe. Acupuncturing the correct combination of acupuncture points helps to restore imbalances, which occur in disorders.

Diagnosis of disease by traditional methods entails the ascertaining of energy imbalances. The therapy requires that transfers of energies be carried out in order to reestablish the normal state of energy balance. Such transfers of energy from one region to another must be accomplished in an orderly sequence, in accordance with certain established traditional principles. Haphazard attempts at energy transfer may result not only in making the patient's condition worse, but also may bring about fresh symptoms and new disorders (the iatrogenic diseases of acupuncture therapy). "Hit or miss" kind of therapeutics has no place whatever, in the rigid regimen of energy transfer therapeutics. An outline of the more important principles of energy transfer follows.

THE PRINCIPLES OF ENERGY TRANSFER IN ACUPUNCTURE THERAPEUTICS

1) When transferring energy, the shortest possible pathway is followed. Tonification (bu) must be used in preference to sedation (xie) as it is a more acceptable procedure for the patient.[2]

2) Vital energy flows in the Channels and Organs in a "clockwise" direction. A backflow does not occur (except to a limited extent in the Coupled Channels). Imbalances in Channels or Internal Organs may be either in the nature of an excess or a deficiency.

3) Adjustment of an imbalance in a pair of Coupled Channels or Coupled Organs may be carried out at their communicating points: the Luo-Connecting points (and also at the Yuan-Source points, used as supplementary points).

4) The Channels and Organs form a separate "closed" energy system from a thermodynamic point of view. If there is a deficiency in one Channel or Internal Organ, then an excess in another, either evident or latent.

5) If a Channel is deficient, it may be corrected by energy drawn from its mother. The mother, in due course, will replenish the temporary deficit so created from the point of excess *via* the natural biorhythmic flow.

6) It the deficient Channel commences in the face or the chest region then the point of entry of its circulating energy is the acupuncture point number one (i.e. in a centrifugal Channel).

7) If the deficient Channel commences in the hand or foot region then the point of entry of energy is the Luo-Connecting point (i.e. in a centripetal Channel).

8) In a deficiency of a Channel, the needling is carried out on the son Channel at the points described at paragraphs 6 or 7 above. The technique (polarity[3]) of stimulation is tonification (bu).

---

2 Less painful.

3 Polarity = increase or decrease of yang energy.

9) Energy may be transferred from one Internal Organ to another along the pathways of the Sheng and/or Ko Cycles using the Five-Shu (Five element) points. (Energy cannot be transferred in the reverse direction of either of these cycles).

10) The Sheng or Ko cycle energy transfers should not be used to treat acute disorders. In acute conditions symptomatic points must first be used to allay the acute presenting symptoms, e.g., in tainting use sedation at Jing-Wel points, in severe pain use the analgesic points such as Hegu (L.I. 4); in an acute attack of bronchial asthma use the Xi-cleft point Kongzui (Lu.6). In a chronic disorder manifest in a single Internal Organ, the point of choice is the Yuan-Source point.

11) The commonest clinical presentation is a deficiency of an Internal Organ together with an excess of its Coupled Organ, or an excess in its Mother Organ.

12) Energy must be so transferred in order that the deficiencies are first corrected. (Note: Excesses must not be dispersed by sedation, but rather transferred to the deficient Internal Organ by tonification of the deficient Internal Organ.)

13) Where the deficiency and excess exist between two Coupled Organs the Luo-Connecting point of the Channel of the Deficient Internal Organ is used. The technique of stimulation used is the tonification (bu) method.

14) Where the deficiency and excess is distributed between two Yin (or two Yang organs) the following procedures may be used:

   a) When the Sheng cycle is used: The Channel pertaining to the deficient Organ is needled. The point selected is that Shu point which corresponds to the excess Element. The technique of stimulation is tonification (bu).

   (b) Energy is transferred along the Ko cycle to any Internal Organ where there is an excess of energy. The incoming energy along the arm of the Ko cycle neutralizes this excess. The Channel of the receiving Internal Organ is needled. The point needled is that Element point which corresponds to the donor Internal Organ. The technique of stimulation is tonification (bu)[4].

15) When treatment is carried out using the Five-Shu points (the Sixty Command Points or the Five Element points) the pulses need to be checked at every stage in order to ensure that the desired energy transfers are, in fact, taking place.

16) If a deficiency (or excess) is discovered only in a single Internal Organ, a "latent excess" (or a "latent deficiency") exists in another Organ, frequently in the coupled Organ or the mother Organ. Often this assumption needs to be made when carrying out treatment.

17) The Horary point may be used in treating a Channel or an Internal Organ disorder at the relevant time, of the day, e.g. Jingqu (Lu. 8.) at 3 a.m. Where there is excess, sedation is used. In insufficiency notification is used. As the relevant time is inconvenient, the diametrically opposite time may be used on the point of the diametrically opposite channel of the Organ Clock (e.g., the water-Urinary Bladder Channel for Metal-Lung disorder) with the opposite technique of stimulation.

18) In checking the pulses for energy imbalances or their correction, it is important to be aware of some of the common clinical pitfalls which may cause normal (physiological) or abnormal variations of the pulses.

   a) Lack of sleep or a change of the diurnal rhythm e.g., jet-lag, night worker, long distance longhaul drivers.

   b) Anxiety of the patient, emotional disturbances.

   c) Full urinary bladder.

   d) Hungry patient, overeating, alcohol intake.

   e) Immediately following sexual intercourse.

   f) Acute illness, inflammatory disorder.

4 Complications may occur.

g) Severs pain due to any cause, shock, exposure to cold.

h) Pregnancy.

i) Drugs.

j) Surgery or other trauma.

k) Anatomical abnormalities.

l) Endocrine disturbances.

m) Senility.

n) Climacteric.

o) Climatic disturbances.

p) Physical exercise and several others.

19) The Bu method is always preferable to xie. The Sheng cycle transfers are preferable to Ko cycle transfers.

20) In transferring energy the Great Law of Bu-Xie has to be strictly adhered to at all times.

THE GREAT LAW OF BU-XIE

When needling is carried out, it is done in conformity with the Great Law of Bu-Xie.

i) **Bu** is used in **Xu disease**.

ii) **Xie** may be used in **Shi disease** with acute symptoms. **Bu** is the reinforcing, or the notification method. It is carried out by weak stimulation at the acupuncture point to increase the energy.

Xie is the reducing, dispersing or the sedation method. It is carried out by strong stimulation at the acupuncture point to decrease the energy.

Xu diseases are Yin
Interior
Cold
Deficient
(Hypofunctional, Hypoactive, disorders).

Shi diseases are Yang Exterior

Exterior

Hot

Excesses

(Hyperfunctional Hyperactive, painful disorders).

The Classical Procedures

Bu	Xie
1) Using a gold needle.	1) Silver needle.
2) Insert during inspiration.	2) Expiration.
3) Along the direction of the energy flow.	3) Against the direction.
4) Rotating anti-clockwise.	4) Clockwise.
5) With little force.	5) Forecfully.
6) Retain long.	6) Short retention.
7) Remove slowly.	7) Rapidly.
8) Closing the hole.	8) Leaving the hole open.
9) Massage the hole.	9) No Massage.

These classical methods are not always strictly adhered to by the modern acupuncturists.

Note: A. The patient preference is Bu because it is a less uncomfortable procedure.

B. The use of the Ko cycle can bring about many complications e.g. impotence following treatment of migraine, headaches after treatment of lung disorders, death following treatment of heart disorder due to eupnoria and so on.

■

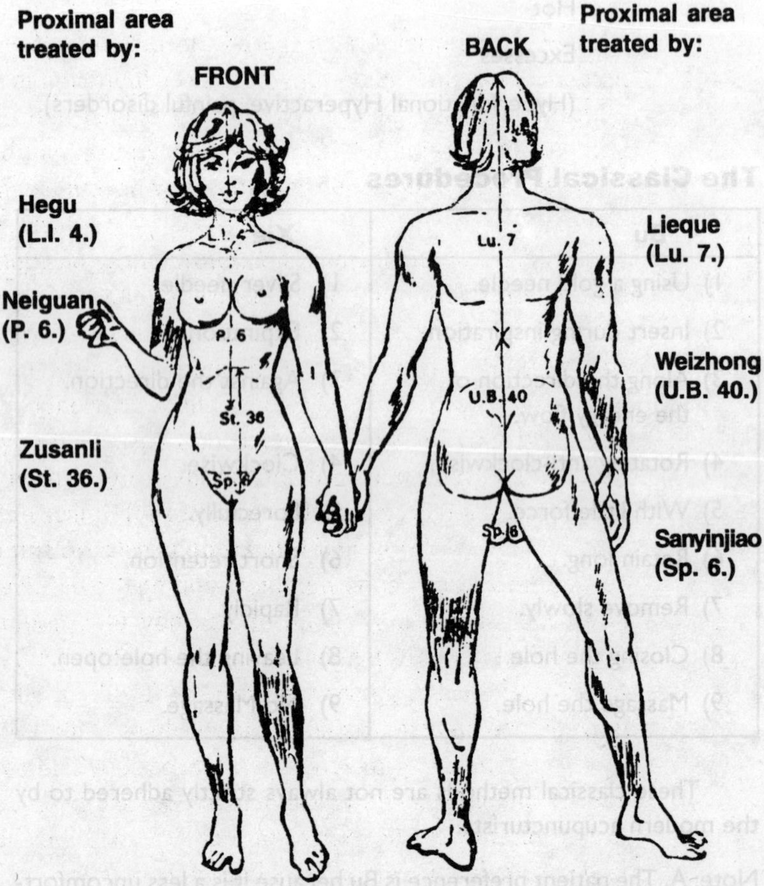

THE PROXIMAL AREAS TREATED BY THE FREQUENTLY USED SIX DISTAL POINTS

PRINCIPLES OF ACUPUNCTURE POINT SELECTION

"One small needle cures a thousand illnesses."

— *Ancient Chinese saying*

To obtain effective results with acupuncture therapy, it is necessary to have a clear idea of the pathways of the Channels and the distribution of the acupuncture points in the body. An acupuncture point occupies a very small circumscribed area of skin, generally not more than a diameter of one millimeter. Accurate anatomical localization is, therefore, very important to obtain the best results in therapy.

When treating a disease, the symptoms and signs should be carefully elucidated in order to determine the nature of the disease and therefore to find out which Organ or Channel is involved. Not infrequently, more than one Organ and several related Channels may be involved.

The following principles are used in the selection of points:

1. **All acupuncture points of a Channel treat diseases occurring along that Channel and also diseases of the corresponding Internal Organ related tissues and of the connected special sense organ**

THE THREE FREQUENTLY USED DISTAL POINTS OF THE UPPER LIMB

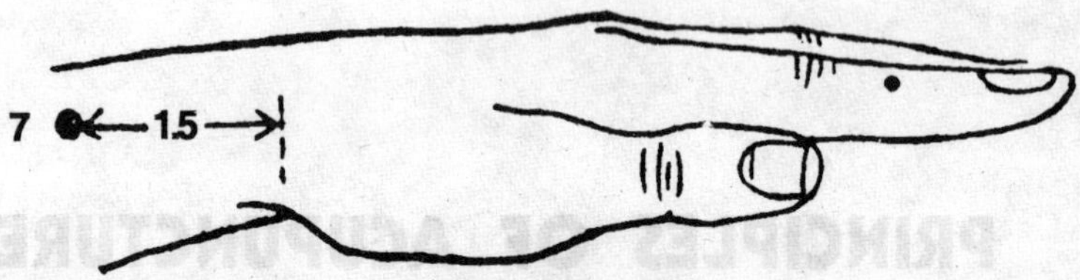

Lieque (Lu. 5.)

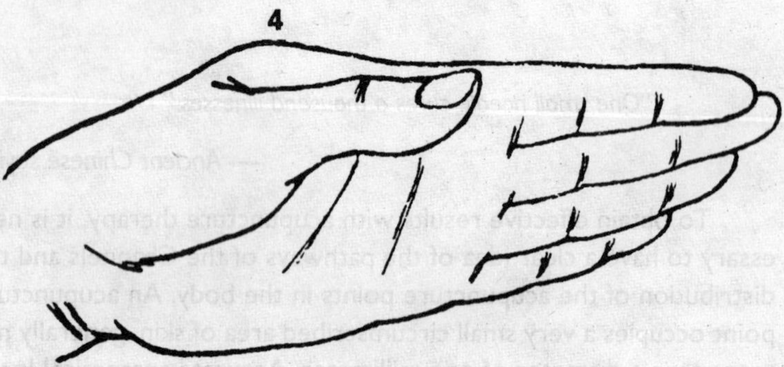

Hegu(L.I. 4.)

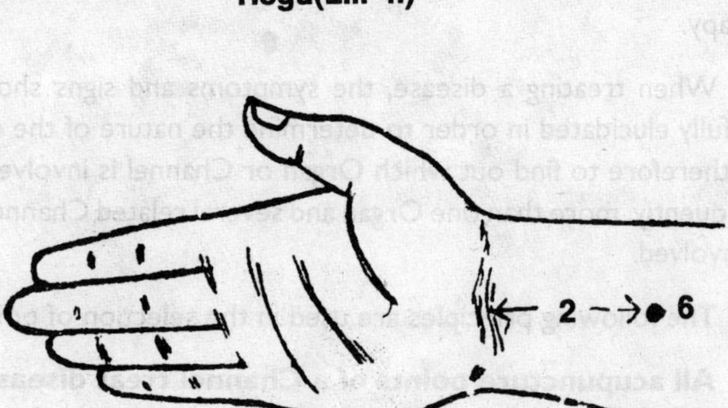

Neiguan (P. 6.)

This is the most important principle. For example, the point Lieque (Lu. 7.) treats arthritis of the wrist, bronchial asthma, rhinitis and skin disorders. (See chapter on The Theories of Traditional Chinese Medicine, where this principle is fully discussed). As a corollary, the acupuncture points of a Channel also treat disorders of the interior-exterior related (Coupled) Channel and its pertaining Organ. The points Lieque (lu. 7.) and Taiyuan (Lu. 9.) may, therefore, be used in treating disorders of the Large Intestine as well as the Lung.

2. All acupuncture points treat diseases of the local and adjacent areas

An acupuncture point has an effect on the area immediately surrounding it, generally an area of about 2-3 centimeters around the points in the limbs, and about half this diameter in the head, neck and trunk. The use of acupuncture points to treat diseases of local and adjacent areas is one of the key principles in the practice of acupuncture therapy. It is the first consideration that should govern the selection of the points for any regional disease. For example, in treating osteoarthritis of the knee, the local points to be selected are those in the immediate vicinity of the knee-joint, i.e. Dubi (St. 35.), Medial-Xiyan (Ex. 32.) and Heding (Ex. 31.). According to authorities such as Y. Omura, the effects of local points are mediated by local reflex arcs causing changes in the regional micro-circulation. Many scientists believe that, irrespective of the precise acupuncture point, similar effects occur if the same dermatome, sclerotome and/or myotome are punctured.

The local points are, by and large, the most effective points in treating a majority of disorders.

3. Points distal to the elbow and distal to the knee treat proximal disorders

The distal areas of the limbs have a much rich innervation and a more complicated network of nerves, than the proximal areas of the limbs. This, perhaps, explains why the Distal points are generally very

THE THREE FREQUENTLY USED DISTAL POINTS OF THE LOWER LIMB

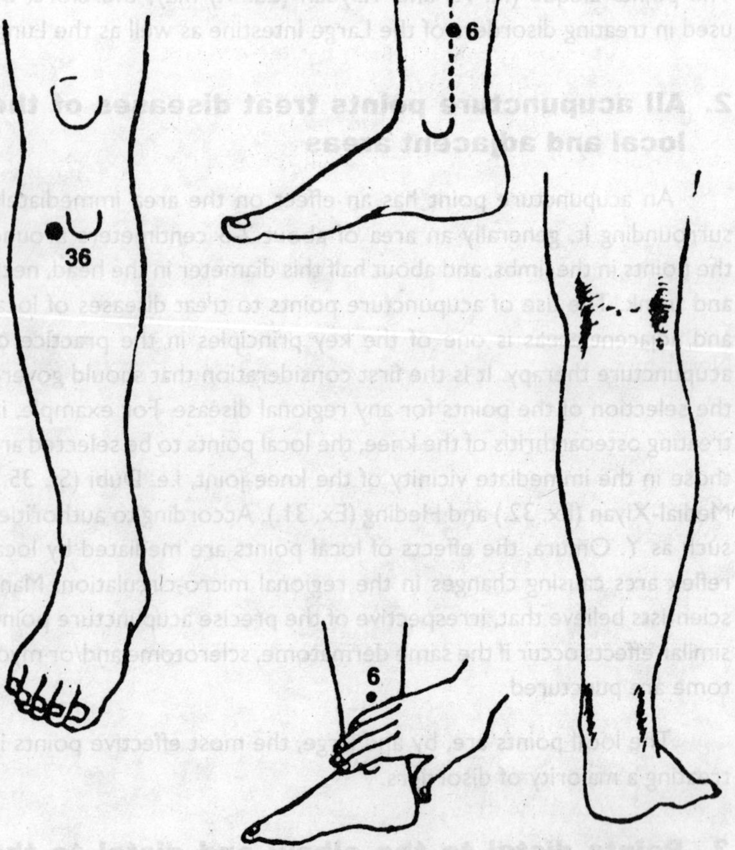

St. 36. Zusanli

Sp. 6. Sanyinjiao

U.B.40. Weizhong

effective. Still, it is a curious fact that a point located in the hand, like Hegu (L.I. 4.), should have distant effects on the face. This is not difficult to understand, however, if one remembers that the hand and face are represented very close to each other in the cerebral cortex.[1]

There are six important frequently used Distal points, three in the upper limb, and three in the lower limb:

Distal Point	Proximal Area Affected
	UPPER LIMB
Hegu (L.I. 4.)	Face and special sense organs front of head and neck.
Lieque (Lu. 7.)	Back of head and neck, back of chest, and lungs.
Neiguan (P. 6.)	Front of chest and upper half of anterior abdominal wall; internal organs of chest, diaphragm, and the internal organs in the upper half of the abdomen.
	LOWER LIMB
Zusanli (St. 36.)	Internal organs of the abdomen.
Weizhong (U.B. 40.)	Low back, urogenital organs.
Sanyinjiao (Sp. 6.)	Perineum, pelvic organs and external genitalia.

(The points Zusanli (St. 36.) and Sanyinjiao (Sp. 6.) are very useful acupuncture points because, apart from their proximal and distal regional effects, they can be used as "notification" points.)

The Distal points are also termed Remote points in some Chinese texts.

1 S. Strauss, Australia, has used thermography to demonstrate these effects.

4. Needling has specific physiological and psychological effects

Modern clinical and laboratory studies have confirmed that the insertion of acupuncture needles into any part of the body produces the following effects:

a) Analgesia.

b) Sedation.

c) Homeostasis.

d) Improvement of the immune mechanisms. Anti-inflammatory effects.

e) Motor effects.

f) Psychological effects.

The insertion of needles into the acupuncture points, themselves, enhances the above effects to a considerably greater degree. At certain acupuncture points these effects are more pronounced than at other points. (However, there are many divergent views today, differing from the traditional belief that there is specificity of action at the acupuncture points).

a) *Analgesia*

Recent research has shown that analgesia occurs with needling due to the raising of the pain threshold. Pain is a symptom of many disorders. The next step, of course, is to relieve the pain. However, in some instances such as in trigeminal neuralgia, herpes zoster and phantom limb pain the symptom of pain itself, is the disease. Some types of pain, like the exquisite pain of childbirth, do not seem to serve any particular purpose.

Acupuncture is the method *par excellence* for the relief of pain and it has limited uses as an anaesthetic agent in surgery. In acupuncture therapy the most effective analgesic points are:

Hegu (L.I. 4.).

Xiangu (St. 43.) or Neiting (St. 44.).

The point Hegu (L.I. 4.), in fact, exhibits all the effects of acupuncture very well. Hegu in Chinese means "the Great Eliminator". It has been given this name because it helps to eliminate a wide spectrum of diseases.

Modern acupuncturists prefer Xiangu (St. 43) to Neiting (St. 44.), as it is a better site for stimulation with a needle.

b) Sedation

Disease causes anxiety. The treatment of any disease, therefore, includes the taking of steps to relieve the patient of anxiety. The following specific points have powerful sedative effects:

Baihui (Du 20.)

Shenmen (H. 7.)

Shenmai (U.B. 62.)

These points are, in fact, a particularly useful combination when treating insomnia and psychosomatic disorders.

The point Baihui (Du 20.) is the governing point of the Du Channel, which in turn governs all other Channels and point.

c) Homeostasis

Homoeostasis is the internal environment of the body in balance. The regulation of such functions as the heartbeat, rate of respiration, body temperature, sleep, appetite, muscle tone, acid-base balance and many other vital parameters, is all geared to delicately balanced homoeostatic mechanisms, mediated either through the nervous system or by chemical transmitters. The autonomic nervous system is a good example of a homeostatic mechanism.

Homeostasis has been found to be one of the most important therapeutic effects of acupuncture needling. With numerous animal experiments performed in the People's Republic of China and in other countries, it has been established that acupuncture needling effects complicated nervous mechanisms and is also associated with the liberation of chemical substances such as acetylcholine, adrenaline, serotonin, endorphins, enkephalins and many others, which could mediate homeostatic and other effects.

The best homeostatic points in clinical practice are as follows:

Quchi (L.I. 11.)

Zusanli (St. 36.)

Sanyinjiao (Sp. 6.)

d) Improvement of the Immune Mechanisms.

For millennia the Chinese have used acupuncture to combat infective disorders. Modern research has shown that certain acupuncture points have the specific effect of stimulating the defence mechanisms of the body, the most powerful of which are:

Dazhui (Du 14.)

Quchi (L.I. 11)

Zusanli (St. 36.)

Sanyinjiao (Sp. 6.)

Today, modern antibiotics are the treatment of choice in infections. However, in cases where there is allergy intolerance or resistance to these drugs, acupuncture may be employed. In chronic infections, where the antibiotics have failed, acupuncture may be useful.

e) Motor effects

Clinically acupuncture is an effective method of treating paralytic disorders. The acupuncture points situated over the motor points are particularly useful in this respect.

5. Certain points on the body surface become tender or act as "trigger points" during disease. They are called "Ah-Shi" points

Some areas of the body become tender particularly in the locomotor disorders, the rheumatic group of diseases and in degenerative conditions like osteoarthitis. These tender points, which are called "*Ah-Shi*" points in acupuncture, should be needled whenever present. "Ah-Shi"[2] in Chinese means "Oh-Yes", this being the verbal reaction of the patient, when the point of tenderness is palpated by the acupuncturist.

There is also another group of points called the "trigger points" that are found in disorders like trigeminal neuralgia. Unlike tender points which give rise only to localized pain, trigger points are also regarded as Ah-Shi points and should be needled. Similarly, the fibrocytic nodules which are often found in locomotor disorders are also considered "Ah-Shi" points. The depth at which the pain is felt. However, when needling Ah-Shi points the anatomy of the area must be considered, to prevent injury to vulnerable structures in that area. Indiscriminate needling of the tender points, especially in the back of the upper half of the trunk, may give rise to serious complications. In one case from a hospital research centre in Stokolm, Sweden, a patient went into severe bradycardia after needling through the triangle of auscultation. (Personal communication from S. Nybecka, Sweden).

6. Certain acupuncture points become painful or exhibit tenderness on palpation when there is disease of the related Organ. They are called "Alarm points"

Alarm points are specific acupuncture points, which become tender in diseases of the related Organ. They are termed Alarm points because they give warning of the presence of, or the impending appearance of disease, of the related Organ. When the disease condition improves, the Alarm points becomes less tender.

These points are therefore used for diagnosis and prognosis, as well as for therapy.

On the anterior aspect of the trunk there are twelve Alarm points corresponding to the twelve Internal Organs. Likewise, there are twelve Alarm points on the trunk. The points at the back are

2 Ah Shi points are also called locus dolenti.

called "Mu-Front" points, while the points at the back are called "Back-Shu" points.[3] It is interesting to note that each of the Back-Shu points is situated almost precisely over the specific paravertebral sympathetic ganglion that is connected with its related Organ; hence it is likely that the functional and anatomical relationship between these points and their related Organ is mediated through the autonomic ganglia of the sympathetic chain.

In therapy these points may be used singly, or in the combination of the Mu-front and Back-Shu points of the affected Organ, without using the Distal points.

The following table is a list of the Mu-Front and the Back-Shu Alarm points:

Mu-Front Point	Internal Organ	Back-Shu Point
Zhongu (Lu. 1.).	Lung	Feishu (U,B. 13.).
Shanzhong (Ren 17.).	Pericardium	Jueyinshu (U.B. 14.).
Jujue (Ren 14.)[4]	Heart	Xinshu (U.B. 15.).
Qimen (Liv. 14.).	Liver	Ganshu (U.B. 18.).
Riyue (G.B. 24.).	Gall Bladder	Danshu (U.B. 19.).
Zhangmen (Liv. 13.).	Spleen	Pishu (U.B. 20.)
Zhongwan (Ren 12.).	Stomach	Weishu (U.B. 21.).
Shimen (Ren 5.).	Sanjiao	Sanjiaoshu (U.B. 22.).
Jingmen (G.B. 25.).	Kidney	Shenshu (U.B. 23.).
Tianshu (St. 25.).	Large Intestine	Dachangshu (U.B. 25.).
Guanyuan (Ren 4.).	Small Intestine	Xiaochangshu (U.B. 27.).
Zhongji (Ren 3.).	Urinary Bladder	Pangguangshu (U.B. 28.).

In addition to the above, there are four Special Alarm points:

Liver:	Zhongdu (Liv. 6.).
Gall Bladder :	Jianjing (G.B. 21).
	Dannang (Ex. 35.).
Vermiform Appendix :	Lanwei (Ex. 33.).

3 All "Back-Shu" points are located in the Urinary Bladder Channel.

4 This point is also spelt as Jugue.

7. There are eight specific acupuncture points called the Eight Influential points which are used to treat diseases of specific tissues

The following eight acupuncture points, in addition to their other effects, treat diseases of certain specific tissues:

Influential Point	Tissue
Shanzhong (Ren 17.)	Respiratory tissue.
Dashu (U.B. 11.).	Bone and cartilage.
Geshu (U.B. 17.).	Blood.
Zhongwan (Ren 12.).	Fu ("hollow") Organs.
Zhangmen (Liv. 13.).	Zang ("solid") Organs.
Taiyuan (Lu. 9.).	Vascular system.
Yanglingquan (G.B. 34.).	Muscle and tendon.
Xuanzhong (G.B. 39.).	Marrow.

Some acupuncturists in the West call these points *correspondence points."*

8. Each of the Twelve Paired Channels has an acupuncture point called the Xi-Cleft point, which treats acute diseases of the Channel and the pertaining Internal Organs

Channel	Xi-Cleft Point
Lung	Kongzui (Lu. 6.).[5]
Large Intestine	Wenliu (L.I. 7.).
Stomach	Liangqiu (St. 34.).[5]
Spleen	Diji (Sp. 8.).
Heart	Yinxi (H. 6.).[5]
Small Intestine	Yanglao (S.I. 6.).
Urinary Bladder	Jinmen (U.B. 63.).
Kidney	Shuiquan (K. 5.).[5]

5 Commonly used Xi-Cleft points.

THE MU-FRONT ALARM POINTS

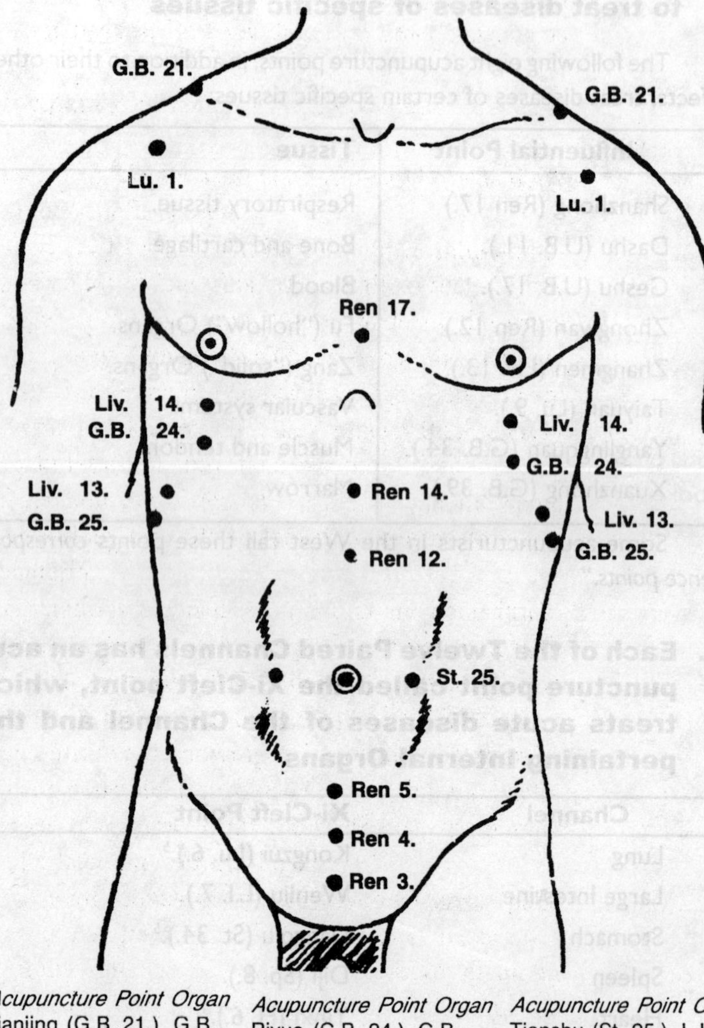

Acupuncture Point Organ	*Acupuncture Point Organ*	*Acupuncture Point Organ*
Jianjing (G.B. 21.), G.B.	Riyue (G.B. 24.). G.B.	Tianshu (St. 25.). L.I.
Zhongfu (Lu. 1.). Lu	Jujue (Ren 14.). H.	Shimen (Ren 5.). S.J.
Shanzhong (Ren 17.). P.	Zhangmen (Liv. 13.). Sp.	Guanyuan (Ren 4.). S.I.
Gimen (Liv. 14). Liv.	Jingmen (Liv. 25.). K.	Zhongji (Ren 3.). U.B.
	Zhong wan (Ren 12.), St.	

Note: The Special Alarm point of Gall bladder at the shoulder is also included.

Pericardium	Ximen (P. 4.).[5]
Sanjiao	Huizong (S.J. 7.).
Gall bladder	Waiqiu (G.B. 36.).
Liver	Zhongdu (Liv. 6.)[5]

To relieve acute disorders very strong manual stimulation is carried out at the Xi-Cleft points to reduce the sieqi. These points are termed *"first-aid points"* by some Western acupuncturists.

9. Each of the Twelve Paired Channels has a point called the *Yuan-Source* point, which treats sub-acute and chronic disorders of the pertaining Organ

The Yuan-Source point is the maximum concentration of the vital energy of the Internal Organ on the Channel. This point may be looked upon as the main sluice gate of an irrigation channel, the Internal Organ being the reservoir.

The Yuan-Source point is connected directly to the Internal Organ by a deep connection. It is also connected to the Coupled Channel at the Luo-Connecting point.

All Yuan-Source points are situated near the wrists or the ankles.

Channel	Yuan-Source Point
Lung	Taiyuan (Lu. 9.).
Large Intestine	Hegu (L.I. 4.).
Stomach	Chongyang (St. 42.).
Spleen	Taibai (Sp. 3.).
Heart	Shenmen (H. 7.).
Small Intestine	Hand-Wangu (S.I. 4.).
Urinary Bladder	Jinggu (U.B. 64.).
Kidney	Taixi (K. 3.).
Pericardium	Daling (P.7.).
Sanjiao	Yangchi (S.J. 4.).
Gall Bladder	Qiuxu (G.B. 40.).
Liver	Taichong (Liv. 3.).

10. There are fifteen named acupuncture points called Luo[6]-Connecting points in the Fourteen Channels (the Spleen Channel has two). These points connect the interior-exterior Channels to each other

A Luo-Connecting point is a point of entrance of vital energy to and from the Coupled Channels. These points also called "junction point" by some Western practitioners.

According to traditional Chinese Medicine, Luo-Connecting points are places where a communication exists between a pair of Yin and Yang Channels, which have what is called an "interior-exterior relationship". By puncturing at these points of communication it is believed that, energy imbalance in the pair of Coupled Channels can be restored to normal or optimal levels.

The collateral Luo-Connecting Channels connect the Coupled Channels from the Luo-Connecting point of one Channel to the Yuan-Source point of the other Channel. Therefore, it is common practice to use the combination of the two Yuan-Source and the two connecting points of a pair of channels in diseases involving the Coupled Channels or Coupled Organs. Thus, whenever there is reason to believe that the disease requiring treatment involves both the interior and exterior related Channels or Organs, the Luo-Connecting points may be used in combination with the Yuan-Source points (e.g. an asthmatic who has severe constipation).

6 Luo in Xgubese means 'the doorx'

The 15 Luo-Connecting Points

Yang (Exterior) Channel	Luo-Connecting Point	Yin (Interior) Channel	Luo-Connecting Point
Large Intestine	Pianli (L.I. 6.)	Lung	Lieque (Lu.7.)
Sanjiao	Waiguan (S.J. 5.).	Pericardium	Neiguan (P. 6.).
Small Intestine	Zhizheng (S.I. 7.)	Heart	Tongli (H. 5.).
Stomach	Fenglong (St. 40.).	Spleen	Gongsun (Sp. 4.). Dabao (Sp. 21.), (the Major Luo point).
Gall Bladder	Guangming (G.B. 37).	Liver	Ligou (Liv. 5.).
Urinary Bladder	Feiyang (U.B. 58.).	Kidney	Dazhong (K. 4.).
Du	Changqiang (Du. 1.).	Ren	Jiuwei (Ren 15).

11. Symptomatic points—Combinations of specific points alleviate symptoms of certain diseases

There are combinations of points some of which have been used from ancient times to treat common disorders. Some of the frequently used points are listed below:

Symptoms	Points Used for Treatment
Asthmatic attack	Tiantu (Ren 22.); Kongzui Lu. 6.).
Abdominal distension	Tianshu (St. 25.); Zusanii (St. 36.).
Cough	Tiantu (Ren 22.); Lieque (Lu. 7.).
Constipation	Tianshu (St. 25.); Zhigou (S.J. 6.).

Convulsions	Renzhong (Du 26.).
Diarrhoea	Gongsun (Sp. 4.); Zusanli (St. 36.) Qihai (Ren 6.); Sanyinjiao (Sp. 6.).
Fever	Dazhui (Du 14.); Quchi (L.I. 11.); Hegu (L.I. 4.).
Hiccough	Neiguan (P. 6.); Geshu (U.B. 17.) Zusanli (St. 36.).
Incontinence (urinary)	Qugu (Ren 2.); Sanyinjiao (Sp. 6.).
Incontinence (rectal)	Changqiang (Du I.); Chengshan (U. B. 57.).
Insomnia	Baihui (Du 20.); Shenmen (H. 7.); Anmian I & II (Ex. 8. & Ex. 9.)
Edema	Shimen (Ren 5.); Shuifen (Ren 9.); Yinlingquan (Sp. 9.); Pishu (U.B. 20.).
Pain in the chest	Shanzhong (Ren 17.); Neiguan (P. 6.).
Phlegm, sputum (excessive)	Fenglong (St. 40.).
Pruritus (allergic)	Dushu (U.B. 16.); Xuehai (Sp. 10.).
Sneezing	Yintang (Ex. I.); Yingxiang (L.I. 20.).
Sweating (excessive)	Yinxi (H. 6.); Fuliu (K.7.); Hegu (L.I. 4.).
Vomiting, nausea	Neiguan (P. 6.); Zusanli St. (36.).

When acute symptoms are exhibited, it is necessary to treat the patient first symptomatically, before a pulse diagnosis is carried out.

12. A disease of one side of the body may be treated by acupuncture points of either side

The Channels on the two sides of the body are connected to each other by the Du, Ren, the Extra Channels and the Collaterals. According to neurology, the activities of both sides of the body are coordinated by the corpus callosum, and at every level below this, in the brain stem and in the spinal cord there are segmental connections. This principle is useful if a particular limb cannot be punctured due to the presence of skin disease, ulceration, swelling, Buerger's disease and varicosity. In such cases, the opposite (contralateral) limb may be used.

If the action of acupuncture is due to humoral mechanisms, such as endorphins, enkephalins, serotonin etc., then too, it is understandable that the side of therapy does not matter.

Some acupuncturists believe however, that when distal points are employed the contralateral side is more effective. It is hypothesized that the representation of the homunculus in the thalamus, in a globular foetal position explains this. The action of the Confluent points is also explained on this basis. This is known as the *Thalamic Neurone Theory of Acupuncture.*

13. The Confluent point of the Eight Extraordinary Channels may he used to treat diseases with mixed symptomatology (complex syndromes)

Since the Eight Extraordinary Channels interconnect the Paired Channels, their symptomatology too should be 'taken into account in therapy. There are eight points belonging to the Twelve Paired Channels situated in the limbs (four in the upper and four in the lower limb) called the Confluent points, the stimulation of which treats diseases related to the Twelve Channels as well as the Extraordinary Channels. Usually diseases or syndromes exhibiting mixed, complex symptomatology are treated by using these points.[7]

The table below illustrates these relationships:

7 Used on the left side in males (Yang side) and the right side in females (Yin side).

The Eight Confluent Point Combinations

Confluent point	Regular Channel	Extra Channel	Indications (area of the body)
Neiguan (P. 6.).	Pericardium	Yinwei	Heart, chest, stomach
Gongsun (Sp. 4.).	Spleen	Chong	
Houxi (S.I. 3.).	Small Intestine	Du	Neck, shoulder,
Shenmal (U.B. 62.).	Urinary Bladder	Yangqiao	back, inner canthus
Waiguan (S.J. 5.).	Sanjiao	Yangwei	
Foot-Linqi (G.B. 41.).	Gall Bladder	Dai	Retroauricular area. Cheek, outer canthus
Liaque (Lu. 7.).	Lung	Ren	
Zhaohai (K. 6.).	Kidney	Yinqiao	Pharynx, chest, lung

Points of the upper extremities may be combined with those of the lower extremities for better therapeutic result. For example, Neiguan (P. 6.) combined with Gongsun (Sp. 4.) is indicated in diseases of the heart, chest and epigastric region. Houxi (S.I. 3.) combined with Shenmai (U.B. 62.) is indicated in diseases of the neck, shoulder, back and inner canthus; Waiguan (S.J. 5.) combined with Foot-Linqi (G.B. 41.) is indicated in disorders of the mastoid region, cheek and outer canthus; while Lieque (Lu. 7.) and Zhaohai (K. 6.) in Combination, are indicated in disorders of the Pharynx, chest and lungs.

The Eight Confluent Points

EXTRAORDINARY CHANNEL AND ITS SYMPTOMATOLOGY	CON-FLUENT POINT	REGULAR CHANNEL
1. DU (The Back Midline Channel). Ano-rectal disorders, Low backache, immune and infective disorders, mental and neurological disorders, oral disorders.	Houxi (S.I. 3.).	Small Intestine
2. REN (The Front Midline Channel). Genito-urinary and gastro-intestinal disorders, heart and lung disorders speech disorders, facial paralysis.	Lieque (Lu. 7.).	Lung
3. CHONG (The Vital Channel. Gastro-intestinal and gynae-cological disorders.	Gongsun (Sp. 4.).	Spleen
4. DAI (The Belt Channel. Abdominal distension, weakness and motor impairment in the lumbar region.	Foot-Linqi (G.B. 41.).	Gall Bladder
5. YANGCHIAO (The yang Moti-lity Channel). Insomnia, paralysis, numbness or muscular, atrophy in the limbs.	Shenmai (U.B. 62.).	Urinary Bladder
6. YINCHIAO (The Yin Motility Channel). Hypersomnia, paralysis, numbness or muscular atrophy of the lower limbs.	Zhaohai (K. 6.).	Kidney
7. YANGWEI (The Yang Regu-lating Channel). Chills and fever.	Waiguan (S.J. 5.)	Sanjiao
8. YINWEI (The Yin Regulating Channel). Upper abdominal and cardiac pain.	Neiguan	Pericar-dium

14. In each of the Twelve Channels there are five points known as the Five Shu points which correspond to the Five Elements

These are known as the Sixty Command Points, and are used principally to bring about energy equilibrium in the Channels. The fundamental concept of traditional Chinese Medicine is that diseases arise from extrinsic and intrinsic factors causing the normal flow of vital energy to be disrupted. The object of acupuncture (as also of all other traditional Chinese therapies) is to restore the normal energy flow and thereby bring the organism to a state of health. The experienced traditional physician is able to identify, mainly with the use of pulse diagnosis, the imbalance of energy in the Organ. Diagnosis was aided by the observation of changes in related areas or tissues and correlating them to the pathological states of the Zang-Fu Organ. Having ascertained which Organs are in disequilibrium and the nature of such disequilibrium, the point or points for puncturing are selected according to the Theory of the Five Elements, which reflects the cyclic flow of energy in the Zang-Fu Organs.

If, for example, the energy is deficient in the Organ Liver (Element: Wood) and the concomitant excess is in the Organ Kidney (Element: Water) then the disequilibrium may be corrected by puncturing the Water point of the Liver Channel. This allows the excess energy to flow through. from the Kidney to the Liver in the Generative or Sheng cycle according to the Mother-Son Law. Similarly, if the excess is discovered in the Lung (Element: Metal), then a puncture would have to be effected on the Metal point of the Kidney Channel after puncturing the water point of the Liver Channel. However, if the excess is in the Large Intestine, the Metal point of the Liver Channel is punctured, as the energy would then flow in the Ko cycle directly to the liver.[8] This is because of the principle that the energy flow in the Ko or destructive cycle changes from Yang to Yin or from Yin to Yang as it reaches the target Organ, thus resulting in its "destructive" activity. (If, on the other hand, the excess is in the Gall Bladder, since this is within the same Element, equilibrium may be

8 The use of the Ko cycle in this manner can cause certain complications.

brought about by puncturing the Luo-Connecting point of the liver. (The Five Shu points are not involved in this transfer).

It will be observed that in the example given here, it is the Channel which is deficient in energy that is first punctured. The principle, follows the ancient maxim that energy should not be wasted; the energy must be gently "drawn" by the deficient Channel, from the Channel having the excess, "as an infant sucks milk from its Mother". The technique of puncturing in all these example is, therefore, the tonification or "bu" or re-enforcing method.

The Sixty Command Points are all located distal to the elbow and distal to the knee.

The technique. of Chinese pulse diagnosis, as a method of detecting energy disequilibrium, is most profitably used in the chronic stages of disease. In the acute stage, the presenting symptoms are treated by specific points or combinations of points which are traditionally prescribed. Strong stimulation, i.e., the "Xie" or reducing method is often used at the main points. For example, for fever the points Dazhui (Du 14.), Quchi (L.I. 1.1.), and Hegu (L.I. 4.). are used with strong hand stimulation at the first and third points' for cardiac pain Shanzhong (Ren 17.), and Neiguan (P. 6.) are used with strong hand stimulation at the latter point; for very acute diarrhoea (as by cholera) the point Gongsun (Sp. 4.) is strongly stimulated.

The presence of acute symptoms, in fact, usually masks the indication of the fundamental energy imbalances in the radial pulses. The traditional Chinese physician, therefore, first treats the acute symptoms and it is only after these have subsided that he makes a careful examination of the pulses. It is then possible, for the expert, to make a fairly accurate assessment of the energy disequilibrium, select the indicated point or points out of the Five Shu points (60 Command points) and carry out puncture so that the energy imbalances are restored.

Discussed below are the Five Shu points of each of the Twelve channels and their general indications, outside of those for. balancing energies as described in the previous page.

1) *Jing-Well point:*

This is always the distal-most point-the first of the Yang or the last point of the Yin Channels of Hand, or the first point of the Yin or the last point of the Yang Channels of foot. All the Jing-Well points are situated near the nails of the fingers or toes, except Yongquan (K.1.), which is situated on the sole of the foot.

The Jing-Well points treat acute emergencies such as fainting, coma, epilepsy, convulsions, cardiac arrest and respiratory arrest. These points may be pressed or pricked to bleed. The forefinger nail of the acupuncturist is usually adequate in treating at Jing-Well points, when needles are not at hand. If a needle is available, Yongquan (K. I.) gives the best results.

The Jing-Well points are situated in the areas where there is a close network of sensory nerves. Stimulation causes a heavy barrage of afferent impulses to 'be generated, thereby resuscitating the patient in the emergency state. The Jing-Well points, therefore, are also known as "Resuscitation points".

The point Renzhong (Du 26.), which is the end point on the skin of the Du Channel, is also very useful in acute emergencies, as acupressure on this point is usually sufficient to revive the patient. The total number of Jing-Well points is, therefore, twenty five.

In using laser-beam therapy, it is common practice to treat at the Jing-Well points of the respective Channels. Jing-Well points lying at the distal-most locations are believed to be the most superficially located points; therefore, this is the situation of choice to introduce external energy such as a laser-beam energy into the body. This is, however, still an experimental, but promising form of therapy.

2) *Yung-Spring point*[9]*:*

This is always the point just proximal to the Jing-Well point; the penultimate point at the extremities.

9 This is spelt Rong-Spring point.

Yung-Spring points are commonly used to treat febrile diseases and other acute disorders.

3) *Shu-Stream point*:

This point is the third or antepenultimate point, located next to the Yung-Spring point, except in the case of the Gall bladder Channel, where it is the fourth point removed[10] from the Jing-Well point.

Shu-Stream points are used mainly in rheumatic disorders, particularly involving the small joints of the hands and feet. Sub-acute and chronic disorders are treated using these points.

4) *Jing-River point*:

This point is always located just proximal to the wrist or ankle.

The Jing-River points are indicated in disorders of the Zang Organs.

5) *He-Sea point*:

This point lies at, or just distal to, the elbow or knee. He-sea points treat a variety of Organ disorders.

Each of the Five Shu points in a Channel is related to one of the Five Elements and follows the generative Sheng cycle from the Jing-Well point to the He-Sea point. The Jing-Well point of the Yin-Channels always corresponds to the Element Wood. (Therefore, in the Yin Channels the Yung-Spring point corresponds to Fire, the Shu-Stream point corresponds to Earth, the Jing-River point corresponds to Metal, and the He-Sea point corresponds to water). The Jing-Well points of the Yang Channels always correspond to the Element Metal. And in the Yang Channels, the Yung-Spring points correspond to water, the Shu-Stream points correspond to Fire and the He-Sea points correspond to Earth.

10 Proximal from.

The following table summarizes these relationships:

The Sixty Command Points of the 12 Channels or the Five Shu Points

YANG	G.B.	S.J.	U.B.	S.I.	St.	L.I.		Liv.	P.	K.	H.	Sp.	Lu.	YIN
Metal	44	1	67	1	45	1	Jing-Well	1	9	1	9	1	11	**Wood**
Water	43	2	66	2	44	2	Yung-Spring	2	8	2	8	2	10	**Fire**
Wood	41	3	65	3	43	3	Shu-Stream	3	7	3	7	3	9	**Earth**
Fire	38	6	60	4	41	5	Jing-River	4	5	7	4	5	8	**Metal**
Earth	34	10	54	8	36	11	He-Sea	8	3	10	3	9	5	**Water**

The Yang Element at each level destroys the Yin Element at the same Shu-point level, as exemplified in the destructive Ko Cycle of the Five Elements.

The *Essentials of Chinese Acupuncture*, Beijing, (1980), discusses an extra set of He-Sea points related to the six Fu Organs:

"The Yang channels have an extra set of He-Sea points known as the Lower He-Sea points. The Lower He-Sea point of the *fu* organs usually give satisfactory results in treating diseases of the six *fu* organs, the reason being that the *fu* organs i.e. stomach, large intestine, small intestine, gall bladder, urinary bladder and *sanjiao* are closely related with the three *Yang* channels of foot, and each has a Lower He-Sea Point. At the same time the three *yang* channels of foot communicate with the three *yang* channels of hand. In treating diseases of the six *fu* organs, the main points selected are the Lower He-Sea Points. For gastric pain and acidity Zusanli (St. 36.) is selected; for dysentery appendicitis, Shangjuxu (St. 37.) is used; Yanglingquan (G.B. 34.) is for pain in the gall bladder, vomiting, etc."

The Lower He-Sea Points of the Six Fu Organs

Yang Channel of the	Fu-Organ	Lower He-Sea Point
Foot-Yangming	Stomach	Zusanli (St. 36.).
	Large Intestine	Shangjuxu (St. 37.).
	Small Intestine	Xiajuxu (St. 39.).
Foot-Shaoyang	Gall Bladder	Yanglingquan (G.B. 34.).
Foot-Taiyang	Urinary Bladder	Weizhong (U.B. 40.).
	Sanjiao	Weiyang (U.B. 39.).

15. The "Mother" and "Son" points of a Channel may be used for tonifying and sedating respectively, the Channel or the pertaining Internal Organs

The "mother point" of a channel has tonifying effect, and is indicated in *xu* syndrome of its related channel, while the "son point" has a reducing effect and is indicated in the *shi* syndrome of its related channel. Hence the maxim: "Reinforce the 'mother' for *xu* syndrome' reduce the 'son' for *shi* syndrome." For example; when the Lung Channel in involved in *xu* syndrome with symptoms of chronic cough, shortness of breath, low voice, sweating and therapy weak pulse, then the reinforcing method on Taiyuan (Lu. 9.) may be prescribed. On the other hand, if the Lung Channel is involved in *shi* syndrome with abrupt onset of cough, dyspnea, hoarse voice, stifling sensation in chest with inability to lie flat, and a superficial and forceful pulse may be present. Chize (Lu. 5.) with the reducing method may then be prescribed.

16. Horary points. (These have been discussed earlier)

17. "Mother" and "son" Points for Reinforcing and Reducing

Channel	Mother point Bu (Reinforcing) (Tonifying)	Son point Xie (Reducing) (Sedating)
Lung Channel of Hand-Taiyin	Taiyuan (Lu.9.)	Chize (Lu. 5.).
Large Intestine Channel of Hand-Yangming	Quchi (L.I. 11.)	Erjian (L.I. 2.).
Stomach Channel of Foot-Yangming	Jiexi (St.41.)	Lidui (St. 45.).
Spleen Channel of Foot-Taiyang	Dadu (Sp. 2.) (Sp. 5.)	Shangqiu
Heart Channel of Hand-Shaoyin	Shaochong (H.9.)	Shenmen (H. 7.).
Small Intestine Channel of Hand-Taiyang	Houxi (S.I. 3.)	Xiaohai (S.I. 8.)
Urinary Bladder Channel of Foot-Taiyang	Zhiyin (U.B. 67.)	Shugu (U.B. 65.).
Kidney Channel of Foot-Shaoyin	Fuliu (K. 7.)	Yongquan (K. 1.).
Pericardium Channel of Hand-Jueyin	Zhongchong (P. 9.)	Daling (P. 7.).
Sanjiao Channel of Hand-Shaoyang	Hand-Zhongzhu (S.J. 3.)	Tianjing (S.J. 10.)
Gall Bladder Channel of Foot Shaoyang	Xiaxi (G.B. 43.)	Yangfu (G.B. 38.)
Liver Channel of Foot-Jueyin	Ququan (Liv. 8.)	Xingjian (Liv. 2.).

THE BACK-SHU POINTS AND THEIR RELATIONSHIPS TO THE SYMPATHETIC OUTFLOW TO THE INTERNAL ORGANS

BACK SHU POINT	ORGAN
U.B. 13 Feishu	Lung
U.B.14 Jueyinshu	Pericardium
U.B. 15 Xinshu	Heart
U.B. 16 Dushu U.B. 17 Geshu	Diaphragm
U.B. 18 Ganshu	Liver
U.B. 19 Danshu	G.B.
U.B. 20 Pishu	Spleen
U.B. 21 Weishu	Stomach
U.B. 22 Sanjiaoshu	Sanjiao
U.B. 23 Shenshu	Kidney
U.B. 24 Qihaishu	
U.B. 25 Dachangshu	Large Int.
U.B. 26 Guanyuanshu	
U.B.27 Ziaochangshu	Small Int.
U.B.28 Pangguangshu	U.B.
U.B. 29 Zhonglushu	
U.B. 30 Baihuanshu	

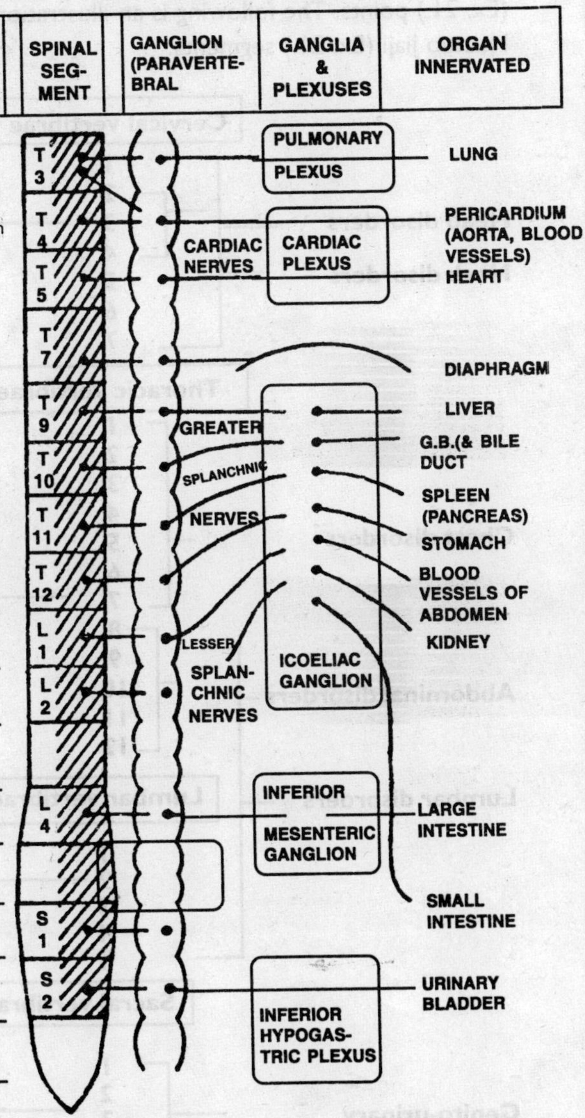

The Back-Shu points are a group of points displaying a segmental arrangement. They form a fairly accurate surface making of the outflow of the sympathetic ganglia to their respective pertaining organs. The Back-Shu points are an interesting example of a holistic meeting point of the chiropracter, osteopath, neurophysiologist, the anatomist and the traditional acupuncturist.

A very useful example is the use of the relevant Huatuo Jioji (Ex. 21.) points. The following is an illustration of the indications of Huatuo Jiaji (Ex. 21.) segments:

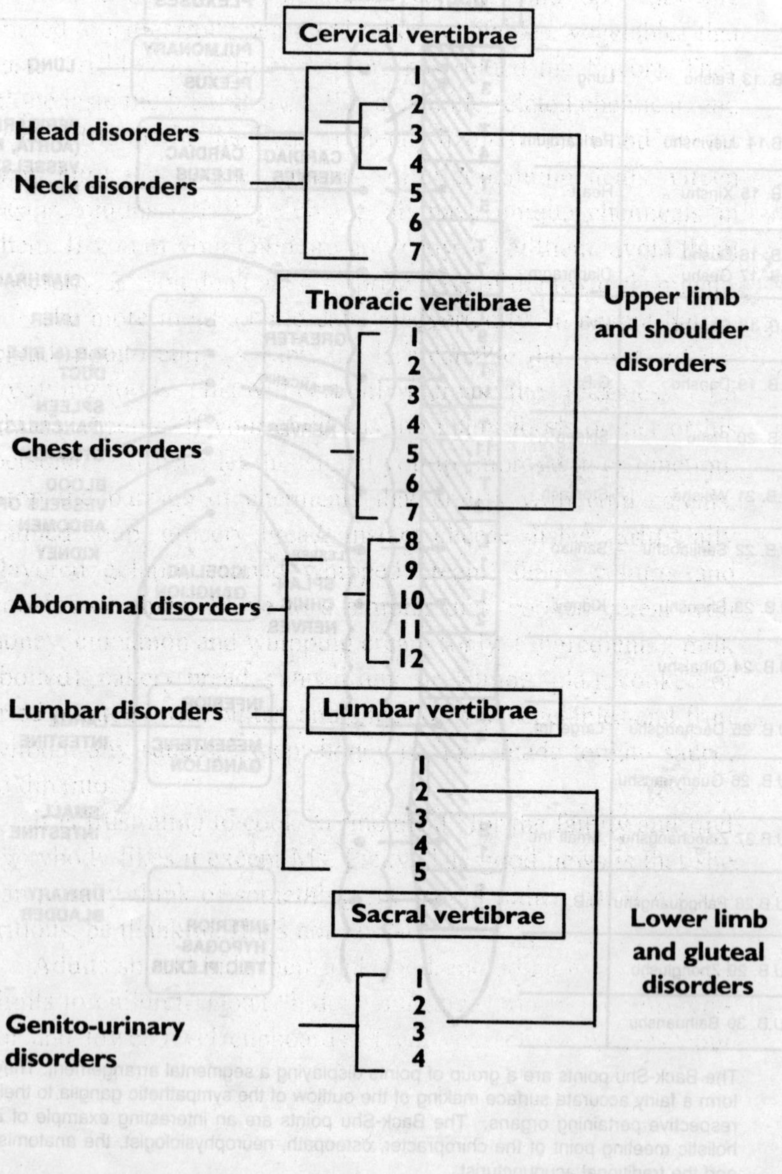

18. Points according to Innervation

Points according to innervation in (a) the same dermatome, (b) the same myotome, (c) the pathway of a nerve (e.g., in sciatica), may be selected in segmental, neurological disorders, e.g., trigeminal neuralgia, herpes zoster, cervical spondylosis, sciatic pain and intercostal neuralgia.

For diseases of the head, trunk, upper and lower limbs, and internal organs, selection of points may be made in areas supplied by the spinal nerves, nerve plexus or appropriate nerve trunk.

THE NOON-MIDNIGHT LAW THE USE OF THE DIAMETRICALLY OPPOSITE POINTS

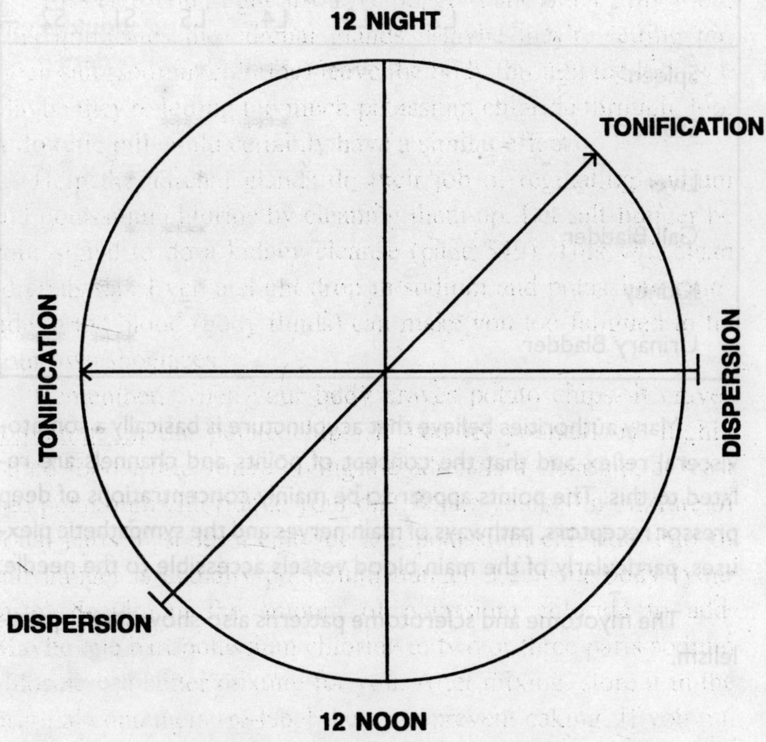

Tonification of an Horary point at the peak hour causes sedation of the diametrically opposite Channel and Organ and vice versa.

TABLE OF DERMATOMES OF ACUPUNCTURE CHANNELS

	C5	C6	C7	C8	T1	T2
Lung	**	***				
Large Intestine		***	**			
Pericardium			***			
Sanjiao			**	***		
Small Intestine				****		
Heart				*	***	
	L2	**L3**	**L4**	**L5**	**S1**	**S2**
Spleen		****	****	*		
Stomach			****	****		
Liver				*	*	
Gall Bladder				****	*	
Kidney			*	*	****	
Urinary Bladder					****	****

Many authorities believe that acupuncture is basically a somato-visceral reflex and that the concept of points and channels are related to this. The points appear to be mainly concentrations of deep pressor receptors, pathways of main nerves and the sympathetic plexuses, particularly of the main blood vessels accessible to the needle.

The myotome and sclerotome patterns also show similar parallelism.

A REVIEW OF THE PRINCIPLES OF ACUPUNCTURE POINT SELECTION FOR THERAPY

Below is a summary of the combinations of points which may be used for selecting points to treat illness, based on the principles described. The particular combination which is eventually selected depends on the nature of the disease, the symptomatology presented, the condition of the patient and, of course, on the experience of the acupuncturist.

1) Painful points:

   a) Ah-Shi points.

   b) Alarm points.

2) Points having specific physiological and psychological effects, e.g., those points having specific analgesic, sedative, homeostatic and immune enhancing properties.

3) Points according to the presenting symptoms.

4) Jing-Well point (Resuscitation Points).

5) Combination of Local points and relevant Distal (Remote) points.

6) Combination of Bank-Shu and Mu-Front points.

7) Points along the affected Channel.

8) Points according to the nerve supply of the diseased area.

9) Influential points (Correspondence points).

10) Yuan-Source points (Source points) in chronic disorders of the Internal Organs.

11) Luo-Connecting points (Junction points) used in imbalances of the coupled Channels or coupled Internal Organs.

12) Combination of Yuan-Source and Luo-Connecting points.

13) Xi-Cleft points (First-Aid points).

14) Confluent points of the Eight Extraordinary Channels.

15) Tonification and Sedation points (Mother and Son Points).

16) Points according to the Four Laws of traditional medicine.

   a) Mother-Son Law.

   b) Husband-Wife Law (used together with pulse diagnosis).

   c) Noon-Midnight Law.

   d) The Theory of the Five Elements (Five Shu points, Command points—points selected by pulse diagnosis).

17) Auriculotherapy (ear acupuncture).

18) Head needle therapy (scalp acupuncture).

19) Other Microsystem acupuncture points:

   a) Face-Nose acupuncture.

   b) Hand acupuncture.

   c) Foot acupuncture.

   d) Wrist-ankle acupuncture.

20) Ancillary methods.

   a) Plum Blossom needle therapy.

   b) Moxibustion.

   c) Laser beam therapy.

   d) Electro-acupuncture. According to Voll (EAV).

   e) Ryodoraku.

   f) Shiatsu.

   g) Reflexotherapy.

   h) Sonotherapy.

   i) Magnetotherapy

   j) Cryotherapy

k) TENS., TCNS.[11]

l) Moratherapy Biotron therapy.

21) Points selected using electro-diagnostic methods.

22) The experience points of each school of acupuncture.

23) Acu-massage (micromassage) points.

24) Periosteal-puncture points.

25) Secret points, strange points, extraordinary points.

26) HOMOEOPUNCTURE: The use of the homoeopathic remedy (simillimum) on the needle. Results appear to be very much better than acupuncture alone.[12]

These different groupings may be used singly or in combination. It must be remembered that Yin and Yang **Distal points** in close proximity are not used together, except when using the Yuan-Source and the Luo-Connecting points in the Coupled Channels.

If the results are inadequate with body acupuncture, ear acupuncture and head needle therapy may be used. Head, ear and body points may be combined in the same patient, when indications exist. Broadly, it has been our experience that body acupuncture is more effective in locomotor disorders, ear acupuncture in disorders of the internal organs such as peptic ulcer and intestinal disorders, and head needle therapy in neurological disorders. However, in all cases, it is best to start with body acupuncture.

Where the traditional methods fail to produce an adequate response, ancillary methods such as moxibustion or laser-beam therapy may be employed.

Acupressure also gives good results, but it is too time-consuming to be used in a busy clinic.

---

11 Transcutaneous electro-neurostimulation.

12 *Reference:* **Clinical Homoeopathy:** Chandrakanthi Press (International), Kalubowila, Sri Lanka (1984), 3rd Edition.

THE INSTITUTE OF ACUPUNCTURE, COLOMBO SOUTH GOVERNMENT GENERAL HOSPITAL, KALUBOWILA, SRI LANKA

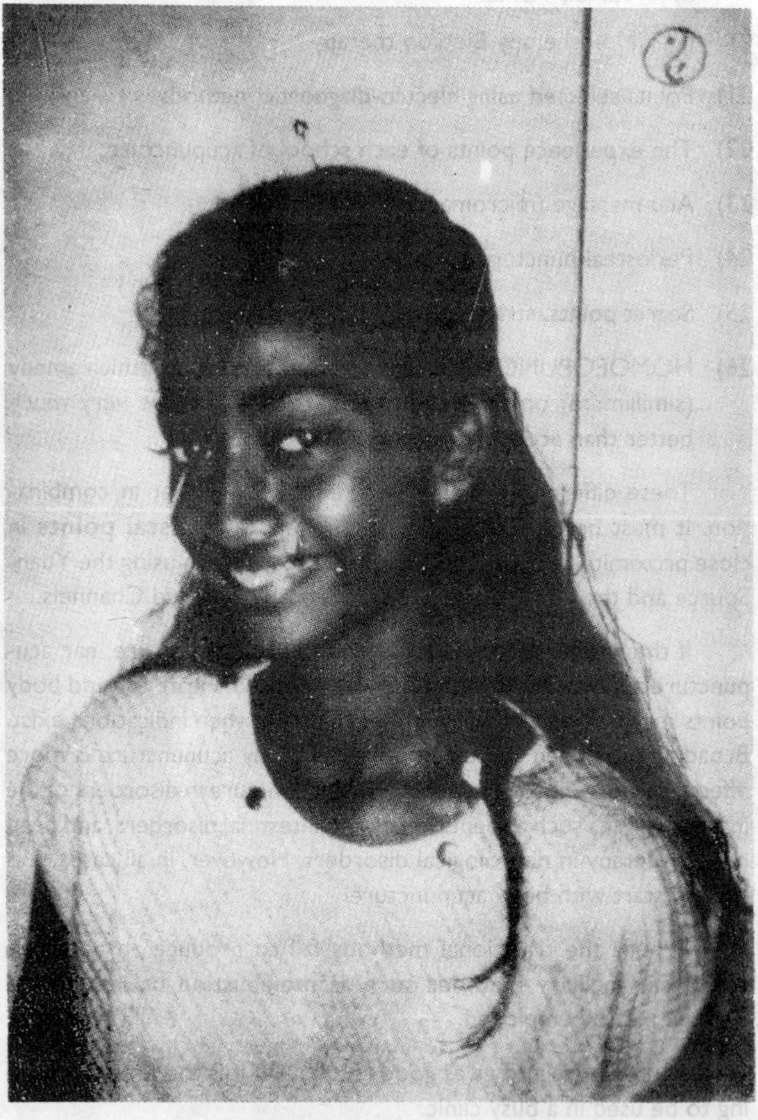

Female, 13 years.
Chronic Rhinitis (Deficiency of Metal)
Treatment: Baihui (Du 20), Yintang (Ex. 1). Yingxiang (L.I. 20), Hegu (L.I. 4), Xuehai (Sp. 10): Homoeopuncture with Pulsatilla c 30. Good result

THE INSTITUTE OF ACUPUNCTURE, COLOMBO SOUTH GOVERNMENT GENERAL HOSPITAL, KALUBOWILA, SRI LANKA

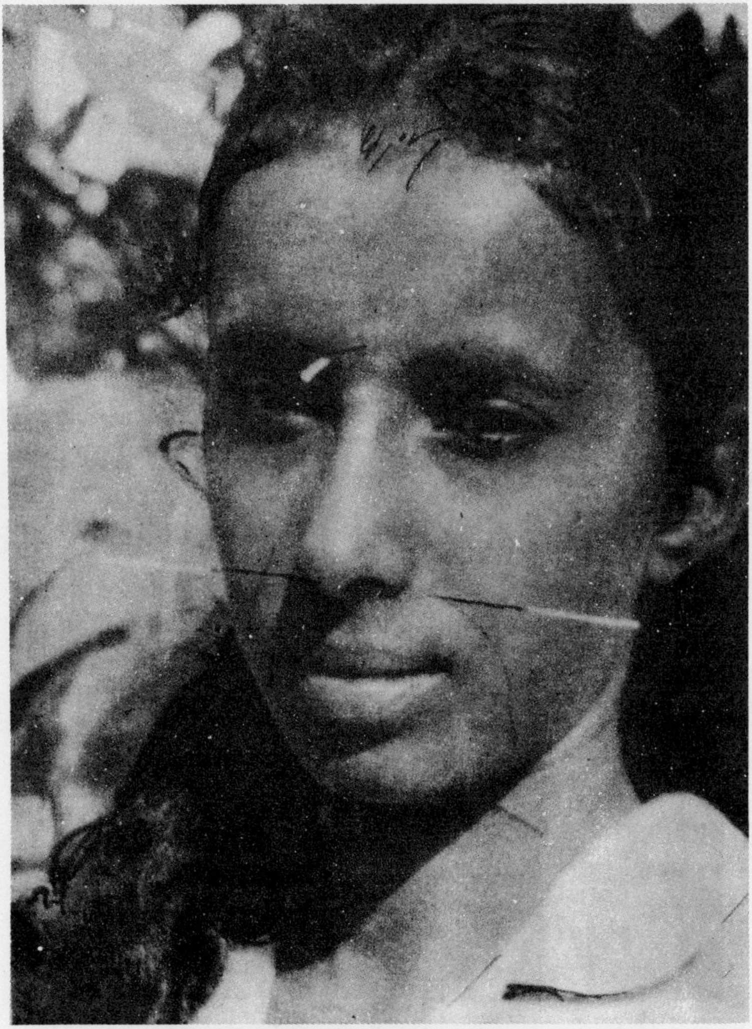

Female, 21 years.
Rhinitis & Chronic Bronchial Asthma (Deficiency of Metal)
Treatment: Baihui (Du 20), Yintang (Ex. 1). Yingxiang (L.I. 20), Shanzhong (Ren 17), Dingchuan (Ex. 17), Lieque (Lu. 7), Fenglong (St. 40). For acute attacks; Tiantu (Ren 22). Kongzui (Lu. 6): Homoeopuncture with Nux vomica c 30, Natrium muriaticum c 30. (3 doses). Result: Cured, after 6 weeks treatment

**THE INSTITUTE OF ACUPUNCTURE,
COLOMBO SOUTH GOVERNMENT GENERAL HOSPITAL,
KALUBOWILA, SRI LANKA**

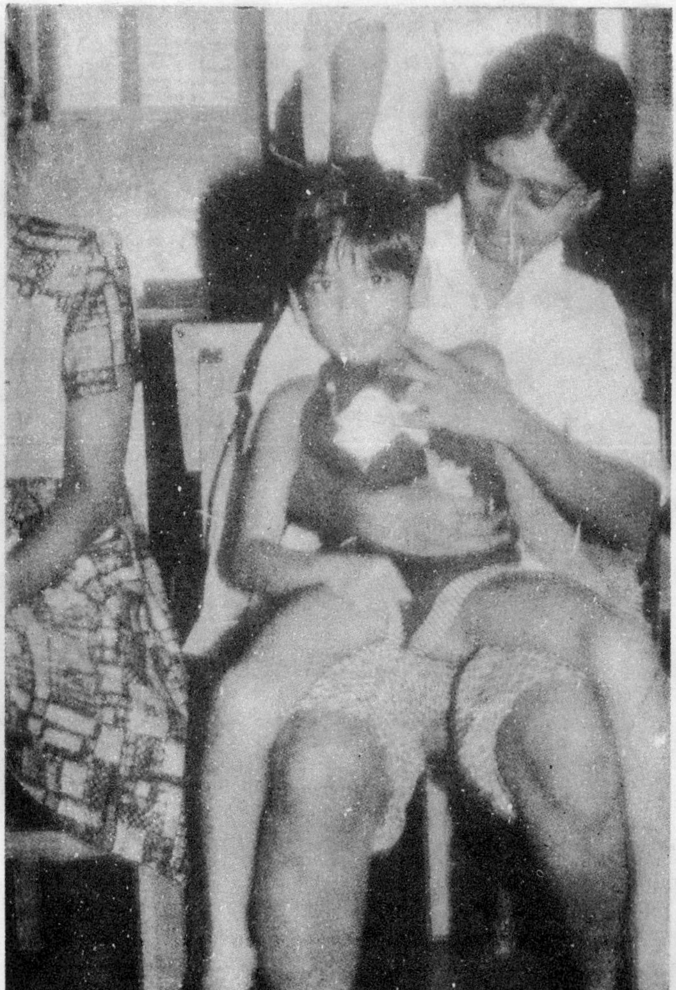

ACUPUNCTURE FOR THE YOUNG

A young patient with cerebral palsy nestling in the ams of his aunt, who is also being treated for an allergic rhinitis.

**THE INSTITUTE OF ACUPUNCTURE,
COLOMBO SOUTH GOVERNMENT GENERAL HOSPITAL,
KALUBOWILA, SRI LANKA**

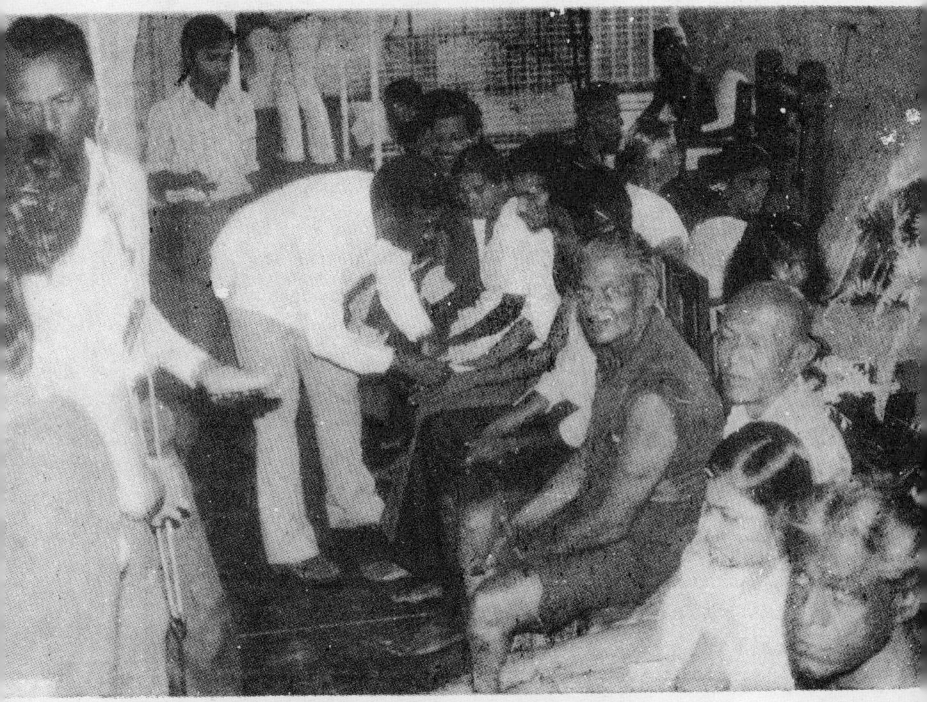

Over 250,000 patients have been treated with Acupuncture at this Institute for the past fifteen years.

SYSTEMATIC THERAPY

In order to obtain the best results, the practitioner of acupuncture must pay careful attention to the following requirements:

a) An accurate diagnosis, using all the methods available.

b) Selection of the most effective acupuncture points following the rules for the selection of points.

c) Accurate location of acupuncture points.

d) Observance of the contra-indications.

e) The use of the correct techniques of insertion and manipulation.

f) Due care at the dangerous points.

g) Observance of proper aseptic procedures.

h) Use of good quality needles

i) *Good rapport with the patient. The is the most important step in obtaining a satisfactory result. Acupuncture is foremost a subjective art, and the treatment should be tailored to suit the needs of each individual patient.*

The acupuncture points to be used may be selected on the basis of one or more of the following different clinical methods:

1) The formulary method.

2) The theories of traditional Chinese medicine.

3) Modern medicine.

4) Newly discovered points.

5) Electrically reactive points.

The first two methods encompass the whole of traditional Chinese acupuncture.

The first, the formulary method, means the selection of specific points or combinations of points which through the observations of successive generations of physicians are known to be effective particular disorders. This includes:

i) Local and Distal points e.g., Touwei (St. 8.) and Neiting (St. 44.) for headache; Tianrong (S.I. 17.) and Hegu (L.I. 4.) for tonsilitis.

ii) Points according to symptoms e.g., Renzhong (Du 26.) for shock.

iii) Specific points e.g., Xuehai (Sp.10.) for allergy.

This method was therefore regarded as an effective means of treatment once the external symptoms of an illness appeared.

As opposed to the first method, the selection of points according to the traditional theories is essentially a matter of the precise regulation of the vital energy ("Qi") circulating in the Channels ("Jing-Luo"). Central to this method is the examination of the pulse, which reveals the disequilibrium of energy. Point selection is then made using the theory of the Five Elements and the Yin-Yang theory. Although other diagnostic procedures such as palpation and observance of external signs were also used, pulse diagnosis was considered the most important. With this method an experienced practitioner was said to be able to detect the onset of an illness long before it manifested itself, and it was primarily for this reason that medicine in ancient China was oriented towards prevention. Unfortunately, pulse diagnosis is a difficult and subjective art and there are only a few practitioners today who are fully conversant in this modality. With the dawn of "scientific acupuncture", pulse diagnosis is infrequently used in modern China.

The third method, the selection of points according to modern medicine, means using those points whose analgesic, sedative, immune-enhancing and psychological effects have been confirmed by modern clinical and laboratory studies, e.g., Dazhui (Du 14.) in chronic infections, or Hegu (L.I. 4.) in pain relief.

Fourth, there are newly discovered points which have been shown to possess specific effects e.g., Neima and Weima (Unnumbered Extra points) which are used to obtain analgesia in perineal and abdominal surgery.

The fifth method, the selection of electrically reactive points, is based on the fact that an acupuncture point is an area of lowered electrical resistance on the skin. When a disorder occurs, the electrical resistance at the related point will be found to be still lower. It is thus easy, with the appropriate apparatus, not only to locate the required point but also to monitor the progress of the therapy as the skin resistance for the point returns to its normal level, as the therapy takes effect. This method is more conveniently carried out in ear acupuncture.

A wide spectrum of common illnesses is described in this section on systematic therapy. The descriptive terminology used here is that of Western medicine. However, it must be kept in mind that the treatment of disease by acupuncture is not based on the aetiological approach of scientific medicine which is totally different. The Western trained physician will, therefore, have to make the necessary mental adjustments when employing acupuncture. With experience it will be realised that the results obtained with acupuncture are not in any way inferior to drug therapy and in most cases, may be, superior.

The point Baihui (Du 20.) is generally employed in all prescriptions, as this point controls and co-ordinates all other points and Channels. It is also an excellent tranquilizer and would therefore be indicated in all disease conditions where there is a psychosomatic overlay to a greater or lesser extent.

During a course of treatment the patient is needled daily, every other day, or at close intervals for 7 to 10 days.[1] At the end of each

1 Does not apply to diseases such as bronchial asthma, epilepsy and neuralgias.

course the patient is given about a week's rest (during which period further improvement may occur). At the end of each rest period the progress should be reviewed and if the improvement exhibited is insufficient, further courses may be administered. During a course, or with each new course of treatment the points may be changed, and new points added or stimulation carried out, depending on the varying symptomatology of each case.

Generally at the first few sittings not more than 2 or 3 needles should be inserted; thereafter, points may be added but no more than 12 to 15 should usually be used. An average of about 6 to 8 needless may be regarded as optimal.[2]

In the majority of disorders the needle is inserted and left in place for 15 to 30 minutes. In chronic intractable painful conditions like trigeminal neuralgia, pain of secondary cancer, or severe migraine, the length of treatment may be prolonged up to 45 minutes or one hour at each sitting, with possibly more than the "normal" number of needles, and with even the employment of strong stimulation.

In acute conditions like diarrhoea, common cold, fever, attack of migraine, sore throat and tonsilitis, the length of each treatment may be short, but it may be carried out several times a day.

In children, very old people and in people who are very sensitive to needling, the non-retention method of needling, acupressure or laser therapy may be employed.

In carrying out therapy it is most important to advise the patient regarding all other important matters such as rest, diet, exercise, physical therapy, rehabilitation, proper habits and other specific advice relevant to each illness. Acupuncture therapy is not an isolated discipline. It is part of an holistic approach of treating the entire individual. The acupuncturist must never fail to remember that he is treating the person and not the disease.

■

2 Some patients who are acupuncture (or endorphia) addicts, like an excess of needles.

DISEASES OF THE NERVOUS SYSTEM

Principles of treatment

Diseases of the nervous system form one of the largest groups of disorders seen in general practice. Their symptomatology is very complex and may range from pain, paralysis and paraesthesia to involuntary movements of various kinds, specific sensory loss and symptoms of autonomic imbalance.

No specific treatment is available in Western medicine in the majority of these diseases and the management consists largely of supportive measures like physiotherapy, administration of vitamins, together with narcotic drugs and analeptics, where necessary. Acupuncture, however, is an extremely helpful modality in the treatment of these diseases. Owing to the powerful analgesic effects of acupuncture it is particularly helpful in allaying pain — a problem which causes much distress in the majority of these patients. In addition, it is possible to obtain a recovery of motor function to a degree which is not attainable with any other form of treatment. Subsidiary complaints like speech disorders, sensory loss and autonomic disturbances are also found to respond very favourably to treatment with acupuncture. The analysis of a neurological disorder entails the elucidation of the anatomical localization and the consequent physio-pathological disturbances which result.

EPILEPSY

This group of disorders is characterised by fits or seizures which are often sudden, usually resulting in loss of consciousness.

a) *Petit Mai:*

The only symptom here is a fleeting loss of consciousness, where the patient (usually a child) may be seen to stare straight ahead into space.

Specific points that may be used in the interim periods for the routine therapy are:

Baihui (Du 20.).	Neiguan (P. 6.).
Yintang (Ex. I.).	Shenmen (H. 7.).
Renzhong (Du 26.).	Shenmai (U.B. 62.).

Mu and Shu points of the Heart and Pericardium.

b) *Grand Mal:*

This is the more common type of fit. It is characterized by an aura, loss of consciousness with generalised convulsions and post epileptic phenomena. Prodromal symptoms are sometimes present and loss of consciousness is often preceded by a sharp scream. Acute fits can be brought under control by acupressure at Renzhong (Du 26.) and, if necessary, needling at Yongquan (K.I.).

Where the patient develops repeated seizures and does not regain consciousness between attacks, the condition is known as "*status epilepticus*". In such cases points selected from the following may be used:

Baihui (Du 20.). and/or	Sishencong (Ex. 6.).
Yintang (Ex. I.).	Xinshu (U.B. 15.).
Anmain I (Ex. 8.).	Neiguan (P. 6.).
Anmian II (Ex. 9.)	Shenmen (H. 7.).

Jizhong (Du 6.).	Hegu (L.I. 4.).
Yaoqi (Ex. 20.).	Shenmai (U.B. 62.).
Fenglong (St. 40.).	Yanglingquan (G.B. 34.).

c) *Jacksonian Fits (Focal Epilepsy):*

Here the seizure begins in one part of the body and may spread to the other muscle groups (sometimes culminating in a grand mal attack). The symptoms sometimes are restricted to an abnormal feeling in a part of the body which may spread to other parts (the so-called sensory epilepsy).

If the patient is seen during a fit, it may be necessary in addition to Renzhong (Du 26.) and Yongquan (K. 1.), to add suitable points lying in the direction of the spread and then stimulating them strongly, in order to stop the fit.

The patient is treated on the following points, daily or every other day for a few months as routine therapy:

Baihui (Du 20.), and/or	Sishencong (Ex. 6.).
Yintang (Ex. 1.).	Neiguan (P. 6.).
Renzhong (Du 26.).	Shenmen (H. 7.).
Fenglong (St. 40.).	Shenmai (U.B. 62.).

Some of the following points may also be added in resistant cases:

Ximen (P.4.).	Quchi (L.I. 11.).
Sanyinjiao (Sp. 6.).	Taichong (Liv. 3.).
Xinshu (U.B. 15.)	Anmian I & II (Ex. 8. and Ex. 9.).

In sensory epilepsy, in addition to Baihui (Du 20.) and Sishencong (Ex. 6.), local points on the scalp, corresponding to the site of the suspected lesion[1] may be used. Local body points corresponding to the region of the sensory disturbance could be added.

1 Surrounding the dragon

d) *Psychomotor (Temporal Lobe) Epilepsy:*

Here the fits are not as severe as in grand mal. Fits may be preceded by an aura of unreality and hallucinations. The following points may be used:

Baihui (Du 20.), and/or	Sishencong (Ex. 6.).
Shuaigu (G.B. 8.).	Shenmen (H. 7.).
Yangbai (G.B. 14.).	Neiguan (P. 6.).
Touwei (St. 8.).	Shenmai (U.B. 62.).

A press needle, placed at the ear point Shenmen,[2] is useful for maintaining continuous stimulation between treatment sessions.

Results obtained with acupuncture in epileptic patients are very promising. In most cases of petit mal the symptoms may be expected to disappear with 10 to 15 treatments. The results are almost equally good in sensory epilepsy and temporal lobe epilepsy. For grand mal, however, 30 or more treatments may be required with weekly reinforcement for about 3 or 4 months or longer. We have also treated a few hundred cases of traumatic epilepsy[3] with good results. The important constraint in treating epilepsies is to take care to eliminate the possibility of a space occupying lesion.

Note: 1) Electrical stimulation is contraindicated, as it might precipitate attacks.

2) All drugs may be completely withdrawn at the commencement of the acupuncture therapy. The vast majority of patients manage so well without medication that even the tailing off the dosage is usually unnecessary. However, where fits of a greater intensity occur within the first few weeks of acupuncture, minimal doses of the earlier drugs may be re-introduced and then withdrawn. The strategy must be explained to the patient before commencing therapy so that his co-operation is fully enlisted.

---

2 Also at ear point Heart.

3 Post-traumatic syndrome responds very well to acupuncture. Homoeopuncture with Arnica montana followed by Natrium sulphuricum is very useful.

3) Embedding of an ear press needle helps to prevent attacks.

PARKINSONISM

The commonest form of parkinsonism is Parkinson's disease. There are however many forms of this disease, which generally affects elderly people. It is mainly a disturbance of voluntary movement caused by the degeneration of the inhibitory nerve fibres in the basal ganglia of the brain. Mental faculties are affected. The disease may be identified by a weakness and spasticity of the face muscles (causing the characteristic mask-like expression), a coarse tremor when at rest (particularly in the hands), a tendency for the mouth to stay open with excessive salivation, rigidity of limbs and the characteristic shuffling gait.

The following points may be used:

Baihui (Du 20.), and/or	Sishencong (Ex. 6.).
Quchi (L.I. 11.).	Zusanli (St. 36.).
Waiguan (S.J. 5.).	Yanglingquan (G.B. 34.).
Shenmen (H. 7.).	Jiexi (St. 41.).
Hegu (L.I. 4.).	Neiting (St. 44.).

Where there is increased salivation, the following points may the added:

Dicang (St. 4.).[4]	Yinlingquan (Sp. 9.).
Chengjiang (Ren 24.).	Jiachengjlang (Ex. 5.).
Lianquan (Ren 23.).	Fenglong (St. 40.).

Usually improvement is slow and 60 or more treatments may be necessary for improvement to commence. A success rate of about 75 per cent may be expected with combined body and ear acupuncture. Some patients may need a minimal dose of medication, in combination with acupuncture. Embedding a press needle helps to alleviate the symptoms.

4 Towards liache (St. 6.)

SPASTIC PARALYSIS, CHOREA, HABIT SPASMS (TICS)

Spastic paralysis is caused by damage to certain brain areas and centres, resulting in the impairment of voluntary movements and presence of muscle spasm. The main indication may be spasm, or lack of co-ordination, or uncontrolled purposeless movements (athetosis), depending on the site of the brain damage. This disorder is often confined to the legs. A rather painful form of recurrent nervous muscular spasm, however, is spasmodic torticollis where, the neck is usually deviated to one side.

Chorea is characterised by uncontrolled jerky movements, involving any part of the body. Sydenham's chorea (rheumatic chorea, St. Vitus' dance) a childhood disorder associated with rheumatic fever. Adults exhibit chorea in a rare hereditary condition known as Huntington's chorea where, in addition to uncontrolled movement, there is progressive mental degeneration.

Habit spasm or tic is an involuntary purposeless movement e.g., shrugging of shoulders, which may earlier have been purposive.

Select from the following points:

Baihui (Du 20.), and/or	Sishencong (Ex. 6.).
Quchi (L.I. 11.).	Yanglingquan (G.B. 34.).
Waiguan (S.J. 5.).	Zusanli (St. 36.).
Shenmen (H. 7.).	Shenmai (U.B. 62.).
Hegu (L.I. 4.).	Neiting (St. 44.).

In spasmodic torticollis the points in the local area may be combined with:

Lieque (Lu. 7.).

Houxi (S.I. 3.). or Yanglao (S.I. 6.).

Yanglingquan (G.B. 34.).

HEADACHES

There are may types of headaches — tension headaches, vascular headaches, post-concussion headaches, headaches due to frontal sinusitis, eye strain and other similar causes.

In all cases of headaches it is advisable to attempt to arrive at a diagnosis before acupuncture is commenced.

The possibility that the headache is due to a cerebral tumour or other space-occupying lesion must be thought of. Conditions like hypertension, constipation, or anxiety, if present, should receive concurrent therapy.

The principle of treatment is to use Local points and Distal points, along the course of the relevant Channels. It should be noted that in all types of headaches the points Baihui (Du 20.) and/or Sishencong (Ex. 6.), together with Hegu (L.I. 4.) as a Distal analgesic point, should be used. If *Ah-Shi* points are present, they should be precisely needled. Migraine headaches respond well to shaochong (H.9.).

a) *Frontal headache:*

Baihui (Du 20.), and/or Sishencong (Ex. 6.).

Local Points:	**Distal Points:**
Ah-Shi points.	Hegu (L.I. 4.).
Shangxing (Du 23.).	Neiting (St. 44.).
Touwei (St. 8.).	Yanglingquan (G.B. 34.).
Yangbai (G.B. 14.).	
Yintang (Ex. 1.).	
Yaiyang (Ex. 2.).	

b) *Temporal headache:*

Baihui (Du 20.). and/or Sishencong (Ex. 6.).

Local Points:	**Distal Points:**
Ah-Shi points.	Neiting (St. 44.).
Touwei (St. 8.).	Foot-Linqi (G.B. 41.).
Shuaigu (G.B. 8.).	Waiguan (S.J. 5.).
Sizhukong (S.J. 23.).	Hegu (L.I. 5.).
Yanglingquan (G.B. 34.).	

c) *Parietal headache:*

Baihui (Du 20.), and/or Sishencong (Ex. 6.).

Local Points:	Distal Points:
Ah-Shi points.	Hegu (L.I. 4.).
Touwei (St. 8.).	Zhongzhi (S.J. 3.).
Shuaigu (G.B. 8.).	

d) Occipital headache.

Baihui (DU.20) and /or	Sisherwng (5x.6)
local points	Distal points.
Ah-shi points	Lieque (Lu.7)
Fenchi (G.B.20)	Kunlun (U.B. 60)

e) *Vertical headache:*

Baihui (Du 20.), and/or	Sishencong (Ex. 6.).
***Ah-Shi* points:**	**Distal Points:**
	Kunlun (U.B. 60.).
	Xingjian (Liv. 2.).
	Yaoshu (Du 2.).

Note: 1) Strong stimulation of acupuncture points in the head area should be avoided. This may aggravate the headache.

2) Where the headache is acute, manual stimulation of Hegu (L.I. 4.) would invariably give almost immediate symptomatic relief.[5]

3) Press needles may be embedded at suitable points in the ear.

INSOMNIA

This is a very common disorder and the causes include any kind of physical discomfort or pain. The points listed below, however, are for the treatment of insomnia due to anxiety and other mental causes:

Baihui (Du 20.), and/or	Sishencong (Ex. 6.).
Anmian I (Ex. 8.).	Neiguan (P. 6.).
Anmain II (Ex. 9.).	Shenmen (H. 7.).
	Shenmai (U.B. 62.).

5 Within about one minute

The following additional points may also be used:

Shenting (Du 24.). Taixi (K. 3.).

Where sleep is disturbed by dreams, the following points may be added:

Xinshu (U.B. 15.). Shendao (Du 11.).

In most cases the disturbed sleep pattern may be corrected after a few treatments. In all cases the cause should be investigated and the patient advised accordingly.

A press needle at Ear, Shenmen is helpful.

MENIERE'S DISEASE, VERTIGO AND TRAVEL SICKNESS

These disorders are casued by dysfunction of the inner ear, involving hearing and balance. In Meniere's disease both these functions are impaired. For further description and points to be used. See under "Ear disorders".

MENINGITIS, ENCEPHALITIS

Meningitis is the inflammation of the meninges (i.e. the three membranes covering the brain and the spinal cord), usually due to some bacterial or virus infection.

Encephalitis refers to inflamation of the brain, generally caused by vithus.

In acute cases it is advisable it establish the identity of the causative organism by examination of the cerebrospinal fluid and to institute the appropriate antibiotic therapy. Acupuncture therapy, however, may be used concurrently to relieve pain and to provide other symptomatic relief, improve immune mechanisms, and thereby reduce the need for prolonged antibiotic therapy. Acupuncture is also particularly useful in cases of viral infections where no specific antibiotics are indicated to where there is hypersensitivity or resistance to antibiotics. In the post-infective period it is useful in dealing with many neurological sequelae.

The points to be used depend on the clinical condition of the patient and the stage of the disease.

In the febrile stage, the following points may be used according to the presenting symptoms:

Baihui (D 20.). and/or sishencong (Ex. 6.).

Points in the region of the headache.

Dazhui (D 14.). Zusanli (St 36.).

Quchi (L.I. 11.). Sanyinjiao (Sp. 6.).

Hegu (L.I. 4.).

For neck rigidity and opisthotonus, the following points may be added:

Yamen (Du 15.).

Other points of the Du and U.B. Channels in the area affected:

Yinmen (U.B. 37.).

Weizhong (U.B. 40.).

Kunlun (U.B. 60.).

For nausea and vomiting, the following points may be used

Neiguam (P. 6.).

Zusanli (St. 36.).

For the neurological sequelae the appropriate points should be used depending on the neurological deficit exhibited.

Usually antibiotics are the first line of choice in the treatment of meningitis. Acupuncture may be used to supplement the drug therapy or where antibiotics cannot be used, on account of the side effects or antibiotic resistance.[6]

FACIAL PARALYSIS (BELL'S PALSY), FACIAL HEMISPASM

In Bell's Palsy one side of the face is paralysed. The cause of facial nerve paresis in these disorders is unknown. It may be due to

6 or in virus infection. Homoeopuncture with a specific nosode may be helpful.

inflammation in the region of the middle ear, probably as a result of exposure to cold or virus infection.

Baihui (Du 20.). and/or Sishencong (Ex. 6.).

Local points (select from affected area of the face):

Yangbai (GB. 14.).
Taiyang (Ex. 2.)
Sibai (St. 2.).
Juliao (St. 3.).
Dicang (St. 4.).
Daying (St. 5.).
Xiaguan (St. 7.).
Quanliao (S.I. 18.).
Jiachenjiang (Ex. 5.).

Distal point:

Hegu (L.I. 4.).

Influential point:

Yanglingquan (G.B. 34.).

Natural recovery occurs rapidly in many cases. In early cases of Bell's palsy recovery may be expected within 6 to 10 sessions of treatment.

In long standing paralysis, the "puncture-through" technique may be tried with the use of long needles:

Dicang (St. 4.). to Jiache (St. 6.).[7]
Yangbai (G.B. 14.). to Yuyao (Ex. 3.).
Tongziliao (G.B. 1.). to Dicang (St. 4.).

Low frequency electrical stimulation, about 3-10 Hertz, is applied at points such as Yangbai (G.B. 14.). and Dicang (St. 4.). High frequency stimulation at 1000-2000 Hertz (dense-disperse) is used usually in intractable cases.

---

7 Catgut embedding may be helpful.

TRIGEMINAL NEURALGIA (TIC DOLOUREUX)

The trigeminal nerve (5th cranial nerve) contains mainly sensory fibres which are in three groups (hence "trigeminal"):

1) the opthalmic nerve (supplying the upper part of the face);
2) the maxillary nerve (supplying the upper jaw area); and
3) the mandibular nerve (supplying the lower jaw area).

In trigeminal neuralgia the patient suffers severe pain in the distribution of one or more branches of the trigeminal nerve. When it is spasmodic, it is associated with a twitching of the facial muscles and is then referred to as "*tic doloureux*".

Treatment is based on the principle of combining *Ah-Shi* Local and Distal points. The selection of the Local points depends on the affected part of the trigeminal nerve:

i) *Opthalmic branch:*

Baihui (Du 20.).

Local points:

Ah-Shi points.
Yangbai (G.B. 14.)
Zanzhu (U.B. 2.).
Taiyang (Ex. 2.).

Distal points:

Hegu (L.I. 4.).
Neiting (St. 44.).

ii) *Maxillary branch:*

Baihui (Du 20.).

Local points:

Ah-Ahi points.
Sibai (St. 2.).
Juliao (St. 3.).
Renzhong (Du 26.).
Xiaguan (St. 7.).
Quanliao (S.I. 18.).
Yingxiang (L.I. 20.).

Distal points:

Hegu (L.I. 4.).
Neiting (St. 44.).

iii) *Mandibular branch:*
Baihui (Du 20.).

Local points:	Distal points:
Ah-Shi points.	Hegu (L.I. 4.).
Yifengjiang (Ex. 5.).	
Dicang (St. 4.) through to	
Jiache (St. 6.).	

When the pain spreads to the area of the external ear, points such as Waiguan (S.I. 5.) may be added.

In the treatment of trigeminal neuralgia it is desirable to use a large number of points on the face and to carry out the treatment daily. When acute pain is present, strong manual stimulation at Hegu (L.I. 4.) should be carried out. The needles on the face may also be gently manipulated every 5 to 10 minutes. In resistant cases the duration of the sittings may be increased from the usual half an hour to 45 minutes or even an hour.[8] Additional body points like Xiangu (St. 43.) may also be introduced for reinforcement. Embedding of press needles in the ear (Facio-mandibular area) and at one or more local *Ah-Shi* points will help to control pain between treatments. Where the patient does not permit the affected side of the face to be needled on account of the severity of the pain, the opposite side of the face may be needled (on the principle that the side of the therapy does not matter).

Acupuncture therapy has been found to be extremely satisfactory. The relief of pain occurs within a few treatments, in most cases. A little paraesthesia may be found as a residual disability. In order to obtain complete recovery the patient may have to be treated or a few months, including self treatment by the patient with electro-stimulation *without needles*, at home.[9]

We have seen six cases of similar neuralgia in the distribution of the glossopharyngeal nerve, the so called glossopharyngeal neural-

8 or more

9 High frequency stimulation at 2,000 Hertz helps to alleviate the pain.

gia. We have treated these cases very successfully using the same principles.

HEMIPLEGIA, HEMIPARESIS

This paralysis of one side of the body caused usually by a cerebrovascular accident (a stroke on the opposite side of the brain). It is important to find out the underlying cause and to eliminate the existence of any space occupying lesion.

In patients who have suffered a stroke the following clinical features may be observed:

a) mental symptoms, e.g., loss of memory, confusion, personality changes;

b) paralysis of the lower two-thirds of the face on the contralateral side;

c) difficulty to speech (aphasia) and of swallowing;

d) paralysis of the contralateral upper limb;

e) paralysis of the contralateral lower limb;

f) spasticity of the affected muscles;

g) loss of sensation in paralysed areas;

h) bed sores, oedema of dependent parts;

i) bladder and bowel symptoms;

j) associated disorders (commonly high blood pressure, diabetes)

The points used depend on the above features. Treatment should be carried out daily or every other day. It should be noted that in all cases of Baihui (Du 20.) and/or Sishencong (Ex. 6.). with Yanglingquan (G.B. 34.). as the Influential point, are used.

a) *Face:*

Baihui (Du 20.) and/or Sishencong (Ex. 6.).

Local points:	Distal point:
(select from):	Hegu (L.I. 4.).

Dicang (St. 4.).
Xiaguan (St. 7.).
Jiache (St. 5.).
Quanliao (S.I. 18.).
Jiachengjiang (Ex. 5.).

Influential point:
Yanglingquan (G.B. 34.).

In case of aphasia, add:

Local points:
Lianquan (Ren 23.).
Tianrong (S.I. 17.).

Distal point:
Tongli (H. 5.).
Specific point:
Hegu (L.I. 4.).
Influential point:
Yanglingquan (G.B. 34.).

b) *Upper limb:*

Baihui (Du 20.) and/or Sishencong (Ex. 6.).

Local points (select from Large Intestine and Sanjiao Channels):

Jianyu (L.I. 15.).
Quchi (L.I. 11.).
Hegu (L.I. 4.).
Baxie (Ex. 28.).
(for paralysis of the fingers)

Jianliao (S.I. 14.).
Waiguan (S.I. 5.).
Zhongzhu (S.J 3.).

Influential point:
Yanglingquan (G.B. 34.).

c) *Lower limb:*

Baihui (Du 20.) and/or Sishencong (Ex. 6.).

Local points (select mainly from Stomach and Gall Bladder Channels):

Biguan (St. 31.).
Femur-Futu (St. 32.).
Zusanli (St. 36.).
Shangjuxu (St. 37.).

Huantiao (G.B. 30.).
Guangming (G.B. 37.).
Qiuxu (G.B. 40.).

Xiajuxu (St. 39.).
Jiexi (St. 41.).
Neiting (St. 44.).
Bafeng (Ex. 36.). (for paralysis of the toes).

Influential point:
Yanglingquan (G.B. 34.).

With the patient in a prone position, suitable regional Huatuojjaji (Ex. 21.) points and points from the lower limb in the Urinary Bladder Channel may also be used.

In cases of dependent oedema of legs and feet, select from the following points:

Local points:
Sanyinjiao (Sp. 6.)
Zhaohai (K. 6.).

Specific points:
Shuifen (Ren 9.).
Shimen (Ren 5.).
Pishu (U.S. 20.).
Yinlingquan (sp. 9.).

Strong stimulation and the obtaining of "*deqi*" at the following points expedites the recovery:

Hegu (L.I. 4.).
Shousanli (L.I. 10.).
Zusanli (St. 36.).
and at other motor points.

Low frequency electrical pulse stimulation also helps to expedite recovery. With 10 to 20 treatment, significant improvement occurs in the majority of cases. The treatment may be combined with moderate exercise therapy. The fitting of orthopaedic appliances, such as foot-drop splints, must be discouraged until the maximum improvement is obtained.

In our experience, acupuncture in the treatment of hemiplegia is more efficacious than drug treatment and physiotherapy. While medication and physiotherapy do not hasten recovery beyond what could be expected from natural remission, acupuncture treatment often results in dramatic improvement in motor functions, even in neglected cases of several years' duration.

BULBAR PALSY

This is a paralysis involving the tongue and the throat muscles and is a common complication of a stroke. Bulbar palsy may also arise as a result of a vascular accident in the brain stem area. Chronic bulbar palsy occurs as a result of motor neurone disease involving the brain stem nuclei, in which event, the prognosis is much less favourable. Acupuncture helps to arrest the progress of this disease.

a) *Swallowing difficulties:*

Baihui (Du 20.).

Local points:	Distal points:
Lianquan (Ren 23.).	Neiguan (P.6.).
Chengjiang (Ren 24.).	Hegu (L.I. 4.).
Renzhong (du 26.).	
Tianrong (S.I. 17.)	Influential point:
Shanzhong (Ren 17.).	Yanglingquan (G.B. 34.).
Neck-Futu (L.I. 18.).	

b) *Excessive salivation:*

Baihui (Du 20.)

Local points:	Distal points:
Dicang (St. 4.).	Hegu (L.I. 4.).
Chengjiang (Ren 24.).	Specific points:
Lianquan (Ren 23.).	Fenglong (St. 40.).
	Yinlingquan (Sp. 9.).

c) Speech *difficulties (aphasia, lisping, stammering, stuttering, slurring and hoarseness*):

Baihui (Du 20.).

Local points:	Distal point:
Lianquan (Re 23.).	Tongli (H. 5.).[10]

10 Tongue is connected to heart.

Dicang (St. 4.).	Influential point:
Chengjiang (Ren 24.).	Yanglingquan (G.B. 34.).

PARAPLEGIA, PARAPARESIS

Paraplegia is paralysis of the lower limbs and the lower half of the trunk caused usually by trauma, inflammation or tumour involving the spinal cord. Partial or total sensory loss in both lower extremities occurs, accompained by urinary and rectal incontinence or retention.

Features typically seen in a paraplegia are:

a) weakness of the trunk below the site of the lesion;

b) weakness or paralysis of the lower limbs;

c) bladder and bowel symptoms;

d) impotence;

e) loss of sensation, paraesthesia;

f) bedsores;

g) oedema of the legs.

In treating paraplegics it is best to use alternatively front and back points on the trunk, and points on the Stomach, Gall Bladder and Urinary Bladder Channels on the lower limbs:

	Front	*Back*
Trunk:	Qihai (Ren 6.).	Alarm points on U.B. Channel
	Guanyuan (Ren 4.).	Huatuojiaji (Ex. 21.) points.
	Zhongji (Ren 3.).	Yaoyangguan (Du 3.).
Legs (select from):		
	Biguan (St. 32.).	Huantiao (G.B. 30.).
	Femur-Futu (St. 31.).	Fengshi (G.B. 31.).
	Zusanli (St. 36.).	Chengfu (U.B. 36.).
	Shangjuxu (St. 37.).	Weizhong (U.B. 40.).
	Xiajuxu (St. 39.).	Chengshan (U.B. 57.).

Jiexi (St. 41.) Kunlun (U.B. 60.).

Xiangu (St. 43.).

Neiting (St. 44.).

Where there is urinary or rectal incontinence, the points specific for these symptoms are used:

Urinary incontinence:

Local points:

Qugu (Ren 2.).

and other Ren Channel points.

Distal points:

Sanyinjiao (Sp. 6.).

Taixi (K. 3.).

Rectal incontinence:

Local points:

Changqiang (Du 1.).

Huiyin (Ren 1.).

Distal points:

Chengshan (U.B. 57.).

Sanyinjiao (Sp. 6.).

Zusanli (St. 36.).

Poliomyelitis (acute anterior poliomyelitis; infantile paralysis) and other disorders causing lower motor neurone paralysis of acute onset

Poliomyelitis is caused by a virus infection which affects the anterior horn cells of the spinal cord and of the brain stem. The virus enters through the gastro-intestinal tract. Paresis or paralysis of the muscles ensues. There is no sensory loss.

In the acute stage of the disease, points are selected according to symptoms:

Diarrhoea:

Tianshu (St. 25.).

Zusanli (St. 36.).

Sore throat:

Tianrong (S.I. 17.).

Neck-Futu (L.I. 18.).

Headache:

Hegu (L.I. 4.).

Vomiting:

Neiguan (P. 6.).

Fever:

Dazhui (Du. 14.).

Quci (L.I. 11.).

Note: No stimulation should be carried out in the acute stage as it may cause further paralysis.

After the acute stage is over and paralysis sets in, points on the paralysed aspect of the body are used with the Influential point Yanglingquan (G.B. 34.).

Paralysis of the diaphragm:

Geshu (U.B. 17.).

Qimen (Liv. 14.).

Paralysis of abdominal muscle:

Liangmen (St. 21.).

Tianshu (St. 25.).

Guilai (St. 29.).

Pishu (U.B. 20.).

Weishu (U.B. 21.).

Paralysis of upper limbs:

Jianyu (L.I. 15.).

Quchi (L.I. 11.).

Waiguan (S.J. 5.).

Wrist drop:

Yanglao (S.I. 6.).

Hegu (L.I. 4.).

Paralysis of lower limbs:

Huatuojiaji (Ex. 21.) points (L. 2 to S. 3.).[11]

Huantiao (G.B. 3. G.).

Yanglingquan (G.B. 34.).

Zusanli (St. 36.).

Shangjuxu (St. 37.).

Foot-drop:

Jiexi (St. 41.).

Kunlun (U.B. 60.).

In chronic poliomyelitis quicker results may be obtained with the use of electrical stimulation. Graduated exercise therapy should also be recommended.

NEUROPRAXIA OF THE LATERAL POPLITEAL NERVE

The chief feature of this disorder is foot-drop.

Select from Local points and also use Yanglingquan (G.B. 34.). Influential point for muscle and tendon:

Baihui (Du 20.) and/or	Sishencong (Ex. 6.).
Local points:	Influential point:
Zusanli (St. 36.).	Yanglingquan (G.B. 34.).
Jiexi (St. 41.).	
Xiangu (St. 43.).	
Neiting (St. 44.).	

Local points of the Gall Bladder Channel are also helpful.

MUSCULAR DYSTROPHIES (MYOPATHIES AND MOTOR NEURONE DISEASE)

There are various types of muscular dystrophy, all of which feature weakness and wasting of certain voluntary muscles. These disorders, many of which are heredofamilial, are not very common.

11 L = Lumbar S = Sacral

There is no specific treatment available apart from general supportive measures. In many cases the prognosis is poor. However, a very fair clinical improvement has been noted in some cases with acupuncture treatment (especially where treatment has commenced early), and arrest of the disease process has been obtained in others. However, there is need for further study and research.

The points used are the Local points, i.e., points on Channels passing over the affected muscles, with Yanglingquan (G.B. 34.) as Influential point, Quchi (L.I. 11.) to obtain homeostasis.

DISORDERS OF THE AUTONOMIC NERVOUS SYSTEM

The autonomic nervous system comprises two components, the sympathetic and the parasympathetic, which reflexively regulate involuntary functions such as heart beat, blood pressure, and digestive activity.

Disorders affecting these systems are characterised by symptoms of autonomic imbalance, i.e., overaction of sympathetic or parasympathetic components. They are very difficult to cure with drugs and are often labelled as being "functional in origin". The symptomatology is complicated by the fact that sometimes more than one of different systems such as cardiovascular, gastro-intestinal, urinary, and reproductive are involved.

These disorders often respond well to acupuncture therapy.

The principles of point selection in those cases are to select the known specific points for the exhibited symptoms add a few Local points (coupled in appropriate cases with one or two Distal points), and to use the main Homeostatic points. For example, in hyperhidrosis (excessive sweating), the following points may be used:

Baihui (Du 20.) and/or Sishencong (Ex. 6.).

Specific points:	Homeostatic points:
Yinxi (H. 6.).	Quchi (L.I. 11.).
Hegu (L.I. 4.).	Zusali (St. 36.).
Fuliu (K. 7.).	Sanyinjiao (Sp. 6.).

Local points:

Laogong (P. 8.).

Shaofu (H. 8.).

Yuji (Lu. 10.).

Yongquan (K. 1.).

(These Local points may be very painful, as they are situated in the palms and soles.)

■

RESPIRATORY DISORDERS

Principles of treatment

The commonly used points for respiratory disorders are contained in the Lung, Ren and Large Intestine Channels.

In the treatment of this group of disorders, whenever infection is present the points Dazhui (du 14.), Quchi (L.I. 11.) and Sanyinjiao (Sp. 6.) may be used, in addition to other specific points which may be indicated according to the symptoms present. Bleeding at a Jing-Well point, e.g., Shaoshang (Lu. 11.) is indicated if there is very high fever due to the infection.

THE COMMON COLD (ACUTE CORYZA)

This is believed to be a virus infection of the mucous membrane of the nose and pharynx. Clinical manifestations are sneezing, running eyes and nose, cough, headache and general malaise. Timely treatment with acupuncture could be useful in avoiding complications like superadded bacterial infection of the mucous membranes, which may lead to bronchitis. The main benefit of acupuncture of course is that it relieves the symptoms. The following points may be used:

Baihui (Du 20.).

Dazhui (Du 14.).

Fengchi (G.B. 20.).

Distal point:

Hegu (L.I.4.).

Further points may be added according to the symptoms present:

Headache:

Taiyang (Ex. 2.).

Touwei (St. 8.).

Blocked nose:

Nose-Heliao (L.I. 19.).

Nasal discharge:

Yintang (Ex. 1.).

Yingxiang (L.I. 20.).

Sore throat:

Shaoshang (Lu. 11.).

Fever:

Dazhui (Du 14.).

Quchi (L.I. 11.).

Cough:

Lieque (Lu. 7.).

When the cold is relieved, the following general tonification points may be needled for a few days to expedite the convalescence:

Qihai (Ren 6.).

Zusanli (St. 36.).

Sanyinjiao (Sp. 6.).

HAY FEVER (ALLERGIC RHINITIS)

This is a common allergic disorder characterised by an acute inflammation of the mucus lining of the nose which may spread to the throat and conjunctiva. This is followed by sneezing and excessive lacrimation. In chronic cases a blocked nose usually occurs.

Baihui (Du 20.).

Local points:

Yintang (Ex. 1.).

Yingxiang (L.I. 20.).

Distal points:

Hegu (L.I. 4.).

Lieque (Lu. 7.).

Specific point for allergy:

Xuehai (Sp. 10.)

When puncturing Yintang (Ex. 1.) the needle should be directed horizontally downwards so that the *deqi* radiates through to the nose. The points Hegu (L.I. 4.). and Lieque (Lu. 7.). should not be needled together on the same side.

Sneezing may be controlled with these Local points and with strong stimulation of Hegu. (L.I. 4.).

The following additional points may be used according to the symptoms:

a) **Blocked nose:**

Nose-Heliao (L.I. 19.).

or

Juliao (St. 3.) through to Yingxiang (L.I. 20)

and

Shangxing (Du 23.) with the needle directed downwards.

b) **Nose bleeding (epistaxis):**

Nose-Heliao (L.I. 19.).

Shangxing (Du 23.).

Suliao (Du 25.).

Renzhong (Du 26.).

Influential point for blood:

Geshu (U.B. 17.).

Influential point for the vascular system:

Taiyuan (Lu. 9.).

Xi-Cleft point of the Lung Channel:

Kongzui (Lu. 6.); Stimulate strongly.

SINUSITIS

This is the inflammation of the mucous membranes of the sinuses of the skull. This is caused by the spread of infection from the nose, inclement weather, and sometimes by allergic states. If left untreated, the condition may become chronic.

Baihui (Du 20.).

Local points:

Yangbai (G.B. 14.).

through to

Yuyao (Ex. 3.).

Quanliao (S.I. 18.).

Distal point:

Hegu (L.I. 4.).

Specific points for infection:

Dazhui (Du 14.).

Quchi (L.I. 11.).

Sanyinjiao (Sp. 6.).

Specific point for allergy:

Xuehai (Sp. 10.).

TONSILLITIS

Inflammation of the tonsils is often a result of bacterial infection and is seen commonly in children and young adults. The onset of the condition is abrupt and is initially severe. Repeated acute attacks may result in chronic tonsillitis.

Baihui (Du 20.).

Local point:

Tianrong (S.I. 17.).

Distal point:

Hegu (L.I. 4.).

Specific points for infection:

Dazhui (Du 14.).

Quchi (L.I. 11.).

Sanyinjiao (Sp. 6.).

For acute tonsillitis use Jing-Well point - Shaoshang (Lu 11.). Bleeding may help.

When there is difficulty in swallowing, stimulation of Hegu (L.I.4.) is very helpful. Strong stimulation at Xi-cleft point Kongzui (Lu.6.) may help.

PHARYNGITIS (SORE THROAT)

Pharyngitis or inflammation of the pharynx may be caused by viral or bacterial infection. Although, usually the problem resolves on its own, but active treatment must be undertaken to prevent the spread of the infection to the surrounding soft tissues or down the respiratory passages, which may cause complications.

Baihui (Du 20.).

Local points:

Tianrong (S.I. 17.).

Lianquan (Ren 23.).

Distal point:

Hegu (L.I.4.).

Specific points for infection:

Dazhui (Du.14.).

Quchi (L.I. 11.).

Sanyinjiao (Sp. 6.).

The use of Taixi (K. 3.) is also helpful. The Kidney Channel is connected internally to the throat.

LARYNGITIS, TRACHEITIS

Laryngitis or acute inflammation of the larynx is usually caused by the spread of infection from the neighboring air passages, such as from a common cold or from an acute bronchitis. Tracheitis refers to the inflammation of the mucous membrane of the trachea, a condition which often accompanies bronchitis.

Baihui (Du 20.).

Local points:

Neck-Futu (L.I. 18.).

Tiantu (Ren 22.).

Distal points:

Hegu (L.I. 4.).

Tongli (H. 5.). – for the hoarse voice.

Specific points for infection may be added.

HOARSE VOICE

This is usually due to damage of the vocal chords caused by overuse of the voice. Those in the speaking trades such as politicians, teachers, and lawyers are specially prone to this disorder.

Baihui (Du 20.).

Local points:

Lianquan (Ren 23.).

Neck-Futu (L.I. 18.).

Tianrong (S.I. 17.).

Dazhui (Du 14.).

Distal points:

Tongli (H. 5.).

Hegu (L.I. 4.).

If the hoarseness persists, the possibility of the presence of a neoplasm must be investigated by laryngoscopy.

BRONCHITIS

The commonest cause of this condition is the downward spread of infection from the nose and the pharynx. The inflammation of the bronchi which results, causes a rapid secretion of mucus from the lining of the bronchi, giving rise to cough. Superadded infection of the bronchi may also occur following bronchitis due to irritants such as dust, tobacco, industrial gases and smoke. Certain infectious diseases, such as whooping cough, may also cause bronchitis as a complication.

Baihui (Du 20.).

Local points:

Zhongfu (Lu 1.).

Feishu (U.B. 13.).

Dazhui (Du 14.).

The following further points may be added according to the specific symptoms exhibited in each case:

Acute bronchitis:

Chize (Lu. 5.).

Hegu (L.I. 4.).

Fever:

Hegu (L.I. 4.).

Dazhui (Du 14.).

Quchi (L.I. 11.).

Sanyinjiao (Sp. 6.).

Sore throat:

Tianrong (S.I. 17.).

Chest pain:

Kongzui (Lu. 6.). with manual stimulation.

Excessive sputum:

Fenglong (St. 40.).

Seasonal attacks of bronchitis are probably caused by an allergen and preventive treatment may be carried out, before its onset, by using such points as:

Xuehai (Sp. 10.).

Dazhui (Du 14.).

Qihai (Ren 6.).

Zusanli (St. 36.).

Sanyinjiao (Sp. 6.).

Moxibustion at these points is also helpful.

COUGH (AS A SYMPTOM)

When the membranes lining the air passages of the lung are infected and inflammed, the secretion of mucus increases causing irritation. Coughing is a reflex action provoked by this irritation. Sometimes, however, coughing may be provoked by inflammation of the trachea and bronchi without expectoration. Regular smoking also gives rise to a chronic smoker's cough.

Baihui (Du 20.).

Local points:

Shanzhong (Ren 17.).

Zhongfu (Lu. 1.).

Feishu (U.B. 13.).

Distal points:

Lieque (Lu. 7.).

Fenglong (St. 40.). (For excessive sputum).

The cause of a chronic cough must always be investigated before treatment is commenced, in order to exclude the possibility of neoplasms, etc.[1]

WHOOPING COUGH (PERTUSSIS):

This is an acute virus infection affecting infants up to about five years of age. It is characterized by a rhinitis accompanied by severe cough which becomes progressively worse and spasmodic, producing the "whooping" sound at the end of a bout of coughing.

1 The avoidance of offending factors such as dust, air-pollution, smoke, and such others is important.

The following points may be used, in addition to those used, for uncomplicated cough described above:

Neiguan (P. 6.).

Chize (Lu. 5.).

Kongzui (Lu. 6.).

BRONCHIAL ASTHMA

This is caused by spasm of the air passages of the lungs, and may arise from allergy, infection, or emotional factors.

In the treatment of this disorder, with acupuncture, a rapid improvement may be expected in the majority of cases. However in the first few days of treatment the response may be uneven, and the patient should be warned about this and reassured. In some cases, the patient may have an aggravation due to the withdrawal of drugs. The necessity of completing at least two or more courses of treatment should be stressed, as some cases are slow to respond.

Difficulty may be encountered with asthmatics who have become dependent on steroids and other drugs. Early, if not immediate, discontinuance of such medications should be encouraged unless it appears that the degree of dependance is very high, in which case, the dosage may be gradually tailed off. The exacerbations of the bronchial asthma during the first few days of therapy are generally due to the withdrawal effects of the medications and should cause no undue alarm. Reassurance is very important to allay the anxiety of the patient. (See page 514 – Homoeopuncture).

a) Acute attack:

Insert a needle at the point Tiantu (Ren 22.). This gives the best relief in an acute attack, but it must be borne in mind that this is one of the Dangerous points and care must be taken to make the insertion precisely (for explanation of the method of insertion, see chapter on description of points on Ren Channel). It is not advisable to stimulate this point. Usually, relief is obtained within five to ten minutes of the insertion.

In some cases it may not be easy to use Tiantu (Ren 22.) during an acute attack. A good alternative is the stimulation of the point Shanzhong (Ren 17.) or the Xi-Cleft point Kongzui (Lu. 6.). In intractable cases Yanglao (S.I. 6.) may be added. Good results may also be obtained by the stimulation of Fuliu (K. 7.) (on the Theory of the Five Elements that Water is the son of Metal).

b) Status asthmaticus:

This, as the name suggests, describes the condition where the patient has a prolonged attack of acute asthma.

In most cases, stimulation of Shanzhong (Ren 17.) together with Kongzui (Lu. 6.), may give quick relief. In resistant cases it may be necessary to needle two or three times a day, using electrical or hand stimulation. In severe intractable cases embedding of catgut at Shanzhong (Ren 17.) or at Dingchuan (Ex. 17.) may be considered. ("Dingchuan" in Chinese means "soothing asthma" and this point has always been used as specific for bronchial asthma).

c) Treatment between attacks:

It is best to commence treatment with a small group of points chosen on the basic principle of combining Local and Distal points:

Baihui (Du 20.).

Local point:

Shanzhong (Ren 17.).

Specific point for soothing asthma:

Dingchuan (Ex. 17.).

Distal point:

Lieque (Lu. 7.).

The following points may be added, thereafter, if any associated symptoms are observed:

Pain and tenderness in the interscapular region:

Feishu (U.B. 13.).

Pain in chest with cough:

Zhongfu (Lu. 1.).

Excessive sputum:

Fenglong (St. 40.).

Low backache:

Shenshu (U.B. 23.).

Palpitation and dyspnea:

Neiguan (P. 6.).

Shenmen (H. 7.).

Abdominal distention:

Tianshu (St. 25.).

Zhongwan (Ren 12.).

Zusanli (St. 36.).

Daheng (Sp. 15.).

Daimai (G.B. 26.).

Eosinophilia:

Sanyinjiao (Sp. 6.).

Geshu (U.B. 17.).

Allergy:

Xuehai (Sp. 10.).

Rhinitis:

Yintang (Ex. 1.).

Yingxiang (L.I. 20.).

Blocked nose:

Nose-Heliao (L.I. 19.).

Treatment may be given daily or every other day. Ten day's treatment comprises one course. A few day's rest may be given and the patient reviewed before a second course of treatment is decided on. A press needle at a suitable body or ear point,[2] helps to prevent or abort attacks.

In the past twelve years, over 6500 cases of bronchial asthma have been treated with acupuncture alone at our clinic. Our clinical assessment shows that about 60% have been cured. The criteria for

2 Ear points: Lung, Shenmen, Dingchuan or Endocrine.

cure are that the patient had no attacks for six months and during this period no medication was given. The rate of relapse is about 5% which seems to arise out of some state of emotional, or physical stress.

When body acupuncture shows no response, we have used ear acupuncture, head needle therapy and moxibustion, in that order. In young children we have obtained good results with laser-beam therapy.

(**Homoeopuncture**—In problematical cases, where the patient has steroids for a long time, it is advisable to administer Nux vomica 30c or 200c in the homoeopathic[3] form to detoxify the patient, as it were. The *Simillimum* may be administered by homoeopuncture, therafter. Refer **Clinical Homoeopathy,** by the present author, Chandrakanthi Press (International) Hospital Road, Kalubowila, Sri Lanka (1984).[4]

■

3 Centesimal potency.

4 Official Printers, Medicina Alternativa.

CARDIOVASCULAR DISORDERS

It has been shown by means of research studies that acupuncture has a number of important regulatory effects on the circulatory system. These effects (which include normalization of heart rate and blood pressure, and lowering of serum cholesterol, triglyceride and lipoprotein levels) together with the analgesic and sedative effects can be utilized, with advantage, in the management of cardiovascular disorders. Electrocardiographic studies done on patients with angina pectoris, arrhythmias, and other similar cardiac complaints have demonstrated beyond doubt, the favourable effects of acupuncture on these disorders. The point Taiyuan (Lu. 9.) the Influential point for the vascular system is helpful in all cardiovascular disorders.

A. CARDIAC DISORDERS

The heart disorders which can be treated with acupuncture include acute coronary insufficiency, myocardial infarction, ischaemic heart disease, cardiac arrythmias, paroxysmal tachycardia, and cardiac neurosis.

In the management of these cases, it is advisable for the acupuncturist to see that the cardiac status of the patient is assessed, from time to time by electrocardiographic and other investigations. A cardiologist's opinion should certainly be sought to follow the progress of such cases. Further, it is absolutely essential that the patient be warned not to overtax himself, even if there is subjective improvement and relief of symptoms. Failure to observe this precaution could lead to serious results. Deaths have occurred due to patients having dramatic relief of symptoms and then over exerting themselves.

The use of acupuncture in this group of disorders merits serious consideration, as the use of drugs alone is not altogether satisfactory with most patients. Nausea, vomiting, anorexia, postural hypertension, and many other side effects are commonly encountered with drug therapy which, more often than not, has to be continued indefinitely.

Principles of treatment

The chief points used are:

Shanzhong (Ren 17.).

Shenmen (H. 7.).

Bipay (U. Ex.).

The following additional points are used for specific symptoms:

1) Pain:

Hegu (L.I. 4.).

Xinshu (U.B. 15.).

Neiguan (P. 6.).

Jueyinshu (U.B. 14.).

Rugen (St. 18.).

2) Shock and collapse:

Renzhong (Du 26.) firm acupressure or strong stimulation with a needle.

Hegu (L.I. 4.).

3) Palpitation, arrythmias:

Baihui (Du 20.).

Neiguan (P. 6.) strong stimulation[1]

Ximen (P. 4.).

1 Electro-stimulation should not be used at point.

4) Nausea, vomiting, hiccough, abdominal distension:

Zusanli (St. 36.).

Neiguan (P. 6.).

Zhongwan (Ren 12.).

5) Insomnia, restlessness, apprehension:

Baihui (Du 26.) and Sishencong (Ex. 6.)

Shenmen (H.7.).

Shenmai (U.B. 62.).

6) Dyspnea, left ventricular failure, cardiac asthma:

Baihui (Du 20.).

Feishu (U.B. 13.).

Dingchuan (Ex. 17.).

Lieque (Lu. 7.).

Yinlingquan (Sp. 9.).

Xi-Cleft point, if the condition is very acute:

Kongzui (Lu. 6.).

For excessive sputum:

Fenglong (St. 40.)

7) Edema of feet and ankles:

Baihui (Du 20.).

Shuifen (Ren 9.).

Shimen (Ren 5.).

Pishu (U.B. 20.).

Yinlingquan (Sp. 9.).

Sanyinjiao (Sp. 6.).

Local points around the ankles.

8) Ascites:

Baihui (Du 20.).

Shuifen (Ren 9.).

Shimen (Ren 5.).

Guanyuan (Ren 4.).

Yinlingquan (Sp. 9.).
Pishu (U.B. 20.).

9) Renal failure:

Baihui (Du 20.).

Local points:

Shenshu (U.B. 23.).
Mingmen (Du 4.).

Distal points:

Taixi (K. 3.).
Sanyinjiao (Sp. 6.).

10) Neurasthenia following coronary heart disease (cardiac-neurosis):

Baihui (Du 20.).

Local points:

Shanzhong (Ren 17.).
Jujue (Ren 14.).
Zhongwan (Ren 12.).

Distal points:

Neiguan (P. 6.).
Shenmen (H. 7.).
Zusanli (St. 36.).
YInlingquan (sp. 9.).

11) Bradycardia:

Baihui (Du 20.).
Neiguan (P. 6.).
Shaochong (H. 9.).
Suliao (Du 25.).

12) Rheumatic heart disease:

Baihul (Du 20.).

Local points:

Points on the chest.

Distal points:

Hegu (L.I. 4.).

Yanglingquan (G.B. 34.).

Zusanli (St. 36.).

Xuanzong (G.B. 39.).

B. VASCULAR DISORDERS:

1) Hypotension (low blood pressure):

Use the General Tonification points:

Qihai (Ren 6.).

Zusanli (St. 36.).

Sanyinjiao (Sp 6.).

2) Hypertension (high blood pressure):

Baihui (Du 20.).

Quchi (L.I. 11.)

Zusanli (St. 36.).

Sanyinjiao (Sp. 6.).

Treat daily or every other day for ten treatments and repeat after an interval of one week, if necessary.

According to traditional Chinese medicine, symptoms commonly associated with high blood pressure are related to the Liver and Kidney. If the response is inadequate after using the above points, one or more of the following points may be added:

Ganshu (U.B. 18.). Back-Shu point of the Liver

Shenshu (U.B. 23.). Back-Shu point of the Kidney.

Taichong (Liv. 3.). Dangerous point,

Xingjian (Liv. 2.).

Taixi (K. 3.).

If the blood pressure is very high, do not use points on the Liver Channel, especially Taichong (Liv. 3.), as an abrupt fall in blood pressure may occur.[2]

2 This may cause a stroke.

In severe hypertension, acupuncture may be combined with drug therapy.

In our experience, acupuncture is effective in controlling mild and moderate cases of hypertension without serious complications. The effects on the systolic pressure is uniformly good, but the fall in diastolic pressure is rather slow and may not drop to the desired level, if it was initially very high. Hence with our present techniques, it cannot be claimed that acupuncture is completely effective in cases of severe hypertension with diastolic pressures of 140 or above. However, it has been observed that even in such cases a substantial reduction of drug dosage is possible. For example, the dosage of methyldopa may be reduced by one-third or even by half. This is an area where we feel that further clinical studies are required for proper evaluation.

Acupuncture is useful in the management of many of the symptoms of hypertension.

a) Headache:

Baihui (Du 20.).
Fengchi (G.B. 20.).
Taiyang (Ex. 2.).
Touwei (St. 8.).
Shangxing (Du 23.).

b) Dizziness, vertigo:

Baihui (Du 20.).
Yintang (Ex. 1.).
Taiyang (Ex. 2.).
Shuaigu (G.B. 8.).

c) Tinnitus:

Baihui (Du 20.).
Ermen (S.J. 21.). } through and through
Tinggong (S.I. 19.). } insertion[3]

3 One needle.

Tinghui (G.B. 2.). } through and through
Yifeng (S.J. 17.). } insertion
Zhongzhu (S.J. 3.).
Foot-Linqi (G.B. 41.).

d) Pain and fullness in the chest:

Baihui (Du 20.).
Neiguan (P. 6.).
Zhigou (S.J. 6.).
Qimen, (Liv. 14.).
Zhangmen (Liv 13.).
Yanglingquan (G.B. 34.).
Jingmen (G.B. 25.).

e) Numbness of the extremities:

Upper limbs:

Waiguan (S.J. 5.).
Quchi (L.I. 11.).
Zhongzhu (S.J. 3.).

Lower limbs:

Yanglingquan (G.B. 34.).
Zusanli (St. 36.).
Sanyinjiao (Sp. 6.).

f) Aphasia:

Baihui (Du 20.).
Yamen (Du 15.).
Lianquan (Ren 23.).
Tongli (H. 5.). On the right side.
Hegu (L.I. 4.). On the left side.

g) Facial paralysis following hypertension:

Points of the Stomach Channel on the face.
Quanliao (S.I. 18.).
Yifeng (S.J. 17.).

3) Thromboangiitis obliterans:

Baihui (Du 20.).
Hegu (L.I. 4.). } on opposite sides.
Taiyuan (Lu 9.). }
Points of Stomach Channel on leg.
Yanglingquan (G.B. 34.).

All points, except Baihui (Du 20.), are stimulated to produce *deqi.*

If there is a gangrenous or ulcerated area, then the opposite leg is needled, in the area corresponding to the diseased area.

4) Peripheral vascular disorders:

The points to be used are the same as for thromboangiitis. The points for polyneuropathy (points along the Large Intestine and Stomach Channels) are also used. For numbness and coldness of hands and feet use:

Hands:
Laogong (P. 8.).
Shaofu. (H. 8.).
Yuji (Lu. 10.).

Feet:
Taixi (K. 3.).
Yongquan (K. 1.).

Influential point:
Taiyuan (Lu. 9.).

The Heart, Pericardium, and Spleen are also involved in the circulation of fluids.

ANGINA PECTORIS

We have obtained good results in angina pectoris using the following points:

Baihui (Du 20.).

Local points:

Mu Pericardium : Shanzhong (Ren 17.).

Shu Heart : Xinshu (U.B. 15.).

Bipay (U. Ex.).

Distal points:

Neiguan (P. 6.).

Shenmen (H. 7.).

Influential point:

Taiyuan (Lu. 9.).

All medications are tailed off as therapy commences.

BLOOD DISORDERS

Acupuncture is being clinically used today in certain blood disorders like pernicious anaeinia, hypoferric anemia, leucopenia, thromocytopenia, purpura, splenic anaemias, and certain other blood dyscrasias. Varying degrees of success have been reported, but there is still no agreement on the best points to use for specific conditions. Research carried out in the People's Republic of China has shown that acupuncture has a normalizing effect on the cellular constituents of the blood, in a number of blood disorders.

Principles of treatment:

a) Use of the Influential point for blood:Geshu (U.B. 17.).

b) Use of the Influential point for marrow:

Xuanzhong (G.B. 39.).

c) Use of the main Tonification points, i.e.,

Qihai (Ren 6.).

Zusanli (St. 36.).

Sanyinjiao (Sp. 6.).

d) Use of points on the Urinary Bladder Channel. This Channel lies close to the vertebral bodies and over the ribs and may therefore be expected to influence marrow function.

e) Use of points on the Du Channel lying over the spine.

f) Use of the Huatuojiaji (Ex. 21.). points.

g) Use of the technique of tapping with the plum blossom needle over the site of the carotid artery. This procedure has been shown to result in an increase of the blood platelets and may, therefore, be used in thrombocytopenic states and also to control haemoptysis.

h) Use of the Homeostatic points, e.g., Quchi (L.I. 11.).

i) Use of the point Baihui (Du 20.), as many Channels are being used.

J) Aquapuncture of vitamin B 12 in weekly doses of 1000 micrograms at Qihai (Ren 6.) is also very helpful in blood disorders, particularly in anaemias.

■

DISORDERS OF THE GASTROINTESTINAL SYSTEM

Principles of treatment

The Stomach and Ren Channels are those commonly used in the treatment of gastrointestinal disorders. The Channels related to these, the Spleen and the Du Channels are also useful. The Back-Shu points of the Urinary Bladder Channel are also effective. A summary of the main points to be used, which are based on traditional Chinese medicine and modern clinical experience, is given below:

a) Zusanli (St. 36.). is the Distal point of choice for normalizing peristaltic activity of the gastrointestinal tract. It is also the best homeostatic point for abdominal disorders.

b) Neiguan P. 6.) is the most effective point for the control of upper abdominal pain and gastrointestinal symptoms like nausea, vomiting, and hiccough.

c) "Alarm" points of the Fu Organs of the gastrointestinal tract:

Zhongwan (Ren 12.).	: Stomach.
Guanyuan (Ren 4.).	: Small Intestine.
Tianshu (St. 25.).	: Large Intestine.
Lanwei (Ex. 33.).	: Vermiform Appendix.

d) "Alarm" points of the liver and gall bladder, as they are associated with gastrointestinal functions:

Zhongdu (Liv. 6.). : Liver.

Dannang (Ex. 35.). : Gall bladder

e) "Alarm" points of the Urinary Bladder Channel (Back-Su points) which correspond to the Organs of the gastrointestinal tract and the related Organs:

Weishu (U.B. 21.). : Stomach.

Dachangshu (U.B. 25.).: Large Intestine.

Xiochangshu (U.B. 27.).: Small Intestine.

Ganshu (U.B. 18.). : Liver

Danshu (U.B. 19.). : Gall bladder.

Pishu (U.B. 20.). : Spleen.

f) Points on the Spleen Channel, as it has an interior-exterior relationship with the Stomach Channel e.g.,

Gongsun (Sp. 4.).
Sanyinjiao (Sp. 6.).
Daheng (Sp. 15.).

g) Local points situated near the origin of the disorder and points adjacent to these.

h) Distal points on Channels which traverse the affected region. The Channels most often used are the Stomach and Spleen Channels. However, the Ren and the Du Channels are also very effective in the treatment of gastrointestinal disorders. When using the Ren and the Du Channels, it must be noted that their Distal points are situated above the neck. Thus, in the treatment of haemorrhoids the point Baihui (Du 20.) could be selected as a Distal point with Changqiang (Du 1.) as a Local point. The point Yinjiao (Du 28.) is another often used Distal point for anorectal disorders.[1]

1 Distal point of Channel.

i) Specific points for certain disorders, e.g.,

Zhigou (S.J. 6.) for constipation;

Neiguan (P. 6.) for nausea and vomiting.

j) Liangqiu (St. 34.), the Xi-Cleft point of the Stomach Channel is indicated in all acute abdominal disorders to relieve pain.

k) Zhongwan (Ren 12.), the Influential point for hollow Organs.

l) Lower He-Sea points.

STOMATITIS, GLOSSITIS:

Stomatitis, or inflammation of the mucous membrane lining of the mouth, may be of several types. The most commonly encountered is gingivitis or inflammation of the gums, which is usually caused by bacterial infection, but may also be due to vitamin deficiencies. In stomatitis associated with nutritional deficiencies, acupuncture therapy should be coupled with proper intake of nourishment.

Thrush is stomatitis caused by infection with the fungus 'candida albicans'. This condition is characterized by a white membrane covering the inside of the mouth and may occur following the prolonged use of antibiotics and steroids.

Allergic reaction to locally applied disinfectants and chemicals such as those found in toothpastes and sweets may also cause stomatitis. It is important to eliminate the offending material. The development of certain multiple ulcers of the mucous membrane of the mouth is termed aphthous stomatitits and is said to be associated with emotional stress.

Glossitis, or inflammation of the tongue, usually accompanies stomatitis resulting from nutritional and vitamin deficiencies. In such cases these deficiencies must be corrected before treatment.

Baihui (Du 20.).

Local points:

Yinjiao (Du 28.).

Jinjin, Yuye (Ex. 10.).

Distal point:

Hegu (L.I. 4.).

Specific points for infection:

Quchi (L.I. 11.).

Dazhui (Du 14.).

Specific point for allergy:

Xuehai (Sp. 10.).

TOOTHACHE

The cause of the toothache needs proper dental attention. To relieve the pain, the following points may be used:

Baihui (Du 20.)

Local points for the upper jaw:

Yingxiang (L.I. 20.).

Quanliao (S.I. 18.).

Xiaguan (St. 7.).

Local points for the lower jaw:

Chengjiang (Ren 24.).

Daying (St. 5.).

Jiache (St. 6.).

Distal points:

Hegu (L.I. 4.).
Neiting (St. 44.). } with strong stimulation.

These points may also be used as analgesia for the extraction of teeth. The points selected depend on the situation of the offending tooth.

DYSPHAGIA (DIFFICULTY OF SWALLOWING)

Most diseases of the esophagus cause dysphagia. It may also be caused by certain diseases of the mouth and pharynx such as stomatitis and tonsillitis. Since, however, dysphagia may be due to causes such as neoplasms (especially in elderly people), the patient must be fully investigated before acupuncture is commenced to eliminate such etiology. Where surgical, radiotherapy, or other treatment has been carried out and the swallowing difficulty still persists, then acupuncture may be tried for symptomatic relief. In treating dysphagia due to motor-neurone disease good results have been obtained by using acupuncture. Dysphagia due to psychosomatic causes, such as hysteria,[2] respond well to acupuncture.

Baihui (Du 20.).

Local points (select from):

Lianquan (Ren 23.).

Tiantu (Ren 22.).

Shanzhong (Ren 17.).

Distal point:

Neiguan (P. 6.).

HIATUS HERNIA

A hernia may be described as the abnormal protrusion of an organ from one compartment of the body into another. Hiatus hernia is a protrusion into the thoracic cavity, through the diaphragm of the stomach or other viscus. This is commonly encountered after middle age. The commonest symptom is heartburn, but regurgitation of food and flatulence may also be often present.

Baihui (Du 20.).

Local points:

Shanzhong (Ren 17.).

Zhongwan (Ren 12.).

Liangmen (St. 21.).

Tianshu (St. 25.).

Weishu (U.B. 21.).

2 Globus hystericut.

Distal points:

Neiguan (P. 6.).

Zusanli (St. 36.).

Since this is a mechanical disorder, acupuncture therapy is not uniformly successful in alleviating the disorder. Where surgery is contraindicated, acupuncture may be used to relieve the symptoms.

HICCOUGH (HICCUP)

This condition is caused by involuntary spasmodic contraction of the diaphragm usually due to local irritation. It may also occur reflexively via the autonomic nerves supplying it. In most cases it stops fairly quickly but if it persists it may exhaust the patient. Hiccough which occurs following surgery can be particularly distressing. General causes like uremia, due ketosis also may cause hiccough.

Baihui (Du 20.).

Local points:

Tiantu (Ren 22.). (No stimulation).

Geshu (U.B. 17.).

Shanzhong (Ren 17.).

Renzhong (Du 26.).

Distal points:

Neiguan (P. 6.). (Strong stimulation)

NAUSEA AND VOMITING

These symptoms occur in a wide variety of diseases. Whatever the cause, the condition must be relieved, unless poisonous toxic material has been ingested.[3]

Baihui (Du 20.).

Local points:

Zhongwan (Ren 12.).

Zhangmen (Liv. 13.).

3 See page 566 for nausea and vomiting of pregnancy.

Distal points:

Neiguan (P. 6.). (Strong manual stimulation).

Zusanli (St. 36.).

GASTRITIS

By gastritis, is meant an inflammation of the inner lining of the stomach, but the term may cover a wide variety of disorders ranging from mild indigestion to more chronic pathology.

In its acute form it may result in severe upper abdominal pain, nausea and vomiting. If there is an accompanying infection there may be fever and diarrhea. The common causes of gastritis are: (i) chemical irritants (e.g. certain drugs); (ii) physical irritants (e.g. hot and spicy food, alcohol); (iii) infection (e.g. from contaminated food); (iv) allergy (e.g., eating shellfish).

Baihui (Du 20.).

Local points:

Weishu (U.B. 21.).

Tianshu (St. 25.).

Influential point:

Zhongwan (Ren 12.).

Distal points:

Zusanli (St. 36.).

Neiguan (P. 6.).

Liangqiu (St. 34.). (Xi-Cleft point).

Sanyinjiao (Sp. 6.).

Additional points according to symptoms:

Infection:

Quchi (L.I. 11.).

Fever:

Dazhui (Du 14.).

Diarrhea:

Shangjuxu (St. 37.).
Xiajuxu (St. 39.).
Gongsun (Sp. 4.).
} Strong manual stimulation.

Flatulence:

Zhangmen (Liv. 13.).
Jingmen (G.B. 25.).
Daimai (G.B. 26.).

(**Note:** Pain due to gastritis should be differentiated from other pains in the upper abdominal area, such as those due to initial pain of onset of appendicitis, or those arising from disorders of other internal organs like the gall bladder and pancreas.)

GASTRIC ULCER, DUODENAL ULCER (PEPTIC ULCER)

This is the destruction of a small area of the lining (mucosa) of the stomach (gastric ulcer) or of the duodenum (duodenal ulcer) by gastric juices (acid-pepsin). Why this should occur is not precisely known.

The main symptom is a cramp-like pain in the upper abdominal area with localized tenderness. In gastric ulcer, the pain is usually felt to the left of the midline, and in duodenal ulcer the pain is felt towards the right side, or in the middle of the upper abdomen radiating upwards Epigastric pain, half to one hour after a meal, is suggestive of a gastric ulcer, and pain two to three hours later suggests a duodenal ulcer.

The pain may sometimes radiate to the back to the region of the eighth to the twelfth dorsal vertebrae where tender points (Alarm points for Stomach and Spleen) may be detected.

Baihui (Du 20.).

Local points (select from):

Liangmen (St. 21.).
Tianshu (St. 25.).

Pishu (U.B. 20.).
Weishu (U.B. 21.).

Influential point:

Zhongwan (Ren 12.).

Distal points:

Neiguan (P. 6.).
Zusanli (St. 36.).
Sanyinjiao (Sp. 6.).

The Back-Shu (Weishu (U.B. 21.)) and the Mu-Front (Zhongwan (Ren 12.)) Alarm points may be used, instead of Local and Distal points.

Where tenderness is observed over area of the dorsal vertebrae, it would be useful to needle the related Huatuojiaji points (Ex. 21.) or the *Ah-Shi* points.

In acute attacks, needling may be performed two to three times a day.

Catgut embedding therapy at Zhongwan (Ren 12.) through to Liangmen (St. 21.). may be tried in chronic cases.

In our experience, acupuncture is not so effective if abdominal surgery has been performed in these conditions.

DYSPEPSIA (INDIGESTION)

This term covers a variety of symptoms which include discomfort or pain, abdominal distension, nausea, diarrhea and constipation. It is usually caused by overeating, or ingesting unsuitable food. It may also be caused by gastritis or gastric ulcer.

Baihui (Du 20.).

Local points (select from):

Liangmen (St. 21.).
Tianshu (St. 25.).
Pishu (U.B. 20.).

Weishu (U.B. 21.).

Shenshu (U.B. 23.)

Influential point:

Zhongwan (Ren. 12)

Distal Points:

Neiguan (P. 6.).

Zusanli (St. 36.).

Sanyinjiao (Sp. 6.).

ABDOMINAL DISTENTION (FLATULENCE)

Flatulence is caused by the distension of the stomach or intestines, due to an excessive accumulation of gas. This symptom is due to a variety of causes such as constipation and gastroenteritis. Mechanical obstruction also may cause distension, in which surgical relief is necessary.

Baihui (Du 20.).

Local points:

Jingmen (G.B. 25.).

Zhangmen (Liv. 13.).

Daimai (G.B. 26.).

Influential point:

Zhongwan (Ren 12.).

Distal points:

Neiguan (P. 6.).

Zusanli (St. 36.).

Sanyinjiao (Sp. 6.).

Taichong (Liv. 3.).

APPENDICITIS:

This is the inflammation of the vermiform appendix caused by an infection or obstruction. The usual symptoms are abdominal pain, nausea, vomiting and fever. There is pain and tenderness in the right iliac fossa. The inflammation of the appendix may resolve giving rise to a subacute or chronic stage, if left untreated. In a small proportion of cases, gangrene or rupture may occur. Therefore, it is always, safer to remove the appendix if the disease is suspected.

In a high proportion of cases, the point Lanwei (Ex. 33.). becomes tender and this may aid the diagnosis. (The point Lanwei (Ex. 33.) is the Alarm point of the vermiform appendix (Lanwei is the Chinese word for the appendix).

Where adequate surgical facilities are not available, such as on the high seas or in remote inaccessible areas or due to other reasons when surgery is contraindicated, conservative therapy combined with acupuncture helps to resolve the inflammation in the vast majority of cases.

Baihui (Du 20.).

Local points:

Ah-Shi points on the abdomen.

Tianshu (St. 25.).

Guilai (St. 29.).

Influential point:

Zhongwan (Ren 12.).

Distal points:

Lanwei (Ex. 33.).

Zusanli (St. 36.).

Analgesic point:

Hegu (L.I. 4.).

Immune-enhancing and anti-infective points:

Dazhui (Du 14.).

Quchi (L.I. 11.).

Sanyinjiao (Sp. 6.).

In the People's Republic of China, several papers have been published describing the treatment of appendicitis with acupuncture alone or in combination with herbal drugs. Many Chinese authorities indicate that acupuncture is an effective therapy for acute appendicitis and that complete resolution takes place in the vast majority of cases.

INTESTINAL PARASITOSIS (HELMINTHIASIS. AMEBIASIS)

Intestinal parasitosis, in the form of worm infestation or amoebiasis of the intestines is common in tropical countries. Symptoms may be absent or consist of pruritus of the anus (threadworm), inflammation of the intestine (tapeworm), gastroenteritis (roundworm), nausea, vomiting and lack of appetite. The patient is likely to suffer from anemia and nutritional disorders, and in many cases eosinophilia may also occur.

Baihui (Du 20.).

Local points:

Daheng (Sp. 15.).

Tianshu (St. 25.).

Influential point:

Zhongwan (Ren 12.).

Distal points:

Zusanli (St. 36.).

Neiguan (P. 6.).

Strong stimulation is carried out at the distal points. As the present day anti-helminthics are extremely effective acupuncture therapy has no place in the routine treatment of helminthiasis, except in the patient who is tolerant or otherwise unfit for modern drug therapy. In ancient times, before effective drug therapy was available, acupuncture provided a harmless method of management of helminthiasis and its complications. However, in the weak, emaciated, malnourished and toxic children (especially in the Third World) it has still a place as an adjuvant or interim therapy.

DIARRHEA, DYSENTERY (BACILLARY, AMEBIC)

Diarrhoea with blood, mucus, abdominal pain, and discomfort is a common symptom of dysentery. It is caused by an infection with a bacillus, amebae, or unsuitable food. Symptoms of amebic dysentery may become chronic and may last for several years.

Baihui (Du 20.).

Local points:

Tianshu (St. 25.).

Qihai (Ren 6.).

Zhongli (Ren 3.).

Distal points:

Zusanli (St. 36.).

Shangjuxu (St. 37.).

Gongsun (Sp. 4.).

Sanyinjiao (Sp. 6.).

Immune enhancing points:

Quchi (L.I. 11.).

Dazhui (Du. 14.).

Strong manual stimulation may be carried out at the Distal points, particularly at Zusanli (St. 36.) and Shangjuxu (St. 37.). After stimulation, the needles may be retained for about 30 minutes. In acute cases the procedure may be repeated 3-4 times a day. In bacterial dysentery, treatment should be continued for one week after disappearance of the symptoms.

The following points may be added according to the symptoms:

Acute abdominal pain:

Liangqiu (St. 34.).

Nausea and vomiting:

Neiguan (P. 6.).

Fever:

Dazhui (Du 14.).

Tenesmus:

Changqiang (Du 1.).

Huiyin (Ren 1.).

Flatulence:

Zhangmen (Liv. 13.).

Jingmen (G.B. 25.).

Daimai (G.B. 26.).

In acute diarrhea, the dehydration and electrolytic imbalance needs to be corrected with infusions. With present day drug therapy being very effective in these conditions, acupuncture only needs to be used as an ancilliary or in cases resistant to medication.

INTESTINAL COLIC

Intestinal colic is due to the complete or partial obstruction of the intestines, which is usually caused by inflammation after ingestion of toxic food. The pain of colic is characteristically intermittent, coming on at regular or irregular intervals. The pain is often severe.

The non-obstructive type of colic responds well to acupuncture. The obstructive type may be due to some mechanical cause and may need surgery.

Baihui (Du 20.)

Local point:

Tianshu (St. 25.).

Distal points:

Zusanli (St. 36.).

Sanyinjiao (Sp. 6.).

Specific point for pain:

Hegu (L.I. 4.). with strong stimulation.

Strong manual stimulation of the Distal points may also be carried out.

CONSTIPATION

Constipation may be described as an infrequent evacuation of the bowels. What constitutes "infrequency" differs from person to person. However, what is important is that there should be regularity of the bowel movement.

Constipation may be due to faulty diet (e.g., insufficiency of 'roughage' and irregularity of meals) or lack of exercise. Psychological factors may also be present. Proper advice on these matters should therefore be given to the patient, if relief obtained from acupuncture is to be maintained.

Constipation could also be a symptom of carcinoma of the large intestine. In majority of cases of constipation, the cause is not known.

If the condition is neglected, it may lead to the cracking of the skin of the anus (and fissure) or the distention of the veins around it (hemorrhoids).

Local points:

Tianshu (St. 25.).

Distal points:

Baihui (Du 20.).
Zhigou (S.J. 6.). } Strong manual stimulation
Zusanli (St. 36.).

Influential point:

Zhongwan (Ren 12.).

HEMORRHOIDS (PILES), ANAL FISSURE

Local points:

Changqiang (Du 1.).
Huiyin (Ren 1.).
Ciliao (U.B. 32.).
Zhibian (U.B. 54.).

Distal points:

Baihui (Du 20.).

Yinjiao (Du 28.).

Sanyinjiao (Sp. 6.).

Jizhong (Du 6.).

Chengshan (U.B. 57.).

PROLAPSE OF THE RECTUM

Local points:

Changqiang (Du 1.).

Huiyin (Ren 1.).

Distal points:

Chengshan (U.B. 57.).

Baihui (Du 20.).

Influential point:

Yanglingquan (G.B. 34.).

HEPATIC, BILIARY, SPLENIC AND PANCREATIC DISORDERS

The liver, gall bladder, biliary tract and the pancreas are functionally related to the digestive tract and to each other. In traditional Chinese medicine, the term "Spleen" includes the pancreatic functions as well. This is why the Spleen Channel is also called the "Spleno-Pancreatic Channel"

Principles of treatment

1) Owing to these inter-relationships, points from the following Channels are frequently used together in the treatment of this group of disorders:

   a) Liver Channel.

   b) Gall bladder Channel.

   c) Spleen Channel.

   d) Stomach Channel.

2) Points from the following Channels are used as they traverse the area of the abdomen:

   a) Urinary bladder Channel.

b) Du Channel.

c) Ren Channel.

3) The Influential point of the Zang Organs, namely:

Zhangmen (Liv 13.).

4) The Back-Shu points of the affected organs:

Ganshu (U.B. 18.).
Danshu (U.B. 19.).
Pishu (U.B. 20.).

5) The Mu-Front points and other Alarm points of the Organs involved in this group of disorders:

Qimen (Liv. 14.)-Mu-Front Alarm point of the Liver.

Riyue (G.B. 24.)-Mu-Front Alarm point of the Gall bladder.

Zhangmen (Liv. 13.)-Mu-Front Alarm point of the Spleen.

Zhongdu (Liv. 6.)-Alarm point of the Liver in the leg.

Dannang (E. 25.)-Alarm point of the Gall bladder in the led.

Jiangjing (G.B. 21.)-Alarm point of the Gall bladder in the shoulder area.

These points are useful in diagnosis as well as in the therapy.[1]

6) The point Liangmen (St. 21.). on the right side lies directly over the gall bladder and is often used in diseases of that organ. On the right side, therefore, this is a Dangerous points and for this reason on that side, the needle should be inserted superficially or directed obliquely.

7) Further points may be used where accompanying symptoms are present:

Pain:

Hegu (L.I. 4.).

Hiccough, nausea, vomiting:

1 Also in prognosis.

Neiguan (P. 6.).

Tiantu (Ren 22.).

Infection:

Dazhui (Du 14.).

Quchi (L.I. 11.).

Sanyinjiao (Sp. 6.).

Abdominal distention:

Tianshu (St. 25.).

Daheng (Sp. 15.).

Zhongwan (Ren 12.).

Daimai (G.B. 26.).

Sanyiniao (Sp. 6.).

Constipation:

Zhigou (S.J. 6.).

Diarrhea:

Gongsun (Sp. 4.).

By making a judicious clinical selection from these specific acupuncture points we have found it possible to manage these disorders satisfactorily. This is a great advantage because in these disorders there is liver damage and patients, therefore, cannot tolerate drug therapy and serious side effects may occur. Acupuncture is free of such complications and is, therefore, recommended as the first line of therapy in these disorders, perhaps combined with minimal doses of drugs where indicated.

HEPATITIS (INFECTIVE HEPATITIS, SERUM HEPATITIS), AMEBIC HEPATITIS:

Hepatitis is an inflammation of the liver cells. There are two acute forms caused by virus infection; infective hepatitits (epidemic jaundice) which is usually transmitted in food contaminated by the faeces of an infected person, and serum hepatitis (homologous serum jaundice) which is transmitted by blood and serum used for transfusions, or more commonly by needles and syringes used on persons suffering from the disease. While both these forms of hepatitis have many common pathological features, there are differences with regard to the incubation period (about 15-50 days for the former and about 15-100 days for the latter) and severity (generally serum hepatitis is more severe).

Generally, about two weeks after the onset of the infection, the patient becomes jaundiced and the skin and the sclera of the eyes turn yellow, the urine becomes dark and the stools become pale. These symptoms may have been preceded by headache, general malaise and gastrointestinal symptoms such as loss of appetite, nausea, vomiting and diarrhea. The liver becomes enlarged and tender.

The duration of the illness varies, and even after the jaundice diappears the patient will continue to feel malaise for some time. Some cases may take up to six months to recover. Relapses also occur. Amebic hepatitis may present in an acute form or as a chronic abscess.

Although the main lesion is in the liver, the disease also affects the gastrointestinal tract, and other organs. Additional points should be selected if these features are present.

Baihui (Du 20.).

Local points (select from):

Qimen (Liv. 14.). (Mu-Front and Back-
Ganshu (U.B. 18.). Shu Alarm points of the Liver)
Riyue (G.B. 24.). (Mu-Front and Back-
Danshu (U.B. 19.). Shu Alarm points of the Gall bladder)
Zhangmen (Liv. 13.). Influential point for Zang Organs.
Daimai (G.B. 26.).
Zhongwan (Ren 12.).
Liangmen (St. 21.).
Pishu (U.B. 20.).
Weishu (U.B. 21.).

Distal points:

Zhongdu (Liv. 6.). (Alarm point of Liver in leg)

Dannang (Ex. 35.). (Alarm point of Gall bladder in leg)

Taichong (Liv. 3.).

Zusanli (St. 36.).

Sanyinjiao (Sp. 6.).

The following points may be added according to the symptoms present:

For fever:

Dazhui (Du 14.).

Quchi (L.I. 11.).

For malaise:

Qihai (Ren 6.).

Zusanli (St. 36.).

Sanyinjiao (Sp. 6.).

For severe jaundice:

Yanglingquan (G.B. 34.).

Since ordinary methods of boiling are insufficient where the virus of hepatitis is concerned, it is advisable to autoclave the needles used on these patients. It is a good practice for such patients to have their own needles reserved for them.

CIRRHOSIS OF THE LIVER

This is a condition of fibrosis which arises as a result of degenerative changes in the liver. It may be due to malnutrition, alcoholism, or as a complication of infections of the liver.

Early cirrhosis responds well to acupuncture. The patient should, however, be given advice regarding a regulated diet and abstention from alcohol.

Selection of points is similar to those for hepatitis as described above. Associated complications such as ascites (fluid in the peritoneal cavity) and enlargement of the spleen should be treated by the use of the following points:

Ascites:

Yinlingquan (Sp. 9.).

Shimen (Ren 5.).

Shuifen (Ren 9.).

Pishu (U.B. 20.).

Enlargement of the spleen:

Local points (select from):

Zhangmen (Liv. 13.).

Qimen (Liv. 14.).

Daimai (G.B. 26.).

Riyue (G.B. 24.).

Liangmen (St. 21.).

Pishu (U.S. 20.).

Distal points:

Sanyinjiao (Sp. 6.).

Yinlingquan (Sp. 4.).

Zusanli (St. 36.).

BILIARY COLIC

This refers to the characteristically intermittent severe pain produced as a result of the obstruction and inflammation of the gall bladder or its bile duct. The pain is felt generally in the upper abdomen with maximal tenderness in the right costal (rib) margin. It may radiate to the right shoulder and the back. Nausea, vomiting, fever, and mild jaundice may also appear.

The more usual forms of this condition are:

i) acute cholecystitis or inflammation of the gall bladder often due to the presence of gall stones (cholelithiasis), which may also cause complete or partial obstruction of the bile duct, and

ii) ascariasis or infestation by roundworm or threadworm of the bile duct, which could be further complicated, by bacterial infection which may in turn cause cholecystits obstructive jaundice and gastrointestinal complications.

Acupuncture treatment is first given for the management of pain. After that the primary cause should be ascertained. Where ascariasis is present, appropriate vermicidal drugs need to be administered. If perforation of the gall bladder has occurred or obstruction to the bile duct is present, surgery will then be indicated. In all cases, the possibility of neoplasms must be excluded.

In acute cases Hegu (L.I. 4.), should first be strongly stimulated to alleviate the pain, together with the Xi-cleft point of the Gall bladder: Waiqiu (G.B. 36.).

The following points may be used as a course of treatment:

Baihui (Du 20.).

Local points (select from):

Riyue (G.B. 24.).

Danshu (U.B. 19.).

Zhangmen (Liv. 13.).

Ganshu (U.B. 18.).

Huatuojiaji (Ex. 21.) of 8-12 dorsal vertebrae

Liangmen (St. 21.).

Also, select from:

Jingmen (G.B. 25.).

Daimai (G.B. 26.).

Qimen (Liv. 14.).

Pishu (U.B. 20.).

Weishu (U.B. 21.).

Distal points:

Hegu (L.I. 4.).

Neiguan (P. 6.).

Dannang (Ex. 35.).

Zhongdu (Liv. 6.).

Zusanli (St. 36.).

Qiuxu (G.B. 40.).

Specific points for infection:

Dazhul (Du 14.).

Quchi (L.I. 11.).

Sanyinjiao (Sp. 6.).

PANCREATITIS

This is an inflammatory condition of the pancreas which may occur in acute, subacute, or in chronic forms.

Acute pancreatitis is a very painful disorder commonly associated with disease of the gall bladder. There may be obstruction of the pancreatic duct as it enters the duodenum due to a gall stone, edema, or spasm, as the pancreatic duct shares a common opening into the duodenum with the bile duct. As a result of this obstruction, bile enters the pancreatic duct and activates the digestive enzymes secreted by the pancreas, which causes the digestion of the pancreatic tissue.

The patient usually suffers from a sudden onset of acute pain in the upper abdomen, often with nausea and vomiting. In severe cases the condition may render the patient unconscious. The pain often radiates to the back, to either shoulder, or to one or both the iliac fossae. As the destructive process of the pancreas continues, the digestive enzymes will leak into the abdominal cavity and cause a chemical peritonitis.

Since the symptoms may resemble perforated peptic ulcer, acute intestinal obstruction, acute appendicitis, or acute myocardial infarction, it is very important that an early diagnosis is made.

The immediate treatment is to control the severe pain by strong stimulation at:

Hegu (L.I. 4.).

Sanyangluo (S.J. 8.).

Neiguan (P. 6.).,

If shock and collapse occur, use:

Jing-Well points, with

Homeostatic points.

Subacute pancreatitis is a less severe condition which may occur as a complication of viral infections such as mumps, influenza, or infective hepatitis. There will be fever, pain, and tenderness in the upper abdominal area.

Points are selected as for chronic pancreatitis (see below), with the following points added for the infection:

Dazhul (Du 14.).

Quchi (L.I. 11.).

Sanyinjiao (Sp. 6.).

Chronic pancreatitis may follow acute or subacute pancreatitis, or be associated with a chronic inflammation of the bile duct, or with the erosion of the pancreas by a chronic peptic ulcer. There may be a history of excessive intake of alcohol.

Pain will be felt in the upper abdominal area and often in the back along the dorsal spine, characteristically about a day after excessive consumption of food or alcohol. Other symptoms include jaundice and diarrhea.

Baihui (Du 20.).

Local points (select from):

Zhongwan (Ren 12.).

Zhangman (Liv 13.) Mu-Front point of Spleen

Pishu (U.B. 20.). Back-Shu point of Pancreas

Tianshu (St. 25.).

Qimen (Liv. 14.).

Ganshu (U.B. 18.).

Distal points (select from):

Neiguan (P. 6.).

Zusanli (St. 36.).

Dannang (Ex. 35.).
Sanyinjiao (Sp. 6.).
Taichong (Liv. 3.).

SPLENOMEGALY:

Splenomegaly, or enlargement of the spleen, is a symptom of many diseases, but it is most commonly caused by malaria. An enlarged spleen may also be encountered in certain chronic infections, anaemia, blood disorders, and in cirrhosis of the liver.

Baihui (Du 20.).
Local points (select from):
Zhangmen (Liv. 13.).
Qimen (Liv. 14.).
Daimai (G.B. 26.).
Riyue (G.B. 24.).
Liangmen (St. 21.).
Pishu (U.B. 20.).
Distal points:
Sanyinjiao (Sp. 6.).
Yinlingquan (Sp. 9.).
Gongsun (Sp. 4.).
Zusanli (St. 36.).

As malaria and Bilharzia were common disorders in ancient China, the traditional physician was familiar with gross enlargements of the spleen.

■

GENITOURINARY DISORDERS

Principles of treatment

Local and Adjacent points along with Distal points are used in treating these disorders.

The Local points are selected principally from the Urinary Bladder, Ren and Du channels, as they run anatomically in close proximity to or traverse the genitourinary system.

The Distal points are usually chosen from the Stomach, Spleen, Kidney and Urinary Bladder Channels, as they too overlie the lower abdominal area.

According to traditional Chinese medicine, disorders of the genitourinary system are most likely to arise from the lack of balance of vital energy in the above Channels. These Channels are in Yin-Yang pairs, having an interior-exterior relationship with each other:

Yin	*Yang*
Ren	Du
Spleen	Stomach
Kidney	Urinary Bladder

The imbalance responsible for these disorders can be corrected by the proper selection of points in the Yin and Yang Channels. In other words, the action of acupuncture in these disorders is primarily homeostatic, even from the point of view of traditional medicine.

Modern research has also shown that it is the balancing of mechanisms like tubular secretion—re-absorption and contraction – relaxation of smooth muscle in the ureters, bladder and sphincters that are most favourably influenced by acupuncture in this group of disorders. (Recent work by Simon Strauss at Monash University, Australia, has demonstrated this normalizing effect in animal experiments).

The Organ and Channel central to, and most directly concerned with the genitourinary system is the Kidney. The traditional Chinese concept of the Kidney meant not only the anatomy and the functions of the kidneys themselves, but also included the adrenal glands (hence the emotion fear being associated with the Kidney), as well as the testes, the ovaries and genital functions.

In genitourinary disorders, before acupuncture treatment, a full investigation is carried out to eliminate neoplastic disorders, mechanical obstructions, renal calculi and, other similar conditions which contraindicate the use of acupuncture.

NEPHRITIS, PYELITIS, PYELONEPHRITIS

Nephritis, or inflammation of the kidneys, may be associated with bacterial infection. Where an infection reaches the kidneys from the bladder via the ureter, the pelvis of the kidney becomes inflammed first and this is known as pyelitis; if the infection then spreads to the kidney tissue it is termed pyelonephritis.

Acute nephritis may take the form of glomerulo-nephritis or anaphylactoid purpura, which are both usually associated with haemolytic streptococci. These conditions often follow a sore throat. After the patient recovers from the sore throat, the following symptoms may appear: Headache, backache, swelling of face and legs and hematuria (blood in urine) with progressive reduction in the output of urine. There may be nausea and vomiting. In anaphylactoid purpura a rash occurs in the skin. There will be protein in the urine, and the blood pressure may rise. It is not the infection from the streptococci, itself, that is thought to result in this condition, but rather that the antibodies formed to destroy the invading streptococci cause an allergic reaction that also damages the kidneys. These factors have to be borne in mind in selecting points for acupuncture.

The causes of chronic nephritis are not precisely known, except perhaps that sometimes, it may develop following an acute nephritis. This condition, which is also called "nephrotic syndrome" is characterized by heavy loss of protein in the urine, edema, and frequently high blood pressure.

Baihui (Du 20.).

Local points (select from):

Shenshu (U.B. 23.).
Dachangshu (U.B. 25.).
Daimai (G.B. 26.).
Mingmen (Du 4.).
Yaoyangguan (Du. 3.).
Guanyuan (Ren 4.).
Zhongji (Ren 3.).

Distal points:

Sanyinjiao (Sp. 6.).
Taixi (K. 3.).

Specific points for infection:

Dazhui (Du 14.).
Quchi (L.I. 11.).

Specific point for allergy:

Xuehai (Sp. 10.).

Specific points for edema:

Shuifen (Ren 6.).
Shimen (Ren 5.).
Pishu (U.B. 20.).
Yinlingquan (Sp. 9.).

HEMATURIA, OLIGURIA ANURIA

Hematuria, or blood in the urine, could be a symptom of kidney or urinary bladder disorder or injury. Blood from the kidney is brownish, while blood from the bladder is reddish. Although this condition may sometimes not have serious significance, it requires early investigation to discover the site of bleeding, as hematuria may occur with calculi or neoplasms of the genitourinary systems as well.

Anuria, or the non-production of urine, is an indication of kidney failure, low pressure in the renal arteries, or more commonly, obstruction of the ureters is the cause.

Baihui (Du 20.).

Local points (select from):

Shenshu (U.B. 23.).

Mingmen (Du 4.).

Yaoyangguan (Du 3.).

Dachangshu (U.B. 25.).

Ciliao (U.B. 32.).

Pangguanshu (U.B. 28.).

Zhibian (U.B. 54.).

Zhongli (Ren 3.).

Guanyuan (Ren 4.)

Qihai (Ren 6.).

Distal points:

Zusanli (St. 36.).

Weizhong (U.B. 40.).

Sanyinjiao (Sp. 6.).

Taixi (K. 3.).

Influential point for the vascular system

Taiyuan (Lu. 9.).

RENAL COLIC

This refers to the spasm of the ureter, often due to a stone (calculus). There is sudden pain in the loin radiating to the groin, and often to the external genitalia. The pain becomes very intense in a few minutes and usually subsides within about two hours but may continue much longer. Sweating and vomiting may occur.

Strong manual stimulation should be administered at:

Hegu (L.I. 4.). and/or

Shuiquan (K. 5.)-Xi-Cleft point of the Kidney Channel, and often dramatic relief from pain is obtained.

After the pain is relieved, the needles should be inserted at the following points:

Baihui (du 20.).

Local points (select from):

Shenshu (U.B. 23.).

Yaoyangguan (Du. 3.).

Dachangshu (U.B. 25.).

Pangguanshu (U.B. 28.).

Ciliao (U.B. 32.).

Zhibian (U.B. 54.).

Distal points:

Zusanli (St. 36.).

Sanyinjiao (Sp. 6.).

Weizhong (U.B. 40.).

Taixi (K. 3.).

Specific point for vomiting:

Neiguan (P. 6.).

The treatment may be repeated daily for a few days, and also at the time of any acute exacerbations. Where indicated, surgical intervention should be undertaken early.

CYSTITIS, URETHRITIS

Cystitis, or inflammation of the urinary bladder, is usually caused by bacterial infection. It is more often found among women, particularly during pregnancy or associated gynecological disorders such as prolapse of the uterus, Recurrent cystitis is often due to stones or crystalline deposits in the urine, but may also be due to a neoplasm.

Frequent and painful micturition which may be foul smelling, cloudy, and occasionally containing blood (hematuria) may occur. There may be fever and excessive sweating due to the infection.

Urethritis, or inflammation of the urethra, is commonly seen as a result of gonorrhoea, but it is also not infrequently caused by catheters left in *situ* over a long time. The treatment is the use of specific antibiotics. Acupuncture may be used for symptomatic relief.

Baihui (Du 20.).

Local points (select from):

Zhongji (Ren 3.).

Guanyuan (Ren 4.).

Ciliao (U.B. 32.).

Distal points (select from):

Sanyinjiao (Sp. 6.).

Yinlingquan (Sp. 9.).

Zusanli (St. 36.).

Weizhong (U.B. 40).

Specific points for infection:

Dazhui (Du 14.).

Quchi (L.I. 11.)

RETENTION OF URINE

In this disorder, accumulation of urine in the bladder occurs and there is an inability to pass it easily, even when the bladder is fully distended. It may be caused by obstructions such as a calculus, prostatic enlargement, or inflammation of the urethra. It may also be due to the interference of the nerve supply of the bladder, such as a fractured spine. Occasionally, psychological factors may be the cause. The proper therapy is to remove any mechanical cause of obstruction surgically. Acupuncture may help in obtaining symptomatic relief.

Baihui (Du 20.).

Local points (select from):

Zhongji (Ren 3.).

Guanyuan (Ren. 4.).

Ciliao (U.B. 32.).

Pangguanshu (U.B) 28.).

Yaoyangguang (Du. 3.).

Distal points:

Sanyinjiao (Sp. 6.).

Yinlingquan (Sp. 9.).

Zusanli (St. 36.).

Weizhong (U.B. 40.).

ENURESIS, NOCTURNAL ENURESIS, (BED WETTING):

Enuresis or urinary incontinence occurs due to an inability to control the sphincters of the bladder. It may be due to such causes as diabetes mellitus, kidney disorder, or paralytic disorders. Its commonest form, however, is bed wetting of children in which, sometimes, psychological causes may be found.

Baihui (Du. 20.).

Local points (select from):

Shenshu (U.B. 23.).

Ciliao (U.B. 32.).

Pangguanshu (U.B. 28.).

Zhongli (Ren 3.).

Guanyuan (Ren 4.).

Qihai (Ren 6.).

Distal points:

Zusanli (St. 36.).

Weizhong (U.B. 40.).

Sanyinjiao (Sp. 6.).

Taixi (K. 3.).

If psychological factors are present, add:

Shenmen (H. 7.).

Shenmai (U.B. 62.).

Nocturnal enuresis in children responds remarkably well to acupuncture. Points in front of the body are used in the first course of treatment; points in the back are used in the second course. We have had uniform success in all cases of bed wetting treated by us with acupuncture.[1]

However, it is essential to ensure that a neurological deficit such as a spina bifida is not present. Some Chinese authorities believe that moxa on the needle at Ciliao (U.B. 32.). is very helpful in curing idiopathic nocturnal enuresis. The needle has to be precisely inserted into the second posterior sacral foramen, and this requires some degree of experience.

■

1 In the idiopathic cases

DISORDERS OF WOMEN

Acupuncture can be usefully applied in a wide range of gynecological and obstetric disorders, as well as during normal childbirth.

Principles of treatment

Points on the Ren Channel are those most commonly used in these disorders. According to traditional Chinese medicine, the Ren Channel is believed to govern the reproductive functions (for which reason this Channel is also called the "Conception Vessel").

Points on the Stomach, Spleen, Urinary Bladder and Kidney Channels are also used as they traverse the area of the genitals.

Before attempting to treat gynecological disorders with acupuncture, however, it is important that a competent gynecologist rules out the presence of malignant or other neoplastic disorders.

A. GYNECOLOGICAL DISORDERS

AMENORRHEA, OLIGOMENORRHEA, IRREGULAR MENSTRUATION:

Amenorrhea means the absence of menstrual periods. Primary amenorrhea refers to the condition where menstruation has not begun, although the girl has reached or passed the age when it should have commenced. It may be an indication of a systematic disorder or of hormonal imbalance. Secondary amenorrhea refers to the condition where a woman of childbearing age, who previously had periods has now stopped having them. If this is not due to pregnancy or menopause it must be regarded as a symptom requiring further investigation, as it is a feature of a wide range of conditions. Common causes of this type of amenorrhea are anemia, debilitating diseases, hormonal imbalances, nervous strain and other emotional disorders. Since this is a symptom, it is necessary that the underlying condition be elicited and treated.

Oligomenorrhea is a form of amenorrhea where there is only an occasional or scanty flow.

The term irregular menstruation is used to describe cases where the periods occur, but in an abnormal manner, e.g., irregularlity of the menstrual cycle, excessive or scanty, prolonged or brief bleeding, or the blood being too dark or clots being formed.

The following points may be used, in addition to any points indicated by the presence of other symptoms:

Baihui (Du 20.).

Local points:

Qihai (Ren 6.).

Guanyuan (Ren 4.).

Shenshu (U.B. 23.).

Guilai (St. 29.).

Ciliao (U.B. 32.).

Distal points:

Sanyinjiao (Sp. 6.).

Zusanli (St. 36.).

Taixi (K. 3.).

DYSMENORRHEA

This refers to excessive pain during the periods. It is felt mainly in the pelvic area, lower abdomen and lower back. Primary dysmenorrhea, which is the more common type, affects girls from the first period or soon after. Neither the cause nor the source of the pain is known and there is no observable pelvic lesion. However, it is likely that there may be an imbalance of the sex hormones in such cases.

Secondary or symptomatic dysmenorrhea occurs in women who have previously had normal periods; it may be caused by a variety of gynecological disorders. The cause of the pain has, therefore, to be first identified and sourced.

Baihui (Du 20.).

Local points:

Qihai (Ren 6.).

Guanyuan (Ren 4.).

Zhongji (Ren 3.).

Zhongwan (Ren 12.).

Ciliao (U.B. 32.).

Distal points:

Sanyinjiao (Sp. 6.).

Zusanli (St. 36.).

Specific points for pain:

Hegu (L.I. 4.).

Neiting (St. 44.).

Specific points for nausea and vomiting:

Neiguan (P. 6.).

Zusanli (St. 36.).

For best results, the acupuncture treatment should be given about a week prior to the commencement of the menstruation. Three or four such monthly treatments usually suffice. Moxibustion may be helpful.

MENORRHAGIA; FUNCTIONAL UTERINE BLEEDING

Menorrhagia or excessive loss of blood during the monthly periods is frequently due to local disorders, such as fibroids. It may also, not uncommonly, be brought on by anxiety and other emotional factors. In severe cases, or if prolonged, it may cause anaemia. It is usually found in women over the age of forty. The possibility of a neoplasm must be excluded. The following points may be used:

Baihui (Du. 20.).

Local points:

Qihai (Ren 6.).

Zhongji (Ren 3.).

Distal points:

Sanyinjiao (Sp. 6.).

Taixi (K. 3.).

Specific point:

Taiyuan (Lu. 9.).

LEUCORRHEA:

This is an excessive discharge of a white or colourless secretion from the vagina. It is a symptom of irritation caused by infections such as candida or trichomonas. Today, there are specific pharmaceutical remedies available for these infections. If they fail, acupuncture may be tried.

Baihui (Du 20.).

Local points:

Daimai (G.B. 26.).

Qugu (Ren 2.).

Shimen (Ren 5.).

Distal points:

Sanyinjiao (Sp. 6.).

Quchi (L.I. 11.).

Zusanli (St. 36.).

SALPINGITIS, ADNEXITIS, CERVICITIS, VAGINITIS AND OTHER PELVIC INFLAMMATIONS

Acute or chronic inflammation of the Fallopian tubes (salpingitis), inflammation of the structures in close proximity to the Fallopian tubes, e.g., ovaries (adnexitis uteri), inflammation of the neck of the womb (cervicitis), inflammation of the vagina (vaginitis) are all the result of infection, usually by bacteria which usually spreads upwards from the vagina.

Prompt treatment with antibiotics is very effective. Acupuncture may however be usefully combined with drug therapy in resistant cases or where the patient is intolerant to drug therapy.

Baihui (Du 20.).

Local points:

Guanyuan (Ren 4.).
Guilai (St. 29.).
Ciliao (U.B. 32.).
Shangliao (U.B. 31.).
Zhongliao (U.B. 33.).
Xialiao (U.B. 34.).

Distal points:

Sanyinjiao (Sp. 6.).
Dazhui (Du 14.).
Quchi (L.I. 11.).
Hegu (L.I. 4.).
Zusanli (St. 36.).

Points according to symptoms:

Shenshu (U.B. 23.)- for low backache.
Daimai (G.B. 26.)- for leucorrhea.

UTEROVAGINAL PROLAPSE

In this condition, the vagina and also the uterus prolapses through the vaginal orifice. It is a common disorder of elderly women due to the weakening of the supporting ligaments and pelvic muscles by frequent pregnancies, chronic cough, or other precipitating causes. Since this is basically a mechanical disorder, relief can be obtained with surgery or a pessary.

Acupuncture, however, can be helpful in many cases of first degree and early second degree prolapse by improving the tone of the supporting pelvic musculature and ligaments. In cases of third degree prolapse, it may not be possible to produce improvement, although the symptoms may be alleviated. In treating cases of prolapse, local infection and erosion must be attended to at the same time.

Baihui (Du 20.).

Local points (select from):

Qihai (Ren 6.).

Weibao (Ex. 15.).

Ciliao (U.B. 32.).

Xialiao (U.B. 34.).

Huiyin (Ren 1.).

Changqiang (Du 1.).

Shangliao (U.B. 31.).

Zhongliao (U.B. 33.).

Distal points:

Sanyinjiao (Sp. 6.).

Zusanli (St. 36.).

Influential point for muscle and tendon:

Yanglingquan (G.B. 34.).

We have carried out vaginal hysterectomy in 641 cases using these points for acupuncture anesthesia. There were 34 failures. In 351 cases adjuvant drugs, such as pethidine (50mg. I.V.) and nitrous oxide were used. The patients were unselected.

PRURITUS VULVAE

Pruritus or itching of the vulva frequently accompanies neurodermatitis. It may also be due to local causes, e.g., worm infestation, vaginitis, and it may arise as a complication of the menopause.

Baihui (Du 20.).

Local points:

Huiyin (Ren 1.).

Changqiang (Du 1.).

Distal points:

Sanyinjiao (Sp. 6.).

Xuehai (Sp. 10.).

Dushu (U.B. 16.).

Quchi (L.I. 11.).

Xinjian (Liv. 2.).

PAIN OF SECONDARY CARCINOMA OF THE CERVIX, UTERUS AND OVARIES:

Acupuncture is particularly useful in relieving the pain of secondary carcinoma of the cervix and other pelvic structures, where surgery and radiation therapy have failed.

The plan of therapy is as follows:

i) Baihui (Du 20.).

ii) Hegu (L.I. 4.) is punctured and manually stimulated very strongly, till most of the pain disappears.

iii) *Ah-Shi* points of the body are located and needled.

iv) Points of the low back such as Shenshu (U.B. 23.). Yaoyangguan (Du. 3.), Dachangshu (U.B. 25.), are needled together with the relevant Distal points like Weizhong (U.B. 40). Electrical pulse stimulation of the dense-disperse pattern is applied at these proximal and Distal points.

A remarkable relief of pain is seen with this therapy.

Embedding needles are applied at the *Ah-Shi* points between treatments.

B. OBSTETRIC DISORDERS

HYPEREMESIS[1]

This term describes the excessive vomiting in pregnancy which may occur in the first trimester. The cause is not known, but psychological factors are probably involved. In very severe cases, the pregnancy may have to be artificially terminated.

Although acupuncture is generally contraindicated in pregnancy owing to the risk of abortion, it may be used with advantage in cases of hyperemesis as it is less damaging to the fetus than drugs.

The points used are:

Neiguan (P. 6.).

Zusanli (St. 36.).

and other Homeostatic points.

Treatment should be given until the symptoms subside. If the symptoms are severe, the patient may the treated two or three times a day.

MALPOSITION OF THE FETUS

The correction of malposition or malpresentation of the fetus in the pelvis is a historical procedure in traditional Chinese medicine.

The commonly used point is Zhiyin (U.B. 67.). Moxibustion was the preferred technique. Alternately, heat was applied with moxa at the head of the acupuncture needle ("moxa on needle").

The procedure has to the repeated daily until the fetal position is corrected. Recent research in China has confirmed that, in fact, correction occurs in a number of cases.

1 Morning sickness responds well to bleeding at Jinjin and Yuye (Ex. 10.). See also Auriculotherapy.

This condition may be caused by many factors. Causes such as contracted pelvis, tumours of the pelvis and congenital abnormalities of the uterus should be managed by other measures.

RELIEF OF PAIN DURING DELIVERY

Acupuncture may be used during childbirth to relieve the pains of delivery. It may also be used in the other events that may occur during delivery such as delayed labour, episiotomy, suturing of the perineum after delivery, caesarean section and the manual removal of the placenta.

The use of acupuncture in the above procedures has distinct advantages. Among them are a less exhausted mother, a better chance of survival for the baby as it is not exposed to narcotics and other drugs during delivery, and a shortened delivery time.

The point to be used at the commencement of labour are:

Baihui (Du 20.).
Hegu (L.I. 4.) with manual stimulation.
Neima (U.Ex.). } with electrical stimulation.
Sanyinjiao (Sp. 6.). }

The needles are placed at the left side only, to allow for the accoucheur to work on the right side of the patient.

If there is delay in the second stage of labour, acupuncture may be used to hasten the delivery by inducing and strengthening the uterine contractions. The points used are:

Hegu (L.I. 4.).
Sanyinjiao (Sp. 6.).
Taichong (Liv. 3.).
Ciliao (U.B. 32.).
Yanglingquan (G.B. 34.).

A large series of deliveries of mothers is being carried out in Sri Lanka using the above procedures. (Cf. "*A Report on Cases of Painless Childbirth with Acupuncture*" –Paper read at the Fifth World Congress of Acupuncture, Tokyo, 1977, by Wilfred S. Perera, F. R. C. S. (Eng.), F. R. C. S. (Edin.), F. R. C. O. G. (Gt. Brit.). Fellow, Sri Lanka Acupuncture Foundation).

AGALACTIA (LACTATION DEFICIENCY)

Inadequate milk supply may be due to almost any kind of ill health after childbirth. The common causes are a sore or cracked nipple, incorrect method of breast feeding, emotional stress, loss of appetite, or insufficient nutrition.

Local point:

Shanzhong (Ren 17.) with the needle directed towards the affected breast-towards Rugen (St. 18.) or Jiquan (H. 1.).

Distal points:

Neiguan (P. 6.).

Hegu (L.I. 4.).

Sanyinjiao (Sp. 6.).

Foot-Linqi (G.B. 41.).

MASTITIS:

Acute mastitis or inflammation of the breast is commonly found in the period just after birth of the baby, in association with a cracked nipple with a super added infection. Symptoms are breast pain and fever, with the affected nipple becoming red and tender. If the fever continues for more than 48 hours, the affected breast swells with the enlargement of the axillary lymph nodes.

Chronic mastitis sometimes occurs when an acute infection of the breast has failed to resolve completely.

Local points:

Shanzhong (Ren 17.) - horizontal insertion, laterally[2]

2 In the direction of the affected breast.

Rugen (St. 18.).

Distal points:

Shaoze (S.I. 1.).

Neiguan (P. 6.).

Taicong (Liv. 3.).

Foot-Linqi (G.B. 41.).

For infection, add:

Dazhui (Du 14.).

Quchi (L.I. 11.).

Sanyinjiao (Sp. 6.).

■

LOCOMOTOR DISORDERS—DISEASES OF SOFT TISSUES, MUSCLES, BONES AND JOINTS

These are the commonest disorders seen in acupuncture practice. It includes muscular and ligamentous sprains and strains, different types of arthritis, spondylosis, spondylitis, and soft tissue lesions like bursitis, tenosynovitis, fibrositis and myositis. These disorders can be mild and self-limiting in their course, or they may become chronic and give rise to progressive degenerative changes. Generally, they are characterized by limitation of movement and the presence of pain which may be acute, subacute or chronic.

The pain is the symptom which bothers the patient most. Mild cases may be relieved within a short period with or without treatment, but the mangement of subacute and chronic cases is often unsatisfactory with heat, exercise, massage, manipulation and other methods of physical medicine. Treatment with prolonged drug therapy may be equally unsatisfactory due to the not infrequent accompaniment of side-effects, and it is doubtful whether these particular drugs have any favourable effect at all on the long term prognosis of the rheumatic group of disorders. However, one frequently finds patients who have been continuously on drugs for many years due to the want of a better alternative.

On the other hand, it has been established on the basis of 'double blind' and other controlled trials that acupuncture is effective to a very large extent in managing these disorders. Our own experience confirms this, and it is acupuncture that has the highest patient acceptance in preference to all other methods of treatment wherever acupuncture is available as an alternative medicine in these diseases.[1]

We believe that acupuncture should not be used as the last line of defence, but as the first line of attack in this group of disorders. By using it at the early stages of the disease it is possible to prevent the many crippling deformities that often develop in these cases. For relieving pain, without causing side-effects, acupuncture is the method *par excellence.* With the population of every country tending to become more geriatric, the treatment of these disorders with acupuncture will become increasingly important in the future, especially in the context of the surging cost of orthodox medical care and the escalation of drug costs.

Principles of treatment

In the treatment of this group of disorders the method best recommended is the use of Local and Adjacent points along with relevant, Distal points. *Ah-shi* points should be detected and needled. The analgesic points Hegu (L.I. 4.). and/or Neiting (St. 44.) are used to alleviate pain. The chief homeostatic point Quchi (L.I. 11.) may be used with Zusanli (St. 36.) and Sanyinjiao (Sp. 6.) which also possess strong homeostatic properties. Likewise, the main sedative points Shenmen (H. 7.) and Shenmai (U.B. 62.) would generally be indicated. Baihui (Du 20.), an important sedative point itself, is usually used in nearly every case as the governing point.

In the following description we have enumerated some of the commonly seen locomotor disorders in regional order for convenience of study. The disorders which have been dealt with are merely some of the representative examples. The acupuncturist selects the points according to the symptomatology presented by the individual

1 The result of combining with homoeopathy as homoeopuncture are overwhelming.

case and varies the therapy, if need be, depending on the response, or the lack of it.

Where bone and cartilage degeneration has occurred, the relevent Influential point, Dashu (U.B. 11.), is used. The point Yanglingquan (G.B. 34.), the Influential point for muscle and tendon, is always used in cases of paralysis, wasting of muscle, and tendon disorders.

A. THE HEAD

Temporo-mandibular Arthritis:

Baihui (Du 20.).

Local points:

Ah-Shi points.

Xiaguan (St. 7.).

Tinghui (G.B. 2.).

Distal points:

Hegu (L.I. 4.).

Waiguan (S.J. 5.).

B. THE NECK

Pain and Stiffness, Torticollis, Cervical Sprain, Cervical Spondylosis, Rheumatoid Arthritis of Cervical Spine:

Baihui (Du 20.).

Local points:

Ah-Shi points

Fengchi (G.B. 20.).

Dazhui (Du 14.).

Huatuojiaji points (Ex. 21.) of the neck area.

Distal points:

Lieque (Lu. 7.).

Xuanzhong (G.B. 39.).

Influential point for bone and cartilage:

Dashu (U.B. 11.).

In cases of very painful and acute stiff neck with difficulty of lateral rotation and flexion, strong manual stimulation should be carried out at Yanglao (S.I. 6.) or Houxi (S.I. 3.). As the latter point is very painful, it is used only in very acute cases.

C. THE CHEST

a) Pain in Dorsal Region, Intercostal Neuralgia, Traumatic chest Pain:

Baihui (Du 20.).

Local points:

Ah-Shi points.

Huatuojiaji points (Ex. 21.) of the dorsal area.

U.B. Channel points of the affected area.

Distal points:

Sanyangluo (S.J. 8.).

Hegu (L.I. 4.).

b) Sprain of Pectoral Muscles:

Baihui (Du 20.).

Local points (select from):

Zhongfu (Lu. 1.).

Rugen (St. 18.).

Qimen (Liv. 14.).

Riyue (G.B. 24.).

Ah-Shi points.

Distal points:

Hegu (L.I. 4.).

Neiguan (P. 6.).

Influential point for muscle and tendon:

Yanglingquan (G.B. 34.).

D. THE BACK OF THE TRUNK

Backache:

In treating backache, it is best to commence therapy with a few points.

Baihui (Du. 20.).

Local points:

Ah-Shi points.

Distal points:

Weizhong (U.B. 40.).

Kunlun (U.B. 60.).

Analgesic point:

Hegu (L.I. 4.).

If degenerative changes in the spine are present:

Deshu (U. B. 11)

Having evaluated the response to the first one or two sittings, further points may be added, if necessary.

a) **Backache in the Dorsal Region:**

Baihui (Du 20.).

Local point:

Ah-Shi points.

Du and U.B. Channel points of the affected area.

Distal points:

Weizhong (U.B. 40.).

Kunlun (U.B. 60.).

Sanyangluo (S.I. 8.).

Yanglao (S.I. 6.).

Analgesic point:

Hegu (L.I. 4.).

b) **Low Backache (Prolapsed disc, with or without sciatica):**

Baihui (Du 20.).

Local points (select from):

Ah-Shi points.

Mingmen (Du 4.).

Yaoyangguan (Du 3.).

Dachangshu (U.B. 25.).

Huatuojiaji points (Ex. 21.), of the region

Ciliao (U.B. 32.).

Zhibian (U.B. 54.).

Distal points (select from):

Weizhong (U.B. 40).

Kunlun (U.B. 60).

Chengshan (U.B. 57.).

Chengfu (U.B. 36.).

Yinmen (U.B. 37.).

Yanglingquan (G.B. 34.).

Taixi (K. 3.).

Sanyinjiao (Sp. 6.).

Of the Distal points, one or two may be selected at each sitting. However, the first two mentioned are those which are most commonly used.

In acute sciatica, Huantiao (G.B. 30.) with stimulation to produce *deqi* is very helpful in relieving pain.

In very acute low backache, Renzhong (Du 26.) may be used to relieve the pain.

c) **Ankylosing Spondylitis:**

Baihui (Du 20.).

Local points:

Ah-Shi points:

Du and U.B. Channel points } in the
Huatuojiaji (Ex. 21.) points } affected region.

Distal points:

Sanyangluo (S.I. 8.).

Weizhong (U.B. 40.).

Kunlun (U.B. 60.)

E. THE LIMBS

Following are the points commonly used in disorders affecting the joints of limbs:

a) **Shoulder:**

Baihui (Du 20.).

Local points:

Jianyu (L.I. 15.).

Jianliao (S.J. 14.).

Jianzhen (S.I. 9.).

Ah-Shi points.

Distal point and analgesic point:

Hegu (L.I. 4.).

At the first sitting, the use of Tiaokou (St. 38.) with fairly strong stimulation is helpful in mobilizing the shoulder. In about 70-80% of cases significant improvement is obtained immediately. (Cf. "*The Use of the Point Tiaokou (St. 38.) in Frozen Shoulder*" BY Pothmann, Stux and Weigel. Dusseldorf, 1979.).

b) **Elbow:**

Baihui (Du 20.).

Local points:

Ah-Shi points.

Chize (Lu. 5.).

Quze (P. 3.).

Shaohai (H. 3.).

Quchi (L.I. 11.).

Distal point and analgesic point:

Hegu (L.I. 4.).

c) **Wrist:**

Baihui (Du 20.).

Local points:

Ah-Shi points.

Daling (P. 7.).

Shenmen (H. 7.).

Taiyuan (Lu. 9.).

Analgesic points:

Hegu (L.I. 4.) of opposite side, and/or

Neiting (St. 44.).

d) **Palms, Carpal Joints:**

Baihui (Du 20.).

Local points:

Ah-Shi points:

Yuji (Lu. 10.).

Laogong (P. 8.).

Shaofu (H. 8.).

Analgesic points:

Hegu (L.I. 4.) of the opposite side, and/or

Neiting (St. 44.).

e) **Sacroiliac Joints:**

Baihui (Du 20.).

Local points:

Ah-Shi points.

Tunzhang (U. Ex.).

Ciliao (U.B. 32.).

Distal points:

Weizhong (U.B. 40.).

Kunlun (U.B. 60.).

Analgesic point:

Hegu (L.I. 4.).

f) **Knee:**

Baihui (Du 20.).

Local points:

Ah-Shi points.

Heding (Ex. 31.).

Xiyan (Ex. 32.).

Dubi (St. 35.).

Weizhong (U.B. 40.).

Distal points:

Neiting (St. 44.).

Kunlun (U.B. 60.).

Analgesic point:

Hegu (L.I. 4.).

Specific point for effusion:

Yinlingquan (Sp. 9.).

Influential point for bone and cartilage:

Dashu (U.B. 11.).

g) **Ankle:**

Baihui (Du 20.).

Local points:

Ah-Shi points.

Kunlun (U.B. 60.).

Taixi (K. 3.).

Zhaohai (K. 6.).

Jiexi (St. 41.).

Qiuxu (G.B. 40.).

Analgesic point:

Hegu (L.I. 4.).

Specific point for swelling:

Yinlingquan (Sp. 9.).

Influential point for bone and cartilage:

Dashu (U.B. 11.).

h) **Foot:**

Dorsum of Foot:

Baihui (Du 20.).

Local points:

Ah-Shi points.

Neiting (St. 44.).

Analgesic point:

Hegu (L.I. 4.).

Sole of Foot:

Baihui (Du 20.).

Local points:

Ah-Shi points

Taixi (K. 3.).

Yongquan (K. 1.).

Analgesic point:

Hegu (L.I. 4.).

I) **Joints of Toes:**

Baihui (Du 20.).

Local points:

Ah-Shi points.

Bafeng (Ex. 36.).

Analgesic point:

Hegu (L.I. 4.).

Some common locomotor disorders affecting the limbs are now discussed:

1) Frozen Shoulder (Capsulitis, Periarthritis):

In this condition, which is commonly found in middle-aged

people, there is pain and limitation of movements at the shoulder joint, often lasting several months.

This condition is often refractory to treatment in diabetic persons and concomitant treatment of the latter disease is indicated. Hypertension may be present in some cases.

The point Tiaokou (St. 38.) should be needled before inserting any other needles, in cases where there is much shoulder immobility. When strong manual stimulation is applied at this point there is often a dramatic increase in the range of movements. The patient should be asked to exercise the shoulder while this manoeuvre is being perfomed.

Baihui (Du 20.).

Local points (select from):

Ah-Shi points.

Jianyu (L.I. 15.).

Jianliao (S.J. 14.).

Jianzhen (S.I. 9.).

Fengchi (G.B. 20.).

Jianquan (U. Ex.).

Jian-Nie-Lin (U. Ex.).

Taner (U. Ex.).

(The first three points are the more commonly used.)

Distal point:

Hegu (L.I. 4.).

Yanglingquan (G.B. 34.) may be added.

2) Tennis Elbow (Lateral Epicondylitis):

This is characterized by pain and stiffness in the extensor muscles of the forearm. It is often met with in tennis players, housewives and in workers who carry heavy loads. There is also pain at the elbow on extension of the wrist and on gripping an object.

Baihui (Du 20.).

Local points:

Ah-Shi points.

Quchi (L.I. 11.).

Shousanli (L.I. 10.).

Distal point:

Hegu (L.I. 4.).

Influential point for muscle and tendon:

Yanglingquan (G.B. 34.).

Manipulation may be very useful.

(In golfer's elbow, points on the medial aspect of the elbow are used).

3) **Stenosing Tenosynovitis at the Radial styloid Process (De Quervain's Disease):**

This condition is indicated by pain just above the wrist and weakness of thumb movements. It is commonly found in middle-aged women who do hard work involving alternate pronation and supination of the forearm, such as washing and wringing clothes.

Baihui (Du 20.).

Local points:

Ah-Shi points.

Lieque (Lu. 7.).[1]

Yangxi (L.I. 5.).

Distal point:

Hegu (L.I. 4.).

Influential point for muscle and tendon:

Yanglingquan (G.B. 34.).

4) **Ganglion of the Wrist:**

This is a cystic mass which appears on the dorsum of the wrist. It is filled with a gelatinous degenerative material.

---

1 Moxa on the needle is very effective.

The best treatment is hot needling. Often with one needling, the condition is resolved when the gummy material escapes.

5) **Median Carpal Compression ("Carpal Tunnel Syndrome"):**

This is caused by compression as the median nerve passes under the flexor retinaculum and results in pain, numbness and tingling in the area of the distribution of this nerve in the hand. It is met most often in middle-aged women, especially during pregnancy.

Drug treatment is often disappointing in these cases. Surgical relief may have to be obtained by dividing the flexor retinaculum. Before deciding on such measures, however, acupuncture should be given a fair trial if there are no objective neurological signs, as it has often been found to be effective. Acupuncture probably acts by reducing the soft tissue inflammation which causes the compression.

Baihui (Du 20.).

Local points:

Ah-Shi points.

Taiyuan (Lu. 9.).

Daling (P. 7.).

Shenmen (H. 7.).

Yuji (Lu. 10.).

Laogong (P. 8.).

Shaofu (H. 8.).

Analgesic points:

Hegu (L.I. 4.) of the opposite side, or

Neiting (St. 44.).

Specific point for swelling:

Yinlingquan (Sp. 9.).

If there are advanced neurological signs, like wasting of the thenar muscles, acupuncture should not be tried. Surgery should then be carried out as soon as possible[2].

2 When in doubt, electroniyography will decide the issue.

6) Dupuytren's Contracture:

This is a disorder caused by the fibrosis of the palmar fascia, with consequent inability to extend the fingers. The condition is most often found among elderly men and is usually progressive.

We have successfully employed acupuncture in a number of cases of early contracture. Acupuncture seems to arrest the process if treatment is commenced early.

Baihui (Du 20.).

Local points:

Ah-Shi points.

Yuji (Lu. 10.).

Laogong (P. 8.).

Shaofu (H. 8.).

7) Interphalangeal Disorders (Rheumatoid Arthritis):

This is often due to rheumatoid arthritis, or Herberden's nodes.

Baihui (Du 20.).

Local points:

Ah-Shi points.

Baxie (Ex. 28.).

Distal point:

Hegu (L.I. 4.).

8) Trigger Finger, Snap Thumb:

There is an inability to straighten the finger or thumb, once flexed. It can only be extended with some force. This is often accompained by a sharp snap. The condition is due to a thickening of the tendon, which prevents its gliding freely inside the synovial sheath.

Baihui (Du 20.).

Local points:

Trigger points.

Ah-Shi points.[3]

---

3 Needle horizontally along the tendon to disrupt the tendon sheath.

Distal point:

Hegu (L.I. 4.).

Influential point for muscle and tendon:

Yanglingquan (G.B. 34.).

As the cause of the triggering is mechanical, results may be disappointing with acupuncture.

9) Osteoarthritis of Hip and Traumatic Disorders of Hip:

Baihui (Du 20.).

Local points:

Ah-Shi points.

Huantiao (G.B. 30.).

Zhibian (U.B. 54.).

Ciliao (U.B. 32.).

Biguan (St. 31.).

Distal points:

Hegu (L.I. 4.).

Neiting (St. 44.).

This condition responds well to acupuncture.

10) Osteoarthritis and other Disorders of the Knee Joint:

The commonest disorder of the knee joint is osteoarthritis in elderly people. Traumatic arthritis and non-mechanical cartilage disorders also respond very well.

Baihui (Du 20.).

Local points:

Ah-Shi points.

Heding (Ex. 31.).

Medial-Xiyan (Ex. 32.).

Dubi (St. 35.).

Xuehai (Sp. 10.).

Liangqiu (St. 34.).

Weizhong (U.B. 40.).

(The first three are the commonly used points)

Distal and Analgesic points:

Hegu (L.I. 4.).

Neiting (St. 44.).

11) **Cramp in Calf Muscles:**

This occurs usually in vascular deficiencies, pregnancy, and in old people. It may also occur in people who are on high doses of diuretics.

Chengshan (U.B. 57.).

12) **Ankle Disorders:**

Acupuncture treatment will be found to be very useful in most disorders affecting the ankle, including sprains, strains and athletic injuries.

Baihui (Du 20.).

Local points:

Ah-Shi points.

Kunlun (U.B. 60.).

Taixi (K. 3.).

Shenmai (U.B. 62.).

Zhaohai (K. 6.).

Qiuxu (G.B. 40.).

Jiexi (St. 41.).

Shangqiu (Sp. 5.).

Analgesic points:

Neiting (St. 44.).

Hegu (L.I. 4.).

13) **Achilles Tendinitis:**

Baihui (Du 20.).

Local points:

Ah-Shi points.

Kunlun (U.B. 60.).

Taixi (K. 3.).

Analgesic points:

Neiting (St. 44.).

Hegu (L.I. 4.).

Influential point for muscle and tendon:

Yanglingquan (G.B. 34.).

14) **Metatarsalgia:**

Baihui (Du 20.).

Local points:

Ah-Shi points.

Points in the affected area.

Bafeng (Ex. 36.).

Analgesic points:

Neiting (St. 44.).

Hegu (L.I. 4.).

15) **Plantar Fasciitis:**

Baihui (Du 20.).

Local points:

Ah-Shi points.

Yongquan (K.I.).

Taixi (K. 3.).

Analgesic point:

Hegu (L.I. 4.).

■

SKIN DISORDERS

Principles of treatment

Most skin disorders respond well to acupuncture treatment[1].

Local points with reference to the lesion, together with points which possess specific properties are selected:

a) Points local and adjacent to the lesion. *The lesion itself is not generally needled, especially if it is ulcerated or excoriated.*

Lasertherapy may be used directly on the affected area.

b) Points of the Lung Channel (Lung is related to the skin), e.g., Chize (Lu. 5.). Bleeding at this point.

c) Points of the Kidney Channel (Kidney is related to head hair).

d) The point Xuehai (Sp. 10.) for its specific anti-allergic properties.

e) The points Dazhui (Du. 14.) and Sanyinjiao (Sp. 6.) for their anti-infective and immune-enhancing properties.

f) The points Baihui (Du 20.) and Shenmen (H. 7.). for their special sedative effects.

---

1 Homoeopuncture is very useful in chronic skin disorders.

g) The point Quchi (L.I. 11.). for its powerful homeostatic effects.

h) For pruritus, strong stimulation of the points Dushu (U.B. 16.) and Xuehai (sp. 10.) are very effective.

i) Where the circulation is poor, Taiyuan (Lu. 9.), the Influential point for the vascular system, is used.

NON-HEALING WOUNDS AND CHRONIC ULCERS OF THE SKIN

These conditions are usually associated with a defective circulation due to varicose veins (which may not always be apparent) or atherosclerosis. Ulcers of this type are commonly found near the ankle. It often follows as injury, even a minor one, such as a scratch or an insect bite. Diabetes mellitus and associated disorders may be present.

Baihui (Du 20.).

Local points:

Points on the Channel or Channels traversing or nearest the ulcer, lying just proximal and/or distal to the lesion.

Points on the contralateral limb or side in the limb or side, in the area corresponding to the site of the lesion.

Taiyuan (Lu. 9.).

Lieque (Lu. 7.).

Specific points for infection:

Dazhui (Du. 14.).

Quchi (L.I. 11.).

Sanyinjiao (Sp. 6.).

FURUNCULOSIS (BOILS), ACNE (PIMPLES)

Furunculosis (collection of boils or furuncles) is caused by infection of the sweat glands or the hair follicles, usually with staphylococci.

Acne is a chronic skin disease affecting the sebaceous glands. These glands become excessively active due to hormonal or other imbalances and cause over-production of sebum, with resulting blocking of their openings. This results in the formation of a plug over a small abscess or pimple of partially dried fatty material. This material is liable to bacterial infection (most commonly Staphyloccus albus and Bacillus acnes). As this disorder is believed to be primarily caused by some imbalance in the body, anxiety and psychological disturbances may aggravate the condition. This disorder is quite common during the period of puberty.

Baihui (Du 20.).

Local points:

Points around the affected area.

Distal points:

Points distal to the affected area.

Hegu (L.I. 4.), if the face is affected.

Immune-enhanching points:

Dazhui (Du 14.).

Quchi (L.I. 11.).

Sanyinjiao (Sp. 6.).

Related Channel points:

Chize (Lu. 5.).

Lieque (Lu. 7.).

WARTS

Warts are a benign overgrowth of the outer layer of the skin. Often they disappear without treatment, but those on the sole of the foot are very painful and may become chronic.

Baihui (Du 20.).

Local points:

Points of the area affected e.g.,

Yongquan (K. 1.) for plantar warts.

Immune-enhancing and Homeostatic points:

Dazhui (Du 14.).

Quchi (L.I. 11.).

Sanyinjiao (Sp. 6.).

Xuehai (Sp. 10.).

Lieque (Lu. 7.). (Lung is related to skin).

As the point Yongquan (K. 1.) is painful, Taixi (K. 3.) may be needled instead, in the first few days of treatment.

URTICARIA (NETTLE RASH, HIVES), ANGIONEUROTIC EDEMA

Urticaria is an allergic reaction of the skin caused by sensitivity to various substances, mostly certain foods, and also to drugs such as aspirin, penicillin or streptomycin taken orally, applied externally, or administered by injection. Itchy weals develop very suddenly on the skin and heal after a few days, but may appear on another part of skin afterwards. The pruritus may be very severe.

Angioneurotic edema is a severe form of urticaria. The swelling becomes severe, affecting the skin of the face, hands or genitals with generalised anaphylactic reaction. The mucous membranes of the nasopharynx and the larynx may be affected causing serious respiratory obstruction and the patient may need urgent intensive care to maintain the potency of the airway.

Baihui (Du 20.)

Local points:

Points close to the site to the reaction.

Specific point for allergy:

Xuehai (Sp. 10.) with strong manual stimulation.

Homeostatic point:

Quchi (L.I. 11.).

Immune-enhancing points:

Dazhui (Du 14.).

Zusanli (St. 36.).

Sanyinjiao (Sp. 6.).

If the attack of urticaria is prolonged, add the following points:

Chize (Lu. 5.).-prick to bleed.

Weizhong (U.B. 40.).- prick to bleed.

Where the urticaria is caused by drug allergy, select from the following points for sedation of the patient:

Sishencong (Ex. 6.).

Shenmen (H. 7.).

Yinxi (H. 6.).

Neiguan (P. 6.).

Ximen (P. 4.). (Xi-Cleft point).

Xinshu (U.B. 15.).

Shenmai (U.B. 62.).

In severe urticaria, strong stimulation of the following specific points usually brings immediate relief:

Dushu (U.B. 16.).

Xuehai (Sp. 10.).

LYMPHANGITIS

Local wounds or other sources of sepsis may spread along the lymph vessels causing them to be inflammed. The regional lymph nodes are also then inflammed. This condition is called lymphangitis. There may be thin red lines in the skin spreading between the wound and the lymph gland.

Swelling of the limb or the affected part may occur. In infestations such as microfilaria, the process become chronic and may result in elephantiasis many years following repeated attacks of lymphangitis.

Baihui (Du 20.).

Local points:

Points along the Channel of the affected area.

Specific points for edema:

Shuifen (Ren 9.).

Shimen (Ren 5.).

Yinlingquan (Sp. 9.).

Pishu (U.B. 20.).

Immune-enhancing points:

Dazhui (Du 14.).

Quchi (L.I. 11.).

Sanyinjiao (Sp. 6.).

ERYSIPELAS

Erysipelas is an acute streptococcal infection of the skin in which there is a spreading inflammation of the skin and subcutaneous tissues. It is accompanied by high fever and sometimes produces severe complications such as pneumonia. Antibiotics usually control the infection. In patients who are intolerant of antibiotics, acupuncture may be used.

Baihui (Du 20.).

Local points:

Points adjacent to the site of the eruption.

For pruritus:

Dushu (U.B. 16.).

Xuehai (Sp. 10.).

Immune-enhancing points:

Dazhui (Du 14.).

Quchi (L.I. 11.).

Sanyinjiao (Sp. 6.).

Influential point for the vascular system:

Taiyuan (Lu. 9.).

Specific points for skin disorders:

Lieque (Lu. 9.).

Chize (Lu. 5.).-bleeding may be carried out.

HERPES ZOSTER (SHINGLES)

Herpes zoster is believed to be caused by the same or similar virus as that which causes chicken pox. At first, there is moderate fever with pain following the path of sensory nerve root originating from the spinal cord or the trigeminal nerve. Then a rash consisting of small vesicles appears along the same path. It usually occurs on the face, chest or abdomen. After a few days, the blisters become crusted and peel off. However, after the herpes attack has subsided there may be persistent severe neuralgic pain in the area supplied by the sensory nerve for months and even years. The pain is usually excrutiating.

Baihui (Du 20.).

Local points:

Ah-Shi points.

Points adjacent to the affected area.

Du Channel points

and

Huatuojiaji (Ex. 21.) points on the corresponding dermatome.

Distal points (select from):

Hegu (L.I. 4.).
Waiguan (S.J. 5.).
Sanyangluo (S.J. 8.).
Houxi (S.I. 3.).
Neiting (St. 44.).

} with strong manual stimulation or with electricity.

Acupuncture is perhaps the best known treatment in the management of this disorder.

ECZEMATOUS LESIONS (DERMATITIS)

This is a non-specific condition arising from the inflammation of the skin, primarily due to any infection, but usually as a result of an allergic reaction in sensitive subjects to substances such as certain foods, and to contact with certain chemicals either directly on the skin or by inhalation. It could also be precipitated by heat, cold, and sunlight. Emotional disturbances also play a part.

Initially a rash appears with severe itching. Then the skin breaks out in small vesicles which then rupture and an exudate forms ("weeping eczema"). At this stage the skin may become infected with bacteria. Pruritus and consequent scratching is liable to spread the infection. The skin may dry up and cracks may appear, or there may be formation of pustules. In the chronic stage, the skin is dry, flaky and may become thickened. The itching and burning sensation may however continue.

Baihui (Du 20.).

Local points:

Points adjacent to (but not within) the affected area.

Specific points:

Dazhui (Du 14.).
Quchi (L.I. 11.).
Lieque (Lu. 7.).
Xuehai (Sp. 10.).

Moderate stimulation at the point Dazhui (Du 14.) and at the other points is used, if the response is inadequate.

In the chronic stage use:

Hegu (L.I. 4.).

For pruritus use:

Dushu (U.B. 16.). } with strong
Xuehai (Sp. 10.). } stimulation.

LEUCODERMA (VITILIGO)

Idiopathic leucoderma is a condition of depigmentation of the skin, occurring in patches or bands. The cause is usually unknown. Secondary leucoderma may follow burns, scars and skin infections.

Local points:

a) Insert a fair number of needles into acupuncture points in the affected area and follow with mild stimulation.

and/or

b) Tap the affected area softly with the plum blossom needle.

Distal points:

Dazhui (Du 14.).

Quchi (L.I. 11.).

Lieque (Lu. 7.).

Xuehai (Sp. 10.).

Sanyinjiao (Sp. 6.).

ALOPECIA AREATA

Alopecia areata is a baldness which appears suddenly in patches, probably following a mental strain or an infective disorder such as typhoid fever. In most cases, the hair grows again in a short time without treatment. Acupuncture may be used in refractory cases to stimulate the regrowth of hair.

Local points:

Baihui (Du 20.).

Sishencong (Ex. 6.). and

A few additional points in the hairless area.

Specific points:

Taixi (K. 3.).

Lieque (Lu. 7.).

Distal points:

Hegu (L.I 4.). (for front of head).

Waiguan (S.J. 5.) (for side of head).

Lieque (Lu. 7.) (for back of head).

Electrical stimulation of the head area along with the Distal points is helpful. Tapping the affected area with the plum blossom needle is also very effective.

PSORIASIS

This is a non-infections skin disease characterized by irregularly shaped, slightly raised red patches with a scaly surface. Elbows, knees, and the scalp are the areas more likely to be affected.

Baihui (Du 20.).

Local points:

points in the affected area.

Homeostatic points:

Quchi (L.I. 11.).

Zusanli (St. 36.).

Sanyinjiao (Sp. 6.).

Specific point for allergy:

Xuehai (Sp. 10.).

Related Channel points:

Lieque (Lu. 7.).

Chize (Lu. 5.).

Tapping the affected area with the plum blossom needle also gives good results. In refractory cases Chize (Lu. 5.) should be bled once or twice a week.

If treatment is carried out for a prolonged period, there will be a noticeable improvement. In a series of 120 cases, complete cure occurred in 60%, while a 10% rate of relapse was recorded in a follow-up period of 4 years. Further, in 10 cases of psoriatic arthritis, cure on the same parameters was seen in 7 cases.

In the acute phase of a skin disorder, strong stimulation at Kongzui (Lu. 6.), the Xi-Cleft point of the Lung Channel, may be helpful. If the scalp is involved, Shuiquan (K. 5.)., the Xi-Cleft point of the Kidney Channel may be strongly stimulated (Kidney is related to head hair).

Note: I. Skin disorders are usually chronic intractable illnesses. Homoeopuncture helps to shorten the period of treatment.

II. Needles around the lesion (surrounding the dragon) or, if the skin is unbroken, needling the area of the lesion attacking the dragon) is helpful.

■

EAR DISORDERS

Principles of treatment

Points Local and Adjacent to the ear are selected along with Distal points on the Sanjiao and Gall bladder Channels. These two Channels circle around the ear and are therefore connected with auditory and balance functions.

According to traditional Chinese medicine, points of the Small Intestine Channel, which ends in front of the ear, are also used as local points. The Kidney is the Organ connected to the ear, Points of the Kidney Channel are, therefore, useful.

DEAFNESS, DEAF-MUTISM

Deafness, or impaired hearing, may be categorised into (a) conductive deafness, and (b) perceptive deafness.

a) Conductive deafness is the result of an obstruction in the transmission of sounds to the inner ear, which may be caused by too much wax in the ear, boils, damage to the ear drum, or otosclerosis (bone formation in the middle ear). The deafness may not be total as the bones of the skull conduct some sound.

b) Perceptive deafness can be the result of a defect in the receiving mechanism in the inner ear, or a disorder in the auditory nerve pathways to the brain. This type of deafness may follow an infection such as mumps or measles, the side-effects of certain drugs (e.g., quinine), or Meniere's disease. The slow impairment of hearing due to old age or the constant exposure to loud noise and congenital deafness also belong to this category.

This classification of deafness should be noted, as acupuncture obviously is less likely to be effective in cases of conductive deafness which is essentially a mechanical disorder.

Deaf-mutism is due to congenital deafness or deafness developing in a child usually following an attack of measles, encephalitis, epidemic meningitis, or drug poisoning. As the child cannot hear he will stop talking and later completely lose his ability to talk. Congenital deafness is found to be less effectively treatable with acupuncture. However, much research is going on in China on the subject of the treatment of deaf-mutism.

Baihui (Du 20.).

Local points (select from):

Ermen (S.J. 21.).
Tinggong (S.I. 19.).
Tinghui (G.B. 2.).
Yifeng (S.J. 17.).
} one needle.

Post-Tinggong (U. Ex.).

Xia-Yifeng (U. Ex.).

Distal points (select from):

Zhongzhu (S.J. 3.).

Foot-Linqi (G.B. 41.).

Waiguan (S.J. 5.).

Yanglao (S.I. 6.).

Houxi (S.I. 3.).

Hegu (L.I. 4.).

For mutism, add:

Yamen (Du 15.).
Lianquan (Ren 23.).
Tongli (H. 5.).

(Note: Yamen (Du 15.) is a Dangerous point)

Satisfactory results are sometimes seen after just a few treatments; however a long course of 60 treatments or more may be required to produce worthwhile results.

TINNITUS

Tinnitus, or the ringing, buzzing or hissing sounds occurring in the ear, have several causes. Disorders of the middle ear, inner ear, or the auditory nerve may produce tinnitus. Wax or other objects in the external auditory meatus, inflammation, drugs (e.g., aspirin) are among the common causes. It can also be caused by inflammation of the middle ear; Meniere's disease, anaemia, old age, trauma vascular degenerative.

Baihui (Du 20.).

Local points (select from):

Ermen (S.J. 21.).
Tinggong (S.I. 19.). } one needle.
Tinghui (G.B. 2.).
Yifeng (S.J. 17.).
Yiming (Ex. 7.).
Fengchi (G.B. 20.).

Distal points (select from):

Zhongzhu (S.J. 3.).
Waiguan (S.J. 5.).
Foot-Linqi (G.B. 41.).

EARACHE

This occurs commonly in ear infections, in trigeminal neuralgia, glossopharyngeal neuralgia and in carcinoma of the cheek. For the symptomatic treatment of the pain, use:

Baihui (Du 20.).

Local points:

Ermen (S.J. 21.).
Tinggong (S.I. 19.) } one needle
Tinghui (G.B. 2.).

Yifeng (S.J. 17.).

Distal points (select from):

Zhongzhu (S.J. 3.).
Waiguan (S.J. 5.).
Foot-Linqi (G.B. 41.).
Hegu (L.I. 4.) with strong manual stimulation.

Immune-enhancing points for infection:

Dazhui (Du 14.).
Quchi (L.I. 11.).
Sanyinjiao (Sp. 6.).

MENIERE'S DISEASE, VERTIGO, TRAVEL SICKNESS, LABYRINTHITIS

These disorders are caused by the dysfunction of the inner ear involving hearing and balance. In Meniere's disease, both these functions are impaired. Attacks of giddiness accompanied by deafness are experienced. As the deafness progresses the attacks of giddiness become less frequent and may disappear altogether when the deafness is complete.

Vertigo is a symptom of many diseases, including Menier's disease, epilepsy, and also of intracranial tumour. The patient feels that his surroundings are rotating.

Travel sickness arises from the disturbance of the balance organs of the inner ear and may result in nausea and vomiting.

Labyrinthitis is the inflammation of the labyrinth of the inner ear consisting of the organs of hearing and balance.

Baihui (Du 20.).

Local points (select from):

Ermen (S.J. 21.).
Tinggong (S.I. 19.). } one needle.
Tinghui (G.B. 2.).

Post-Tinggong (U. Ex.).

Xia-Yifeng (U. Ex.).

Distal points (select from):

Waiguan (S.J. 5.).
Zhongzhu (S.J. 3.).
Yanglao (S.I. 6.).
Foot-Linqi (G.B. 41.).
Taicong (Liv. 3.).
Hegu (L.I. 4.).

Specific points for nausea and vomiting:

Neiguan (P. 6.).
Zusanli (St. 36.).

Results are satisfactory in most cases; better results are however obtained with the use of electro-acupuncture. Satisfactory results have also been obtained in some patients especially children using laser-therapy.

NOSE DISORDERS

See under "Respiratory Disorders".

■

EYE DISORDERS

Principles of treatment

Local and Adjacent points combined with Distal points are used.

a) Local and Adjacent points are those within and around the orbital cavity.

b) Distal points may be selected on the following principles:

i) The point Hegu (L.I. 4.). which is the main Distal point for the face and the special sense organs.

ii). Points along the Liver Channel. According to traditional Chinese medicine, disorders of the eye relate to a dysfunction of the Liver (or the Gall bladder), or as the traditional Chinese theories state, "the Liver opens to the eye".

iii) Points along the Gall bladder Channel, firstly because it is paired with the Liver Channel, and secondly because it begins its course near the eye.

iv) Points along the Urinary Bladder Channel, because it begins its course near the eye, and also because some of its points which lie on the back of the trunk have specific connections with the Liver (Ganshu (U.B. 18.)) and with the Gall bladder (Danshu (U.B. 19.)).

v) Certain Distal points of the Gall bladder and the Urinary Bladder Channels are specific for eye diseases.; e.g., Guangming (G.B. 37.) for visual disorders; Chengshan (U.B. 58.) for ophthalmoplegia.

CONJUNCTIVITIS, THERMAL BURNS OF THE EYE

The conjunctiva is the transparent membrane covering the inner surface of the eyelids and the front of the eyeball. Conjunctivitis is the inflammation of this membrane. Symptoms include pain, soreness and redness of the eyes with tearing and aversion to bright light (photophobia).

When infection is present, antibiotics and steroids are preferable. However, acupuncture can be used in resistant or chronic case of conjunctivitis.

Baihui (Du 20.).

Local points:

Taiyang (Ex. 2.) (prick to bleed).

Jingming (U.B. 1.).

Sizhukong (S.J. 23.).

Chengqi (St. 1.).

Tongziliao (G.B. 1.).

Fengchi (G.B. 20.).

Distal points:

Hegu (L.I. 4.).

Taichong (Liv. 3.).

Immune-enhanching points:

Dazhui (Du 14.).

Quchi (L.I. 11.).

Sanyinjiao (Sp. 6.).

BLEPHARITIS, HORDEOLUM (STYE)

Blepharitis and hordeolum are terms for the inflammation of the margin of the eyelid mostly due to bacterial (staphylococcus) infection. Hordeolum affects particularly a sebaceous gland at the hair follicle of an eyelash and a small pustule is formed. Surgical drainage helps to resolve the condition. However, if there is repeated blepharitis, acupuncture may be helpful.

Baihui (Du 20.).

Local points (select from):

Yuyao (Ex. 3.).

Sizhukong (S.J. 23.).

Jingming (U.B. 1.).

Tongziliao (G.B. 1.).

Distal points:

Hegu (L.I. 4.).

Guangming (G.B. 37.).

Taichong (Liv. 3.).

Immune-enhancing points:

Dazhui (Du 14.).

Quchi (L.I. 11.).

Sanyinjiao (Sp. 6.).

MYOPIA, ASTIGMATISM, SQUINT (STRABISMUS) and DIPLOPIA

Myopia or short-sightedness is the inability to focus on distant objects. In astigmatism the lens and the cornea are not perfectly spherical so that an object will appear distorted. A squint (which is usually congenital) is caused by inco-ordinated action of one or more muscles of the eyeball. A squint which appears in adult life is usually due to the paralysis of one of the nerves of the eye muscles, due to damage, irritation or compression of that nerve. This type of squint results in double vision or diplopia. Diplopia may also arise due to intracranial causes; therefore, a proper neurological examination must be made and a diagnosis established before embarking on acupuncture.

Baihui (Du 20.).

Local points (select from):

Chengqi (St. 1.).

Qiuhou (Ex. 4.).

Jingming (U.B. 1.).

Tongziliao (G.B. 1.).

Fengchi (G.B. 20.).

Distal points (select from):

Hegu (L.I. 4.).

Yanglao (S.I. 6.).

Yangxi (L.I. 5.).

Guangming (G.B. 37.).

Yiming (Ex. 7.).

Feiyang (U.B. 58.)[1].

RETINITIS, DETACHED RETINA, OPTIC NERVE ATROPHY

The lens of the eyeball focuses the images onto the retina, which forms part of the optic nerve. Inflammation of the retina, or retinitis can be caused by many diseases, e.g., kidney disorders, diabetes, hypertension, eclampsia, blood disorders and syphills. A detached retina may occur due to injury or it may sometimes occur spontaneously. In both these conditions, impairment of vision follows. Where surgical or conservative therapy has failed, acupuncture may help.

Baihui (Du 20.).

Local points (select from):

Chengqi (St. 1.).

Qiuhou (Ex. 4.).

Zanzhu (U.B. 2.).

Yangbai (G.B. 14.).

Fengchi (G.B. 20.).

1 Especially useful in paralysis of ocular muscles together with Touwel (St. 8.) and Yanglingquan (G.B. 34.).

Yaiyang (Ex. 2.).

Distal points (select from):

Hegu (L.I. 4.).

Yanglao (S.I. 6.).

Yangxi (L.I. 5.).

Guangming (G.B. 37.).

Ganshu (U.B. 18.).

Sanyinjiao (Sp. 6.).

Taichong (Liv. 3.).

Homeostatic points:

Quchi (L.I. 11.).

Zusanli (St. 36.).

Although this is in fact a mechanical type of disorder, good results have been reported with acupuncture. The improvement of macular vision following acupuncture is probably due to the reflex increased vascular supply.

CATARACT

This is the loss of transparency of the lens of the eye with consequent impairment of vision. It is commonly due to the ageing process, but the condition could be hastened by diabetes, hypertension, arteriosclerosis and other degenerative conditions.

A good response may be obtained in early cataract with acupuncture treatment.

Baihui (Du 20.).

Local points (select from):

Chengqi (St. 1.).

Taiyang (Ex. 2.).

Yangbai (G.B. 14.).

Qiuhou (Ex. 4.).

Zanzhu (U.B. 2.).

Distal points:

Hegu (L.I. 4.).

Quchi (L.I. 11.).

Taichong (Liv. 3.).

OPHTHALMOPLEGIA

This is a paralysis affecting the external muscles of the eye. Most cases respond well.

Baihui (Du 20.).

Local points (select from):

Touwei (St. 8.) with needle directed towards the centre of the pupil.

Jingming (U.B. 1.).

Zanzhu (U.B. 2.).

Chengqi (St. 1.).

Qiuhou (Ex. 4.).

Tongziliao (G.B. 1.).

Fengchi (G.B. 20.).

Sizhukong (S.J. 23.).

Distal points:

Hegu (L.I. 4.).

Feiyang (U.B. 58.)

Influential point for muscks

Yanglingquan (G.B.34.)

GLAUCOMA

This is a disorder where there is an increase of the pressure of the fluid (aqueous and vitreous humour) in the eyeball. It may be caused by the over-secretion of this fluid, but is more commonly the result of blocking of the fine outlet channels which lead the fluid back into the veins. When the glaucoma is of acute onset, there will be severe headache accompanied with nausea and vomiting. The vision will be impaired. There will be blurring of vision with red eyes and sometimes swollen eyelids. In the commoner chronic type of glaucoma, the onset of the disease is insidious and may pass unnoticed until the optic nerve is damaged.

Results of acupuncture treatment have been very satisfactory, except in late cases.

Baihui (Du 20.).

Local points (select from):

Chengqi (St.1.)
Qiuhou (Ex. 4.)
Taiyang (Ex.2.).
Yangbai (G.B. 14.)
through to
Yuyao(Ex. 3.).
Fengchi (G.B. 20.).
Zanzhu (U.B.2.)

Distal points:

Hegu (L.I.4.).
Ganshu (U.B. 18.).
Taichong (Liv. 3.).

Specific points for nausea and vomiting:

Neiguan (P. 6.).
Zusanli (St. 36.).

Specific points for edema:

Shuifen (Ren 9.).
Shimen (Ren 5.).
Yinlingquan (Sp. 9.).
Pishu (U.B. 20.).

NIGHT BLINDNESS

The primary cause of this condition is the deficiency of Vitamin A or its provitamins. The deficiency may be either dietitic or some disorder of metabolism and insufficiency of its formation. Vitamin A helps to produce visual purple (rhodopsin) carried in the rods of the retina which are sensitive to light.

Baihui (Du 20.).

Local points (select from):

Chengqi (St. 1.).

Yangbai (G.B. 14.).

Qiuhou (Ex. 4.).

Zanzhu (U.B. 2.).

Taiyang (Ex. 2.).

Distal points:

Hegu (L.I. 4.).

Guangming (G.B. 37.).

Taichong (Liv. 3.).

Homeostatic points:

Quchi (L.I. 11.).

Zusanli (St. 36.).

Sanyinjiao (Sp. 6.).

Note: Acupuncture is particularly useful in relieving pain in eye disorders. G. M. Greenbaum (Australia) has effectively used his analgesic effect in carrying out surgery for cataract and strabismus. We have successfully tried out the points used by him in corneal graft surgery (keratoplasty).

■

ENDOCRINE DISORDERS

Acupuncture is known to have effects on the hypothalamic-pituitary-adrenocortical axis. Physiological effects such as an increase in the thickness of the adrenal cortex, increase in the circulating blood levels of ACTH and an increase in the urinary excretion of 17-Ketosteroids occur after acupuncture needling. No doubt, other complex humoral mechanisms are also called into play. The discovery of endorphins and enkephalins have added a whole new dimension to the acupuncture phenomenon.

Principles of treatment

a) Use of points of the Ren and Stomach Channels situated in lower abdominal area.

b) Use of points of the Urinary Bladder Channel in the low back area.

c) Use of the main Tonification points especially where there is under-activity of gland function.

d) Use of the points of the Kidney Channel (in traditional Chinese medicine the Kidney includes the adrenal glands, the testes and the overy).

e) Use of the point Jianjing (G.B. 21.), which is a specific endocrine point that may be used in all endocrine imbalances.

f) Use of Quchi (L.I. 11.), the main homeostatic point of the body.

HYPOGONADISM, SUB-FERTILITY

Hypogonadism denotes the failure of the functions of one or both of the testes, being the production of spermatozoa and the secretion of androgens (i.e., hormones which control the secondary sex characteristics, such as the distribution of hair and the deepening of the voice). When this condition occurs before puberty, the external genitalia and the secondary sex characteristics fail to develop. If it occurs after puberty, there will be a gradual loss of pubic hair and the external genitalia will atrophy. Fatigue, loss of initiative and loss of sex drive are common symptoms.

Baihui (Du 20.).

Local points:

Qugu (Ren 2.).

Zhongji (Ren 3.).

Guilai (St. 29.).

Guanyuan (Ren 4.).

Tonification points:

Qihai (Ren 6.).

Zusanli (St. 36.).

Sanyinjiao (St. 6.).

Distal point:

Taixi (K. 3.).

We have had the opportunity of treating several cases of hypogonadism, both male and female. In several of these cases hormonal therapy had been given over a number of years, with no visible improvement. After a few course of acupuncture therapy, rapid progress was observed in several cases as shown by the growth of facial hair in males and the pubic hair in both sexes. Marked improvement in libido was also reported by several of these patients. (In treatment of impotence in men similar points were used with good results).

MASCULINIZATION SYMPTOMS IN WOMEN

Just as the testes in the male produces androgens or the male sex hormone, the ovary in the female produces the female sex hormone or estrogens. However, both testes and ovary produce hormones of each variety, but in the male the testes produces more of androgens and conversely in the female there is more estrogen. (This is an excellent example of a Yin-Yang relationship.)

Thus masculinization symptoms in women may mean that there is too much androgen being produced.

However, another gland, the adrenal cortex, also produces sex hormones, especially androgens. The cause of masculinization must therefore be elucidated with particular attention being paid to the possibility of the presence of tumours affecting the adrenal cortex and causing the over-production of androgens.

Baihui (Du 20.).

Local points (select from):

Qihai (Ren 6.).

Points in the lower abdomen in the Ren Channel.

Points in the lower abdomen in the Stomach Channel.

Points in the low back area in the Urinary bladder Channel.

Distal points:

Kidney Channel points.

Sanyinjiao (Sp. 6.).

Homeostatic points:

Quchi (L.I. 11.).

Zusanli (St. 36.).

GYNECOMASTIA

This is an enlargement of the mammary gland in the male. The enlargement is usually bilateral, but a unilateral enlargement may also occur. It is due to endocrine disorder which may result in symptoms which include impotence and atrophy of the testicle. Liver disease may also cause gynecomastia.

Baihui (Du 20.).

Local points:

Rugen (St. 18.).

Shanzhong (Ren 17.).

Distal points:

Zusanli (St. 36.).

Sanyinjiao (Sp. 6.).

Foot-Linqi (G.B. 41.).

Homeostatic point:

Quchi (L.I. 11.).

GOITER

Goiter is an enlargement of the thyroid gland. The swelling may be:

a) simple, i.e., not associated with the under-activity (hypothyroidism) or over-activity of the gland (hyperthyroidism);

b) malignant (not frequent);

c) associated with hyperthyroidism-known as toxic goiter (also Graves' disease, thyrotoxicosis);

d) associated with hypothyroidism (myxedema).

The common forms of this disease are simple goiter and toxic goiter.

Simple goiter may arise from a lack of iodine in the diet. The gland is then stimulated to hypertrophy in an attempt to secrete more thyroxine, the principal hormone of this gland. Large goiters, besides being unsightly, may compress the neighboring structures such as the trachea, veins, nerves and cause symptoms.

Hyperthyroidism is characterised by an increase in the basal metabolic rate. The patient becomes irritable, loses weight and has an increased pulse rate. It is a disease found commonly in adult females. The thyroid is usually uniformly enlarged and is not as large as in a simple goiter.

Baihui (Du 20.).

Local points:

Neck-Futu (L.I. 18.).

Jianjing (G.B. 21.).

or

Local "hot needle" therapy,

Distal point:

Hegu (L.I. 4.).

In solitary adenomas, the most effective treatment is hot needling. We have carried out hot needling in 400 solitary adenomas of the thyroid with satisfactory regression of the tumour in 92% of the cases. In two cases, there was mild local cellulitis as a complication of this therapy.

The "hot needle" is specially made for this purpose with silver mixed with a little platinum to make it durable. The technique of using this needle is extremely important. The needle is held to the flame and heated till it is red hot and then swiftly and precisely inserted into the lump *and removed with the same movement.* The needle stays in the body only for a fraction of a second. The lump is subjected to cauterisation from inside by the heat of the needle and slowly regresses. In cases where it is necessary to carry out thyroidectomy, acupuncture may be employed as the anaesthesia.

DIABETES MELLITUS

This is a condition in which there is faulty carbohydrate metabolism due to an insufficiency of insulin. The deficiency may arise out of a faulty utilization of this hormone as well. It is a disease which more usually afflicts persons who have passed middle age, and more so if they are obese. If the disease comes on earlier in life it could be expected to be more severe.

As acupuncture has a homeostatic action, needling at any point tends to correct this disease. The patient is exposed to some danger of hypoglycemic attack if the acupuncturist treats him for an unrelated condition while the patient continues to take the usual dose of insulin or oral anti-diabetic preparation. It is therefore important to inquire from every patient whether he is having any other disorder for which he is taking medication. Similar complications may arise in the case of hypertension. Diabetics and hypertensives who are undergoing acupuncture therapy for other disorders should, therefore, have their medication tailored to the level of hyperglycemia (glycosuria) or the degree of hypertension respectively.

Generally, mild and moderate diabetics respond well to acupuncture therapy. Together with exercise and dietetic advice, the vast majority of patients could live free of medication or with lesser doses of the drugs.

Baihui (Du 20.).
Jiaosun (S.J. 20.).
Neck-Futu (L.I. 18.).
Jianjing (G.B. 21.).
Quchi (L.I. 11.).
Sanyinjiao (Sp. 6.).
Zusanli (St. 36.).
Dazhui (Du 14.).
Zhangmen (Liv. 13.).
Taichong (Liv. 3.).

A press needle at the pancreas point of the (left) ear is helpful.

OBESITY OF ENDOCRINE ORIGIN

This is similar to the treatment carried out for obesity as described under management of addictions in the section on "Psychiatric Disorders". The cause of the obesity must be determined and suitable dietetic advice should be given.

■

PSYCHIATRIC DISORDERS

Acupuncture has proved beneficial in many forms of psychiatric illnesses and mental disorders such as neurasthenia, psychoneuroses, schizophrenia, depression, behaviour problems of children, drug addictions, mental states associated with old age, epilepsy and space occupying lesions of the brain. These disorders are being successfully treated in China with the used acupuncture, supplemented in some cases with herbal therapy and drug therapy at dosage levels usually less than used in the Western countries.

Principles of treatment

The most useful points in our experience are the following:

Baihui (Du 20.).

Shenmen (H. 7.).

Neiguan (P. 6.).

Shenmal (U.B. 62.).

In addition to the above points, certain points along the Du Channel and the Shu points of the Heart and the Pericardium are beneficial in certain cases.

Other points may be added when special symptoms are present. For example:

Insomnia:

Anmian I (Ex. 8.).

Anmian II (Ex. 9.).

Fits:

Renzhong (Du. 26.).

Yanglingquan (G.B. 34.).

Depression and vegetative states like presenile dementia:

Zusanli (St. 36.).

Sanyinjiao (Sp. 6.).

Qihai (Ren 6.).

Hyperexcitability and anxiety:

Baihui (Du 20.).

Shenmen (H. 7.).

Forgetfulness:

Shendao (Du 11.)

Auditory hallucinations:

Local points:

Ermen (S.J. 21.).
Tinggong (S.I. 19.).
Tinghui (G.B. 2.).
} one needle.

Distal points:

Zhongzhu (S.J. 3.).

or

Waiguan (S.J. 5.).

Foot-Linqi (G.B. 41.).

The selection of points in psychiatric conditions requires much specialized knowledge and clinical acumen in evaluating the patient's condition. Treatment should be given daily, or every other day, until the condition is controlled; this may take 20 sittings or more, and booster treatments should be given every week for some months. The acupuncture therapy is usually tried in our clinic without drug therapy. However, we believe it can also be profitably combined with drug therapy, where indicated.

The following are some typical examples of the treatment given in some psychiatric disorders:

NEURASTHENIA

A much misused term, it is generally used as a label for lassitude not attributable to any recognised organic illness. It is often encountered in persons having anxiety neurosis and tension states with tiredness as the main symptom. Other associated symptoms are nervousness, irritability, anxiety, depression, insomnia, headaches, and sexual disorders. The main points to be used are:

Baihui (Du 20.).
Shenmen (H. 7.).
Shenmai (U.B. 62.).

These are combined with other points according to the symptoms presented, e.g.,

Headache:
Baihui (Du 20.).
Fengchi (G.B. 20.). (occipital headache).

Palpitations:
Neiguan (P. 6.).

Abdominal complaints:
Zusanli (St. 36.).

Sexual disorders:
Qugu (Ren 2.).
Guanyuan (Ren 4.).
Sanyinjiao (Sp. 6.).

HYSTERIA

This is a condition which is wholly psychological in origin, characterized mainly by disassociation (i.e., apparent cutting off of one part of the mind from the other). There is a diversity of symptoms, e.g., tics, paralysis, fits, which do not seem to accord with any positive findings on physical examination.

Baihui (Du 20.).

Shenmen (H. 7.).

Shenmai (U.B. 62.).

Depending on the symptoms present, the following additional points may be used with strong stimulation:

Renzhong (Du 26.).

Neiguan (P. 6.). through to

Waiguan (S.J. 5.).

Hegu (L.I. 4.).

Taixi (K. 3.).

If the condition becomes acute, use a Jing-Well point preferably Yongquan (K. 1.), with very strong stimulation.

SCHIZOPHRENIA

Schizophrenia (or "a split mind") is a type of functional psychosis or mental derangement characterized by a pattern of symptoms such as delusions (e.g., of the patient's own importance, persecution by others), disorders of thought, hallucinations (usually of hearing), and general lassitude. It occurs mainly in young and middle aged persons.

Select from : Baihui (Du 20.).

Shenmen (H. 7.).

Shenmai (U.B. 62.).

Renzhong (Du 26.).

Dazhui (Du 14.).

Xinshu (U.B. 15.).

Fenglong (St. 40).

Anmian I (Ex. 8.).

Anmian II (Ex. 9.).

In resistant cases, electrical stimulation may be used at the following points:

Hegu (L.I. 4.).

Shenmen (H. 7.).

For this purpose, mild electrical stimulation at the rate of about five pulses per second may be given daily for two weeks. It may be continued thereafter with one week's rest and review.

If auditory hallucinations are present, the following specific points may be used:

Local points:

Ermen (S.J. 21.).
Tinggong (S.I. 19.). } one needle.
Tinghui (G.B. 2.).

Distal points:

Zhongzhu (S.J. 3.).

or

Waiguan (S.J. 5.).

Foot-Linqi (G.B. 41.).

MENTAL DEPRESSION

This may be described as a disorder of mood which is deeper and longer than what would be normally expected from that particular person. There is a general impairment of all mental processes and of physical functions such as appetite, sleep, sex and work.

In what is called reactive depression, the patient reacts to external events to a greater extent and for longer than the circumstances warrant. Where the reasons for the misery seem to arise from within the patient himself, it is referred to as endogenous depression. It should be noted that severe depression may be a symptom of other more serious mental illness like maniac-depressive psychosis.

Baihui (Du 20.)

Shenmen (H. 7.).

Neiguan (P. 6.).

Shenmai (U.B. 62.).

Qihai (Ren 6.).

Zusanli (St. 36.).

Sanyinjiao (Sp. 6.).

A press needle at Ear Shenmen may help to thwart suicidal tendencies.

SEXUAL IMPOTENCE, EJACULATIO PRAECOX[1]

The absence of sexual drive in the male may be due either to organic or more usually to psychological factors. When it is due to organic factors (e.g., diabetes mellitus, alcoholism, tabes dorsalis) the underlying cause may have to be treated first.

Ejaculatio praecox or the too early emission of semen during intercourse may be a precursor to impotence and is associated with a general debility of the patient.

Select from:

Baihui (Du 20.).

Qugu (Ren 2.).

Zhongji (Ren 3.).

Guanyuan (Ren 4.).

Qihai (Ren 6.).

Mingmen (Du 4.).

Shenshu (U.B. 23.).

Zusanli (St. 36.).

Sanyinjiao (Sp. 6.).

Taixi (K. 3.).

Ququan (Liv. 8.).

See page 71.

1 Premature ejaculation.

DRUG AND OTHER ADDICTIONS

The treatment of drug addiction with acupuncture is an experimental field with much promise. The pioneering work of H.L. Wen and S. Y. C. Cheung at the Neuro-surgical Unit of the Kwong Wah Hospital, Kowloon, Hong Kong, has shown that relieving the drug withdrawal syndrome and counteracting drug addiction can be successfully done with acupuncture.

The following is a summary of the methodology used by the author for relieving several types of addictions. Electrical pulse stimulation is carried out in all cases. In between sittings press needles are placed in the relevant ear (auriculotherapy) points.

ADDICTION	POINTS USED:	FREQUENCY OF THERAPY
a) Drugs		*In-patients:*
	Baihui (Du 20.).	One hour 3 times a day for
	Shenmen (H. 7.).	3 days; then one hour daily
	Hegu (L.I. 4.)	for 5 days.
	Houxi (S.I. 3.).	*Out patients:*
	Neiguan (P. 6.).	Half hour daily for 10 days
	Waiguan (S. J. 5.).	and review.
	Ear pt. Lung.	
b) Food		*Out-patients:*
(Obesity)	Baihui (Du 20.).	Half hour daily for 10 days
	Shenmen (H. 7.).	and review.
	Ear pt. Stomach	Dietetic advice given.
		Exercise program.
c) Alcohol		
	Baihui (Du 20.).	Same as for drugs in
	Shenmen (H. 7.).	above for both in-patients
	Ear pt. Mouth	and out-patients treatment.
	Ear pt. Stomach	
	Ear pt. Liver	

d) Smoking		*Out-patients:*
	Baihui (Du 20.).	Half hour daily for 10 days
	Shenmen (H. 7.).	and review.
	Ear pt. Lung	
	Ear pt. Large Intestine.	
e) Betel chewing		*Out-patients:*
	Baihui (Du 20.).	Half hour daily for 10 days
	Shenmen (H. 7.).	and review.
	Ear pt. mouth.	
f) Glue sniffing		*Out-patients*
	Baihui (Du. 20.)	Half hour daily for 10 days
	Shenmen (H.7.)	and review.
	Ear point.	
	Internal Nose	

Note: Press needles must be retained at an appropriate point in the ear throughout the period of treatment (the needle being replaced at a new ear point every four to seven days.).

Wen and Cheung have recently adopted a method in which they commence with a three and half hour sitting using similar points and electrical simulation. They believe that the maximal elevation of the body's own endogenous opiates helps as a booster to commence the therapy. Better long term results are claimed using this newer technique. The results of this new technique have not yet been published.

Psychological supportive therapy is important to obtain good results.

By far the best results for the treatment of addictions are obtained with acupuncture. Relapses are common.

■

DISORDERS OF CHILDREN

Principles of treatment

Acupuncture may be used on children, including infants, on the same principles as for diseases of adults. It will be found that acupuncture is very effective in many children's disorders, the response to treatment being quicker and more positive.

However, there are special problem in using acupuncture in children. Unlike in the case of an adult, it may not be easy to obtain the co-operation of the patient. Children are generally averse to needling and a greater degree of tact and skill is required of the acupuncturist. Playfully distracting the child's attention, and skill in the painless insertion technique are the keys to carrying out the treatment in an acceptable manner. Force or compulsion should never be used.

For these reasons the ancillary methods such as acupressure, electro-acupuncture without needles, the plum blossom needle and lasertherapy may be used without any diminution in effectiveness. Where needles are used, the thinner gauges are preferred, e.g., gauge 32, and the degree of stimulation should be kept at moderate to low levels.

Some common examples of the use of acupuncture in pediatrics are now described.

INFANTILE CONVULSIONS, FEBRILE FITS

The most effective way of controlling a fit is to apply firm finger pressure at the point Renzhong (Du 26.). Pressure is exerted in an obliquely upward direction for a short time. The fit in most instances ceases almost instantly. If the fit is severe, this point may be strongly stimulated (sedation) with a needle and the following points added according to the severity of the condition:

Yongquan (K. 1.). (stimulate strongly with a needle).
Shaoshang (Lu. 11.) } (prick to cause
Shixuan (Ex. 30.) } bleeding).

After consciousness is regained, further points may be used according to the presenting symptoms:

High fever:
Dazhui (Du 14.).
Quchi (L.I. 11.).
Clouded sensorium:
Neiguan (P. 6.).
Taichong (Liv. 3.).
Meningismus:
Fengchi (G.B. 20.).
Respiratory depression:
Suliao (Du 25.).
Cough:
Lieque (Lu. 7.).
Excessive sputum:
Fenglong (St. 40.).

In appropriate conditions drug therapy in suitably reduced dosages may be combined with acupuncture.

EPILEPSY, REPETITIVE FITS

In treating epileptiform disorders, it is best to discontinue drugs and start with daily treatment.

Baihui (Du 20.).
Yintang (Ex. I.).
Renzhong (Du. 26.).
Shenmen (H. 7.).
Shenmai (U.. 62.).
Yaoqi (Ex. 20.).

Very good results may be obtained in idiopathic epilepsy without the use of drugs.

A press needle in the ear helps to prevent attacks.

BEHAVIOUR DISORDERS

As these disorders are predominantly due to psychological factors, the main sedative points are used.

Baihui (Du 20.).
Sishencong (Ex. 6.).
Neiguan (P. 6.).
Shenmen (H. 7.).
Yanglingquan (G.B. 34.).
Shenmai (U.B. 62.).

NOCTURNAL ENURESIS

Treatment may be considered for bed-wetting by children over three years of age. Intermittent bed-wetting could be due to inflammation of the urinary passages, but more often the cause may be neuromuscular inco-ordination with a psychological overlay. However, before commencement of acupuncture treatment, it will be useful to ascertain whether the condition is not due to spina bifida, diabetes mellitus, or kidney disease. Generally, very good results are obtained with acupuncture in this condition.

Baihui (Du 20.).

a) **Points on front of trunk (select from):**

Local points:

Guanyuan (Ren 4.).

Zhongji (Ren 3.).

Qugu (Ren 2.).

Guilai (St. 29.).

Distal points:

Zusanli (St. 36.).

Sanyinjiao (Sp. 6.).

b) **Points on back of trunk (select from):**

Local points:

Shenshu (U.B. 23.).

Yaoyangguan (Du 3.).

Ciliao (U.B. 32.).

Zhibian (U.B. 54.).

Distal points:

Weizhong (U.B. 40.).

Kunlun (U.B. 60.).

The above points may be used in different combinations, e.g., (i) many local points without Distal points; (ii) Local and Distal points; (iii) combined Mu-Front and Back-Shu points.

Many Chinese acupuncturists believe that the point Ciliao (U.B. 32.) is specific for this disorder. The use of Moxibustion at the Urinary Bladder points is particularly useful in this condition. An often used technique is to heat with moxa a needle inserted at Ciliao (U.B. 32.). This is known as the moxa on needle technique.

PYREXIAS

High fever in children occurs due to a variety of causes. When a child is moribund and toxic, the response to drugs in high fevers is not always satsifactory. Acupuncture is known to bring down the fever often dramatically.

The points used are:

Dazhui (Du 14.).

Quchi (L.I. 11.).

Hegu (L.I. 4.).

Strong stimulation at Dazhui (Du 14.). relieves the fever, often in a matter of minutes.

Many other disorders may be encountered in pediatric practice which can be treated with acupuncture. Infectious diseases like whooping cough, mumps, influenza and poliomyelitis; respiratory ailments like allergic rhinitis, sinusitis and bronchial asthma; hypothyroidism, deaf-mutism, hypogonadism, diarrhea, and rheumatism are some examples. The acupuncture treatment of these diseases are described in the relevant sections of this book.

■

ACUTE DISORDERS

EMERGENCY MEASURES

Acupuncture is eminently suitable for use in a wide variety of emergency conditions. Not only is it quicker in producing the desired results, but owing to the absence of side-effects it has a distinct advantage over drug therapy. Its greatest advantage, especially in emergencies, is that as a mode of therapy it is available at all times. For even if a needle is not at hand, acupressure may be employed with satisfactory results in most cases, and if skillfully administered, with hardly any diminution in effectiveness. Moreover, in conditions where sophisticated intensive care therapy is required, acupuncture may be used as the first line of therapy till the patient is transported to a hospital.

Principles of treatment

a) The use of Jing-well points for all acute emergencies.

b) The use of the point Hegu (L.I. 4.) and the other important Distal points for the rapid relief of pain.

c) The use of the *Ah-Shi* points for localized pain.

d) The use of Xi-Cleft points in acute conditions involving any of the internal Organs.

e) The use of the specific points for symptoms, e.g., the point Neiguan (P. 6.). for vomiting, Tiantu (Ren 22.) for hiccough.

f) The use of Baihui (Du 20.) which has a controlling effect on all the Channels and points in addition to its calming and sedative actions.

A few representative example of therapy in these conditions are given below:

The unconscious patient:

Renzhong (Du 26.) with strong acupressure.

If response is inadequate:

Renzhong (Du 26.)
Yongquan (K. 1.). } strong needle manipulation.

The same points are useful in respiratory distress of the new-born.

Heat stroke:

Renzhong (Du 26.) with strong acupressure.

Hegu (L.I. 4.).

Neiguan (P. 6.). with moderate stimulation.

Zusanli (St. 36.).

Epileptic attack, hysterical attack, febrile fit:

Renzhong (Du 26.) with firm acupressure.

If attack is severe:

Renzhong (Du 26.)
Yongquan (K. 1.) } Strong needle manipulation.

Shaoshang (Lu. 11.)
Shixuan (Ex. 30.). } Prick to cause bleeding.

Xi-Cleft point:

Yinxi (H. 6.) with strong stimulation.

Severe headache:

In all cases of headache, the principal point to be used is Hegu

(L.I. 4.). with strong manual stimulation. A needle is also inserted at Baihui (Du 20.) to sedate the patient.

The following additional points may be used depending on the localization of the pain:

a) Frontal headache:

Local points:

Ah-Shi points.

Yintang (Ex. I.).

Yangbai (G.B. 14.).

Distal point:

Neiting (St. 44.). or Xiangu (St. 43.) } with strong stimulation.

b) Temporal headache:

Local points:

Ah-Shi points.

Taiyang (Ex. 2.).

Sizhukong (S.J. 23.).

Distal points:

Waiguan (S.J. 5.). Foot-Linqi (G.B. 41.) } with strong stimulation.

c) Parietal headache:

Local points:

Ah-Shi points.

Shuaigu (G.B. 8.).

Touwei (St. 8.).

Distal points:

Zhongzhu (S.J. 3.). Waiguan (S.J. 5.) } with strong stimulation.

d) Vertical headache:

Local points:

Shishencong (Ex. 6.).

Ah-Shi point.

Distal points:

Yongquan (K. 1.) } with strong
Kunlun (U.B. 60.) } stimulation.

e) Occipital headache:

Local points:

Ah-Shi points.

Fengchi (G.B. 20.).

Tianzhu (U.B. 10.).

Distal points:

Lieque (Lu. 7.) } with strong stimulation.
Yanglao (S.I. 6.) }

After the pain has been alleviated it is important to elicit, where possible, the cause of the headache and to treat it early.

High fever:

Specific points:

Dazhui (Du 14.) with strong stimulation.

Quchi (L.I. 11.).

Hegu (L.I. 4).

Shock:

Renzhong (Du 26.).

Yongquan (K. 1.).

Homeostatic points:

Quchi (L.I. 11.).

Zusanli (St. 36.).

Sanyinjiao (Sp. 6.).

Acute eye disorders

(e.g., thermal burns, acute conjunctivitis):

Baihui (Du 20.).

Local points:

Point around the eye (no stimulation).

Distal points:

Hegu (L.I. 4.) } with strong manual
Xiangu (St. 43.) } stimulation.

Acute ear disorders

(e.g., earache, acute labyrinthitis, vertigo):

Baihui (Du 20.).

Local points:

Ermen (S.J. 21).

Tinggong (S.I. 19.).

Tinghui (G.B. 2.).

Distal points:

Hegu (L.I. 4.) with strong manual stimulation.

Zhongzhu (S.J. 3.).

Foot-Linqi (G.B. 41.).

Acute nose disorders (e.g., epistaxis, acute rhinitis):

Baihui (Du 20.).

Local points:

Shangxing (Du 23.).

Suliao (Du 25.).

Nose-Heliao (L.I. 19.).

Distal points:

Hegu (L.I. 4.).

Influential point for vascular disorders:

Taiyuan (Lu. 9.).

Xi-Cleft point of Lung Channel:

Kongzui (Lu. 6.) with strong stimulation.

Acute attack of bronchial asthma:

Baihui (Du 20.).

Specific point:

Tiantu (Ren 22.)-no stimulation.

Xi-Cleft point of Lung Channel:

Kongzui (Lu. 6.) with strong stimulation.

Influential point for respiratory disorders:

Shanzhong (Ren 17.) with stimulation.

Acute attack of hiccough:

Neiguan (P. 6.) } with stimulation.
Zusanli (St. 36.) }

Tiantu (Ren 22.)-no stimulation.

Geshu (U.B. 17.).

Acute coronary insufficiency (angina pectoris):

Baihui (Du 20.).

Jing-Well point:

Shaochong (H.9.)-prick to cause bleeding

Local point:

Bipay (U. Ex.).

Distal points:

Neiguan (P. 6.).

Shenmen (H. 7.).

Mu-Front point of the Pericardium:

Shanzhong (Ren 17.).

Xi-Cleft point of the Heart Channel:

Yinxi (H. 6.).

Acute gastritis:

Baihui (Du 20.).

Local points:

Zhongwan (Ren 12.).

Tianshu (St. 25.).

Distal points:

Neiguan (P. 6.).

Zusanli (St. 36.).

Xi-Cleft point of the Stomach Channel:

Liangqiu (St. 34.).

Gastro-enteritis, acute diarrhea:

Baihui (Du 20.).

Local point:

Tianshu (St. 25.).

Distal point:

Zusanli (St. 36.) with strong stimulation

Specific point:

Gongsun (Sp. 4.) with strong stimulation

Nausea, vomiting:

Baihui (Du 20.).

Local points:

Jinjin, Yuye (Ex. 10.)-prick to cause bleeding.

Specific points:

Neiguan (P. 6.). } with strong stimulation.

Zusanli (St. 36.). }

Acute abdominal pain, intestinal colic:

Baihui (Du 20.).

Local points:

Tianshu (St. 25.).

Zhongwan (Ren 12.).

Distal points:

Neiguan (P. 6.) Strong manual

Zusanli (St. 36.). stimulation.

Specific point for pain:

Hegu (L.I. 4.) with strong stimulation

Acute appendicitis:

Specific point:

Lanwei (Ex. 33.) with strong stimulation

Distal point:

Zusanli (St. 36.).

Specific point for pain:

Hegu (L.I. 4.).

Biliary colic:

Baihui (Du 20.).

Specific point:

Liangmen (St. 21.)-not on the right side.

Specific point for pain:

Hegu (L.I. 4.) with strong stimulation.

Special Alarm point of Gall bladder:

Dannang (Ex. 35.).

Renal colic:

Baihui (Du 20.)

Specific point:

Shenshu (U.B. 23.).

Specific point for pain:

Hegu (L.I. 4.) with strong stimulation.

Xi-Cleft point of Kidney Channel:

Shuiquan (K. 5.) with strong stimulation

Acute sciatica, acute low back pain:

Baihui (Du 20.).

Local points:

Ah-Shi points.

Huatuojiaji (Ex. 21.) points in the affected region.

Huantiao (G.B. 30.).

Specific point for pain:

Hegu (L.I. 4.) with strong stimulation.

Distal points:

Weizhong (U.B. 40.).

Kunlun (U.B. 60.).

Renzhong (Du 26.).

Acute retention of urine:

Baihui (Du 20.).

Local points:

Zhongji (Ren 3.).

Qugu (Ren 2.).

Distal points:

Sanyinjiao (Sp. 6.).

Taixi (K. 3.).

Moxibustion on the Ren Channel points on the abdomen below the umbilicus is also useful.

Acute dysmenorrhea:

Baihui (Du 20.).

Local points:

Guanyuan (Ren 4.).

Zhongji (Ren 3.).

Distal points:

Zusanli (St. 36.).

Sanyinjiao (St. 6.).

Specific points for Pain:

Hegu (L.I. 4.)
Neiting (St. 44.) } with strong stimulation.

Specific points for nausea and vomiting:

Neiguan (P. 6.).
Zusanli (St. 36.). } with strong stimulation.

Post-operative pain:

Baihui (Du 20.).

Specific points for pain:

Hegu (L.I. 4.)
Neiting (St. 44.). } with strong stimulation.

For the head and neck area:

Quanliao (S.I. 18.).

TRADITIONAL CHINESE THERAPEUTICS

(EXAMPLE OF THE TREATMENT OF SOME COMMON DISEASES USING TRADITIONAL THEORY)[1]

"Health and disease are the crest and nadir of life"

-King Buddhadasa, Royal Acupuncturist and Surgeon of Sri Lanka. (200 A.D.)

WINDSTROKES (APOPLEXY, STROKE)

Etiology:

The causative factor of this disease is usually the stirring wind arising from hyperactivity of *yang* in the Liver accompanied with disturbances of the *zang-fu* organs, *qi* and blood, imbalance of *yin* and *yang* and dysfunctions in the channels and collaterals. Another cause is endogenous wind caused by phlegm-heat after regular over-indulgence in alcohol and a fatty diet.

1 Differentiation of syndrome.

Differentiations:

There are two types of windstrokes according to the degree of severity:

(1) The severe type of cases where the *zang-fu* organs are affected, showing signs and symptoms in the channels, the collaterals and the viscerae.

(2) The mild type where only the channels and collaterals are affected. The signs and symptoms pertain only to the channels and collaterals.

(1) *The severe type*—the *zang-fu* organs being affected—may be subdivided into (a) tense syndrome and (b) flaccid syndrome.

(a) Tense syndrome: Sudden collapse, coma, staring eyes, fists and jaws clenched, redness of the face and ears, gurgling with sputum, coarse breathing, retention of urine and constipation, a wiry and rolling forceful pulse.

(b) Flaccid syndrome: Coma, hands relaxed and mouth agape, eyes closed, pallor, profuse drops of sweat over the head and face, snoring. There may be incontinence of faeces and urine, cold limbs and a feeble pulse.

Comparison of the leading signs and symptoms of tense and flaccid syndromes of windstrokes (apoplexy)

Tense syndrome	*Flaccid syndrome*
Eyes open	Eyes closed
Clenched jaws	Mouth agape
Clenched fists	Relaxed hands
Anhidrosis	Hidrosis
Continence of urine, constipation	Incontinence of urine and faeces
Wiry, rolling and forceful pulse	Feeble pulse

(2) *The mild type*—(channels and collaterals are disordered):

Symptoms and signs are chiefly those of the sequelae of the severe type, which involve the channels and collaterals. There are also primary cases without affliction of the *zang-fu* Organs. Manifestations are hemiplegia or deviation of the mouth due to the motor impairment.

Treatment:

(1) *The severe type*—(*Zang-Fu* Organs disordered)

(a) *The tense syndrome:*

Method: To promote resuscitation by applying the reducing method to points of the Du Channel and the Jing-Well Points.

Prescription:

Renzhong (Du 26.).

Baihui (Du 20.).

The 12 Jing-Well Points of both hands:

(Lu. 11., H. 9., P. 9., L.I. 1., S.J. 1., S.I. 1.),

Yongquan (K. 1.).

Points according to the signs and symptoms:

Clenched jaws:

Jiache (St. 6.).

Xiaguan (St. 7.).

Hegu (L.I. 4.).

Gurgling with excessive sputum:

Tiantu (Ren 22.).

Fenglong (St. 40.)

Aphasia and stiffness of the tongue:

Yamen (Du 15.).

Lianquan (Ren 23.).

Tongli (H. 5.).

Rationale:

Renzhong (Du 26.) and Baihui (Du 20.) regulate the *qi* of the Du Channel, effecting resuscitation. Bleeding the twelve Jing-Well Points of both hands may eliminate heat of the upper portion of the body, thus causing the endogenous wind to subside. Yongquan (K. 1.) conducts the heat downwards. This method is known as selecting points of the lower portion of the body to treat diseases of the upper parts of the body.

When the acute crisis is over, points may be chosen according to symptoms, such as Jiache (St. 6.), Xiaguan (St. 7.) and Hegu (L.I. 4.) for the clenched jaws. This method is known as combining the local and distal (remote) points according to the courses of the channels, because the large Intestine Channel and Stomach Channel traverse the cheek. Tiantu (Ren 22.) and Fenglong (St. 40.) are effective in soothing *Taqi* (breath) and resolving sputum. Yamen (Du 15.) and Lianquan (Ren 23.) are local and adjacent points of the tongue. Tongi (H. 5.), the Luo (Connecting) Point of the Heart Channel, may relieve stiffness of the tongue because functionally the tongue is related to the Heart.

b) *The flaccid syndrome:*

Method : To reconstitute the *yang* and prevent the collapsing state by applying moxibustion to point of the Ren Channel.

Prescription:

Qihai (Ren 6.).
Guanyuan (Ren 4.).
Shenjue (Ren 8.).

Rationale:

These three points are the main points for emergency measures to restore vital functions. Continuous indirect moxibustion with salt may bring about an improvement.

If it is difficult to decide whether the syndrome is of the tense or the flaccid type, it is not advisable to bleed the twelve Jing-Well

Points of the hand, but it is desirable to apply acupuncture to Renzhong (Du 26.) for regaining consciousness, and Zusanli (St. 36.) to readjust the vital functions.

(2) *The mild type*—(channels and collaterals only are disordered).

The hemiplegia which occurs may be mild or severe, and the stroke may be on either side of the body. At the beginning, the affected limbs may be weak; later, they become stiff, which finally leads to motor impairment. There may be dizziness and dysphasia.

Method: Readjust the *qi* (vital energy) and blood circulation, and remove obstruction from the channels and collaterals by puncturing the points of the Yang Channels of the affected area as the main points. Points of the healthy side may also be combined. Puncture the healthy side first and then the affected side. Moxibustion may be applied as a supplement. The manipulation used is the tonifying method. The *bi* and *wei* syndromes, which may result as complications, also need to be treated later. Exercise therapy, postural drainage, massage and manipulation are very useful ancillary methods in treating strokes.

Prescription:

Head Region:

Baihui (Du 20.).
Fengfu (Du 16.).
Tongian (U.B. 7.).

Upper Extremity:

Jianyu (L.I. 15.).
Quchi (L.I. 11.).
Waiguan (S.J. 5.).
Hegu (L.I. 4.).

Lower Extremity:

Huantiao (G.B. 30.).
Yanglingquan (G.B. 34.).
Zusanli (St. 36.).
Jiexi (St. 41.).

Rationale:

Wind, being a *yang* pathogenic factor, usually invades the upper and exterior parts of the body, Baihui (Du 20.), Fengfu (Du 16.) and Tongian (U.B. 7.) are used to eliminate pathogenic wind of the upper parts of the body. Since *yang* channels dominate the exterior part of the body, the acupuncture points are chosen mainly from these to readjust the *qi* and blood of the body and to promote the smooth circulation in the channels and collaterals of both the upper and lower parts of the body.

Facial paralysis : This can be treated with Local and Distal points together with Yanglingquan (G.B. 34.). an influential point.

Prophylactic measures:

Senile patients with deficiency of *qi* and excessive sputum or with manifestations of hyperactivity of *yang* of Liver such as dizziness and palpitation may sometimes present symptoms of stiffness of the tongue, slurred speech and numbness of the fingers. These are prodromal signs of windstroke. Prophylactic measures entail paying attention to diet, daily activities. and avoiding excesses of all types. Frequent moxibustion on Zusanli (St. 36.) and Xuanzhong (G.B. 39.) may prevent windstrokes.

Note: Windstroke is the equivalent of cerebrovascular accidents of modern medicine. This group of diseases include cerebral haemorrhage, embolism and subarachnoid hemorrhage.

After the acute stage is over, there may be sequelae such as hemiplegia, monoplegia, dysphasia or aphasia and also mental changes.

It is important to investigate the frequent causative factors, as described in Western medicine, such as:

(1) Diabetes mellitus.

(2) Hypertension.

(3) Intracranial lesions and malformations.

(4) Rheumatic heart diseases.

(5) Thrombosis, embolism.

(6) Trauma.

(7) Birth injury.

These etiologies have their traditional Chinese equivalents.

SYNCOPE (YIN EXCESS OF THE HEAD REGION)

Etiology:

Onset of syncope is due mainly to disorders caused by emotional disturbances and exhaustion. Such a condition causes derangement in *qi* of the channels, which in turn hinders the *qi* and blood of the twelve channels in their ascent to the head, preventing the *yang qi* from reaching the ex-remities. This leads the nutrient *qi* and defensive *qi* out of their normal routes of circulation of the head region.

Differentiation:

Xu type: Shallow breathing, mouth agape, sweating, pallor, cold extremities, deep, feeble and thready pulse.

Shi type: Coarse breathing, rigid extremities, clenched jaws, deep and forceful pulse.

Treatment:

Method : Promote resuscitation and mental clarity by puncturing points of the Du and Pericardium Channels as the main points. Reducing method for the *shi* type and reinforcing method for the *Xu* type is used.

Prescription:

Renzhong (Du 26.).
Zhongchong (P. 9.).
Hegu (L.I. 4.).
Taichong (Liv. 3.).

Secondary points:

Bu type:

Baihui (Du 20.).

Qihai (Ren 6.).

Zusanli (St. 36.).

Apply acupuncture combined with moxibustion.

Shi type:

Laogong (P. 8.).

Yongquan (K. 1.).

Rationale:

Renzhong (Du 26.) and Zhongchong (P. 9.) are points for resuscitation. Hegu (L.I. 4.) and Taichong (Liv. 3.) may relieve clenching of the jaws and mental cloudiness and invigorate the circulation of *qi* and Blood. Laogong (P. 8.) and Yongquan (K. 1.) promote a clear mind and dissipate heat. Baihui (Du 20.), Zusanli (St. 36.) and Qihai (Ren 6.) reconstitute the *qi* and re-establish the *yang*.

Ear acupuncture points:

Heart.

Subcortex.

Adrenal.

Ear-Shenmen.

Method—Strong stimulation (electrically or acupressure).

Note: This condition includes simple fainting, postural hypotension, sunstroke, hypoglycemia and hysteria, as described in modern medicine.

YANG EXCESS OF THE HEAD REGION (HEADACHES)

Etiology:

The head is where all the *yang* channels of the hand and foot meet. Attack of endogenous or exogenous factors may cause headaches due to derangement of *qi* and Blood in the head and retardation of the circulation of *qi* in the channels that traverse the head.

Headache such as in a common cold is caused by exogenous pathogenic factors. Headache of endogenous origin, called "headwind" is intermittent, protracted and intractable. Pain occurs on either side of the head. It may be of the *shi* or *xu* type, the former due mainly to hyperactivity of *yang* of the Liver and the latter due to deficiency of *qi* and blood.

Differentiation:

Headache is differentiated according to its locality and its supplying channels. Pain at the occipital region and nape, for example, is related to Urinary Bladder Channel of Foot-Taiyang; pain at the forehead and supraorbital region relates to the Stomach Channel of Foot-Yangming; pain at the temporal region of both sides or only one side relates to the Gall bladder Channel of Foot-Shaoyang, and that at the parietal region is related of Liver-Channel of Foot-Jueyin.

Shi type : Violent boring pain may be accompanied by dizziness, irritability, a bitter taste in the mouth, nausea, suffocating feeling in the chest, hypochondrium pain, a sticky tongue coating and a wiry pulse.

Xu type : Onset is mostly due to strain and stress. The pain is insidious. It may be agitating or mild, and responds to warmth and pressure. The accompanying signs and symptoms are usually lassitude, palpitation, insomnia, a pale tongue and a weak pulse.

Treatment:

Method : To dispel wind, remove obstruction in the channels and collaterals and regulate the *qi* and blood by puncturing the points of the local area combined with points of the distal (remote) areas. The reducing method is for the *shi* type, and the reinforcing method or tapping with a cutaneous needle is for the *xu* type.

Prescriptions:

Occipital headaches:

Fengchi (G.B. 20.).

Kunlun (U.B. 60.).

Houxi (S.I. 3.).

Frontal headaches:

Touwei (St. 8.).

Yintang (Extra. 1.).

Shuaigu (G.B. 8.).

Waiguan (S.J. 5.).

Foot-Linqi (G.B. 41.).

Parietal headaches:

Baihui (Du 20.).

Houxi (S.I. 3.).

Zhiyin (U.B. 67.).

Taichong (Liv. 3.).

Points according to the signs and symptoms:

Hyperactivity of *yang* of the Liver:

Xingjian (Liv. 2.).

Yanglingquan (G.B. 34.).

Deficiency of the qi and Blood:

Qihai (Ren 6.).

Zusanli (St. 36.).

Rationale:

The above prescriptions are formulated by combining the local points with the distal points according to the location of the headache and the channel affected.

Occipital headaches-points of Taiyang Channels of Hand and Foot.

Frontal headaches-points of Yangming Channels of Hand and Foot.

Unilateral headaches-points of Shaoyang Channels of Hand and Foot.

Parietal headaches-points of Taiyang Channels Hand and Foot together with those of Jueyin Channel of Foot.

These prescriptions have the effect of removing the obstruction of the channels and collaterals, regulating the *qi* and blood and relieving the pain.

Plum-Blossom needle tapping and cupping methods:

Main points: Area along L.I. to S. 4,[1] is tapped.

Supplementary points:

Fengchi (G.B. 20.).

Taiyang (Extra 2.).

Yangbai (G.B. 14.).

Method : Tap on the area from L.1. to S.4. Then tap on the local area and the area where the affected channels pass through. In acute pain, Taiyang (Extra. 2.). and Yangbai (G.B. 14.) may be tapped until slight bleeding occurs. Then apply cupping. (Small cups should be used).

Ear acupuncture points:

Subcortex,

Forehead,

Occiput,

Kidney,

Gall bladder.

Method : Insert needles and manipulate intermittently. For persistent headache, stimulate the needles continuously for 5 minutes to cause strong deqi. Also, needles may be embedded at the sensitive (reactive) points for 1-7 days.

---

1 Lumbar 1 to Sacral 4.

Note: Yang deficiency of the head region may also cause headaches. A differential diagnosis is derived from pulse diagnosis and from the signs and symptoms.

Headaches occur in a variety of diseases according to modern medicine e.g., internal organ disorders, neurological disorders, psychosis, ear, nose and throat disorders. Acupuncture gives gratifying results in migraine, and in vascular and functional headaches.

YANG EXCESS OF THE FACE (TRIGEMINAL NEURALGIA)

This is a transient, paroxysmal burning pain of the facial region which is supplied by the trigeminal nerve. This disease is caused by a yang excess of the face area.

Treatment:

Prescription:

Upper : Pain in the 1st (opthalmic) branch:

Yangbai (G.B. 14.).

Taiyang (Extra. 2.).

Zanzhu (U.B. 2.).

Waiguan (S.J. 5.).

Middle : Pain in the 2nd (maxillary) branch:

Sibai (St. 2.).

Nose-Juliao (St. 3.).

Renzhong (Du 26.).

Hegu (L.I. 4.).

Lower : Pain in the 3rd (mandibular) branch:

Xiaguan (St. 7.).

Jiache (St. 6.).

Chengjiang (Ren 24.).

Neiting (St. 44.).

Ear Acupuncture points:

Forehead.

Sympathetic Nerve.

Ear-Shenmen.

Auricular points corresponding to the painful areas.

Reactive points.

Method : Rotate the needles for several minutes, or embed them at the sensitive points.

DIZZINESS AND VERTIGO (KIDNEY DYSFUNCTIONS)

Etiology:

Dizziness and vertigo may be explained in modern medicine, as a derangement of the sense of equilibrium. Clinically, such symptoms are usually present in Meniere's syndrome, labyrinthitis, otosclerosis, hyper-or hypotension, neurasthenia, and the post-traumatic syndrome.

According to traditional Chinese medicine these disorders may be due to:

(1) An upward attack of the hyperactive *yang* of the Liver due to an insufficiency of water to nourish the wood (dysfunction of the Kidney affecting the Liver).

(2) Retention of damp-phlegm, which causes mental cloudiness.

(3) Deficiency (*Xu*) of the *qi* and the Blood, which causes insufficiency of the "sea of marrow" in the head. (The brain is known as sea of marrow in traditional Chinese medicine.)

Differentiation:

The presenting symptoms are giddiness and blurring of vision with vertigo and a tendency to fall.

(1) Upward attack of hyperactive *yang* of Liver: Besides the main symptoms, there appears tinnitus, a flushed face, nausea, backache, redness of the tongue, proper and a wiry, rapid pulse.

(2) Retention of damp-phlegm : The complications are fullness and a suffocating sensation of the chest and epigastric region, nausea and vomiting, profuse sputum, anorexia, a white and sticky coated tongue and a rolling pulse.

(3) Deficiency (*Xu*) of *qi* and Blood : The complications are listlessness, lassitude, palpitation, insomnia, and a pulse without much force.

Treatment:

(1) An upward attack of the hyperactive *yang* of the Liver:

Method : Points from the Jueyin (Liver) Channel and the Shaoyin (Kidney) Channel are selected as the main points to nourish yin and pacify *yang*. Reinforcing or reducing methods may be used as indicated. The severity of the disease determines the choice of therapy.

Prescription:

Shenshu (U.B. 23.).
Taixi (K. 3.).
Ganshu (U.B. 18.).
Xingjian (Liv. 2.).
Fengchi (G.B. 20.).

Rationale:

Application of the reinforcing method at Shenshu (U.B. 23.) and Taixi,(K. 3.) tonifies the Kidney, while the application of the reducing method to Ganshu (U.B. 18.), Xingjian (Liv. 2.) and Fengchi (G.B. 20.) pacifies the *yang* of the Liver.

(2) Retention of damp-phlegm:

Method: Resolve the phlegm and eliminate the damp by applying the reinforcing and reducing methods to the Back-Shu, Front-Mu and Luo-Connecting Points of the Spleen and Stomach.

Prescription:

Pishu (U.B. 20.).
Zhongwan (Ren 12.).
Fenglong (St. 40.).
Neiguan (P. 6.).
Touwei (St. 8.).

Rationale:

The application of the reinforcing method to Pishu (U.B. 20.), the Back-Shu Point of the Spleen, and Zhongwan (Ren 12.), the Front-Mu Point of the Stomach, strengthens the functions of the Spleen and Stomach to eliminate the damp. Fenglong (St. 40.) the Luo (Connecting) Point of the Stomach has the function of resolving phlegm when the reducing method is applied. Touwei (St. 8.) is an effective point for dizziness. Neiguan (P. 6.) normalises the Stomach and stops the vomiting.

(3) Deficiency (*Xu*) of the *qi* and the Blood.

Method: Points of the Ren, Taiyang (Urinary Bladder) and Yangming (Stomach) Channels are selected as the main points. The reinforcing method is applied. Moxibustion may also be used.

Prescription:

Guanyuan (Ren 4.).
Pishu (U.B. 20.).
Sanyinjiao (Sp. 6.).
Zusanli (St. 36.).

Rationale:

Guanyuan (Ren 4.) strengthens the vital energy. Pishu (U.B. 20.), Sanyinjiao (Sp. 6.) and Zusanli (St. 36.) invigorate the Spleen and Stomach, the sources of *qi* and Blood.

Plum-Blossom (Tapping) needle method:

Taiyang (Extra. 2.),
Yintang (Extra. 1.),
Huatuo Jiaji (Extra. 21.).

Method : Treat once or twice daily with moderate stimulation. Five to seven treatments constitute a course.

Ear acupuncture points:

Select from:

Forehead.
Heart.
Sympathetic Nerve.
Ear-Shenmen.
Kidney.
Endocrine.
Adrenal.
Occiput.

Method : Select 2-4 points in each treatment. Retain the needles for about 30 minutes. Treatment may be given daily, five to seven treatments comprise a course. A press needle may also be implanted intradermally.

FACIAL PARALYSIS (WEI SYNDROME OF THE FACE)

Etiology:

The onset of this disease is due to the derangements of the *qi* and blood. Malnutrition of the channels is then caused by the invasion of the channels and collaterals in the facial region by pathogenic wind, cold or phlegm.

Differentiation:

The clinical manifestations are an incomplete closing of the eye, lacrimation, drooping of the angle of the mouth and salivation. The patient has an inability to frown, raise the eyebrow, close the eye, blow out the cheek, show the teeth or whistle. There may also be pain in the mastoid region or headache. The tongue is coated white. The pulse is superficial.

Treatment:

Method : Eliminate the wind and remove the obstruction of the collaterals by applying mild stimulation with the needles to points of the Yangming Channels of Hand and Foot as the main points.

Prescription:

Yifeng (S.J. 17.).
Dicang (St. 4.).
Jiache (St. 6.).
Yangbai (G.B. 14.).
Taiyang (Extra. 2.).
Hegu (L.I. 4.).
Quanliao (S.I. 18.).
Xiaguan (St. 7.).

Manipulation: Select 3-5 points at one sitting. The method of horizontal penetration of two points may be used in penetration of Dicang (St. 4.) horizontally towards Jiache (St. 6.). Daily treatment is carried out at the commencement of the course of treatment. The following points are selected according to the signs and symptoms:

Headache:

Fengchi (G.B. 20.).

Profuse sputum:

Fenglong (St. 40.).

Difficulty in frowning and raising the eyebrow:

Zanzhu (U.B. 2.).

Sizhukong (S.J. 23.).

Incomplete closing of the eye:

Zanzhu (U.B. 2.).

Jingming (U.B. 1.).

Tongziliao (G.B. 1.).

Yuyao (Extra. 3.).

Sizhukong (S.J. 23.).

Difficulty in sniffing:

Yingxang (L.I. 20.).

Deviation of the philtrum:

Renzhong (Du 26.).

Inability to show the teeth:

Nose-Juliao (St. 3.).

Tinnitus and deafness:

Tinghui (G.B. 2.).

Twitching of the eyelids and the mouth:

Taichong (Liv. 3.).

Tenderness at the mastoid region:

Head-Wangu (G.B. 12.).

Rationale:

Combination of Hegu (L.I. 4.), and Taichong (Liv. 3), the respective Yuan (Source) Points of the Large Intestine and Liver Channels are effective in eliminating pathogenic wind in the head and face regions. Tinghui (G.B. 2.) and Head-Wangu (G.B. 12.) are useful in eliminating the wind and clearing the ear. Jiache (St. 6.), Xiaguan (St. 7.). Dicang (St. 4.), Nose-Juliao (St. 3.), Quanliao (S.I. 18.), Yangbai (G.B. 14.), Tongziliao (G.B. 1.), Zanzhu (U.B. 2.), Sizhukong (S.J. 23.), Jingming (U.B. 1.), Yingxiang (L.I. 20.), and Renzhong (Du 26.) are all local points of the affected channels. They have the effect of eliminating the wind and invigorating the circulation in the channels and collaterals.

Moxibustion : In long-standing cases, the warming needle or mild moxibustion may be applied. The points are Taiyang (Extra. 2.), Jiache (St. 6.), Dicang (St. 4.), Nose-Juliao (St. 3.) and Xiaguan (St. 7.). Two or three points may be used at each treatment, with heat applied to each for 2-3 minutes.

Cupping : Cupping may be used as an adjunct method to acupuncture. The affected side may be treated with small cups.

Note: This disease is the same as peripheral (lower motor neuron facial paralysis) or Bell's palsy of modern medicine.

SUNSTROKE (EXTRINSIC EXCESS HEAT DISORDER)

Etiology:

This is due to the invastion of the body by summer heat, damaging the *qi* and *yin* and causing extreme fatigue from prolonged exposure to the sun.

Differentiation:

Sunstrokes may be divided into the mild and severe types. The clinical features are:

(1) The mild type : Headache, sweating, hot skin, coarse breathing, dry tongue and mouth, thirst, with a superficial full, and rapid pulse.

(2) The severe type : Headache, thirst, shallow breathing followed by sudden collapse, loss of consciousness, sweating with a deep and forceless by sudden collapse, loss of consciousness, sweating with a deep and forceless pulse.

Treatment:

(1)The mild type:

Method : Eliminate the summer heat by application of the reducing method of stimulation to points selected from the Du. Jueyin (Pericardium), and Yangming (Large Intestine) Channels as the main points.

Prescription:

Dazhui (Du 14.).
Daling (P. 7.).
Weizhong (U.B. 40.).
Hegu (L.I. 4.).
Quchi (L.I. 11.).
Jinjin, Yuye (Extra. 10.).

Rationale:

Dazhui (Du 14.) eliminates heat. Daling (P. 7.) reduces the fire of the heart. Pricking Weizhong (U.B. 40.) to cause bleeding dispels the summer heat. Hegu (L.I. 4.) and Quchi (L.I. 11.) are the two main antipyretic points. Pricking and bleeding Jinjin, Yuye (Extra. 10.) may relieve the dry mouth and the thirst.

(2) The severe type:

Method : Reduce the heat and re-establish consciousness by applying the reducing method to points of the Du Channel as the main points.

Prescription:

Renzhong (Du 26.).
Baihui (Du 20.).
Weizhong (U.B. 40.).
Shixuan (Ex. 30.).

Rationale:

Renzhong (Du 26.) and Baihui (Du 20.). are used to promote resuscitation and mental clearness respectively. Weizhong (U.B. 40.) and Shixuan Ex. 30.) will reduce the Summer heat.

MALARIA (EXTRINSIC HUMID HEAT AND DAMP DISORDER)

Etiology:

Malaria is known today as quotidian malaria, tertian malaria and quartan malaria, according to the interval between the attacks. In ancient times these rhythmic attacks were described. In chronic cases there may be enlargements felt in the right and left hypochondria.

Onset of the disease is mostly due to derangement of the nutrient *qi* and the defensive *qi* (weiqi) caused by humid heat and damp attacking the Shaoyang Channel, complicated with an epidemic factor. The main manifestations are alternate chills and fever.

Differentiation:

Chills are usually present at the beginning of the seizure, followed by fever with symptoms and signs of headache, flushed face and thirst. After the attack, the fever subsides and there is general sweating. There may be a stifling feeling in the chest and the hypochondrium regions, a bitter taste in the mouth, yellow, sticky, thinly coated tongue, a wiry and rapid pulse.

Treatment:

Method : The treatment mainly aims at regulating the Du Channel and harmonizing the Shaoyang Channels. If chills are the dominant symptom during the attack, acupuncture and moxibution may be used simultaneously. If fever is the dominant symptom, acupuncture only is used. Treatment is given two hours prior to the expected time of the symptoms.

Prescription:[1]

Dazhui (Du 14.). This is the main point.

Taodao (Du 13.).

Foot-Linqi (G.B. 41.).

1 This is the classic prescription used by the Red Army acupuncturists during The Great Revolution in China.

Houxi (S.I. 3.).
Janshi (P. 5.).

Supplementary points:

High fever-Quchi (L.I. 11.), needling with the reducing method, (strong stimulation).

A mass in the right hypochondrium-Zhangmen (Liv. 13.)-Huangmen (U.B. 51.). Apply acupuncture at the former point and moxibustion at the latter point.

In a severe attack with delirium and mental cloudiness-Prick the twelve Jing-Well Points of the hand (Lu. 11., H. 9., P. 9., L.I. 1., S.J. 1., S.I. 1.). Bleeding is carried out.

Ear-acupuncture points:

Adrenal.
Subcortex.
Endocrine.
Sanjiao.
Spleen.

Rationale:

Dazhui (Du 14.) and Taodao (Du 13.) will remove the obstruction in the Du Channel and therefore harmonize *yin* and *yang*, while Foot-Linqi (G.B. 41.) harmonizes the *qi* of the Shaoyang Channels. Houxi (S.I. 3.) disperses the exterior heat, and Jianshi (P. 5.) eliminates the interior heat. When both the exterior and interior heat subside, the coordination of nutrient *qi* and defensive *qi* (vital functions) is obtained. This checks the disease.

Method : Treatment may be given 1-2 hours before the attack successively for three days. Retain needles for one hour. For recurrent cases, add the auricular point Spleen.

AN EXCESS EXTRINSIC LUNG DISORDER (THE COMMON COLD)

Etiology:

Causative factors are exogenous wind-cold or wind-heat which hinders the dispersing action of the lung. Low defensive vital activity of the superficial portions of the body is a contributory cause. The type of cough discussed here, occurs frequently in the common cold, acute and chronic bronchitis and pneumonias.

Differentiation:

(1) The common cold due to wind-cold : Chills, fever, dry skin, headache, nasal obstruction, rhinitis, and aching of joints. There may also be itching of the throat, and cough. Tongue coating is thin and white and the pulse is superficial and tense.

(2) The common cold due to wind-heat: Fever, intolerance of wind, sweating, distended sensation in the head, thirst, hacking cough, dry, congested and sore throat, thin and yellowish tongue coating, a superficial and rapid pulse.

Treatment:

(1) *Wind-cold type of the common cold:*

Method : To eliminate the wind relieve the exterior symptoms by applying the reducing method to points of the Du, Taiyang and Shaoyang Channels as the main points.

Prescription :

Fengfu (Du 16.).

Fengmen (U.B. 12.).

Fengchi (G.B. 20.).

Lieque (Lu. 7.).

Hegu (L.I. 4.).

Fuliu (K. 7.).

Points according to the signs and symptoms:

Headache:

Taiyang (Ex. 2.).

Nasal obstruction:

Yingxiang (L.I. 20.).

Rationale:

Fengfu (Du 16.), Fengmen (U.B. 12.) and Fengchi (G.B. 20.) with stimulation alleviate the headache by eliminating wind and relieving the exterior symptoms. Lieque (Lu. 7.), the Luo (Connecting) Point of the Lung Channel, is used in treating disorders of the head, neck, and relieving the nasal obstruction. Hegu (L.I. 4.) and Fuliu (K. 7.) help to cause sweating and relieve the exterior symptoms. Taiyang (Ex. 2.) and Yingxiang (L.I. 20.) are local points used to eliminate pathogenic wind in the scalp and facial region.

(2) Wind-heat type of the common cold:

Method : To eliminate the wind and heat by applying needling with the reducing method to points of the Du and Shaoyang Channels as the main points.

Prescription:

Dazhui (Du 14.).
Fengchi (G.B. 20.).
Waiguan (S.J. 5.).
Hegu (L.I. 4.).
Shaoshang (Lu. 11.).

Rationale:

Dazhui (Du 14.) is a point where the Du Channel and all the *yang* channels meet. Fengchi (G.B. 20.), Waiguan (S.J. 5.) and Hegu (L.I. 4.) eliminate the wind and heat. Pricking Shaoshang (Lu. 11.) to cause bleeding eliminates wind-heat in the Lung Channel and allays the symptoms of the sore throat.

Prophylaxis:

Application of moxibustion to Fengmen (U.B. 12.) or Zusanli (St. 36.) daily helps prevent a common cold when this disease is prevalent in the area. Acupuncture and moxibustion were often used in ancient times as a preventive.

LUNG DEFICIENCY (CHRONIC COUGH)

Etiology:

Causative factors may be exogenous or endogenous such as wind-cold or wind-heat which attack the lung, preventing it from performing its functions of dispersing Endogenous factors are (1) dryness of its descending function, and (2) *xu* (deficiency) of the *yang* of the Spleen leading to accumulation of damp and the formation of phlegm.

Differentiation:

(1) Invasion by exogenous pathogenic factors:

(a) Wind-cold type : Chills, fever, headache, nasal obstruction and choking cough. The tongue has a thin white coating and the pulse is superficial.

(b) Wind-heat type : Fever without chills, thirst, cough with purulent thick sputum, yellow tongue coating, and superficial rapid pulse.

(2) Endogenous pathogenic factors:

(a) Dryness of the lung to *xu* (deficiency) of *yin:* Dry cough with a scanty sputum, dry or sore throat. There may be bloody sputum or even hemoptysis, afternoon fever, and a malar flush. A red tongue with a thin coating and feeble rapid pulse may be present.

(b) *Xu* (Deficiency) of *yang* of the Spleen: Cough with excessive sputum which becomes severe in winter, anorexia, listlessness, thick, sticky, slippery, whitecoated tongue. The pulse is usually deep and slow.

Treatment:

(1) Invasion by exogenous pathogenic factors:

Method : Points are mainly selected from the Taiyin (Lung) and Yangming (the Large Intestine) Channels to activate the dispersing functions of the Lung and to relieve the exterior symptoms. For wind-cold type, acupuncture may be combined with moxibustion; for the wind-heat type acupuncture only is used.

Prescription:

Lieque. (Lu. 7.).

Flegu (L.I. 4.).

Feishu (U.B. 13.).

Chize (Lu. 5.).

Rationale:

Lieque (Lu. 7.) and Hegu (L.I. 4.), the combination of Yuan (Source) and Luo (Connecting) Points, are used to eliminate the wind and relieve the exterior symptoms. Feishu (U.B. 13.) activates the dispersing function of the Lung, Chize (Lu. 5.) clears the Lung and thereby relieves the cough.

(2) Endogenous factors:

(a) Dryness of the Lung due to *xu* (deficiency) of *yin:*

Method : The Back-Shu and Front-Mu Points of the Lung are used as the main points to tonify the *yin* and activate the descending function of the Lung. Points are punctured superficially. Moxibustion is not advisable.

Prescription:

Feishu (U.B. 13.).

Zhongfu (Lu. 1.).

Lieque (Lu. 7.).

Zhaohai (K. 6.).

Secondary points for hemoptysis:

Kongzui (Lu. 6.).

Geshu (U.B. 17.).

Rationale:

Feishu (U.B. 13.), and Zhongfu (Lu. 1.), a combination of Back-Shu and Front-Mu Points, are used to regulate the respiratory tract. Lieque (Lu. 7.) and Zhaohai (K. 6.), a pair of Confluent Points, may ease the throat through their action of tonifying the *yin* and activating the descending *qi* of the Lung. Kongzui (Lu. 6.), the Xi-Cleft Point of the Lung and Geshu (U.B. 17.), the Influential Point for Blood, are used to achieve an hemostatic effect.

(b) Xu (deficiency) of Yang of Spleen:

Method : The Back-Shu Point of the Spleen and the Front-Mu Point of the Stomach are taken as the main points to strengthen the Spleen and resolve the sputum. Apply needling with the reinforcing method combined with moxibustion.

Prescription:

Pishu (U.B. 20.).

Zhongwan (Ren 12.).

Zusanli (St. 36.).

Feishu (U.B. 13.).

Gaohuangshu (U.B. 43.).

Fenglong (St. 40.).

Rationale:

Pishu (U.B. 20.), Zhongwan (Ren 12.) and Zusanli (St. 36.) strengthen the Spleen and Stomach to eliminate damp and resolve the phlegm. Application of moxibustion to Feishu (U.B. 13.) and Gaohuangshu (U.B. 43.) activates and gives warmth to the *qi* of the Lung.

Cupping method:

Main points:

Fengmen (U.B. 12.).

Feishu (U.B. 13.).

Plum-Blossom method : Tap along the Du and Urinary Bladder Channels on the upper part of the trunk till the skin becomes red.

Ear Acupuncture points:

Main points:

Dingchuan.

Spleen.

Method : Treatment is given once daily or every other day. Needles are retained for about 30 minutes. A course may be 5-10 treatments. Press needles may also be used.

IMBALANCE OF THE LUNGS (BRONCHIAL ASTHMA)

Etiology:

There are two main types of bronchial asthma: the *xu* type and the *shi* type. *Shi* type asthma results from the dysfunction of Lung due to an invasion by exogenous wind-cold or disturbance of phlegm-heat. *Xu* type asthma is due to (1) *xu* (weakness) or deficiency of the Lung, or (2) *xu* (weakness) of the Kidney which fails to perform its function of receiving *qi* (air) thereby creating an excess of the Lung.

Differentiation:

(1) *Shi type:*

(a) Wind-cold : Cough with thin sputum, shortness of breath. Usually there are accompanying symptoms of fever, chills, anhidrosis, a white coating of the tongue, and a superficial pulse.

(b) Phlegm-heat : Rapid and coarse breathing, stifling sensation in the chest, thick purulent sputum, thick yellowish coating on the tongue, and a rapid, rolling forceful pulse.

(2) *Xu* type : (Deficiency of Lung or Kidney).

(a) *Xu* of Lung : Short and quick breathing, weak and low voice, sweating and weak pulse.

(b) *Xu* of Kidney (Deficiency of kidney) : Asthma, dyspnea upon exertion, chillness with cold extremities, deep thready and feeble pulse.

Treatment:

(1) *Shi type:*

Method: For asthma due to wind-cold, points of the Lung Channel are taken as the main points to eliminate wind and cold and soothe the asthma. For asthma due to phlegm-heat, points of the Stomach Channel are taken as the main points to resolve phlegm and soothe the asthma. Puncture with the reducing method for both types. Moxibustion may be added for the former type of disorder.

Prescription :

(a) Wind-cold:
Feishu (U.B. 13.).
Lieque (Lu. 7.).
Hegu (L.I. 4..

(b) Phlegm-heat:
Fenglong (St. 40.).
Tiantu (Ren 22.).
Chize (Lu. 5.).
Dingchuan (Soothing Asthma) (Extra. 17).

Rationale:

Feishu (U.B. 13.) activates the *qi* of the Lung. Lieque (Lu. 7.) and Hegu (L.I. 4.) eliminate the wind and cold. Fenglong (St. 40.), a Distal point, combined with Tiantu (Ren 22.), a Local point, relieves breathing difficulties and resolves the phlegm. Chize (Lu. 5.), He-Sea Point of the Lung Channel reduces the heat in the Lung to soothe the asthma.

(2) *Xu* type:

Method : Reinforce the *qi* (vital energy) of the Lung and Kidney. Puncture with the reinforcing (tonification) method. Moxibustion is advisable.

Prescription :

(a) *Xu* of Lung:

Feishu (U.B. 13.).

Taiyuan (Lu. 9.).

Zusanti (St. 36.).

(b) *Xu* of Kidney:

Shenshu (U.B. 23.).

Mingmen (Du 4.).

Shanzhong (Ren 17.).

Qihai (Ren 6.).

Secondary points:

Chronic persistent asthma:

Shenzhu (Du 12.).

Gaohuangshu (U.B. 43.).

Xu of Spleen:

Zhongwan (Ren 12.).

Pishu (U.B. 20.).

Rationale:

Applying moxibustion to Feishu (U.B. 13.) reinforces the *qi* of the Lung. According to the theory of the five elements, both Taiyuan (Lu. 9.), the Shu-Stream Point of the Lung Channel and Zusanli (St. 36.), the He-Sea Point of the Stomach Channel, are related to the element earth. Puncturing these two points strengthens the Lung (metal) through invigorating the Spleen (earth) and Stomach (earth). Shenshu (U.B. 23.) and Mingmen (Du 4.) reinforce the *qi* (vital energy) of the Kidney. Qihai (Ren 6.) is an essential point for strengthening *qi.* Shanzhong (Ren 17.), the Influential Point dominating *qi.* of respiration, is for regulating *qi* and soothing asthma. Application of indirect moxibustion with garlic to Shenzhu (Du 12.) and Gaohuangshu (U.B. 43.) help relieve chronic asthma. Application of moxibustion to Zhongwan (Ren 12.) and Pishu (U.B. 20.) strengthens the *qi* (vital energy) of the Spleen.

Ear acupuncture points:

Ear acupuncture may be applied during the attack as well as for the interim period of treatment.

Main points:

Lung.

Kidney.

Adrenal.

Sympathetic Nerve.

Dingchuan.

Method : Select 2-3 points each time, or puncture the tender points. Needles are retained for about 30 minutes. After about 10-15 sittings 3-5 days rest may be given before starting another course of treatment.

DISHARMONY OF THE HEART AND OTHER ORGANS (INSOMNIA)

Etiology:

Common causative factors are:

(1) *xu* of Spleen and Blood insufficiency resulting from anxiety.

(2) flaring of the Heart fire due to insufficiency of *yin* in the Kidney causing disharmony of Heart and Kidney.

(3) upward disturbance of the Liver fire resulting from mental depression.

(4) retention of phlegm-heat due to indigestion (Stomach excess).

Differentiation:

(1) *Xu* of Spleen and Blood insufficiency : Difficulty in falling asleep and disturbed sleep accompained by palpitation, poor memory, lassitude, listlessness, anorexia, sallow complexion, and a thready weak pulse.

(2) Disharmony of the Heart and Kidney : Irritability and insomnia accompanied by dizziness, tinnitus, low back pain, seminal emission, leucorrhea and a rapid, weak pulse.

(3) Upward disturbance of the Liver fire : Mental depression, quick temper and dream-disturbed sleep accompained by headache, distending pain in the costal and hypochondriac regions, a bitter taste in the mouth and a wiry pulse.

(4) Dysfunction of the Stomach : Insomnia accompanied by fullness and suffocating feeling in the epigastric region, abdominal distention, belching, and a full forceful pulse.

Treatment:

Method : Points are mainly selected from the Heart Channel to calm the Heart and thereby to soothe the mind (Brain).

Xu of Spleen and Blood insufficiency : Apply needling with the reinforcing method. Moxibustion is used in combination.

Disharmony of the Heart and Kidneys : Apply needling with mild stimulation.

Upward disturbance of the Liver fire : Apply needling with the reducing method.

Dysfunction of the Stomach : Apply needling with the reducing method.

Prescription :

Shenmen (H. 7.).

Neiguan (P. 6.).

Sanyinjiao (Sp. 6.).

Points according to the different syndromes:

Xu of Spleen and Blood insufficiency:

Pishu (U.B. 20.).

Xinshu (U.B. 15.).

Yinbai (Sp. 1.), (moxibustion with small moxa cones).

Disharmony of the Heart and Kidney:

Xinshu (U.B. 15.).

Shenshu (U.B. 23.).

Taixi (K. 3.).

Upward disturbance of the Liver fire:

Ganshu (U.B. 18.).

Danshu (U.B. 19.).

Head-Wangu (G.B. 12.).

Dysfunction of the Stomach:

Weishu (U.B. 21.).

Zusanli (St. 36.).

Rationale:

Shenmen (H. 7.) is the Yuan (Source) Point of the Heart Channel, Neiguan (P. 6.) the Luo (Connecting) Point of the Pericardium Channel, and Sanyinjiao (Sp. 6.) the Crossing Point of the Liver, Spleen and Kidney Channels. Combining these three points calms the Heart and soothes the mind (Brain). Pishu (U.B. 20.) and Xinshu (U.B. 15.) are used because the Spleen controls the Blood, and the Heart produces Blood. Yinbai (Sp. 1.). is the Jing-Well Point of the Spleen Channel. Moxibustion using small moxa cones at this point treats dream-disturbed sleep and nightmares. Combination of Xinshu (U.B. 15.), Shenshu (U.B. 23.), and Taixi (K. 3.) adjusts the disharmony of the Heart and Kidney. Combination of Ganshu (U.B. 18.), Danshu (U.B.

19.) and Head-Wangu (G.B. 12.) reduces the upward disturbance of the Liver and Gall bladder. Weishu (U.B. 21.) and Zusanli (St. 36.) are used to promote the digestion in the Stomach and relieve the distension.

Remarks:

(1) *Plum-Blossom method* : Tap on Sishencong (Extra. 6.) and Huatuojiaji (Ex. 21.) lightly from above downwards 2-3 times at one sitting. Give treatment once daily or every other day. Ten treatments constitute a course. Continue treatment regularly till symptoms subside.

(2) *Ear Acupuncture points:*

Subcortex.
Ear-Shenmen.
Kidney.
Heat.

Method : Select 2-3 points each time. Needles are retained for about 30 minutes or embedded for 3-5 days.

EXCESS OF HEART (PALPITATION, ANXIETY)

Etiology:

(1) Deficiency of *qi* and Blood due to mental disturbances or fright caused by anxiety.

(2) Disturbance of the Heart by the stirring of endogenous phlegm fire.

(3) Perversion of harmful fluid due to dysfunction of the Heart. In mild cases, palpitation may be intermittent; in severe cases, there may be a continuous, throbbing sensation in the chest.

Differentiation:

(1) Insufficiency of *qi* and Blood: Pallor, shortness of breath, general weakness, disturbed sleep, dizziness, blurring of vision, pale

flabby tongue with teeth marks on its margin and a thready forceless pulse.

(2) Stirring of endogenous phlegm-fire: Irritability, restlessness, dream-disturbed sleep, yellow coating on the tongue and a rolling rapid pulse.

(3) Retention of harmful fluid : Expectoration of mucoid sputum, fullness in the chest and epigastric region, lassitude, a white coating on the tongue, and wiry, rolling pulse.

Treatment:

Method : Apply strong manual stimulation at the Back-Shu and Front-Mu Points of the Heart as the main points, to sedate the Heart.

Prescription:

Xinshu (U.B. 15.).
Juque (Ren 14.).
Shenmen (H. 7.).
Neiguan (P. 6.).

Points according to the syndromes:

(1) Insufficiency of *qi* and blood:

Qihai (Ren 6.).
Pishu (U.B. 20.).
Weishu (U.B. 21.).

(2) Stirring of endogenous phlegm-fire:

Fenglong (St. 40.).
Yanglingquan (G.B. 34.).

(3) Retention of harmful fluid:

Guanyuan (Ren 4.).
Sanjiaoshu (U.B. 22.).
Zusanli (St. 36.).
Shanzhong (Ren 17.).

Rationale:

Xinshu (U.B. 15.) and Juque (Ren 14.), the Back-Shu and Front-Mu Points of the Heart, Shenmen (H. 7.), the Yuan (Source) Point of the Heart Channel, and Neiguan (P. 6.), the Luo-Connecting Point of the Pericardium Channel, all have the properties of regulating *qi* and Blood of the Heart and acting as a tranquilizer. Qihai (Ren 6.) strengthens *qi*. Pishu (U.B. 20.) and Weishu (U.B. 21.) adjust the functions of the Spleen and Stomach, where the *qi* and blood is produced. Applying acupuncture or moxibustion at Guanyuan (Ren 4.), Shanzhong (Ren 17.) and Zusanli (St. 36.) will strengthen the Spleen, invigorate *yang* and eliminate harmful fluids. Sanjiaoshu (U.B. 22.) regulates the upper, middle and lower *jiao* and promotes the transportation of water. Fenglong (St. 40.) and Yanglingquan (G.B. 34.) eliminate the phlegm-fire in the Stomach.

Ear acupuncture points:

Ear-Shenmen.

Heart.

Sympathetic Nerve.

Subcortex.

Small Intestine.

Methods : Select 2-3 points in each treatment and give moderate stimulation. Needles are retained for 15-20 minutes. Treatment is given every other day. About 10-15 treatments constitute a course. A 3-5 days interval between the courses of treatment is given to the patient.

Note: Palpitation and anxiety, according to Western medicine may be symptoms present in neurosis, functional disorders of the autonomic nervous system, and cardiac arrhythmias of diverse origins.

HEART DYSFUNCTIONS (DEPRESSIVE AND MANIC MENTAL DISORDERS)

Etiology:

Depressive mental disorders are usually caused by the retardation of *qi* and the accumulation of phlegm resulting from mental depression. Manic disorders may be caused by:

(1) A *qi* stasis due to a circulatory defect, which elicits fire and causes formation of phlegm.

(2) An excessive heat in the Stomach hindering the descent of harmful *qi* which results in the accumulation of heat disturbing the mind (Brain).

Differentiation:

(1) Depressive mental disorder: Gradual onset, mental depression and dullness at the initial stage, followed by gradual dysphasia, aphasia, or muteness, hypersomnia and anorexia. The tongue is thinly or moderately coated. The pulse is wiry and thready.

(2) Manic mental disorder : Sudden onset, preceded by irritability, peevishness, impaired sleeping and poor appetite. This is followed by mania demonstrated by shouting, yelling, tearing off the clothes, running around and sleeplessness. The tongue is yellow and sticky. The pulse is usually wiry, rolling and rapid.

Treatment:

Method : Points from the Du Channel and Hand-Jueyin (Pericardium) Channel are selected as the main points to calm the Heart and mind (Brain) and restore the mental clarity. For depressive mental disorders, apply needling with the tonification method. Moxibustion may be applied according to the deficiency diagnosed. For mania, use the reducing (sedation) method of needling.

Prescription:

Renzhong (Du 26.).

Shaoshang (Lu. 11.).

Yinbai (Sp. 1.).
Daling (P. 7.).
Shenmai (U.B. 62.).
Fengfu (Du 16.).
Jiache (St. 6.).
Chengjiang (Ren 24.).
Laogong (P. 8.).
Shangxing (Du 23.).
Quchi (L.I. 11.).

Points for manic cases with extreme heat: Prick all the 12 Jing-Well Points on the hand (Lu. 11., H. 9., P.9., L.I. 1., S.J. 1., S.I. 1.) to cause bleeding and thereby to reduce heat.

Rationale:

Renzhong (Du 26.), Shaoshang (Lu. 11.) and Yinbai (Sp. 1.) are effective points for re-establishing mental clarity dispelling the heat and suppressing mania. Daling (P. 7.), the Yuan-Source Point of the Pericardium Channel, and Laogong (P. 8.), the Ying-Spring Point of the Pericardium Channel, are used to reduce the heat in the Pericardium Channel. Shenmai (U.B. 62.), Fengfu (Du 16.) and Shangxing (Du 23.) Dispel the heat in the Yangqiao Channel and Du Channel to tranquilize the mind. Jiache (St. 6.) and Quchi (L.I. 11.) dissipate the heat from the Hand and Foot-Yangming Channels.

Ear Acupuncture points:

Sympathetic Nerve.
Ear-Shenmen.
Heart.
Liver.
Subcortex.
Endocrine.
Stomach.
Occiput.

Method : Select one or two points at each sitting.

Note: Depressive and manic mental disorders correspond to the depressive and manic types of schizophrenia and psychosis of modern medicine.

DYSFUNCTION OF THE STOMACH (GASTRITIS, PEPTIC ULCER, NAUSEA, VOMITING)

Etiology:

Vomiting is due to the dysfunction of the Stomach in digestion and transportation. The *qi* of the Stomach ascends instead of descending. Causative factors are:

(1) Over-eating and retention of cold and fatty foods.

(2) Perversion of the *qi* of the Liver due to anger affecting the functions of the Stomach.

(3) Weakness of the Spleen and Stomach *qi*.

Differentiation:

(1) Retention of food : Epigastric and abdominal distension with pain, acid fermented vomitus, belching, anorexia, constipation, and foul gas. The tongue has a thin, sticky coating, the pulse wiry.

(2) Invasion of the stomach, by qui of Liver - vomiting, acid regurgitation, continual belching, distending pain in hypochondrium region. The tongue has a thin, shicky, coating, the pulse wiry.

(3) Weakness of the Spleen and Stomach : Sallow complexion, vomiting after eating a very full meal, lack of appetite, slightly loose stools, general lassitude, forceless pulse, thinly coated, sticky tongue.

Treatment:

Method : Points of the Stomach Channel are the main points. When retention of food or invasion of the Stomach by *qi* of Liver is faulty, needling is given with the reducing method. For weakness of Spleen and Stomach, needling is given with the reinforcing method combined with moxibustion.

Prescription :

Zusanli (St. 36.).

Zhongwan (Ren 12.).

Neiguan (P. 6.).

Gongsun (St. 4.).

Secondary points:

(1) Retention of food:

Tianshu (St. 25.).

(2) Invasion of the Stomach by *qi* of the Liver:

Taichong (Liv. 3.).

(3) Weakness of the Spleen and the Stomach:

Pishu (U.B. 20.).

(4) Cyclical vomiting:

Jinjin, Yuye (Extra. 10.).

Rationale:

Zusanli (St. 36.). is the He-Sea Point of the Stomach Channel and Zhongwan (Ren 12.) is the Front-Mu Point of the Stomach. The two points when used together are effective in readjusting the Stomach and subduing the ascending *qi*. Neiguan (P. 6.) and Gongsun (Sp. 4.), a pair of Confluent Points, treat the feeling of fullness in the chest and the Stomach. Stimulation of Tianshu (St. 25.) relieves intestinal obstruction. Needling Taichong (Liv. 3.) with the reducing method activates the functions of the Liver. Needling Pishu (U.B. 20.) with the reinforcing method, strengthens the Spleen. Pricking Jinjin, Yuye (Extra. 10.) to cause bleeding is a symptomatic method of treating Stomach dysfunciton.

■

DYSFUNCTION OF THE STOMACH AND DIAPHRAGM (HICCUP, HICCOUGH)

Etiology:

(1) Failure of *qi* of the Stomach to descend caused by irregular food intake and stagnation of *qi* of the Liver.

(2) Ascending of *qi* of Stomach caused by an attack of cold.

Differentiation:

(1) Retention of food and stagnation of *qi* : Epigastric and abdominal distension, hiccups, yellowish sticky coated tongue, rolling forceful pulse. There may be distending pain in the chest and hypochondrium, irritability and a wiry forceful pulse.

(2) Attack by pathogenic cold : Slow but forceful hiccough which may be alleviated by hot drinks; white moist tongue coating, slow pulse.

Treatment:

Method : Points are mainly selected from the Foot-Yangming (Stomach) Channel to regularize the functions of the Stomach, subdue the ascending *qi* and relieve hiccups. In cases due to retention of food and stagnation of *qi*, needling with the reducing (sedation) method is advisable. For cases due to cold, acupuncture should be combined with moxibustion.

Prescription:

Zusanli (St. 36.).
Zhongwan (Ren 12.).
Neiguan (P. 6.).
Geshu (U.B. 17.).
Tiantu (Ren 22.).

Points for the different syndromes:

(1) Retention of food and stagnation of *qi*:
Neiting (St. 44.).

Taichong (Liv. 3.).

Juque (Ren 14.).

(2) Attack by pathogenic cold:

Shangwan (Ren 13.).

Rationale:

Zusanli (St. 36.), Zhongwan (Ren 12.), and Neiguan (P. 6.) help to relieve the sensation of fullness in the chest and activate the *qi*. Geshu (U.B. 17.) and Tiantu (Ren 22.) subdue the ascending *qi*. Neiting (St. 44.) normalises the Stomach and relieves the stagnation. Taichong (Liv. 3.) readjusts the *qi* of the Liver. Juque (Ren 14.) relieves the chest and diaphragm to allay hiccups. Application of moxibustion to Shangwan (Ren 13.) warms the Spleen and the Stomach and thereby eliminates the cold.

Ear acupuncture points:

Ear-Shenmen.

Diaphragm.

Subcortex.

Method : Give strong stimulation. Needles are retained for about an hour.

DISHARMONY OF THE STOMACH (EPIGASTRIC PAIN)

Etiology:

(1) Irregular meals which injure the Spleen and the Stomach.

(2) Imbalance of the Stomach by perversion of Liver *qi* due to mental depression.

(3) *Xi* of the Stomach with stagnation of cold.

Differentiation:

(1) Retention of fluid : Distention and pain in the epigastrium, pain

after eating, aggravated on abdominal pressure, belching with fetid odor, anorexia, thick sticky coated tongue with a deep, forceful pulse.

(2) Attack on Stomach by Liver *qi* : Paroxysmal pain in the epigastrium, distending pain in the hypochondrium region. There may be nausea, acidity, abdominal distension and anorexia. The pulse is deep and wiry.

(3) *Xu* of Stomach with stagnation of cold : Dull pain in the epigastrium, general lassitude, regurgitation of thin fluid, pain which may be alleviated by pressure and warmth, thin white coated tongue, a deep slow pulse.

Treatment:

Method : The principle of treatment is to pacify the Stomach and relieve the pain by a combination of Local with Distal points. For cases due to retention of food or attack on the Stomach by Liver *qi*, acupuncture with the reducing method is advisable. Needles are retained for about 30 minutes. For cases with *xu* of the Stomach and stagnation of cold, acupuncture with the tonification method combined with moxibustion is recommended.

Prescription:

Zusanli (St. 36.).
Zhongwan (Ren 12.).
Neiguan (P. 6.).

Points for the different syndromes:

(1) Retention of food:
Zhangmen (Liv. 13.).
Neiting (St. 44.).

(2) Attack on Stomach by Liver *qi:*
Taichong (Liv. 3.).
Qimen (Liv. 14.).

(3) *Xu* of Stomach with stagnation of cold:

Qihai (Ren 6.). Indirect moxibustion with ginger.

Pishu (U.B. 20.).

Gongsun (Sp. 4.).

Rationale:

Zusanli (St. 36.), the He-Sea Point of the Stomach Channel, and Zhongwan (Ren 12.), the Front-Mu Point of the Stomach, possess the effect of sedating the Stomach and relieving the pain. Neiguan (P. 6.) communicates with the Yinwei Channel, relaxes the chest and stops the vomiting. Zhangmen (Liv. 13.) and Neiting (St. 44.) Promote digestion and relieve epigastric fullness. Needling Qimen (Liv. 14.) and Taichong (Liv. 3.) with the reducing method helps promote the functions of the Liver, regulates *qi* and relieves the distension and pain. Application of moxibustion to Gongsun (Sp. 4.) and Pishu (U.B. 20.) strengthens the Spleen, pacifies the Stomach, dispels cold and relieves pain. Indirect moxibustion of Qihai (Ren 6.) with ginger is the most suitable method to treat chronic gastric pain due to cold, as ginger and moxa together have the property of dispelling cold.

Cupping method : Cupping is applied with large or medium-sized cups to the upper abdomen or the Back-Shu Points for about 10 minutes.

Ear acupuncture points:

Stomach.

Sympathetic Nerve.

Subcortex.

Duodenum.

Note: Epigastric pain described here is a symptom of gastric and peptic ulcer, gastritis, neurosis, and diseases of the Liver, Gall bladder and Pancreas.

Method : Select 2-3 points for each treatment. Needles are retained for about 30 minutes. 10-15 treatments constitute a course; 2-3 days rest is given before starting the next course.

DISHARMONY OF THE ABDOMINAL ZANG-FU IN THE MIDDLE BODY CAVITY (ABDOMINAL PAIN)

Etiology:

Causative factors:

(1) Accumulation of cold is due to an invasion of exogenous pathogenic cold and endogenous cold due to eating an excess of unsuitable cold food.

(2) Retardation of *qi* is due to the retention of food impairing the functions of transportation of the Stomach and Intestines.

Differentiation:

(1) Internal accumulation of cold : Sudden violent pain which responds to warmth; loose stools, white coated tongue and a deep tense pulse.

(2) Retention of food : Epigastric and abdominal distention and pain which may be aggravated by pressure, foul belching and acidity. Abdominal pain may be aggravated by pressure, accompained by diarrhoea relieved after defecation. The tongue is sticky : the pulse is rolling.

Treatment :

Method : Local and Distal points relevant to the diseased region and the involved channels are selected with the purpose of dispelling cold and relieving stagnation. When cold accumulates, apply both acupuncture and moxibustion. In cases of retention of food, needling with the reducing method is applied.

Prescription:

Pain above the umbilicus:

Gongsun (Sp. 4.).

Huaroumen (St. 24.).

Xiawan (Ren 10.).

Pain around the umbilicus:

Shuiquan (K. 5.).

Qihai (Ren 6.).

Tianshu (St. 25.).

Pain in the lower abdomen:

Sanyinjiao (St. 6.).

Guilai (St. 29.).

Guanyuan (Ren 4.).

Rationale:

As the region above the umbilicus relates to the Spleen, Gongsun (Sp. 4.), the Luo-Connecting Point of the Spleen Channel, combined with the local points Huaroumen (St. 24.) and Xiawan (Ren 10.) adjust the functions of the Spleen and Stomach. The umbilical region relates to the Kidney: Shuiquan (K. 5.), the Xi-Cleft Point of the Kidney Channel, combined with the local points Qihai (Ren 6.) and Tianshu (St. 25.) are prescribed. The three *yin* channels of the foot pass through the lower abdomen: Sanyinjiao (Sp. 6.), the Crossing Point of the three foot-*yin* channels, combined with the local points Guilai (St. 29.) and Guanyuan (Ren 4.) are selected.

Note: Various diseases such as disorders of the organs in the abdominal cavity and urogenital organs in the pelvic cavity of the female, intestinal parasitic diseases and functional disorders, may be accompained by the symptom of abdominal pain. Acute disorders, such as acute appendicitis, intestinal obstructions, acute peritonitis and perforation, or peptic ulcer will also cause similar symptoms. If acupuncture is applied, strict observation of the patient is necessary and other therapeutic measures such as surgery should be available, if indicated.

DYSFUNCTIONS OF THE DIGESTIVE TRACT AND ASSOCIATED ORGANS (DIARRHEA)

Etiology:

Causative factors of acute diarrhea are:

(1) Dysfunction of the digestive tract due to unsuitable food and the invasion of exogenous cold-damp;

(2) Invasion of damp-heat in summer or autumn. Chronic diarrhea is due to *xu* (insufficiency) of *yang* of Spleen and Kidney affecting the functions of transportation and transformation of the food.

Differentiation:

(1) *Acute diarrhea:*

(a) Cold-damp: Watery diarrhea with abdominal pain and borborygmos, chilliness which responds to warmth, absence of thirst, a pale tongue with a white coating and a deep, slow pulse.

(b) Damp-heat: Diarrhea with yellow, hot, loose and foetid stools, accompanied by abdominal pain, a burning sensation in the anus, scanty brownish urine, yellow sticky coated tongue, and a rolling and rapid pulse. There may be fever and thirst.

(2) *Chronic diarrhea:*

(a) Xu (insufficiency of Yang of Spleen): Loose stools with undigested food, epigastric and abdominal distention, anorexia, lassitude, thin whitish coated tongue, thready forceless pulse.

(b) *Xu* (insufficiency of *yang* of Kidney): Slight abdominal pain, borborygmos and diarrhea with pain several times each day. Cramps in the abdomen and lower extremities, a whitish coated tongue and a deep, forceless pulse.

Treatment:

Method: The Back-Shu and Front-Mu Points of the Large Intestine are the main points for treatment. For the cold-damp type, apply needling with the tonification method combined with direct moxibustion (or indirect moxibustion with ginger). For the damp-heat type, apply needling with the reducing method. Moxibustion may be the main treatment for the *xu* syndrome of *yang* of the Kidney.

Prescription :

Tianshu (St. 25.).
Dachangshu (U.B. 25.).
Zusanli (St. 36.).

Points for the different syndromes:

(1) Cold-damp:
Zhongwan (Ren 12.).
Qihai (Ren 6.).

(2) Damp-heat:
Neiting (St. 44.).
Yinlingquan (Sp. 9.).
Hegu (L.I. 4.).

(3) *Xu* of *yang* of Spleen:
Pishu (U.B. 20.).
Zhangmen (Liv. 13.).
Taibai (Sp. 3.).
Zhongwan (Ren 12.).

(4) *Xu* of *yang* of Kidney:
Shenshu (U.B. 23.).
Mingmen (Du 4.).
Taixi (K. 3.).
Guanyuan (Ren 4.).
Baihui (Du 20.).

Rationale:

Tianshu (St. 25.) and Dachangshu (U.B. 25.), the Front-Mu and Back-Shu Points of the Large Intestine are effective in adjusting the transporting functions of the Large Intestine and relieving the diarrhea. Zusanli (St. 36.) is used to strengthen the transporting functions of the Spleen and Stomach. Application of acupuncture and moxibustion dispels the cold of the Spleen and Stomach. Needling Neiting (St. 44.), Yinlingquan (Sp. 9.) and Hegu (L.I. 4.) with the reducing method eliminates the damp-heat in the Large Intestine. Application of acupuncture and moxibustion to Pishu (U.B. 20.), Zhangmen (Liv. 13.) and Taibai (Sp. 3.), the Back-Shu, Front-Mu and Yuan-Source Points of the Spleen respectively, together with Zhongwan (Ren 12.), the Front-Mu Point of the Stomach, invigorates the *yang* of the Spleen, promotes the transporting functions and relieves the diarrhea. Shenshu (U.B. 23.) Mingmen (Du 4.) and Taixi (K. 3.) are able to warm and invigorate the *yang* of the Kidney.

Note: Diarrhea according to traditional Chinese medicine, includes diarrhea appearing in acute and chronic enteritis, dyspepsia, intestinal parasitic diseases, diseases of the pancreas, liver and biliary tract, disorders of endocrine origin, as well as diarrhea due to psychosomatic causes is described in Western medicine.

DYSFUNCTIONS OF THE LARGE INTESTINE (DYSENTERY)

Etiology:

This disease is usually caused by disorders of the Intestines and Stomach due to the invasion of damp-heat or cold-damp and the intake of contaminated food.

Differentiation:

The main clinical types of dysentery are:

(1) The Damp-heat type : Abdominal pain, tenesmus, white with red streaked (or mainly red) mucus in stool. There may be accompanying symptoms of high fever, nausea and vomiting. The tongue is frequently yellow, sticky and coated; the pulse is rolling and rapid.

(2) The Cold-damp type: Scanty defecation of white mucus stained stools. The patient responds to warmth and dislikes the cold. There is usually accompanying symptoms of fullness in the chest and epigastrium, abdominal pain, loss of taste, absence of thirst, a white, sticky, coated tongue and a deep, slow pulse.

(3) Chronic dysentery: Prolonged persistent dysentery or recurrent dysentery occurs. In addition, there may be lassitude, a sallow complexion, feeling of cold, anorexia and a deep, thready pulse.

Treatment:

Method: The Front-Mu and the inferior He-Sea Points of the Large Intestine are the main points to relieve the stagnation and promote the smooth transportation. For dysentery of the Damp-heat type, apply needling with the reducing (sedation) method; for that of cold-damp type, apply needling with tonification together with moxibustion; while for chronic dysentery, needling is given with the reinforcing method combined with moxibustion (moxa on the needle).

Prescription:

Tianshu (St. 25.).

Shangjuxu (St. 37.).

Hegu (L.I. 4.).

Points for the different syndromes and symptoms

(1) Damp-heat type:

Quchi (L.I. 11.).

Neiting (St. 44.).

Yinlingquan (Sp. 9.).

(2) The Cold-damp type:

Zhongwan (Ren 12.).

Qihai (Ren 6.).

Sanyinjiao (Sp. 6.).

(3) Chronic dysentery:

Pishu (U.B. 20.).

Weishu (U.B. 21.).

Zhongwan (Ren 12.).

Zusanli (St. 36.).

(4) Tenesmus:

Zhonglushu (U.B. 29.).

(5) Prolapse of the rectum:

Baihui (Du 20.).

Rationale:

It is recorded in the *Nei Jing* that for diseases of the *Fu* organs, He-Sea Points are recommended. Therefore Shangjuxu (St. 37.), the Inferior He-Sea Point of the Large Intestine, Tianshu (St. 25.), and Hegu (L.I. 4.) are used as the main points to relieve stagnation in the intestines. Needling Neiting (St. 44.), Quchi (L.I. 11.) and Yinlingquan (Sp. 9.) with the reducing method eliminates damp-heat. Application of moxibustion at Zhongwan (Ren 12.) and Qihai (Ren 6.) warms the Spleen and Stomach to dispel cold.

Sanyinjiao (Sp. 6.) strengthens the Spleen and disperses damp. Applying acupuncture with either the reinforcing or reducing methods as indicated; and frequent moxibustion to Pishu (U.B. 20.), Zhongwan (Ren 12.) and Zusanli (St. 36.) warms the Spleen and Stomach and also eliminates intestinal stagnation.

Note: Dysentery according to traditional Chinese medicine includes acute and chronic forms of both the bacillary and amoebic types of dysentery as described in Western medicine.

JAUNDICE (DYSFUNCTIONS OF THE BILE CIRCULATION)

Etiology:

Dysfunctions of the Spleen and Stomach in transporting and transforming, leads to an internal accumulation of damp which impedes the normal excretion of bile causing a yellowish discoloration of the skin. There are two types of jaundice:

(1) the *yang* type in which damp-heat is dominant.

(2) the *yin* type in which cold-damp is dominant.

Differentiation:

Jaundice is characterized by yellow sclera, skin and urine. Yellow with lustre indicates the *yang* type, while lustreless yellow indicates the *yin* type of disorder.

Jaundice of the *yang* type is usually accompanied by fever, a heavy sensation in the body, thirst, fullness in the abdomen, a yellow, sticky, coated tongue, a wiry and rapid pulse.

Jaundice of the *yin* type is usually accompanied by a heavy sensation in the body, lassitude, somnolence, absence of thirst, a thick white coated tongue and a deep slow pulse.

Treatment:

Method : Points are selected mainly from the Taiyin (Spleen), Yangming (Stomach) and Shaoyang (Gall bladder) Channels. Needling with the reducing method is recommended for treating jaundice of the *yang* type, as the principle is to dispel the damp-heat. In treating jaundice of the *yin* type, the principle is to dispel damp by warming the Spleen and Stomach. Needling is carried out daily by combining the tonification method with moxibustion.

Prescription:

Yinlingquan (Sp. 9.).

Zusanli (St. 36.).

Riyue (G.B. 24.).

Danshu (U.B. 19.).

Yanggang (U.B. 48.).

Zhiyang (Du 9.).

Points for the different clinical types:

Yang type:

Penetration of Taichong (Liv. 3.) towards Yongquan (K. 1.).

Yanglingquan (G.B. 34.).

Yin type:

Pishu (U.B. 20.).

Zhangmen (Liv. 13.).

Rationale:

Yinlingquan (Sp. 9.) and Zusanli (St. 36.) strengthens the Spleen to deperse the damp. Riyue (G.B. 24.), Danshu (U.B. 19.), Zhiyang (Du 9.) and Yanggang (U.B. 48.) are essential points for the treatment of jaundice. Taichong (Liv. 3.) and Yanglingquan (G.B. 34.) eliminate the heat in the *yang* type of jaundice. Application of moxibustion to Pishu (U.B. 20.) and Zhangmen (Liv. 13.) in the *yin* type disperses the cold-damp.

Note: Jaundice, as discussed here, is seen in the acute infective hepatitis of Western medicine, and in Gall bladder and Liver disorders.

LIVER AND GALL BLADDER DYSFUNCTIONS (HYPOCHONDRIUM PAIN)

Etiology:

The Liver Channel supplies the costal and hypochondrium region. Emotional depression from various causes may depress Liver functions causing insufficient circulation of *qi* in the channels resulting in costal and hypochondrium pain. Traumatic injuries such as a sprain or contusion may also cause hypochondrium pain due to blood stasis in the collaterals.

Differentiation:

Stagnation of *qi:* Pain in the costal and hypochondrium regions, fullness in the chest, a bitter taste and a wiry pulse. The severity of symptoms varies with the emotional state.

Stagnation of Blood : Fixed stabbing pain in the hypochondrium region, pain intensified on pressure and palpation, purplish petechiae on the tongue and a wiry pulse.

Treatment:

Method : Points are selected mainly from the Foot-Jueyin and Shaoyang Chanels to ease the Liver and remove the obstruction in the collaterals. Needling with the reducing method is applied for both types.

Prescription:

Yanglingquan (G.B. 34.).

Zhigou (S.J. 6.).

Qimen (Liv. 14.).

Points for the different clinical types:

Stagnation of *qi*:

Ganshu (U.B. 18.).

Qiuxu (G.B. 40.).

Stagnation of blood:

Geshu (U.B. 17.).

Xingjiang (Liv. 2.).

Rationale:

The Shaoyang Channels supply the lateral aspect of the body, therefore Zhigou (S.J. 6.) and Yanglingquan (G.B. 34.) are used to relieve pain by regulating the *qi* of the Shaoyang Channels. Qimen (Liv. 14.), the Front-Mu Point of the Liver Channel, eases the Liver and relieves the pain in the hypochondrium area. Ganshu (U.B. 18.) and Qiuxu (G.B. 40.) promote the functions of the Liver and regulate circulation of *qi*. Sanyinjiao (Sp. 6.) and Geshu (U.B. 17.) activate the blood circulation and thereby remove the stasis.

Ear-acupuncture points:

Chest.

Ear-Shenmen.

Liver.

Gall bladder.

Method: Select 2-3 points on the affected side. Needles are retained for 20-30 minutes. Treatment is given during the painful period.

Note: Hypochondrium pain is seen in diseases of the Liver and Gall bladder, sprain of the hyochondriac region, intercostal neuralgia and costochondritis.

KIDNEY AND URINARY BLADDER DYSFUNCTIONS (LOW BACK PAIN)

Etiology:

(1) Retention of pathogenic wind, cold, damp in the channels and collaterals.

(2) *Xu* (deficiency) of *qi* of the Kidney.

(3) Stagnation of *qi* and blood in the lumbar region due to sprain or contusion caused by trauma.

Differentiation:

(1) Cold-damp : Low-back pain usually occurs after exposure to pathogenic wind, cold and damp. Clinical manifestations are pain in the dorso-lumbar region and stiffness of the muscles, limiting extension and flexion of the back. The pain may radiate down-

wards to the buttocks and lower extremities and the affected area usually feels cold. Pain may become intensified in rainy weather.

(2) *Xu* (insufficiency) of *qi* of the Kidney : The onset is insidious, and the pain is mild but protracted, with lassitude and weakness of the lumbar region and knees. Symptoms are intensified after strain and stress and alleviated by bed rest.

(3) Trauma : The patient gives a history of trauma directed to the lumbar region. Clinical manifestations are pain and rigidity in the low-back area. The pain is continuous and aggravated by pressure and by movements of the body.

Treatment:

Method: The points are mainly selected from the Du and Foot-Taiyang (Urinary Bladder) Channels to promote the circulation of *qi* and Blood, relax the muscles and to activate the collaterals. Both acupuncture and moxibustion are carried out for the cold-damp type. In case of *xu* (insufficiency) of *qi* of Kidney, apply needling with stimulation by the reinforcing method and moxibustion. For traumatic low back pain, needling with the sedation (reducing) method is applied. Pricking to cause bleeding also may be carried out.

Prescription:

Shenshu (U.B. 23.).
Yaoyangguan (Du 3.).
Feiyang (U.B. 58.).

Secondary points:

Xu (Insufficiency) of *qi* of the Kidney:

Mingmen (Du 4.).
Zhishi (U.B. 52.).
Taixi (K. 3.).

Sprain in the lumbar region:

Renzhong (Du 26.).
Weizhong (U.B. 40.).

Rationale:

Shenshu (U.B. 23.) increases the *qi* of the Kidney. Yaoyangguan (Du 3.) is a local point. Feiyang (U.B. 58.) the Luo (Connecting) Point of the Urinary Bladder Channel is a Distal point effective in the treatment of low back pain. Combination of the above three points gives the effect of relaxing the soft tissues and activating the blood circulation. For backache due to cold-damp a needle with moxa is applied to Shenshu (U.B. 23.) and Yaoyangguan (Du 3.) to dispel the cold-damp channel and relieve pain. For low back pain due to *xu* (insufficiency) of the *qi* of the Kidney, Mingmen (Du 4.), Zhishi (U.B. 52.) and Taixi (K. 3.) are selected for tonifying the essence of the Kidney. Renzhong (Du 26.) is selected according to the principle of selection of upper points for disorders of the lower areas. Pricking Weizhong (U.B. 40.) to cause bleeding is an effective method to treat traumatic low back pain and rigidity.

Ear acupuncture points:

Kidney,
Lumbar Vertebrae,
Sacral Vertebrae,
Ear-Shenmen,
Sympathetic Nerve.

Method : Select 2-3 points for each treatment. Needles are retained for about 30 minutes. Treat once daily or every other day. Needles may also be embedded for 3-5 days.

Note: Low back pain may be seen in renal diseases, rheumatic locomotor diseases, strains or traumatic injuries of the lumbar region, as described in Western medicine.

EXCESS OF FLUID (EDEMA ASCITES)

Etiology:

Obstruction of the fluid passages in the three *jiao* (the upper, middle and lower portions of the body cavity) is due to derangements of the Lung, Spleen and Kidney caused by the invasion of the Lung by the wind and cold or *xu* (insufficiency) of *yang* in Spleen and Kidney. This results in the overflow of excess fluid into the tissue space without circulating.

Differentiation:

Shi (Excess) type : The onset is usually abrupt. Generally edema appears first on the head, face or lower extremities. The skin has a lustre. Accompanying symptoms and signs are cough, asthma, fever, thirst, scanty urine and low back pain. The pulse is superficial or rolling and rapid.

Xu (Insufficiency) type : The onset in insidious. Edema first appears on the dorsum of the foot or eyelids, then over the entire body. Accompanying symptoms and signs are pallor, backache, general weakness, abdominal distension, loose stools and a deep thready pulse.

Treatment:

Method: For edema of the *shi* type, acupuncture is applied at points to strengthen the dispersing function of the Lung and promoting the circulation of water. After the exterior pathogenic factors are eliminated, the method of treatment is similar to that for edema of the *xu* type. Points for warming and tonifying the Spleen and Kidney may also be applied.

Prescription:

Shi type:

Lieque (Lu. 7.).

Hegu (L.I. 4.).

Pianli (L.I. 6.).

Yinlingquan (Sp. 9.).

Pangguanshu (U.B. 28.).

Xu type:

Pishu (U.B. 20.).

Shenshu (U.B. 23.).

Shuifen (Ren 9.).

Qihai (Ren 6.).

Sanyinjiao (Sp. 6.).

Zusanli (St. 36.).

Weiyang (U.B. 39.).

Points according to the symptoms:

Edema of the face:

Renzhong (Du 26.).

Constipation with abdominal distension:

Fenglong (St. 40.).

Edema of the feet and ankles:

Foot-Linqi (G.B. 41.).

Shangqiu (Sp. 5.).

Rationale:

Sweating is desirable in edema above the waist. Lieque (Lu. 7.) and Hegu (L.I. 4.) are used to promote perspiration and the relief of the exterior symptoms by activating the *qi* of the Lung. For edema below the waist, diuresis is recommended. Pianli (L.I. 6.) and Yinlingquan (Sp. 9.) are used to cause diuresis in order to eliminate the damp. Pangguanshu (U.B. 28.) regulates the function of the Urinary Bladder in excreting fluid. Application of moxibustion to Pishu (U.B. 20.) and Shenshu (U.B. 23.) for edema of the *xu* (insufficiency) type eliminates damp and fluid through warming and tonifying the *yang* of both the Spleen and the Kidney. Moxibustion applied to Shuifen (Ren 9.) produces a diuretic effect, while at Qihai (Ren 6.) it tonifies the Organ *qi*. Needling Weiyang (U.B. 39.), the Inferior He-Sea Point of *Sanjiao*, removes the obstruction from the fluid passages. Needling

Zusanli (St. 36.) and Sanyinjiao (Sp. 6.) with the reinforcing method strengthens the functions of the Spleen and the Stomach in order to eliminate damp.

Note: Edema is commonly seen in acute and chronic nephritis, malnurition, cardiac failure and in anaemias as described in Western medicine.

KIDNEY AND URINARY BLADDER DYSFUNCTIONS (NOCTURNAL ENURESIS)

Etiology:

Enuresis in children over three years of age and in any adult is considered pathological. The causative factor is insufficiency of the *qi* of the Kidney and inability of the Urinary Bladder to control the act of urination.

Differentiation:

There is involuntary urination during sleep with dreams. In protracted cases, there are accompanying symptoms of sallow complexion, anorexia, and lassitude.

Treatment:

Method: The Back-Shu and Front-Mu Points of the Urinary Bladder and Kidney are the main points for tonification of *qi* of the Kidney. Acupuncture with the reinforcing method or moxibustion is recommended.

Prescription:

Shenshu (U.B. 23.).

Pangguanshu (U.B. 28.).

Zhongji (Ren 3.).

Sanyinjiao (Sp. 6.).

Dadun (Liv. I.).

Point for the different symptoms:

Enuresis with dreams:

Pishu (U.B. 20.).

Anorexia:

Zusanli (St. 36.).

Rationale:

The Kidney and Urinary Bladder are externally-internally related Organs. The Back-Shu Points of the two organs, together with Zhongji (Ren 3.), the Front-Mu Point of the Urinary Bladder, adjust the function of the two Organs. Moxibustion applied to Sanyinjiao (Sp. 6.) the Crossing Point of the three *yin* channels of the foot and Dadun (Liv. 1.), the Jing-Well Point of the Liver Channel which curves around the public region can warm and remove the obstruction Channels to enhance their therapeutic effects.

Ear acupuncture points.

Kidney.

Urinary Bladder.

Brain Point.

Subcortex.

Method : Select 2-3 points for each treatment. Needles are retained for 20-30 minutes. Treatment is given once every other day. Needles may also be embedded for 3-5 days.

Note: Enuresis may be due to organic disease such as deformity of the urinary tract, spina bifida, organic cerebral diseases, oxyuriasis of the urinary tract. In these cases, the primary disease should be treated.

RETENTION OF URINE

Etiology:

(1) Accumulation of damp-heat in the Urinary Bladder which disturbs its function of excreting urine.

(2) Traumatic injuries or surgical operations on the lower abdomen in which the *qi* of the channels is damaged.

(3) Insufficiency of the *yang* of the Kidney which results in disability of the Urinary Bladder to excrete urine.

Differentiation:

The symptoms of the 3 main types are as follows:

(1) Accumulation of damp-heat in the Urinary Bladder: Hot scanty urine or retention of urine, distension of the lower abdomen, thirst but with no desire to drink. There may be constipation. The tongue is red with a yellow coating on the posterior third. The pulse is thready and rapid.

(2) Damage of the *qi* of the channels : Dribbling of urine or complete retention of urine, distension and pain in the lower abdomen, thready rapid pulse, petechia over the tongue.

(3) Insufficiency of the *yang* of the Kidney : Dribbling of foul smelling urine, pallor, listlessness, pain and weakness in the lumbar region and knees, pale tongue, thready pulse especially weak at the proximal position.

Treatment:

Method: In accordance with the principle of treating acute symptoms first in case of an emergency, the Front-Mu Point of the Urinary Bladder should be chosen as the main point to promote urination. In treating the first two types, needling with the reducing method is advisable. For retention of urine due to insufficiency of *yang* of the Kidney, needling should be carried out with the reinforcing method combined with moxibustion.

Prescription:

Zhongji (Ren 3.).

Sanyinjiao (Sp. 6.).

Weiyang (U.B. 39.).

Points for the different clinical types:

Accumulation of damp-heat in the Urinary Bladder.

Yinlingquan (Sp. 9.).

Damage of the *qi* of the channels:

Xuehai (Sp. 10.).

Insufficiency of the *yang* of the Kidney:

Baihui (Du 20.).

Guanyuan (Ren 4.).

Rationale:

Zhongji (Ren 3.) the Front-Mu Point of the Urinary Bladder, combined with Sanyinjiao (Sp. 6.) can normalise the functions of the Urinary Bladder. Weiyang (U.B. 39.) the inferior He-Sea Point of *Sanjiao*, promotes circulation of water and fluids. Yinlingquan (St. 9.) eliminates damp heat. Xuehai (Sp. 10.) activates the channels and collaterals. Moxibustion when applied to Guanyuan (Ren 4.) strengthens the *qi* of the Kidney to promote urination. Application of moxibustion to Baihui (Du 20.) is a method of selection of upper points for disorders of the lower regions of the body.

DISTURBANCES OF SEMINAL EMISSION

Etiology:

Seminal emission may be involuntary, or during dreams (nocturnal emission). The former is mainly due to anxiety or excessive indulgence which leads to weakness of the Kidney and excess of fire in the Heart. Involuntary emission also results from long illness. Excessive sexual activity may cause exhaustion of the essence of the Kidney. Loss of *yin* affects *yang* which leads to uncontrolled emission.

Differentiation:

(1) Nocturnal emission : "Morning-after" dizziness, palpitation, listlessness, lassitude, scanty yellow urine, red tongue and a thready rapid pulse.

(2) Involuntary emission : Frequent emission, pallor, listlessness, pale tongue and a deep, feeble, forceless pulse.

Treatment:

Method : For nocturnal emission, apply acupuncture with the reducing method to points of the Hand-Shaoyin (Heart) Channel and reinforcing method to points of the Foot-Shaoyin (Kidney) Channel. For involuntary emission, apply acupuncture with the reinforcing method together with moxibustion to points mainly selected from the Foot-Shaoyin (Kidney) and Ren Channels.

Prescription:

(1) *Nocturnal emission:*
Shenmen (H. 7.).
Xinshu (U.B. 15.).
Taixi (K. 3.).
Zhishi (U.B. 52.).

(2) *Involuntary emission:*
Shenshu (U.B. 23.).
Dahe (K. 12.).
Sanyinjiao (Sp. 6.).
Guanyuan (Ren 4.).
Qihai (Ren 6.).

Rationale:

For treating nocturnal emission, Shenmen (H. 7.) and Xinshu (U.B. 15.) are punctured with the reducing method to lessen the fire of the Heart and Zhishi (U.B. 52.) and Taixi (K. 3.) with the reinforcing method to tonify the *qi* of the Kidney. For treating involuntary emission, Shenshu (U.B. 23.), Dahe (K. 12.) and Sanyinjiao (Sp. 6.) are punctured with the reinforcing method to strengthen the function of the Kidney in controlling emission. Guanyuan (Ren 4.) and Qihai (Ren 6.) are two important tonification points of the Ren Channel. Moxibustion is applied to these two points to strengthen the original *qi*.

Ear acupuncture points:

Seminal Vesicle.

Endocrine.

Liver.

Kidney.

Method : Select 2-4 points for each treatment. Needles are retained for 10-30 minutes. Treatment is given once daily or every other day; or needles may be embedded for 3-5 days.

IMPOTENCE, FRIGIDITY (DEFICIENT KIDNEY YANG)[2]

Etiology:

Impotence is usually due to damage of the Kidney *yang* resulting from repeated seminal emission or excessive sexual activity. It may also be due to damage of the *qi* of the Heart, Spleen and Kidney resulting from emotional factors such as fright and anxiety.

Differentiation:

Impotence is characterized by a failure of erection. In cases of insufficiency of *yang* of Kidney, there may be pallor, dizziness, blurring of vision, listlessness, soreness of the lumbar region and kness, frequency of urination and a deep thready pulse. If it is complicated by damage to the *qi* of the Heart and Spleen, palpitation and insomnia may be present.

Treatment:

Method : Apply acupuncture with the reinforcing method plus moxibustion to points selected from the Ren and Kidney Channels to tonify the *yang* of the Kidney.

---

2 Male impotence and frigidity in women are similarly treated.

Prescription:

Guanyuan (Ren 4.).

Mingmen (Du 4.).

Shenshu (U.B. 23.).

Taixi (K. 3.).

Baihui (Du 20.).

Points for damage of the qi of Heart and Spleen:

Xinshu (U.B. 15.).

Shenmen (H. 7.).

Sanyinjiao (Sp. 6.).

Rationale:

Moxibustion applied to Guanyuan (Ren 4.) tonifies the original *qi*, Mingmen (Du 4.), Shenshu (U.B. 23.) and Taixi (K.3.) are used to strengthen the *yang* of the Kidney. Moxibustion at Baihui (Du. 20.) can reinforce *yang qi*. Xinshu (U.B. 15.). Shenmen (H. 7.) and Sanyinjiao (Sp. 6.) are used to tonify the *qi* of the Heart and Spleen.

Ear acupuncture points:

Seminal Vesicle (Uterus in the case of frigidity).

External Genitalia.

Testis.

Endocrine.

Method : Select 2-4 points for each treatment. Needles are retained for 10-30 minutes. Treatment is given once daily or every other day; or needles may be embedded for 3-5 days.

BI SYNDROMES (PAINFUL LOCOMOTOR DISORDERS)

Etiology:

Bi means obstruction of the circulation of *qi* and blood, which usually results from an invasion of the intermediate network of channels and collaterals by wind, cold and damp. This obstruction arises due to weakness of defensive *qi* when one is wet with perspiration and exposed to humid wind in damp places or wading in water. There are different types of *bi* syndromes, such as wandering *bi* (in which wind predominates), painful bi (in which cold predominates), fixed *bi* (in which damp predominates) and febrile *bi* (in which wind, cold and damp turn into heat).

Differentiation:

The chief symptom of *bi* syndromes is arthritis. There may also be muscular pain and numbness. In prologed cases, contracture of the extremities, or even swelling or deformity of the joints may be present.

(1) *Wandering bi :* This type is characterized by a wandering pain in the joints of the extremities with a limitation of movement. There may be sweating and fever, a thin sticky coated tongue, a superficial and rapid pulse.

(2) *Painful bi :* Arthralgia responds to warmth and is aggravated by cold. There is no local inflammation. A thin white coated tongue and a deep wiry pulse may be present.

(3) *Fixed bi :* Numbness of the skin and muscles, heavy sensation of the body and extremities, arthralgia with fixed pain, attacks provoked by cloudy or wet weather. White sticky, coated tongue; deep, slow pulse.

(4) *Febrile bi :* Arthralgia with local redness, swelling and tenderness in which one or several joints are involved. Accompanying symptoms are fever and thirst. Yellow coated tongue, rolling rapid pulse.

Treatment:

Method : Local and Distal points are selected from the *yang* channels supplying the diseased areas for the purpose of eliminating wind, cold and damp. Wandering *bi* is mainly treated with needling; painful *bi* with moxibustion and needling as an adjuvant. For severe pain, the use of intradermal (embedding) needles or indirect moxibustion with ginger is recommended. Fixed *bi* is treated with both acupuncture and moxibustion. Warming the needle (moxa on a needle) is also advisable. Febrile *bi* is treated by needing with the reducing method.

Prescription:

Pain in the shoulder joints:

Jianyu (L.I. 15.).

Jianliao (S.J. 14.).

Jianzen (S.I. 9.).

Gaoguang (U.B. 43.).

Pain in the elbows:

Quchi (L.I. 11.).

Chize (Lu. 5.).

Tianjing (S.J. 10.).

Waiguan (S.J. 5.).

Hegu (L.I. 4.).

Pain in the wrists:

Yangchi (S.J. 4.).

Yangxi (L.I. 5.).

Yanggu (S.I. 5.).

Waiguan (S.J. 5.).

Numbness and pain in the fingers:

Houxi (S.I. 3.).

Sanjian (L.I. 3.).

Baxie (Extra 28).

Pain in the hip joints:

Huantiao (G.B. 30.).

Yinmen (U.B. 37.).

Femur-Juliao (G.B. 29.).

Pain in the knee joints:

Lianqiu (St. 34.).

Dubi (St. 35.).

Medial Xiyan (Extra (32).

Yanglingquan (G.P. 34.).

Xiyangguan (G.B. 33.).

Yinlingquan (Sp. 9.).

Numbness and pain in the legs:

Chengshan (U.B. 57.).

Feiyang (U.B. 58.).

Pain in the ankles:

Jiexi (St. 41.).

Shangqiu (Sp. 5.).

Qiuxu (G.B. 40.).

Kunlun (U.B. 60.).

Taixi (K. 3.).

Numbness and pain in the toes:

Gongsun (Sp. 4.).

Shugu (U.B. 65.).

Bafeng (Extra 36.).

Pain in the lumbar region:

Yaoyangguan (Du 3.).

Muscular points (for polymyositis):

Houxi (S.I. 3.).

Shenmai (U.B. 62.).

Dabao (Sp. 21.).

Geshu (U.B. 17.).

Yanglingquan (G.B. 34.).

Points according to the signs and symptoms:

Fever:

Dazhui (Du 14.).

Deformities of the joints:

Dashu (U.B. 11.).

Rationale:

The above prescriptions are formulated by selection of local points according to the courses of channels to relax the muscles, remove the obstruction from the channels and collaterals, regulate *qi* and blood. and eliminate the pathogenic factors.

Note: *Bi* syndromes are seen in rheumatic fever, rheumatic arthritis, rheumatoid arthritis, collagen disorder and gout.

WEI SYNDROMES (PARALYSIS)

(e.g. *Infantile paralysis, poliomyelitis, upper or lower motor neurone paralysis*).

Etiology:

Causative factors are:

(1) Malnutrition of the tendons due to exhaustion of body fluids caused by an invasion of the Lungs by exogenous pathogenic wind-heat.

(2) Lesion of the tendons due to accumulation of damp-heat which affects the Yangming Channels.

(3) Malnutrition of the tendons due to loss of the essences and *qi* of Liver and Kidney caused by a prolonged illness or sexual excesses.

Differentiation:

Wei syndromes are characterized by muscular flaccidity or atrophy of the extremities with motor impairment.

(1) *Heat in the Lungs :* This usually occurs during or after a febrile disease, accompanied by cough, irritability, thirst, scanty brownish urine, red tongue with yellow coating, and a thready rapid pulse.

(2) *Damp-heat :* The accompanying symptoms and signs are sallow complexion, listlessness and cloudy urine. There may be a hot sensation in the soles of the feet. A yellow and sticky coated tongue with a forceful pulse may be present.

(3) *Insufficiency of essences of the Liver and Kidney :* The accompanying symptoms are soreness and weakness of the lumbar region, seminal emission, hypospermia, leucorrhea, dizziness and blurring of vision, red tongue and thready rapid pulse.

Treatment:

Method : Main points are selected from the Yangming Channels to promote circulation of *qi* in the channels and nourish the tendons and bones. When heat in the Lung or damp-heat is responsible, needle with the reducing method to dissipate heat. Moxibustion is contraindicated. In case of insufficiency of essence[3] of the Liver and Kidney, needle with the reinforcing method. Since the process of treatment is prolonged, the method of puncturing both sides may be applied. Puncture the normal side first and then the affected side.

Prescription:

Upper limb:

Jianyu (L.I. 15.).

Quchi (L.I. 11.).

Hegu (L.I. 4.).

Waiguan (S.J. 5.).

Lower limb:

Biguan (St. 31.).

Zusanli (St. 36.).

Jiexi (St. 41.).

3 Essence: hormonal secretions.

Huantiao (G.B. 30.).

Yanglingquan (G.B. 34.).

Xuanzhong (G.B. 39.).

Points for the different types of syndromes:

Heat in the Lungs:

Chize (Lu. 5.).

Feishu (U.B. 13.).

Damp-heat:

Pishu (U.B. 20.).

Yinlingquan (Sp. 9.).

Insufficiency of the essencess of Liver and Kidney:

Ganshu (U.B. 18.).

Shenshu (U.B. 23.).

Rationale:

These prescription are based on the *Nei Jing*. Select points only from Yangming for treating *wei* syndromes. Yanglingquan (G.B. 34.) and Xuanzhong (G.B. 39.), the two Influential Points dominating respectively the tendons and marrow, are added to enhance the effect of nourishing the tendons and bones. Feishu (U.B. 13.) and Chize (Lu. 5.) are used to dissipate heat in the Lung, and Pishu (U.B. 20.) and Yinlingquan (Sp. 9.) to eliminate the damp-heat. Moxibustion combined with acupuncture is applied after the heat subsides. Ganshu (U.B. 18.) and Shenshu (U.B. 23.) are used to tonify the Liver and Kidney. As *wei* syndromes require a long period of treatment, it is necessary to maximize the patient's co-operation and confidence. Applying the plum-blossom with the tapping method along the channels of the diseased area is helpful.

The principles involved in treating infantile paralysis are similar to that for other *wei* syndromes. The corresponding Huatuojiaji Points (Extra. 21.) may be added. In paresis of the extensor aspect, points from the *yang* channels of the extensor aspect are advisable: while in those cases with paresis of the flexors, modern acupuncture allows points on the *yin* channels of the flexor to be selected. During convalescence, acupuntures should be the main treatment, with light and superficial manipulation. Moxibustion may be applied in addition to needling.

Note: *Wei* syndromes are seen in upper and lower motor neurone paralysis, muscular dystrophies, myasthenia gravis, periodic paralysis and hysterical paralysis.

HYSTERIA (FIRE IMBALANCE)

Etiology:

Hysteria is a mental disturbance caused by excessive fire resulting from frustration or depression of the Heart.

Differentiation:

Various psychotic symptoms such as melancholy without an obvious reason, agitation, paraphobia, palpitation, irritability and somnolence may cause hysteria. There may be a sudden onset of a suffocating sensation, hiccup, aphonia or convulsions. The pulse is wiry and thready. In severe cases, there may be loss of consciousness and syncope.

Treatment:

Method: The Front-Mu and Yuan-Source Points of the Heart Channel are selected as the main points to tranquilize the patient. Needling is carried out with the reducing method.

Prescription:

Juque (Ren 14.).

Shenmen (H. 7.).

Sanyinhuao (Sp. 6.).

Points according to the presenting signs and symptoms

Suffocating sensations:

Neiguan (P. 6.).

Shanzhong (Ren 17.).

Hiccup:

Gongsun (Sp. 4.).

Tiantu (Ren 22.).

Aphonia:

Tongli (H. 5.).

Lianquan (Ren 23.).

Convulsions:

Hegu (L.I. 4.).

Taichong (Liv. 3.).

Loss of consciousness and syncope:

Renzhong (Du 26.).

Yongquan (K. 1.).

Rationale:

Juque (Ren 14.) and Shenmen (H. 7.), the Front-Mu and Yuan-Source Points of the Heart Channel, together with Sanyinjiao (Sp. 6.) of the spleen Channel, constitute the main prescription for the purpose of nourishing the blood and tranquilization. Neiguan (P. 6.) and Shanzhong (Ren 17.) are used to relieve the suffocating sensation. Gongsun (Sp. 4.) and Tiantu (Ren 22.) conduct the *qi* down-wards to stop the hiccup. Tongli (H. 5.) and Lianquan (Ren 23.) relieve aphasia. Hegu (L.I. 4.) and Taichong (Liv. 3.) adjust the Liver to relieve convulsions. Renzhong (Du 26.) and Yongquan (K. 1.) restore consciousness as these are Jing-Well points.

Ear acupuncture points:

Heart.

Kidney.

Subcortex.

Ear-Shenmen.

Stomach.

Sympathetic Nerve.

Method : Select 2-3 points at each treatment. Strong stimulation is given.

Note: Hysteria described in this section corresponds to hysteria in modern medicine. However there are different forms of hysteria, some of which may relate to other diseases in traditional Chinese medicine such as Kidney excess.

AMENORRHEA (DEFICIENCY OF YIN IN THE LOWER JIAO)

Etiology:

There are various causative factors. The main factors are blood stasis and blood exhaustion. Amenorrhea due to blood stasis is usually caused by mental depression or invasion by cold during menstruation. Amenorrhea due to Blood exhaustion most commonly results from deficiency of the Liver, Spleen and Kidney Channels caused by chronic illness or Blood depletion due to repeated pregnancies.

Differentiation:

(1) Blood stasis : Sudden onset, distension and pain in the lower abdomen aggravated by pressure. There may be a mass felt in the lower abdomen and pelvis on palpation. A deep wiry pulse may be present.

(2) Blood exhaustion : Delayed menstruation usually accompanied by a sallow complexion, dry skin, listlessness, anorexia, loose stools, white coated tongue and a forceless pulse.

Treatment:

(1) *Blood stasis type:*

Method: Points are mainly selected from the Ren, Spleen and Liver Channels to remove the stasis. Needling is given with the reducing method.

Prescription:

Zhongji (Ren 3.).
Xuehai (Sp. 10.).
Sanyinjiao (Sp. 6.).
Xingjian (Liv. 2.).
Guilai (St. 29.).
Ciliao (U.B. 32.).
Hegu (L.I. 4.).

Rationale:

Zhongji (Ren 3.) is a point where the Ren Channel and the three *yin* channels of the foot meet. Ciliao (U.B. 32.) and Guilai (St. 29.) are local point used to remove blood stasis of the uterus. Hegu (L.I. 4.) and Sanyinjiao (Sp. 6.) adjust the *qi* and Blood. Xingjian (Liv. 2.) releases *qi* of the Liver. Xuehai (Sp. 10.) activates blood circulation and promotes the menstrual flow.

(2) *Blood exhaustion type:*

Method : Points from the Ren Channel and Back-Shu Points are the main points used to adjust and nourish the Liver, Spleen and Kidney. Needling is given with the reinforcing method. Moxibustion may be used in combination with needling.

Prescription:

Select from:

Ganshu (U.B. 18.).
Pishu (U.B. 20.).
Shenshu (U.B. 23.).
Tianshu (St. 25.).
Zusanli (St. 36.).
Sanyinjiao (Sp. 6.).

Rationale:

Qihai (Ren 6.) is a point used for tonification. Ganshu (U.B. 11.), Pishu (U.B. 20.) and Shenshu (U.B. 23.) activate the functions of the Liver, Spleen and Kidney. Zusanli (St. 36.) and Sanyinjiao (Sp. 6.) are Distal points of the related channels. Tianshu (St. 25.) is an adjacent point used to regulate the Spleen and Stomach, the sources of *qi* and Blood formation.

DYSMENORRHEA (EXCESS OR DEFICIENCY OF YANG IN THE LOWER JIAO)

Etiology:

Dysmenorrhea is generally of two types:

(1) Dysmenorrhea of *shi* (excess) is due to the coagulation of Blood in the uterus resulting from emotional disturbances such as obsession, worry, melancholy and anger, invasion of cold, or due to excessive of cold drinks during menstruation.

(2) Dysmenorrhea of *xu* (deficiency) is caused by insufficiency of *qi* and Blood and dysfunction of the Extraordinary Chong and Ren Channels.

Differentiation:

(1) *Shi type :* Premenstrual cramps in the lower abdomen aggravated on pressure. This radiates to the lower back and thighs, gradually diminishing after the onset of menstruation; mentstrual flow is dark purplish in colour, with clots. The pulse is wiry.

(2) *Xu type :* Lower abdominal pain at the later days of menstruation on post-menstruation. Mild but persistent pain responding to warmth and pressure, menstrual flow scanty and pinkish in colour. In severe cases, there may be palpitations and dizziness. The pulse in thready and forceless.

Treatment:

(1) *Shi type:*

Method : Points are mainly selected from the Ren Channel and the Spleen Channel to activate the Blood circulation and remove obstruction from the channels, Needling is given with the reducing method. For cases due to the cold nature, moxibustion is advisable.

Prescription:

Zhongji (Ren 3.).
Xuehai (Sp. 10.).
Diji (Sp. 8.).
Hegu (L.I. 4.).
Daju (St. 27.).

Rationale:

Xuehai (Sp. 10.) activates the blood circulation. Diji (Sp. 8.), the Xi-Cleft Point of the Spleen Channel, when combined with Hegu (L.I. 4.), is indicated in painful menstruation. Zhongji (Ren 3.) and Daju (St. 27.) are local points to remove blood stasis and relieve the pain.

(2) *Xu type:*

Method : Points from the Ren Channel and the Back-Shu Points of the Spleen and Kidney are taken as the main points to adjust and strengthen *qi* and Blood. Needling is given with the reinforcing method and combined with moxibution.

Prescription:

Guanyuan (Ren 4.).
Pishu (U.B. 20.).
Shenshu (U.B. 23.).
Zusanli (St. 36.).
Sanyinjiao (St. 6.).

Rationale:

Moxibustion applied to Guanyuan (Ren 4.) warms and strengthens the original *qi.* Pishu (U.B. 20.) and Shenshu (U.B. 23.) regulate and promote the functions of the Spleen and Kidney. Zusanli (St. 36.) and Sanyinjiao (Sp. 6.) are Distal points used to strengthen the Spleen and Stomach, the sources of blood formation.

Ear acupuncture points:

Ovary.

Ear-Shenmen.

Endocrine.

Uterus.

Method : Manipulate the needles intermittently with moderately strong stimulation until the pain is alleviated.

MENORRHAGIA, POST-PARTUM HEMORRHAGE, UTERINE HEMORRHAGE

Etiology:

Causative factors are:

(1) Physical or mental strain which injures the Spleen.

(2) Dysfunction of the Spleen in conducting Blood, caused by impairment of Liver function due to extreme anger[4].

(3) Dysfunction of the Extra-Ordinary Chong and Ren Channels caused by the invasion of the Uterus (an extraordinary) organ by pathogenic cold or heat.

Differentiation:

Uterine haemorrhage may be of abrupt onset, profuse or lingering and scanty; or the two conditions may occur alternately. Other symptoms are dizziness, fatigue, low back pain and general weakness.

(1) *Heat in the Blood:* The blood is bright red with a foul odor. Irritability, rapid pulse, and a yellow coated tongue are common symptoms.

(2) *Deficiency of qi:* The blood is pinkish and dull, there is cold in the lower abdomen, usually with chillness, pallor of the face and lips and a deep slow pulse.

4 Pre-menstrual symdrome is also a related disorder.

Treatment:

Method:

(1) *Heat in the Blood* : Treatment is aimed at eliminating heat to stop the bleeding. Needling is given mainly with the reducing method.

(2) *Deficiency of qi* : Treatment is aimed at regulating the Extraordinary Chong and Ren Channels. Needling is given with the reinforcing method, together with moxibustion.

Prescription:

Guanyuan (Ren 4.).

Yinbai (Sp. 1.).

Point for the different types:

(1) Heat in the Blood:

Taichong (Liv. 3.).

Rangu (K. 2.).

(2) Deficiency of *qi*:

Baihui (Du 20.).

Yangchi (S.J. 4.).

Rationale:

Guanyuan (Ren 4.) regulates the functions of the Extraordinary Chong and Ren Channels. Yinbai (Sp. 1.) a point of the Spleen Channel, is used to invigorate the functions of the Spleen in circulating Blood. Uterine bleeding can be treated with moxibustion at these two points. Taichong (Liv. 3.), the Yuan-Source Point of the Liver Channel, promotes Liver functions and regulates the vital energy. When combined with Rangu (K. 2.), the Ying-Spring Point of the Kidney Channel, they eliminate heat and cool the Blood. Applying moxibustion to Baihui (Du 20.) raises the *yang qi* of the Du Channel. Yangchi (S.J. 4.), the Yuan-Source Point of the Sanjiao Channel, promotes the functions of the Chong and Ren Channels in controlling Blood.

Any massive bleeding should be immediately checked. If bleeding is lingering, observe whether there is blood stagnation, if there are purplish clots in the blood, and if abdominal pain is aggravated when pressure is applied and alleviated after bleeding. Hegu (L.I. 4.) combined with Sanyinjiao (St. 6.), may be used to activate the Blood circulation and remove the stagnation.

Ear acupuncture points:

Uterus.
Subcortex.
Endocrine,
Kidney.
Spleen.

Needles are retain for 1-2 hours and manipulated intermittently.

Note: Uterine haemorrhage as described here also corresponds to functional uterine haemorrhage due to derangement of the ovaries. Organic diseases of the genital system should be excluded before embarking on acupuncture or moxa therapy.

LEUCORRHEA (DYSFUNCTIONS OF THE LOWER JIAO)

Etiology:

Leucorrhea refers to a persistent mucus discharge in the absence of menstruation. Causative factors are dysfunctions of the Extraordinary Ching and Ren Channels and weakness of the *qi* of the Dai Channel due to an insufficiency of *qi* and downward diffusion of damp-heat.

Differentiation:

Leucorrhea may be differentiated between a white or yellow discharge.

(1) White discharge is due to insufficiency of *qi* and presence of damp. It is thin and whitish with an odor.

(2) Yellow discharge is due to the downward infusion of damp-heat. It is pinkish or deep yellow with a fetid odor.

Both conditions may be accompanied by low back pain, dizziness and lassitude.

Treatment:

Method : Main points are those from the Dai and Spleen Channels for regulating *qi* and Blood and eliminating damp heat. Acupuncture with the reinforcing method (plus moxibustion) is applied for white discharge and the reducing method is applied for yellow discharge.

Prescription:

Daimai (G.B. 26.).
Wushu (G.B. 27.).
Qihai (Ren 6.).
Sanyinjiao (Sp. 6.).

Points for the different symptoms:

(1) White discharge:
Ciliao (U.B. 32.).
Shenshu (U.B. 23.).
Baihuanshu (U.B. 30.).

(2) Yellow discharge:
Zhongji (Ren 3.).
Ligou (Liv. 5.).
Yinlingquan (Sp. 9.).

Rationale:

Qihai (Ren 6.) is used to regulate the *qi* of the Chong and Ren Channels. Dai (G.B. 26.) and Wushu (G.B. 27.), being the Crossing Point of the Dai and Gall bladder Channels, have the property of strengthening the Dai Channel and are indicated in treating leucorrhea. Sanyinjiao (Sp. 6.) regulates the three *yin* channels of foot to eliminate damp-heat. Shenshu (U.B. 23.) strengthens the *qi* of the Kidney and is efficacious for tonic purposes. Ciliao (U.B. 32.) and Baihuanshu (U.B. 30.) are local points. Zhongji (Ren 3.), Crossing Point of the Ren Channel and the Liver Channel, and Ligou (Liv. 5.), the Luo-Connecting and the Liver Channel, when used in combination, can reduce the fire of the Liver. Yinlingquan (Sp. 9.) strengthens the Spleen to eliminate damp-heat.

Note: Leucorrhea as described in this section refers to inflammations of the genitourinary system such as vaginitis, cervicitis, endometritis, and other non-specific infections of the pelvic organs.

MORNING SICKNESS[5]

Etiology:

Vomiting in the early stage of pregnancy is mainly due to a general weakness of Stomach *qi* as a reaction to the fetus.

Differentiation:

Nausea and vomiting occur after about one month of pregnancy. Vomiting may take place immediately after food or at the sight or smell of food. The accompanying symptoms are fullness in the chest, dizziness, blurring of vision and lassitude.

Treatment:

Method: The points selected are mainly from the Foot-Yangming (Stomach) and Hand-Jueyin (Pericardium) Channels. These inhibit vomiting by sedating the Stomach *qi*. Needling is given with mild stimulation.

5 Also pre-eclampsia.

Prescription:

Zusanli (St. 36.).

Neiguan (P. 6.).

Shangwan (Ren 13.).

Rationale:

Zusanli (St. 36.) calms the ascending *qi* of the Stomach. Neiguan (P. 6.) relieves vomiting by easing the discomfort of the chest. Shangwan (Ren 13.), a local point, is indicated in treating fullness in the epigastric region.

Ear acupuncture points:

Liver.

Stomach.

Ear-Shenmen.

Sympathetic Nerve.

Method : Treatment is given once a day; or needles may be embedded for 3-5 days. Massaging the points where needles are embedded enhances their therapeutic effect.

LACTATION INSUFFICIENCY

Etiology:

Causative factors are:

(1) Poor health and deficiency of *qi* Blood.

(2) Massive loss of blood during childbirth.

(3) Mental depression affecting the Liver.

Differentiation:

Scanty or absence of milk secretion after childbirth, or continuous decrease in quantity during lactation. In the *xu* type, the accompanying symptoms are palpitation, lassitude and low viscosity milk. In the *shi* type, there appears fullness of the chest, anorexia, retention of milk and pain in the hypochondrium.

Treatment:

Method:

(1) *Xu type* : Needling is given with the reinforcing method, combined with moxibustion.

(2) *Shi type* : Needling is given with the reducing method.

Prescription:

Rugen (St. 18.).

Shanzhong (Ren 17.).

Shaoze (S.I. 1.).

Secondary points for the different types:

(1) *Xu type:*

Pishu (U.B. 20.).

Zusanli (St. 36.).

(2) *Shi type:*

Qimen (Liv. 14.).

Neiguan (P. 6.).

Rationale:

Rugen (St. 18.) is a point of the Stomach Channel and also a local point. Shanzhong (Ren 17.) is the Influential Point dominating *qi*. Moxibustion applied at these two points warms the *qi* and Blood and activates the circulation. Some effect may also be obtained by puncturing these two points horizontally towards the breasts to cause radiating *deqi* sensations in the local area. Shaoze (S.I. 1.) is an empirical point for promoting lactation. Pishu (U.B. 20.), the Back-Shu Point of the Spleen, and Zusanli (St. 36.) the He-Sea Point of the Stomach, regulate the functions of Blood and milk formation in the Spleen and Stomach. Qimen (Liv. 14.) the Front-Mu Point of the Liver regulates the functions of the Liver to relieve the pain of the hypochondrium. Neiguan (P. 6.) eases the chest and relieves depression to allow the flow of milk.

INFANTILE CONVULSIONS (ENDOGENOUS WINDS, YIN EXCESS)

Etiology:

Infantile convulsions may be of the acute or chronic types.

(1) Acute convulsions. Causative factor is endogenous wind caused by extreme heat due to phlegm. This is usually caused by an invasion of exogenous wind-cold accompanied by accumulation of undigested food in the Stomach. Acute febrile disease may also lead to acute convulsions.

(2) Chronic convulsions. This is usually due to weakness (yin excess) of Spleen and Stomach after any chronic illness.

Differentiation:

(1) Acute convulsions. High fever, coma, upward staring eyes, clenched jaws, tetanic contractions, opisthotonos, cyanosis and a rapid pulse.

(2) Chronic convulsions : Emaciation, pallor, lassitude, lethargy with half-closed eyes, intermittent convulsions, cold extremities, loose stools with undigested food, profuse clear urine and a deep feeble pulse.

Treatment:

(1) *Acute convulsions:*

Method : Elimination of the heat and wind by applying needling with the reducing method mainly to points of the Du Channel. Moxibustion is contraindicated.

Prescription:

Shixuan (Extra. 30.).
Yintang (Extra. 1.).
Renzhong (Du 26.).
Quchi (L.I. 11.).
Taichong (Liv. 3.).

Secondary points for the different signs and symptoms:

Coma:

Laogong (P. 8.).

Yongquan (K. 1.).

Protracted convulsions:

Xingjian (Liv. 2.).

Yanglingquan (G.B. 34.).

Kunlun (U.B. 60.).

Houxi (S.I. 3.).

Continuous high fever:

Dazhui (Du 14.).

Hegu (L.I. 4.).

Rationale:

Pricking and bleeding at Shixuan (Extra. 30.) eliminates the heat. Yintang (Extra. 1.) promotes relaxation, Renzhong (Du 26.) is effective in resuscitation. Quchi (L.I. 11.) eliminates the heat of the Yangming Channels. Needling Taichong (Liv. 3.) with the reducing method calms the wind of the Liver. Laogong (P. 7.) and Yongquan (K. 1.) are important points for emergency treatment which eliminate heat. Xingjian (Liv. 2.) and Yanglingquan (G.B. 34.) are used for reducing Phlegm. Kunlun (U.B. 60.) is a point of the Urinary Bladder Channel which communicates with the brain; Houxi (S.I. 3.) communicates with the Du Channel. Puncturing these points together is effective in clearing mental cloudiness and relieving convulsions. Dazhui (Du 14.), the Crossing Point of all the *yang* channels, and Hegu (L.I. 4.) the Yuan-Source Point of the Hand-Yangming Channel are used to relieve excess heat in the *yang* channels.

(2) *Chronic convulsions:*

Method : To strengthen the Spleen and Stomach by applying acupuncture and moxibustion at points of the Ren and Foot-Yangming (Stomach) Channel as the main points.

Prescription:

Zhongwan (Ren 12.).
Guanyuan (Ren 4.).
Zusanli (St. 36.).
Zhangmen (Liv. 13.).
Yintang (Extra 1.).

Rationale:

Zhangmen (Liv. 13.), Zhongwan (Ren 12.) and Zusanli (St. 36.) are used to readjust the functions of the Spleen and Stomach. Moxibustion on Guanyuan (Ren 4.) strengthens the original *qi* (vital force). Moxibustions at Yingtang (Extra. 1.) checks the convulsions.

Note: Acute convulsions may be due to infections of the central nervous system and toxic encephalopathies, such as epidemic meningoencephalitis and toxic pneumonia. Acupunture tends to reduce the fever and spasticity but specific diagnosis is imperative in order to give proper treatment using antibiotics if necessary.

Chronic convulsions are usually due to prolonged chronic vomiting and diarrhea, metabolic disturbances, malnutrition, or chronic infections of the central nervous system.

INFANTILE DIARRHEA (EXOGENOUS FOOD DISORDERS)

Etiology:

Causative factors are indigeston due to improper nursing with contaminated milk and irregular feeding resulting in weakness of the infant's Spleen and Stomach. It may also be combined with undue exposure to exogenous cold.

Differentiation:

Abdominal distension, borborygmus, intermittent abdominal pain relieved after diarrhea. More than ten stools a day with strong fetid odor may occur. Tongue is sticky and coated; the pulse is deep and forceless.

Treatment:

Method : To normalise the functions of the Spleen and Stomach by applying acupuncture to points of the Foot-Yangming (Stomach) Channel as the main points. Needling is given with the even-movement method. The needle is usually not retained.

Prescription:

Zhongwan (Ren 12.).
Tianshu (St. 25.).
Shangjuxu (St. 37.).
Sifeng (U. Extra.).

Exogenous cold:

Hegu (L.I. 4.).

Rationale:

Zhongwan (Ren 12.), the Front-Mu Point of the Stomach and also the Confluent Point of the *Fu* organs, regulates the *qi* (vital functions) of the Stomach. Tianshu (St. 25.) and Shangjuxu (St. 37.), the Front-Mu Point and the Inferior He-Sea Point of the Large Intestine, when used in combination, adjust the function of the intestines to relieve the diarrhea. Sifeng (U. Extra.) are empirical points in the treatment of digestive disturbance in infants; they have the effects of promoting digestion, relieving abdominal distension, and strengthening the Spleen and Stomach.

MUMPS (EXTRINSIC HEAT DISORDER)

Etiology:

Causative factor is the accumulation of heat in the Large Intestine and Sanjiao Channels due to the invasion of seasonal epidemic factors and an upward attack of the heat of the Stomach.

Differentiation:

Onset combines chills and fever with redness and swelling of the parotid region on one or both sides. In severe cases, the symptoms are thirst, constipation, deep yellow urine, a sticky coated tongue, and a superficial rapid pulse.

Treatment:

Method : To disperse the heat and wind by applying superficial puncture with the reducing method to points of the Large Intestine and Sanjiao Channels as the main points.

Prescription:

Waiguan (S.J. 5.).
Yifeng (S.J. 17.).
Jiache (St. 6.).
Quchi (L.I. 11.).
Hegu (L.I. 4.).

Rationale:

Waiguan (S.J. 5.) eliminates heat from the Sanjiao Channel. Quchi (L.I. 11.) and Hegu (L.I. 4.) eliminate heat from the Large Intestine Channel. Yifeng (S.J. 17.) and Jiache (St. 6.) are local points used to remove obstruction from the affected channels supplying the parotid region in order to relieve the swelling and pain.

Note: Pricking the ear apex and facio-mandibular area with a three-edged needle to cause bleeding is also effective in treating mumps and relieving the painful symptoms.

URTICARIA (EXTRINSIC FOOD DISORDER)

Etiology:

Causative factor is heat in the Blood complicated with exogenous wind attacking the superficial layer of the muscles or an accumulation of heat in the Stomach and Intestines due to intake of a food to which the patient is unaccustomed.

Differentiation:

Abrupt onset with itching wheals of various sizes. There may be accompanying abdominal pain, constipation and a superficial rapid pulse. Acute conditions subside quickly, while recurrences are frequent when the disease becomes chronic.

Treatment:

Method : To disperse wind and eliminate the heat in the Blood by puncturing with the reducing method at points of the Spleen and Large Intestine Channels as the main points.

Prescription:

Xuehai (Sp. 10.).
Sanyinjiao (Sp. 6.).
Quchi (L.I. 11.).
Hegu (L.I. 4.).

Abdominal pain:

Zusanli (St. 36.).

Rationale:

Xuehai (Sp. 10.) and Sanyinjiao (Sp. 6.) eliminate damp heat in the Blood. Quchi (L.I. 11.) and Hegu (L.I. 4.) relieve itching and wheals through eliminating wind-heat. Zusanli (St. 36.) soothes the Stomach and Intestines to relieve abdominal pain.

Ear acupuncture points:

Endocrine.
Lung.
Adrenal.

Method : Needles are retained for about an hour, with intermittent manipulation.

ERYSIPELAS, HERPES ZOSTER (EXOGENOUS HEAT)

Etiology:

Causative factor is the invasion of the Large Intestine Channel by exogenous wind-heat or damp-heat which injures the Blood. The main site of occurrence is the trunk and the face. It may, however, spread over the entire body.

Differentiation:

The onset is with chills and fever, followed by the sudden appearance of deep red cloudy patches diffusely spreading over the skin with clear demarcation and burning pain. The accompanying symptoms and signs are irritability, thirst, constipation, brownish urine, a rapid pulse and a thick coated tongue.

Treatment:

Method : Eliminate heat in the Blood by puncturing with the reducing method, or pricking to cause bleeding to points of the Large Intestine Channel as the main points.

Prescription:

Quchi (L.I. 11.).
Hegu (L.I. 4.).
Weizhong (U.B. 40.).
Quze (P. 3.).
Xuehai (Sp. 10.).

Needling is done with the reducing method. Puncturing the Huatuojiaji points (Extra. 21.) corresponding to the site of lesion is also advisable.

Rationale:

Quchi (L.I. 11.) and Hegu (L.I. 4.) eliminate the heat of the Large Intestine. Venous pricking at Weizhong (U.B. 40.) and Quze (P. 3.) eliminates heat in the Blood.

Note: Erysipelas of the lower limbs may also be treated by pricking the affected area with the three-edged needle or tapping with the cutaneous needle to cause bleeding. Toxic heat may be relieved but care should be taken to avoid infection; therefore good sterilization should be carried out before puncturing.

Herpes Zoster occurs mainly in the lumbar and hypochondrium regions, with small vesicles forming a girdle. Severe burning pain with redness and hotness of the skin are characteristic of the disease. It is an Exterior-heat disorder. Herpes Zoster of the face area can be extremely painful.

FURUNCLE AND LYMPHANGITIS (TOXIC EXCESS HEAT)

Etiology:

(1) Endogenous toxicity due to the extreme heat of the viscera caused by fatty and spicy food.

(2) Stagnation of *qi* and Blood resulting from the invasion of toxic exogenous factors during the late summer.

Differentiation:

A furuncle may occur on the head, face or extremities. If first appears like a grain of millet, with a hard base. Pain or a tingling sensation may be present. A blister or pustula, yellowish or purplish in colour and hard as a nail is formed, usually accompanied by chills and fever. If it occurs at the extremities with a red thread-like line running proximally, it is known as lymphangitis.

Treatment:

Method : Apply needling with the reducing method or pricking to cause bleeding to points of the Du and Large Intestine Channels as the main points. For lymphangitis, prick with the three-edged needle to cause bleeding at 2-inch intervals along the inflammed area proximally towards the focus.

Prescription:

Lingtai (Du 10.).
Shenzhu (Du 12.).
Ximen (P. 4.).
Hegu (L.I. 4.).
Weizhong (U.B. 40.).

Rationale:

Lingtai (Du 10.) is an empirical point for the treatment of furuncles. Shenzhu (Du 12.), being a point of the Du Channel, readjusts the *qi* of all the *yang* channels. Ximen (P. 4.), the Xi-Cleft Point of the Pericardium Channel is effective in treating acute diseases. Hegu (L.I. 4.) eliminates the exogenous pathogenic factors from the exterior portion of the body. Weizhong (U.B. 40.) is effective in clearing heat and toxins from the blood. Using these two points together allays inflammation. Pricking to cause bleeding disperses toxin and heat from the blood.

ACUTE MASTITIS

Etiology:

Causative factor is retention of milk in the breast caused by mental depression affecting the *qi* of the Liver or stagnation of toxic heat in the Stomach Channel.

Differentiation:

Onset is redness, swelling, heat and pain in the breast, accompanied by chills, fever, nausea, irritability and thirst. The pulse is wiry and rapid.

Treatment:

To regulate the *qi* of the Liver and Stomach Channels, relieve depression and eliminate heat by applying needling with the reducing method to points of the Liver. Gall bladder and Stomach Channels. Moxibustion may be used in combination.

Prescription:

Taichong (Liv. 3.).
Foot-Linqi (G.B. 41.).
Shanzhong (Ren 17.).
Jianjing (G.B. 21.).
Rugen (St. 18.).

Chills and fever:

Hegu (L.I. 4.).
Waiguan (S.J. 5.).

Distending pain in the breasts:

Yingchuang (St. 16.).

Rationale:

Taichong (Liv. 3.) promotes the Liver function. Foot-Linqi (G.B. 41.) helps the swelling of the breast. Shanzhong (Ren 17.) relieves the feeling of pressure in the chest. Jianjing (G.B. 21.) and Rugen (St. 18.) promote circulation of *qi* to stop the pain. Hegu (L.I. 4.) and Waiguan (S.J. 5.) reduce fever. Yingchuang (St. 16.) is punctured obliquely to soften the lump in the breast and to promote the milk flow.

Ear acupuncture points:

Chest.
Adrenal.

Ear-Shenmen.

Subcortex.

Method : Puncture two points at each treatment with moderate stimulation. Needles are left in place for 30 minutes. Give treatment once daily.

GOITER

Etiology:

This is an endemic disease whose causative factors are:

(1) Blood stasis and accumulation of phlegm due to obstruction of *qi* caused by anxiety or mental depression.

(2) Stagnation of *qi* in the neck due to an invasion by any of the six exogenous pathogenic factors.

Diffirentiation:

Swelling of the neck, which may be accompanied by stuffiness in the chest, palpitation, shortness of breath, and oxopthalmos. The pulse is wiry and rolling.

Treatment:

Mothod : To activate blood and *qi* circulation and remove stasis and lumps by puncturing with the reducing method at points of the Sanjiao, Large intestine and Stomach Channels as the main points.

Prescription:

Naohui (S.J. 13.)

Tianding (L.I. 17.).

Tianrong (S.I. 17.).

Tiantu (Ren 22.).

Hegu (L.I. 4.).

Zusanli (St. 36.).

Depression of qi of Liver:

Shanzhong (Ren 17.).

Taichong (Liv. 3.).

Rationale:

Naohui (S.J. 13.), a point of the Sanjiao Channel has the effect of dispersing the stagnant *qi* and phlegm in the goiter because *Sanjiao* dominates the *qi* of the whole body. Tianding (L.I. 17.), Tianrong (S.I. 17.) and Tiantu (Ren 2.) are located at the neck; puncturing these three points promotes the circulation of *qi* and Blood in the local area so as to disperse the stagnant *qi* and Blood. Hegu (L.I. 4.) and Zusanli (St. 36.) are distal points pertaining respectively to the Hand- and Foot-Yangming Channels which pass through the neck. They are used to direct the circulation of *qi* and Blood.

Ear acupuncture points:

Endocrine.

Ear-Shenmen.

Neck.

Method : Give moderate stimulation. Needles are retained for 30 minutes. Treatment is given once daily or every other day. About 12-15 treatments constituţe a course.

Note: (1) Goiter as described in this section corresponds to simple goiter and hyperthyroidism.

(2) Hot needle therapy in benign solitary adenoma is a very effective form of therapy.

SPRAIN AND STRAIN (QI AND BLOOD OBSTRUCTION IN SOFT TISSUES)

Etiology:

Locai congestion caused by obstruction of *qi* and Blood in the soft tissues due to an awkward posture of the body, sudden twisting or falling during physical exertion.

Differentiation:

Local soreness, distension and pain, or mild redness and swelling. Movement is limited or painful.

Treatment:

Method : Ah-Shi Points are the main points used to ease the tendons and activate blood circulation. Local and distal points of the involved channels may be combined. Apply needling plus moxibustion to the former and needling to the latter.

Prescription:

Ah-Shi Points.

Regional points:

Neck:

Tianzhu (U.B. 10.).

Houxi (S.I. 3.).

Shoulder joint:

Jianjing (G.B. 21.).

Jianyu (L.I. 15.).

Elbow joint:

Quchi (L.I. 11.).

Hegu (L.I. 4.).

Wrist joint:

Yangchi (S.J. 4.).

Waiguan (S.J. 5.).

Hip joint:

Huantiao (G.B. 30.).

Yanglingquan (G.B. 34.).

Knee joint:

Dubi (St. 35.).

Neiting (St. 44.).

Ankle joint:

Jiexi (St. 41.).

Qiuxu (G.B. 40.).

Kunlun (U.B. 60.).

Rationale:

Local and distal points selected from the involved areas help promote the circulation of *qi* and Blood in the channels and collaterals. Moxibustion on the local points warms and promotes circulation of *qi* and Blood to relieve swelling and pain.

Note: Needling may be applied to the normal side at the area corresponding to the affected area. When manipulating the needle, instruct the patient to move the sprained joint gently. Alleviation of pain will result.

DEAFNESS AND TINNITUS

Etiology:

Deafness and tinnitus may be divided into two types: the *xu* and the *shi*. The *shi* type is usually due to the upward migration of the *sieqi* of the Liver and Gall bladder which affects the sense of hearing. The *xu* type is usually due to lowering of the *qi* of the Kidney, which fails to ascend.

Differentiation:

(1) *Shi type:* Tinnitus (continuous ringing in the ears unrelieved by pressure), deafness. The accompanying symptoms and signs are distension and a heavy sensation of the head, nasal obstruction, bitter taste in the mouth, hypochondrium pain, sticky coated tongue, and a rolling rapid pulse.

(2) *Xu type:* Tinnitus (intermittent ringing in the ears which becomes aggravated after stress which is somewhat alleviated by pressure).

Deafness : Gradual onset of deafness.

The accompanying symptoms and signs are dizziness, blurring of vision, low back pain, lassitude and a thready pulse.

Treatment:

Method:

(1) *Shi type* : To restore the sense of hearing by puncturing with the reducing method at points of the Sanjiao and Gall bladder Channels as the main points.

(2) *Xu type* : To strengthen the Liver and Kidney by puncturing with even movements plus moxibustion at points of the Kidney and Liver Channels.

Prescription:

Yifeng (S.J. 17.).

Ermen (S.J. 21.).

Tinghui (G.B. 2.).

Yemen (S.J. 2.).

Xiaxi (G.B. 43.).

Hand-Zhongzhu (S.J. 3.).

Secondary points:

(1) *Shi type:*

Upward perversion of *qi* of the Liver and Gall bladder:

Xingjian (Liv. 2.).

Foot-Linqi (G.B. 41.).

Sudden deafness:

Tianyou (S.J. 16.).

(2) *Xu type:*

Lowering of the *qi* of Kidney:

Shenshu (U.B. 23.).

Mingmen (Du 4.).

Taixi (K. 3.).

Insufficiency of *yin* of Liver and Kidney:

Taichong (Liv. 3.).

Sanyinjiao (Sp. 6.).

Rationale:

Yemen (S.J. 2.), Xiaxi (G.B. 43.), Yifeng (S.J. 17.), Ermen (S.J. 21.), Tinghui (G.B. 2.) and Hand-Zhongzhu (S.J. 3.) are selected as the main points because the Hand-and Foot-Shaoyang Channels (Sanjiao and Gall bladder Channels) pass through the ear regions. Xingjian (Liv. 2.) and Foot-Linqi (G.B. 41.) are used to regulate the *qi* of the Liver and Gall bladder Channels. Tianyou (U.B. 16.) is a local point used for treatment to sudden deafness. Shenshu (U.B. 23.) Mingmen (Du 4.) and Taixi (K. 3.) strengthen the *qi* of the Kidney. Sanyinjiao (Sp. 6.) and Taichong (Liv. 3.) nourish the Yin of the liver and kidney to reduce the Xu fire (the presence of which is due to insufficiency of *yin*).

Ear acupuncture points:

Ear.

Internal Ear.

Ear-Shenmen.

Kidney.

Endocrine.

Occiput.

Method : Select 2-3 points at each treatment. Needles are retained for 20-30 minutes at each treatment, which is given every other day. About 10-15 treatments make a course.

Note: Tinnitus and deafness may be present in various diseases. Those most often encountered in acupuncture practice are due to nerve defects.

CONGESTION, SWELLING, AND PAIN OF THE EYE (EXOGENOUS HEAT, LIVER AND GALL BLADDER DYSFUNCTIONS)

Etiology:

(1) Invasion of exogenous wind-heat.

(2) Upward disturbance of the Liver and Gall bladder.

Differentiation:

Congestion, swelling, pain, and burning sensation of the eyes, photophobia, lacrimation and a sticky discharge.

(1) Invasion of exogenous wind-heat : Headache, fever and superficial rapid pulse.

(2) Upward disturbance of fire of Liver and Gall bladder : Bitter taste in the mouth, irritability with feverish sensation, constipation, wiry pulse.

Treatment:

Method : Distal and local points are used in combination to disperse the wind-heat. Needling is given with the reducing method.

Prescription:

Hegu (L.I. 4.).

Jingming (U.B. 1.).

Fengchi (G.B. 20.).

Taiyang (Extra. 2.).

Xingjian (Liv. 2.).

Upward disturbance of fire of the Liver and Gall bladder:

Taichong (Liv. 3.).

Guangming (G.B. 37.).

Rationale:

Hegu (L.I. 4.) and Fengchi (G.B. 20.) disperse wind-heat. Jingming (U.B. 1.), a point where the Urinary Bladder and Stomach Channels meet, eliminates heat in the diseased area. Xingjian (Liv. 2.), a specific point, also eliminates heat in the diseased area. Xingjian (Liv. 2.), the Ying-Spring Point of the Liver Channel, reduces the heat of the Liver. Pricking Taiyang (Extra 2.) to cause bleeding enhances the effect of reducing the heat. Taichong (Liv. 3.), the Yuan-Source Point of the Liver Channel is selcted because the Liver is related to the eye. As there is an external-internal relation between the Liver and Gall bladder, Guangming (G.B. 37.), the Luo-Connecting Point of the Gall bladder Channel is used to reduce the fire of the Liver and Gall bladder.

Ear acupuncture points:

Liver.

Eye.

Ear Apex.

Method : Treatment is given once daily with needles retained for 15 to 20 minutes and the ear apex pricked to let out 2-3 drops of blood. About 3-5 treatments make a course.

Note: The condition corresponds to acute conjunctivitis in the pathology of modern medicine.

RHINORRHEA, RHINITIS, SINUSITIS

Etiology:

(1) Invasion of the exterior of the body by wind-cold which when accumulated turns into heat blocking the nose.

(2) Damp-heat of the Gall bladder Channel which goes upwards and accumulates in the nose.

Differentiation:

Nasal obstruction, loss of the sense of smell, yellow fetid nasal discharge accompanied by cough, dull pain, tenderness, and heaviness of the frontal region of the head, red tongue with a thin yellow coating, wiry rapid pulse.

Treatment:

Method : To disperse the heat of the Lung by puncturing with reducing method at points of the Lung and Large Intestine Channels as the main points.

Prescription:

Lieque (Lu. 7.).

Hegu (L.I. 4.).

Yingxiang (L.I. 20.).

Yintang (Extra. I.).

Headache:

Fengchi (G.B. 20.).

Taiyang (Extra. 2.).

Rationale:

Lieque (Lu. 7.) eliminates pathogenic wind by activating the dispersing function of the Lung. Hegu (L.I. 4.) and Yingxiang (L.I. 20.) reduce the heat of the Lung by regulating the *qi* of the Large Intestine Channel. Yintang (Extra. I) a local point at the nose, has the effect of reducing heat by removing the obstruction in the nose. Fengchi (G.B. 20.) eliminates the wind and reduces the heat so as to relieve headache. Taiyang (Extra. 2.) is an important point for the treatment of headaches.

Ear acupunture Points:

External Nose.

Internal Nose.

Forehead.

Method : Give moderate stimulation. Needles are retained for 10-15 minutes. About 10-15 treatments make a course.

Note: Rhinorrhea as described in this section corresponds to chronic rhinitis and chronic sinusitis of modern medicine.

EPISTAXIS (ASCENDING HYPERACTIVE FIRE)

Etiology:

Extravasation of blood due to:

(1) Ascending wind-heat of the Lung or fire of the Stomach which disturbs the nose.

(2) Insufficiency of *yin* causing hyperactivity of fire, which exhausts the *yin* of the Lung.

Differentiation:

(1) Excess of heat in the Lung and the Stomach: Epistaxis is accompanied by fever, cough, thirst, constipation and a superficial rapid pulse.

(2) Hyperactivity of fire due to insufficiency of *yin:* Epistaxis accompanied by malar flush, dryness of the mouth and a feverish sensation in the palms and soles. In severe cases there may be afternoon fever and a thready rapid pulse.

Treatment:

Method : Reduce the heat and stop bleeding by puncturing with the reducing method for the heat-excessive type and even movement for *yin* insufficient type at points of the Large Intestine and Du Channels.

Prescription:

Hegu (L.I. 4.).

Shangxing (Du 23.).

Points for the different clinical manifestations:

Heat of the Lung:

Shaoshang (L.I. 11.).

Heat of the Stomach:

Neiting (St. 44.).

Hyperactivity of fire due to insufficiency of *yin:*

Taixi (K. 3.).

Rationale:

The Large Intestine Channel is externally-internally related to the Lung Channel and links with the Stomach Channel, so Hegu (L.I. 4.) is used to reduce the heat of the three channels to stop bleeding. The Du channel is the confluence of all the *yang* channels, and Shangxing (Du 23.) is used to reduce the excessive *yang* of the Du Channel which causes hyperactivity of heat. Shaoshang (Lu. 11.), the Jing-Well Point of the Lung Channel is used to reduce the heat of the Lung. Neiting (St. 44.), the Yung-Spring Point of the Stomach Channel, is effective in reducing fire in the Stomach. Taixi (K. 3.), Yuan-Source Point of the Kidney Channel, has the effect of tonifying *yin* and reducing heat.

Ear acupuncture points:

Internal Nose.

Ear-Shenmen.

Sympathetic Nerves.

Method : Give moderate stimulation. Treatment is given 1-2 times a day, with needles retained for 15-20 minutes each session, with 4-6 treatments making a course.

Note: Epistaxis may be caused by trauma, nasal diseases, or systemic diseases such as diseases of blood, cardiovascular diseases and acute febrile infectious diseases. In addition to acupuncture treatment, other therapeutic measures should be adopted according to the primary cause.

TOOTHACHE

Etiology:

(1) Flaring up of the accumulated heat of the Stomach and Intestines together with invasion of exogenous pathogenic factors.

(2) Flaring up of *xu* fire due to an insufficiency of *yin* of Kidney.

Differentiation:

(1) Wind-heat: Gingival swelling and pain, thirst and preference for cold beverages, constipation, red tongue with yellow coating, and a rapid pulse.

(2) *Xu of Kidney:* Intermittent dull pain, loose teeth, red tongue, and a thready rapid pulse.

Treatment:

(1) Wind-heat:

Method : To reduce heat and relieve pain by puncturing with the reducing method at points mainly selected from the Large Intestine and Stomach Channels.

Prescription:

Hegu (L.I. 4.).
Xiaguan (St. 7.).
Jiache (St. 6.).
Fengchi (G.B. 20.).

Rationale:

Hegu (L.I. 4.) on the contralateral side is used to disperse the pathogenic heat of the Large Intestine Channel. Neiting (St. 44.), the Yung-Spring Point of the Stomach Channel pertains to water in the five Elements, so it is used to reduce the fire of the Stomach. Fengchi (G.B. 20.) has the effect of eliminating wind and reducing the fire. Xiaguan (St. 7.) and Jiache (St. 6.) are local points.

(2) *Xu of Kidney:*

Method : To nourish *yin* and reduce fire by puncturing with even movement (moderate stimulation) at points of the Stomach Channel as the main points.

Prescription:

Taixi (K. 3.).
Jiache (St. 6.).
Xiaguan (St. 7.).

Rationale:

Teeth relate to the Kidneys and are situated where the Stomach Channel and the Large Intestine Channel travel through, thus Taixi (K. 3.) is effective in nourishing *yin* of the Kidney and reducing *xu* fire. Jiache (St. 6.) and Xiaguan (St. 7.) relieve pain by regulating the *qi* of the channels.

Note: Toothache as described in traditional medicine includes acute and chronic pulpitis, dental caries and periodontal abscess of modern medicine.

SORE THROAT

Etiology:

Sore throat is divided into two types: the *shi* and the *xu*.

(1) *Shi type :* Invasion of the larynx and pharynx by exogenous pathogenic wind-heat, or flaring up of the accumulated heat of the Lung Channel and the Stomach Channel.

(2) *Xu type :* Flaring up of *xu* fire, due to insufficiency of *yin* of the Kidney.

Differentiation:

(1) *Shi type :* Abrupt onset with chills, fever and headache, congested and sore throat, thirst, constipation, red tongue with a thin yellow coating, and superficial rapid pulse.

(2) *Xu type :* Gradual onset without fever or with low fever, intermittent sore throat, dryness of the throat which usually becomes aggravated by night, feverish sensation in the palms and soles, uncoated red tongue, and thready rapid pulse.

Treatment:

(1) *Shi type:*

Method : To eliminate wind and heat by puncturing with the reducing method at points of the Large Intestine and Stomach Channels as the main points.

Prescription:

Shaoshang (Lu. 11.).
Hegu (L.I. 4.).
Neiting (St. 44.).
Tianrong (S.I. 17.).

Rationale:

Pricking Shaoshang (Lu. 11.) to let out a small amount of blood clears the heat of the Lung and relieves pain. Hegu (L.I. 4.) disperses exterior pathogenic factors of the Lung Channel. Neiting (St. 44.), the Yung-Spring Point of the Stomach Channel, reduces heat in the Stomach. Tianrong (S.I. 17.), a local point is used to promote circulation of *qi* and blood in the local area is effective in relieving sore throat.

(2) *Xu type:*

Method : To nourish the *yin* and reduce *xu* fire by puncturing with the reinforcing method at points of the Kidney Channel as the main points.

Prescription:

(a) Taixi (K. 3.).
Yuji (Lu. 10.).
(b) Zhaohai (K. 6.).
Lieque (Lu. 7.).

These two prescriptions may be used alternatively every other day.

Rationale:

Taixi (K. 3.) is the Yung-Spring Point of the Kidney Channel which travels to the pharynx and tongue. Yuji (Lu. 10.) is the Yung-Spring Point of the Lung Channel. Combination of the two nourishes *yin* and reduces fire. Zhaohai (K. 6.) and Lieque (Lu. 7.), one of the pairs of the Eight Confluent Points, relieves sore throat by reducing *xu fire*.

Ear acupuncture points:

Pharynx.

Tonsil.

Spleen.

Method : Puncture 2-3 points at each treatment with moderate stimulation. Needles are retained for an hour. Treatment is given once daily. About 3-5 treatments make a course. Prick the small vein in the back of the ear to let out a small amount of blood.

Note: Sore throat as described in this section includes acute tonsillitis, acute and chronic pharyngitis in the pathology of modern medicine.

THE ANCILLARY TECHNIQUES OF ACUPUNCTURE

A. MECHANICAL METHODS

(1) Acupressure
(2) Massage
(3) Exercise Therapy
(4) Periosteal Acupuncture
(5) Surgical Suture Embedding
(6) Three-edged Needle Bleeding Therapy
(7) Plum-Blossom Therapy
(8) Embedding Needle Therapy
(9) Relaxation Therapy
(10) Reflexotherapy (Zonal Therapy)
(11) Penetration Puncture
(12) Strong Stimulation Techniques
(13) Cupping

B. HYDROTHERAPY

Aquapuncture (Point Injection Therapy).
Homoeopuncture

C. HEAT

(1) Hot Needle
(2) Moxibustion
(3) Radiant Heat (Electrical Moxa), Microwave
(4) Akabane Method (A Diagnostic Procedure)

D. COLD (Cryopuncture)

E. LIGHT Laser Beam Therapy (Laserpuncture), Chromotherapy (Colour Therapy)

F. SOUND Sonopuncture, ultrasonic Therapy

G. ELECTROTHERAPY

(1) Electro-acupuncture, (Electro-anesthesia), (E.S.A.). (E.P.S.) Stimulation-induced anestheia (SIA),

(a) Low Frequency	continuous
(b) High Frequency	discontinuous
(c) Ultra High Frequency	dense-disperse

(2) T.E.N.S., T.C.N.S. (Transcutaneous Electro-Neuro-Stimulation)

(3) Dorsal Column Stimulation

(4) Voll Acupuncture (EAV), Biotron, Moratherapy and Vega

(5) Ryodoraku (Nakatani)

H. MAGNETISM Magnetotherapy

I. ANCILLARY REMEDIES Ginseng, Homoeopathy (Homoeopuncture)

J. MEDITATION, PSYCHOTHERAPY, TAI-CHI-CHUAN, YOGA, MASSAGE & MANIPULATION

K. NUTRITION

THE ANCILLARY TECHNIQUES OF ACUPUNCTURE

"Medicine is the Mother of all sciences"

-Sir William Osler

The practice of acupuncture throughout its long history has been carried out using many ancillary and allied techniques. Some of these methods are of great antiquity and are discussed in the two thousand year old classic, the *Huang Di Nei Jing* (Yellow Emperor's Classic of Internal Medicine) and other ancient classical texts. Others are of more recent vintage, being a spin-off of the Cultural Revolution and after in the Peoples' Republic of China. The older techniques too have been revised and modernized to keep abreast with the other recent advances in acupuncture therapy. However, all these special ancillary techniques, both old and new, are based on the same principles of acupuncture used to treat, disorders. It is only in the materials used and the methodology of their applications that they are different from one another. Some of these methods have become highly specialized. Intensive research into the different aspects of their usefulness, as regards their curative powers, is being carried out today in institutions like the Academies of Traditional Medicine in Peking and Shanghai, and the Departments of Acupuncture and Moxibustion in several medical faculties in the Peoples' Republic of China.

A. MECHANICAL METHODS

1. Acupressure,
2. Remedial Massage,
3. Exercise Therapy.

Acupressure is a very useful form of acupuncture therapy particularly in emergencies in the field, when needles are not available. It is the first line of treatment in acute emergencies accompanied by shock and collapse or unconsciousness. The procedure is to apply firm finger-pressure in an obliquely upward direction at the point Renzhong (Du. 26.) or other Jing-Well points. Acupressure at certain points may be used in tooth extractions or other minor surgery, such as an incision of an abscess or the suture of a superficial injury.

Acupressure forms the basis of the martial arts (karate judo, jujitsu, etc.). Remedial massage was a recognized modality of treatment during the Han and Tang dynasties and was taught as a popular subject in the ancient medical schools. Later it declined in popularity but has now been revived as an auxiliary method of therapy. There are two chief methods of massage - the An-mo consisting of 'pressing and rubbing' and the *Tui-na* method consisting of 'thrusting and rolling'. In Sri Lanka too, acupressure at command points (nilas) is used in the treatment of disease by traditional practitioners who are conversant with this art. The mahout (elephant keeper) is able to control the elephant by prodding him at specific acupuncture points with the 'henduwa'-a long metal rod. The elephant has 89 known acupuncture points.

Exercise therapy usually follows massage. It is widely practiced by the Chinese, both in health and disease. The content and scope of the exercises are much wider and sophisticated than today's modern physiotherapy regimen prescribed for patients. The ancient Chinese traditional physician on account of his preventive outlook always prescribed exercises for his clients in order to keep them healthy. Tai-Chi[1] is a special Chinese exercise routine, recommended for everyone young and old. Tai-Chi exercises brings the body into harmony with the universe.

---

1 Tai-Chai-Chuan

4. Periosteal Acupuncture

In this technique a filiform needle is inserted over a bone to touch the periosteum and then lifting and thrusting are carried out. This procedure is also known as "*periosteal pecking*". This method was first described by Felix Mann of U.K. and later developed by others such as Geoff Greenbaum[2] in Australia. It is particularly effective in chronic arthritic disorders. The tip of the coracoid process is a very effective point to be pecked in a frozen shoulder. The small joints of the hands and feet in rheumatoid arthritis are relieved of morning stiffness and pain with this procedure. Periosteal acupuncture at the Ah-Shi points where the bone is subcutaneous, is also helpful in low-backache. A fair degree of mobilization of the spine is also possible in ankylosing spondylitis using this procedure.

Periosteal acupuncture is contraindicated in the presence of acute inflammation and in sensitive individuals with a low threshold for pain. It is also contraindicated in the pain of malignant disease. If inexpertly carried out, periosteal puncture may aggravate the symptoms.

5. Surgical Suture Embedding Therapy

This method of treatment was developed during the 1965-70 period of the Cultural Revolution in China. The object of this treatment is to cure or alleviate diseases by producing prolonged stimulation at one or more acupuncture points by embedding a length of sterile catgut at these points. It has been found effective in resistant cases of bronchial asthma, gastric and duodenal ulcer, impotence, pain in the lumbosacral region, sacroiliac strain, other chronic locomotor diseases and for the sequelae of anterior poliomyelitis and similar disabilities.

The best method of embedding is to use a lumbar- puncture needle through which a piece of catgut, about 1 cm, long has been threaded. The needle is introduced through the skin. Then through

2 Greenbaum has demonstrated that periosteal pecking at the middle of the infrascapular fossa relieves intractable brachalgia.

the stylet, the catgut is pushed into the tissues and the needle is withdrawn. In an alternative method, the catgut is embedded in the deeper tissues after a surgical incision. The latter method is more invasive.

Points commonly selected for embedding therapy are:-

a) For bronchial asthma: Shanzhong (Ren 17.), Dingchuan (Ex. 17.).

b) For gastric and duodenal ulcers: Zhongwan (Ren 12.) through to Shangwan (Ren 13.), Weishu (U.B. 21.) through to Pishu (U.B. 20.).

c) For impotence: Qugu (Ren 2.).

d) For lumbar muscle strain: Yaoyangguan (Du 3.), Shenshu (U.B. 23.) *Ah-Shi* points.

e) Lumbo-sacral pain: Yaoyangguan (Du 3.), Dachangshu (U.B. 25.) through to Guanyuanshu (U.B. 26.) and the interpace S 2/3.

f) Sacro-iliac strain: Yaoyangguan (Du 3.), Dachangshu (U.B. 25.) through to Guanyuanshu (U.B. 26.), Chengfu (U.B. 36.), and the interpace Sacral 2/3. spines.

This therapy should not be carried out on little children, old and debilitated patients, and on diabetics. Scrupulous asepsis must be observed throughout the procedure.

6. The Three-edged Needle Bleeding Therapy:

The three-edged needle is a special type of needle having a triple cutting edge which is used to cause bleeding or to perform sacrification at certain acupuncture points. Bleeding of such points may be used for the purpose of resuscitation in acute emergencies, or it may be used as a curative measure in certain diseases.

In emergencies and acute conditions like convulsions, coma, unconsciousness, shock and collapse, cardiorespiratory distress, drowning, high fever and other emergencies, it is best to bleed the Jing-Well points of the extremities by the 'prompt pricking method'. In this method, the pricking is done very swiftly to a depth of about

0.1 cun and a few drops of blood are squeezed out from the point. In the treatment of diseases like dyspepsia or malnutrition in children, tonsilitis, conjunctivitis, and the chronic psoriatic type of skin disorders, another method called the 'slow pricking method' is employed. Slow pricking is usually done at points like Chize (Lu. 5.) and Weizhong (U.B. 40.), for skin diseases. The procedure adopted is to make a superficial vein over the selected acupuncture point prominent by constricting it proximally: it is then pricked slowly. The needle is punctured through the wall of the vein. After withdrawing the needle slowly, the tourniquet is released and the bleeding is arrested by applying firm pressure with a piece of sterile cotton wool at the site of the puncture. (In modern acupuncture, a syringe and an intravenous needle are usually used for the same purpose.).[3]

Except for the fact that it seems to work, the rationale for this type of blood-letting in the treatment of diseases is not clearly understood. According to some workers, skin disorders, are generally due to 'excess lung' and bleeding, which is a sedation method, helps to reduce this excess. The amount of blood drawn off is very small and the procedure has nothing in common with the medieval Western practice of 'blood-letting' in which copious amounts of blood were withdrawn from the patient (based on the theory of 'plethora' or 'excess blood'.). Nor is it related to the practice of venesection or 'raktha mokshana' of classical ayurveda, where bleeding is carried out on the course of any superficial vein. However, it has been widely practised in Sri Lanka where it is called 'nila vida ley hareema' meaning *'blood-letting after puncturing an acupuncture point"*. Some clinical tests on this indigenous form of 'acu-blood-letting' are now being conducted in collaboration with knowledgeable practitioners of the traditional system of acupuncture of Sri Lanka. This method is contraindicated in diabetics, very old people and in persons suffering from blood dyscrasias.

3 The blood may be injected at Dazhui (Du 14.) to enhance the immunity and/or at Xuchai (Sp. 10), which is an anti-allergic point. Only one drop is injected at each point.

7. Plum-blossom tapping:

The plum-blossom needle is a very useful device, especially when treating young children who may not take kindly to the insertion of filiform needles, as well as very old and debilitated persons. It is a very old method, which has been mentioned in the *Ling Shu* section of the *Huang Di Nei ling*. The plum-blossom needle is made up of a long 'stem' (handle) and a 'holder' to which are attached 5 or 7 fine needles. These are known as the five star or seven star needles respectively. These needles cover an area of about I square centimetre. The technique used is to tap the selected region with this instrument using the wrist movement only. The tapping should be done rapidly and precisely with the tip of the points striking the skin perpendicularly. According to the condition of the patient, the degree of force exerted in tapping may be light, medium, or heavy. In the case of children, debilitated, old, and nervous patients, only light tapping should be employed. Heavy tapping should be used only in cases where the skin sensation is dull or when the patient is suffering from a very painful condition. Medium tapping will do in most other cases.

The indications for plum-blossom needle tapping are certain types of skin conditions (such as alopecia areata, leucoderma, neurodermatitis, and erysipelas), asthma, migraine, neuralgia, arthritis, hemiplegia, chronic gastritis, and chronic gynecological disorders. It is also a very useful procedure for 'breaking up' areas of stiffness and tender subcutaneous nodules which often appear in the musculoskeletal and rheumatic disorders.

In skin diseases like alopecia and leucoderma, the affected areas should be tapped until slight redness occurs. After several such treatments are administered, it is common to see re-growth of hair and re-pigmentation, which are probably due to the stimulation of the dormant hair follicles and the dormant melanin layer. Injury to the skin should be avoided when tapping.

In small children suffering from bronchial asthma, good results are obtained by tapping along the course of the Lung Channel and on the Front-Mu and Back-Shu Points of the lung. In migraine, neuralgia and arthritis, tapping should be performed over the painful areas and the affected points. Likewise in hemiplegia, tapping should be done over the course of the channels of the paralysed area of muscles.

For diseases of the Internal Organs and the nervous system, tapping should be performed at the corresponding Huatuojiaji (Ex. 21.) points of the back. Alternatively, the Back-Shu Points on the Urinary Bladder Channel corresponding to the Organ concerned may be used. For example, in Liver disorders, tapping should be done at the point Ganshu (U.B. 18.), which is the Back-Shu Point of the liver. The site of tapping may also be selected on the basis of the therapeutic properties possessed by various specific points. For instance the points Zusanli (St. 36.) and Neiguan (P. 6.) may be used for chronic gastric disorders, while the point Zhongdu (Liv. 6.) may be used for diseases of the Liver. Another commonsense principle is to use local points for the diseases of local and adjacent areas. Thus, tapping may be carried out at the lumbosacral region for low backache, at the neck for stiff neck and at the intercostal spaces for diseases of the chest wall such as sprain or strain of the chest muscles and or intercostal neuralgia.

In using the plum-blossom needle, proper attention should be paid to the disinfection of the instrument before use. Plurn-blossom needles made out of plastic cannot be sterilized using an autoclave as the plastic will be damaged. The tips of the needles should be examined, from time to time, to ensure that they are even and sharp.

Contraindications are trauma, acute inflammations or the presence of varicose veins, cutaneous ulcers, severe edema, or burns, and infections of the skin such as scabies. In diabetics and those suffering from polyneuropathy and poor peripheral circulation, plum-blossom needling should be avoided.

8. Embedding Needle Therapy (Dermal Embedding Needles):

Also called the press needle, intradermal needle and implanted needle, they come in several shapes depending on their use.

(i) The thumbtack type :- This looks like a small thumbtack. The body of the needle is in the form of a small circle, about 3 mm. in diameter and its tip stands out at right angles to the circle. It penetrates to a depth of 2-3 mm. It is most commonly used in ear acupuncture.

(ii) The "fish tail" type :- This is similar to the thumbtack type except that its shaft lies at the same plane as its body. This needle is used on certain body acupuncture points for continuous stimulation. It is inserted horizontally under the skin and then fixed with adhesive tape.

Both these types of needles are indicated in chronic conditions like bronchial asthma, epilepsy, and in painful conditions like migraine. They may be kept in place for up to seven days and are therefore useful in providing mild stimulation of an acupuncture point between treatment sessions. In warm weather, it is advisable to change the needle in about half this time.

(iii) The spherical press needle (ball bearing type):- Used for the same purpose, this newer style is becoming more popular nowadays as it is safer. It consists of tiny stainless steel ball, which is fixed on the skin at the acupuncture point with adhesive tape.

(iv) The muscle embedding needle :- These are slightly longer than the fish tail type and are used to allay very intractable pain conditions, like phantom limb pain, or the pain of secondary cancer. The muscle embedding needle is left *in situ* at local painful points in the muscle (*Ah-Shi* points) for a few days.

After the needles are in place, intermittent stimulation is carried out by the patient himself, by pressing on the needle for a few minutes several times a day, hence they are also called 'press needles'. The thumbtack and fishtail types should be removed after one week in temperate countries. In the tropics, where there is much sweating, and the possibility of infection is greater, the removal should be earlier. The spherical press needles are much safer and may be left *in situ* for a few weeks. Aseptic precautions must however be scrupulously observed in order to prevent perichondritis of the auricular cartilage which can be a very serious complication. Embedding of needles is indicated in the treatment of chronic conditions like bronchial asthma, drug addictions, obesity, migraine, low-backache, pain of malignant diseases and travel sickness. If there is the slightest discomfort with an embedding needle, it should be immediately removed and the ear examined carefully in a good light.[4]

9. Relaxation Therapy :

A special relaxation method for spastic muscles has been recently discovered using electrical stimulation at points Jizhong (Du 6.) and Yaoqi (Ex. 20.). In paraplegia, cerebral palsy, transverse myelitis and other spastic states this is very effective. Relaxation therapy has also been used to obtain relaxation of muscles during abdominal surgery. Gabriel Stux of Dusseldorf has shown that electro-acupuncture with needling at these points helps to relieve the spasticity of cerebral paisy in the upper motor neurone disorders such as strokes. In the Peoples' Republic of China it was shown that by using these points, muscular relaxation was obtained during abdominal surgery. At the Institute of Acupuncture, Sri lanka, using a combined method of acupuncture anaesthesia (acusthesia) it was shown that significantly less muscle relaxants are required during surgery when these points are used. This has been confirmed in Shanghai.

10. Reflexotherapy or Zonal Therapy:

This is a form of combined acupressure and acumassage used on the foot acupuncture zones. The use of a suitable cream to reduce friction makes this a very pleasant form of therapy. It is particularly helpful in little children and elderly people. When carried out properly, it is a very acceptable form of therapy. In Europe and North America, reflexotherapy or zonal therapy is usually performed by para-medical practitioners as this is a non-invasive procedure. It is

4 The adhesive tape used may also cause sensitivity reactions.

useful in chronic painful disorders such as low-backache, migraine, and dysmenorrhea. Bronchial asthma in little children also responds very well to this form of therapy. The tenderness of the respective zones may be used to diagnose internal organ disorders.

Many designs of acupressure pegs made of wooden, bamboo, jade, silver and other exotic materials are available in some countries, However, the trained therapist's fingers are, perhaps, the most effective.[5]

11. Penetration Puncture:

This is an old needle technique improved during the Cultural Revolution. The object of the method is to obtain maximal effect from two or more acupuncture points with a single needle insertion. It is named *'penetration puncture'* or *'puncturing-through technique'* because the needle inserted at one acupuncture point is made to penetrate or puncture through to another point or points in its path. For example the points Ermen (S.J. 21.), Tinggong (S.I. 19.), and Tinghui (G.B. 2.), which treat many ear diseases, may be punctured through with only one needle inserted at Ermen (S.J. 21.). Besides economising on time and needles, this causes less inconvenience to the patient and it is also believed to result in potentizing the combined effects of the points. Another example of penetration puncture is in needling Dicang (St. 4.) through to Jiache (St.6.) using a long needle, in cases of facial paralysis, facial hemispasm, and trigeminal neuralgia.

Sometimes, actual penetration of the second point is not carried out, but the needle is merely directed towards the latter location for some distance. An example of this is the puncturing Neiguan (P. 6.), through towards Waiguan (S.J. 5.) as is done in acupuncture anaesthesia.

Hegu (L.I. 4.) towards Laogong (P. 8.), with manipulation, is an important example of penetration that will relieve any acute pain.

5 Rolfing along the Channels is becoming a popular procedure in the west.

12. The Strong Stimulation Technique:

Strong stimulation is the rapid manipulation of the needle by means of a combined manoeuvre involving simultaneous rotation together with a lifting and thrusting movement. This method is invaluable in the treatment of acutely painful conditions (and excess disorders), where immediate relief is desirable. This is also known as the *'sedation method'* or *xie method.*

To perform strong stimulation, the needle should be inserted into the selected point with its tip embedded deep in the underlying muscle. Rotation ('twirling') of the needle at a rate up to about 200 rotations per minute and with an arc of not more than 180 degrees is carried out. This may be combined with simultaneous lifting and thrusting movements of the needle at a rate of up to 200 per minute, the range of the lift-thrust being about 0. - 0.2 centimetres. The stimulation should be continued until the acupuncture sensation (*deqi*) is felt and is repeated if necessary. Strong stimulation may also be carried out electrically using a voltage of about 10 volts and a frequency of over 200 pulses per second. In very severely painful disorders and during surgery, a frequency of up to 2000 Hertz may be employed. (The Medicina Alternativa Stimulator is able to deliver these frequencies). One observes however, that the results with hand manipulation are often better. Hence it is strongly recommended that every acupuncturist should familiarize himself with the manual technique. The art of acupuncture depends on a painless insertion and the correct manipulation techniques.

Relief of pain by means of strong stimulation may be very dramatic in its effects on the patient, as well as on the onlookers. Acute pain as well as pain of long-standing duration which has resisted all previous therapies may be effectively relieved by this simple procedure. The most popular explanation at present is that strong stimulation sets up a stream of nerve impulses which compete with the pain impulses, thereby 'closing the sensory gate' for pain transmission.[6] Another method of 'strong stimulation' has recently been ex-

6 Prolonged relief is due to humoural mechanisms.

perimented with in the People's Republic of China for the treatment of patients with motor dysfunction. In this method, longitudinal incisions about 1.5 to 2.0 cm. long are made under local anaesthesia or acupuncture anaesthesia at selected points on the affected limbs. After separating the muscles from each other by using blunt forceps, the nerves should be identified and massaged gently with the same forceps. Thereafter strong stimulation should be applied using blunt vascular forceps, the nerves being vibrated rhythmically with small amplitude, but high frequency. Vibration should be kept up for about 1 minute, and after a rest period it should be repeated 3 to 5 times until sensations of tingling, burning, or distension are felt by the patient. Manipulation must be extremely gentle to avoid causing shock and damage to nerves and blood vessels. The order in which the various points are stimulated should follow a definite pattern, like 'chasing from the proximal points to the more distal points on the same limb'. Thus in the lower limb, the order of stimulation should be Huantiao (G.B. 30.), Yanglingquan (G.B. 34.), and Zusanli (St. 36.). The nerves that are commonly stimulated at these points are as follows-

Upper Limb:

JianZhen (S I. 9.),	:	Radial, ulnar, median.
Quchi (L.I. 11.).	:	Radial, median.
Hegu (I.I. 4.), through to Laogong (P. 8.).	:	Branches of radial, median, ulnar.

Lower Limb:

Huantiao (G.B. 30.).	:	Superior gluteal, sciatic.
Yanglingquan (G.B. 34.).	:	Peroneal, anterior tibial.
Zusanli (St. 36.).	:	Anterior tibial.

In order to produce prolonged stimulation, a piece of sterilized catgut may be embedded intramuscularly at the site of incision before it is closed. The treatment should be followed up with massage, exercises, physiotherapy, acupuncture, and the injection of B complex vitamin in order to assist recovery.

Owing to the heavy demands on our time in clinical work and training programmes, we have not been able to explore the technique of direct stimulation as described above. However we have been treating a large number of patients with long standing motor dysfunctions by means of strong stimulation at the above points after simple insertion of thick needles and the results are remarkably good. We believe that the light functional recovery which occurs in these cases is explained on the basis of *'The Motor-Gate Theory'*.

Strong stimulation may also be carried out by inserting long, thick needles along the channels. This is particularly useful for paraplegia where such insertions are carried out along the course of the Stomach Channels or Urinary Bladder Channels.[7]

Strong stimulation of acupuncture points, both for the relief of pain and for the improvement of motor functions is a significant advance in medical treatment for the rehabilitation of the pain-ridden patient and those afflicted with crippling motor disorders. It has no doubt great therapeutic potential and is being extensively used in pain clinics, rehabilitation units, and physiotherapy departments.

13. Cupping:

Cupping is a method of stimulating the acupuncture points or areas by applying suction through a hollow vessel in which a partial vacuum has been artificially created. This procedure induces blood stasis or even blister formation at the site, thereby stimulating the acupuncture points.

In ancient times, this method of treatment was called the *'horn method'* (*chio-fa*). An animal horn with the tip cut off was inverted over the selected site and suction applied through the hole at the top. After the air was sucked out, the hole was plugged with the finger and the horn kept in position for some time. Later on these horns were replaced by vessels made of bamboo, burnt clay, glass, or ceramic. Today elegant spherical glass jars are used.

7 Korean acupuncturists have demonstrated the usefulness of 10 inch needles inserted along the channels.

The method of cupping most commonly used today is to soak a cotton ball attached to a stick in alcohol, after which it is ignited circled in the interior of the jar quickly and then withdrawn. Immediately after, the jar is swiftly cupped over the skin surface. The partial vacuum so created helps the cup attach itself to the skin area by suction. It requires a swift technique to do this correctly and painlessly.

Cupping is an effective method of treating low backache, sprains and soft tissue injuries whenever the response to acupuncture and other forms of treatment is slow or inadequate. Cupping of the chest is also perfomed to encourage the elimination of secretions from the lungs. Combined with postural drainage and deep breathing exercises, this procedure is very helpful.

Contraindications to cupping:

High fever, convulsions, very sensitive and inflamed skin areas, regions covered with much hair, pregnancy, infectious diseases, and the presence of ulcers and abscesses are contraindications to cupping. It is also best avoided in nervous patients.

B. HYDROTHERAPY

Acupuncture (Point-injection Therapy):

Point-injection therapy is a modern technique that combines traditional medicine and Western medicine. It consists of the injection of certain therapeutic drugs or distilled water into the acupuncture points, preferably at those points which exhibit pathological changes or are manifestations of positive reaction to disease. The Back-Shu Points or Mu-Front Points, Alarm Points and the Ah-Shi Points are where such reactions are usually found and they are commonly used for this form of therapy. When injected, a definite 'needle sensation' may be produced at these points, due to the physical and chemical stimulation. The protracted stimulation which results is said to increase the body resistance to disease thereby promoting curative effects. In the case of narcotics like morphine and pethidine (dolantin) and tranquillizers like chlorpromazine, it has been found that a very much smaller dosage than usual may be used to produce sedation. Hydrotherapy is often used in premedication before acupuncture anaesthesia in China. Fractional doses such as 1½ g (5mg) of morphine are claimed to be sufficient for premedication, using the method of point injection therapy.[8]

The best points to use, as mentioned above, are those which show some form of reaction as determined by inspection and palpation. However, points on the hand and feet areas where the muscle layer is thin should be avoided wherever possible. Before the treatment is given, it is best to explain to the patient that certain normal reactions (like sensations of numbness, soreness, heaviness, and distension at the site of the injection and some degree of lassitude) are to be expected. After routine disinfection at the selected point, the injection should be administered after drawing back the plunger and checking to ensure that no blood appears in the barrel of the syringe. The speed of the injection should be moderate. In asthenic patients with chronic diseases the injection should be given even slower, and the concentration of the drug should be very low. In more robust patients, the injection may be faster and the drug concentration higher.

Drugs used for injection should be easily absorbable and be free of side-effects and have certain stimulating properties. Those most commonly used are the B vitamins, C, and distilled water[9]. Placental extracts, antibiotics, and certain herbal drugs are also used. In the case of drugs with allergenic properties, sensitivity tests must be carried out before use. The treatments should be administered once daily or every other day. Seven to ten treatments usually comprise one course. The interval between two courses should be 5 to 7 days. Good results are reported in the locomotor disorders with acupuncture points corresponding to the motor points of the paralysed muscles.

---

8 Potentized homoeopathic preparations on medicated needles are very effective (Homoeopuncture).

9 The water may be energized with the similimum (Moratherapy, Biotrom).

C. HEAT

1. Hot Needle Therapy:

Hot needling is another ancient technique which was updated during the Cultural Revolution. It is a good example of how creative thinking in the realm of traditional medicine leading to the emergence of simple, yet effective, methods of treatment where the results compare very favourably with those obtained by sophisticated medical and surgical procedures.

The method of hot needling was discovered several thousands of years ago. The present practice is to take a firm sharp *Yuan-li* needle, make it red hot in a flame, thrust in to the affected part, and withdraw it very quickly. The disorders which may be successfully treated include benign small adenoma of the thyroid, "ganglion" of the wrist, Baker's cysts, lipoma and other types of benign lumps. The procedure is very simple; the results are magnificent, but the methodology must be learnt supervised through practice in a clinic.

2. Moxibustion:

Moxibustion has been widely used in China and in several other Eastern countries since prehistoric times. Moxibustion is the therapeutic method of treating diseases by burning 'moxa-wool' or generating similar forms of heat on or near-specific acupuncture points. It is a very ancient form of treatment, perhaps even pre-dating acupuncture. There are references to it in the Huang Di Nei Jing, and according to some authorities it was practiced as far back as the Stone Age, and may even have antedated the use of stone needle acupressure. From prehistoric times, acupuncture and moxibustion have been practiced together as complementary forms of therapy, often on the same patient, hence the name "acupuncture-moxibustion" or *Zhen-Jiu* (or 'acumoxy') in Chinese. In Sri Lanka too, these modalities were closely related and acupuncture-moxibustion is called vidum-pilissum. In Sri Lanka moxibustion is widely used on farm animals, particularly on cattle.[10] In moxibustion, the points used are anatomically the same as for acupuncture, but the therapeutic indications are some-what different and there is also some divergence regarding the Forbidden Points in the two procedures. For example, the umbilicus is commonly used for moxibustion, whereas it is absolutely forbidden for acupuncture. Moxibustion is generally indicated in chronic bronchitis, chronic bronchial asthma, chronic diarrhea, arthritis, and whenever there has been an inadequate response to acupuncture in Yin (*Xu*)[11] diseases. According to recent research carried out in Japan, it is possibly more effective than needle acupuncture in improving the body's resistance to disease by its action on the immune-enhancing mechanisms. This is probably a result of the tissue injury created by the intense heat due to the burning moxas. More work remains to be done to elucidate the mechanism of action in this healing method.

The term 'moxibustion' is derived from the Japanese name 'mogusa' for the mugwort plant whose botanical name is *Artemisia Vulgaris.* Moxa-wool is made by grinding the sun-dried leaves of the plant into a fine wool. The Sinhalese name for this plant is val kolondu. Moxa leaves have a characteristic smell. They are used as a cooking spice. Moxa is an essential ingredient in the stuffing of the Martinmas goose, a choice delicacy of the German cuisine.

Moxas may take various forms - balls, cones, cigars and sticks of different sizes, ranging from that of a cherry seed to a Cuban cigar. Using these preparations, moxibustion can be carried out in many different ways:

(i) **Direct Moxibustion:** In direct moxibustion a small moxa-cone is placed directly on the skin surface at an acupuncture (moxibustion) point and then ignited. There are two forms of this method:-

a) *Scarring Moxibustion:* The moxa is allowed to burn out completely on the skin. This results in the formation of a blister and is not used very much today for obvious reasons,

10 Traditional Chinese acupuncture is used in Sri Lanka by many Veterinary Surgeons to treat domestic and farm animals, including elephants.

11 All yin diseases due to a yang deficiency.

although it is said to be very effective in certain chronic seasonal allergies. In the People's Republic of China, intractable cases of allergic bronchial asthma seem to respond very well to this form of therapy.

b) *Non-Scarring Moxibustion:* A cone is ignited at the top, placed on the point and removed as soon as a sensation of scorching with slight pain is felt. The procedure may be repeated several times until there is redness and congestion at the site. Usually 3 to 5 cones are applied during a single session and this is repeated daily or every other day. If performed carefully, this method is quite safe and there is no blistering or scarring.

(ii) **Indirect Moxibustion:** In indirect moxibustion a slice of ginger, a slice of garlic or a thin layer of salt is placed over the point before introducing the moxa. Alternatively, an ignited moxa stick may be used to warm the point from a distance of about 3-5 cm. The lighted end of the stick may also be brought briefly into contact with the diseased area and immediately withdrawn. This movement is repeated at intervals of a few seconds. It is known as the *"sparrow pecking method"* of moxibustion. Another method is to warm the head of an acupuncture needle inserted at the site, with a piece of lighted moxa firmly fixed to its handle. Sometimes electrical methods of heating are employed, in which case it is called 'electrical moxibustion'. This is a modern innovation. In one design of an instrument manufactured by M/S. MBB of West Germany, radiant heat emanates from an electrically heated sapphire head. The heat generated is similar to that of moxibustion. We have found that this is a fairly effective method in many Yin disorders. Refer to Radiant heat therapy (Electrical Moxa).

Contraindications to moxibustion: Moxibustion should not be applied to areas with much hair, near special sense organs, the facial region, near large blood vessels, areas of sensory loss, or poor circulation, the scalp, or on mucous membranes, and ulcerated areas. Points Fengfu (Du 16.) and Yamen (Du 15.) on the neck are contraindicated for moxibustion. Moxibustion should not be used on little children, nervous, debilitated, diabetic and mentally deficient patients. Moxibustion is absolutely contraindicated in Yang disorders and in deaf-mutes.

BOTANICAL DESCRIPTION OF THE PLANT USED FOR MOXIBUSTION

Moxa is a latinized form of *Mogusa*, the Japanese name for this plant.

Botanical Description:

Perennial, leaves alternate, deeply pinnatisect, heads very small, inspicate inflorescences, involucre ovoid. bracts few, imbricate, inner very obtuse, membraneous, receptacle naked; flowers all tubular, outer row female, fertile, disk flowers few bisexual, anther bases obtuse; style branches bisexual; flower short, truncate, with tuft of hair at end; achene very small, oblong, striate, pappus.

150 species; 27 are described in "*Flora of British India*". Only the species "*Vulgaris*" is found in Sri Lanka. It is likely that the species "*Artemisia Vulgaris*" was imported here in ancient times and grown in herbaria for moxibustion.

Species Description:

Artemisia Vulgaris Linneus: Perennial semi-shrubby, stems erect, 2-3 feet, virgate slightly cottony; leaves numerous, 2-4 inches, broadly oval in outline, very deeply pinnatisect, the upper segments large, the lower very small, and the basal ones stipule-like, all again cut into narrow acute micronate segments, pilose or glabrous above, densely cottony - pubescent, and white beneath, uppermost lancellate, entire; heads solitary or two or three together, sessile or stalked in axile of leaves and forming long spicate leafy inflorescences, outer inflorescences scales slightly pubescent.

COMMON NAMES FOR THE ARTEMISIA VULGARIS (MOXA PLANT)

Bengali	-	Nagadona
Chinese	-	Ai, Jiu.
Deharadun	-	Samri, Sami.
English	-	Fleabane, India Wormwood, St. John's Wort, Mugwort.
Hindi	-	Dona, Majtari, Mastaru, Muguduna, Gathivana.
Japanese	-	Yomogi, Mogusa.
Kannada	-	Dovana, Manjipatri.
Kashmiri	-	Tithwan.
Malaya	-	Ai, Chiai, Kheengai, kiai, Ngai.
Malayalam	-	Appa.
Marathi	-	Dhor-Davana, Gathona.
Nepali	-	Titapat.
Punjabi	-	Afsunthin, Banjiru, Buimadaran, Chambra, Puujan, Tarkha, Tataur, Ubusha.
Sanskrit	-	Nagadamani, Nilpushpa, Sara – parni, Sugandha, Barha, Barhikusum, Barhipushpa Granthika, Granthiparna, Granthiparnake, Guchhakar, Gutthaka, kakapushpa, Kukura, Shuka, Shukabarha, Shukachhada, Shukapuccha.
Sinhala	-	Val Kolondu
Tamil	-	Machibattiri, Tarunama, Marikilondu, Thavanam.
Telgu	-	Davanamu, Mashiparti.
Oriya	-	Doyona, Gondhermaro, Nagodoyona.

Location:

Roadside and waste places, rather common, but only as an escape from gardens. Flowers brownish, yellow and small in size.

Throughout temperate Asia and Europe. The Chinese emigrants to North America have introduced this species on the American continent for moxibustion. Not endemic in Africa, Australia, and South America.

In Sri Lanka this plant now grows wild by the roadside in the Kandyan areas.

3. Radiant Heat (Electrical moxa):

Many different designs of electrical equipment are available where the generation of heat is similar to that of the burning moxa. In one design made by Messrs. MBB of the Federal Republic of Germany, the heat is generated by an electrically heated sapphire head. We have used this equipment for over 10 years and find it a convenient alternative to traditional moxa therapy.

4. Akabane method (a diagnostic method):

This is a method invented by Akabane of Japan around the turn of the century in order to determine the imbalance of energy in the channels. The lightened end of a Joss-stick is placed quickly on the Jing-Well points until the threshold of heat is felt. With the advent of sensitive acupunctoscopes this method is now largely historical.

D. COLD (CRYOACUPUNCTURE, CRYOPUNCTURE)

There are many new designs of electrical instruments where cold is applied to the acupuncture points. This is known as cold therapy, cryoacupuncture, or cryopuncture. Good results have been reported by using this method in acute sprains, particularly at the *Ah-Shi* points.

LASER BEAM THERAPY

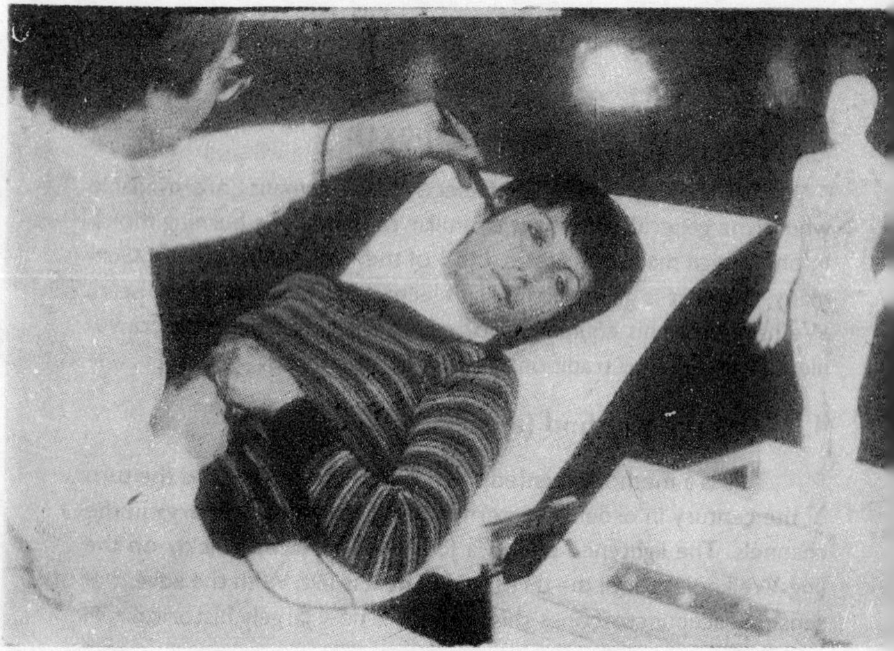

Laser beam therapy may be used at the Jing-Well points, Ah-shi points, Local and Distal points, or to sweep all the channels in the direction of the energy flow. Laser beam therapy at auricular points (as shown above) is also an effective method of treatment.

E. LIGHT

Laser Beam Therapy:

A laser is a beam of monochromatic, coherent, monophasic, light energy. The word *"laser"* is an acronym for *Light Amplification by Stimulated Emission of Radiation.*

Entities capable of vibration, such as atoms or molecules, may assume an energetically "excited" state. Many of these states have a "lifetime" considerably above the normal limit of about 10 secs. If a light wave of a given wavelength falls on an atom or molecule in the excited state, the system returns to the ground state and the radiation emitted reinforces the source of light.

Lasers are a new innovation in the scientific scene in medicine. The theory of lasers was first suggested by Professor Albert Einstein in 1917. However until recently, a laser could not be constructed until the correct equipment and technology was available. In fact, so many uses for lasers had been invented before the equipment was built, that lasers were cynically termed *"a solution chasing the problem!"* In the late 1950's the practical possibility of an optical laser was demonstrated by two workers, Schawlow and Townes. The first ruby laser was made by Theodore Kaiman of the Hughes Aircraft Company, U.S.A., in 1963. The heart of this first laser was a cube of synthetic ruby. It is now possible to construct lasers based on solids, gases or liquids as the emitting source. Helium-Neon (HeNe) lasers are the most widely used in acupuncture therapy today.[12]

Technological research has developed many different laser-active media. The nature of the media determines the fundamental properties of a laser beam. One of the main distinguishing characteristics between the many laser active media is the state of its aggregation. Among the gaseous lasers are the HeNe laser, the argon. CO_2 and krypton lasers.

The three essential physical properties of a laser beam are monochromaticity, coherence and small divergence.

12 Gallium is used in Infra-red Lasers.

Monochromaticity describes radiation which spectrographically forms a very narrow (spectral) line. In the production of a laser beam this entails that only one definite wavelength is amplified and caused to radiate.

On both sides of the laser medium there are resonator mirrors, one of which is only half-silvered. Radiation produced in the laser medium by the action of the pumping energy can travel only along an axis which is determined by these resonator mirrors. When the radiation has been sufficiently amplified by repeated to and fro passage along this axis, it escapes through the partially silvered resonator mirror. This radiation constitutes the laser beam proper.

Lasers were hailed as a tremendous advance because of the special properties of the light which they emit. A common source of light, like an electric bulb or a flame, produces a wide spectrum radiation, which is emitted spontaneously. In a laser, the material that is emitting the light is stimulated to radiate by external energy. The conditions are more controlled and the light has more specific properties. A simple way in which to explain this difference is that in ordinary light, radiation is emitted in a random fashion like a group of people hitting the water at one end of a swimming pool with paddles out of tune with one another and creating lots of little ripples. In a laser, the light from each other molecule comes out in an orderly and regulated way as if a group of oarsmen were hitting the water at the same time so that each wave is added up with all the others to form a much larger and continuous series of waves. This orderly property is called coherence and all the light waves sent out by a laser have the same wave-length and frequency. This means that the light is emitted in an almost parallel beam which can travel great distances, without diffusing appreciably. The colour of the laser radiation, therefore, has a particular purity that does not normally occur in nature.

The basic property of the laser beam, namely the small divergence, is of particular practical importance. In the laser- active material only the pathways of beams in the neighbourhood of the axes undergo amplification. The emerging beams are therefore substantially parallel. Minimum divergence therefore means, in practice, maximum parallelism. In this way it is possible to obtain foci of extremely small diameters perhaps in the range of 3 to 10 wavelengths.

When an electron drops from a configuration of higher energy to one of lower energy, the surplus energy appears as radiation, partly electromagnetic and partly acoustic or vibrational. The electromagnetic radiation from any one type of electronic configuration always has the same frequency. In a heated solid however, many different types of electronic configurations are possible and light is emitted at many different frequencies. The specific difference between a conventional light source and a laser lies in the extent to which the emission of surplus energy can be controlled.

Lasers are primarily used in Western medicine for their thermal effect. In a laser, intensive electromagnetic energy can be concentrated with in a very small area producing a burning or cutting effect, which can be utilized for various surgical procedures.

Laser is being used today in medical technology for surgery, diagnosis, and stimulation therapy (or acupuncture).

In surgery, the treatment of retinal detachment has long been an established practice. In addition to this, endoscopic surgery stands out as a future domain of the laser beam. In addition to the treatment of internal haemorrhages, there is the treatment of small tumours and polyps. Favourable results are being reported in dermatological surgery and neurosurgery and also for ear, nose, and throat surgery and gynecological surgery, especially in cases that permit a vaginal approach.

While the surgeon applies high intensity laser energy for its cauterising effect; weak intensity lasers of specific wave lengths stimulate biological functions. Laser radiation is used for its destructive, "antibiotic effect", in surgery. The biotic effect is used for what Inyushin of the U.S.S.R. calls *"light vitamins"*. This therapy is based on the principle of bio-resonance. It is a consequence of new developments in biophysical research in the soviet Union and West Germany.[13]

13 Akumed, MBB, LAWO.

Although the radiation of various frequencies of light have biological effects, the effects due to different frequencies partially counteract or cancel each other. Ordinary sources of light possess a heterogenous mixture of different frequencies, therefore no pronounced biological reactions occur with such radiators. A laser beam is characterized by a monochromatic, polarized, monophasic radiation in a much sharper frequency-band than can be obtained from other sources of light.

The sharpest frequency-band is obtained from gas lasers. Inyushin and his co-workers in Alma Alta, U.S.S.R. discovered that the Helium-Neon laser is the optimal light source for this phototherapy.

The wave length of the Helium-Neon laser is in the vicinity of 6328 Angstrom units, (the red part of the visible spectrum.)[14] Red light of this frequency has known biological effects. It is generally found to have vitalizing effects on living tissue. For this reason, radiation with the red Helium - Neon laser is used for a variety of therapeutic purposes such as promoting wound healing, encouraging healing of skin grafts, skin diseases, and in blood disorders. In laboratory animals whose bone marrow has been destroyed, lasers encourage re-formation. In agronomy it has been shown that this kind of laser radiation may be used to energize seeds, thus making the sprouts grow faster.

According to some authorities in the U.S.S.R., the red laser acts on the "biological plasma" by a resonance effect to strengthen its energetic state. Thus it acts like a "light vitamin" at the bioenergetic level.

Some of the actions of laser beams on living tissue are also observed on inanimate material. The properties on materials irradiated may be described on an increasing physical scale as follows:

a) absorption,

b) dispersion (scattering),

c) local warming of the tissues.

14 632.8 nanometers.

d) dehydration or withering of the tissues,

e) denaturation of protein, i.e. coagulation,

f) thermolysis (carbonization) and

g) evaporation.

The magnitude of the effect on irradiated tissues depends on two factors, namely:

- the duration of the irradiation, and
- the laser power used.

In acupuncture we deal on the bioenergetic system of acupuncture channels and points. The traditional system of acupuncture is utilized in combination with the new bioenergetic technique of laser therapy. The research in Alma Ata[15] has shown that the acupuncture points are specific points of energy exchange between the living organism and the surrounding environment and that the application of laser therapy to acupuncture points has specific advantages whereby significant results are obtained in a variety of diseases. Biophysical experiments have demonstrated that the bioenergy produced by laser radiation of acupuncture points is conducted along bioenergetic channels similar to the accepted traditional acupuncture channels, thus providing new evidence both for the physiological significance of the acupuncture points and the channels.

The acupuncture points are specific points in the bioenergetic sense. This is indicated by experimental findings that the conductance of various forms of energy, like heat, light, sound and electricity is greater in the area of the point than in the surrounding areas of the skin. The acupuncture system is apparently not only a bioelectrical (cosmic) energy and information are being transferred in the form of electromagnetic radiation. As with the bioelectrical properties of this system, the protobiological properties may also be utilized both for therapeutic and diagnostic purposes.

In medical therapy at Alma Ata. a Helium-Neon laser is used with an output of 25 milliwatts. Radiation of acupuncture points for

15 U.S.S.R.—Medicina Alternativa was established in Alma Ata in 1962

a few seconds is used for stimulation, while a longer exposure of 30-120 seconds is used for sedation. The penetration depth of the Alma Ata laser in human tissues is about 5 mm. The treatment is given in dark rooms and the patient is kept in darkness for some time after treatment to reduce the counteracting effects of other frequencies of light. Local radiation of affected areas is used for local disorders.

The advent of laser acupuncture opens very promising vistas for acupuncture as a bioenergetic medicine.

Recently Chinese researchers have carried out major surgery using laser anaesthesia.

Laser-Beam Equipment and Procedure:

In our clinical practice we have treated about 12000 cases with laser beam therapy. We have found it quite useful, particularly in children.[16]

The apparatus used in our clinic is designed for two functions. The first function is the location of an acupuncture point using the phenomenon of higher electrical conductivity of the skin at the acupuncture point (as indicated by a microammeter as well as an acoustical device that signals when the measuring electrode touches the point). Then the apparatus is switched to its second function: the generation of a laser beam is emitted through the same hand piece that contains the measuring electrode, and the acupuncture point is directly irradiated. The period of treatment at each point may range from one second to one minute.

Only a few points are treated per session. The points usually selected are the Distal points, especially the end points of the Channels at the extremities, the Jing-Well points, which are treated bilaterally. Proximal points may also be used. Baihui (Du 20.) is generally not used. The intensity of the laserbeam is very low so that there is no danger of damage to the skin, the underlying tissues or the patient's eyes. We have found that the use of laser directly on the eye for eye disorders is a very effective form of therapy.

16 Laser was used routinely for the first time on patients at Kalubowila in 1974.

With the ammeter in the apparatus it is possible to monitor the skin conductivity of the points treated. As the treatment progresses and the patient begins to improve, a gradual normalization of skin conductivity may be noted, indicating the restoration of functional and energetic balance.

The theoretical basis of this therapy comes from the discovery by certain researchers that the living organism has mechanisms for receiving, storing, and even emitting electromagnetic waves in the optical region. The red part of the visible spectrum is said to be capable of the highest level of transmission and the skin is believed to function as an optical filter for its absorption by the underlying connective tissue. This is how a red light laser beam is able to penetrate the skin more efficiently. Laser beam therapy is therefore distinguishable from electro-acupuncture in that, while in the latter, the stimulation brings about effects on cells due to electrical current and micro-coagulations, in the former the stimulation, is caused solely by the absorption of light radiated through the skin.

In laserbeam therapy, the indications are generally the same as in conventional acupuncture. It is claimed that "deqi" is occasionally elicited and when this happens, a fast response may be expected. Particular success has been reported in the treatment of chronic ulcers and non- healing wounds. Good results are also said to be obtained in diseases associated with symptoms of the Yin type of disorders. Neuralgia on the other hand shows a positive reaction when the ear points are treated. We have on record a patient who regularly faints when laser beam is applied to her. In our experience a wide range of diseases including bronchial asthma, the locomotor diseases and migraine have been helped using this technique.[7]

Although this technique seems to be a fruitful development, much work still has to he done to clarify its theoretical basis so that its full potential may be understood and applied.

17 Laser therapy is used worldwode in cosmetic therapy.

ELECTRO-ACUPUNCTURE STIMULATOR

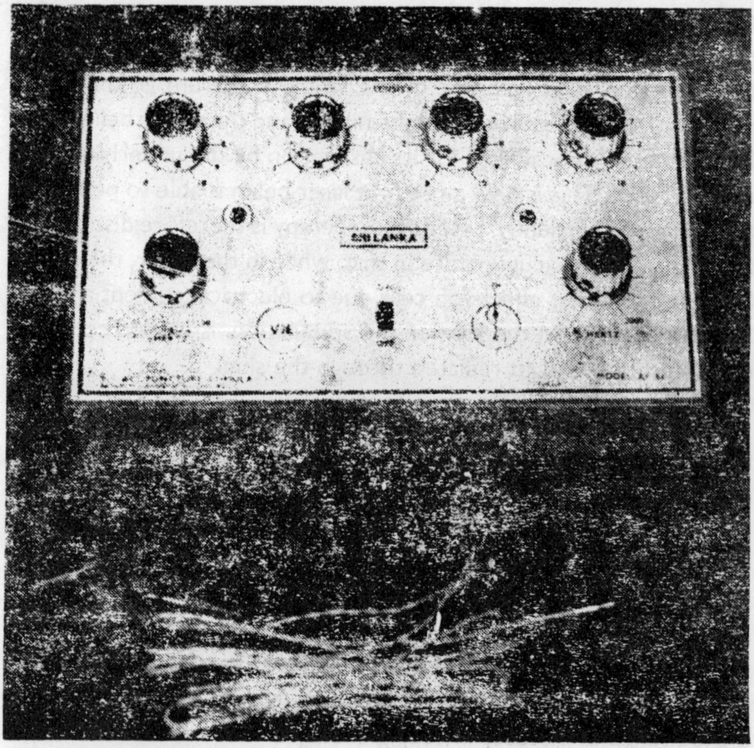

The Medicina Alternativa Stimulator (Made in Sri Lanka)
Suitable for therapy, TENS and anaesthesia.

F. SOUND THERAPY

Sonopuncture:

Sonopuncture is the name given to the recently developed technique of stimulating acupuncture points by means of supersonic waves (waves travelling faster than the speed of sound) and ultrasonic waves. Many advantages are claimed for this new form of therapy and sonic stimulators have already made their appearance in the North American market. While this "non-invasive procedure" may turn out to he a useful development, the possibility of some damage at the cellular level exists from "breaking the sound barrier'. Much research is being done in the U.S.S.R. on sonopuncture. However, more work needs to be done to evaluate this method.

G. ELECTROTHERAPY (E.P.S., S.I.A., E.S.A.).[18]

I. Electro-acupuncture, Electro-anaestheisa.
(See the Chapter on the History of Electro-anaesthesia).

a) Low Frequency

b) High Frequency

c) Ultra-High Frequency

Stimulation of the needle by electricity is a modern innovation in acupuncture. Although manual stimulation is superior to electrical stimulation, the latter has certain advantages such as convenience, time savings, and less traumatization of the tissues. It is also preferred by children.

Electroacupuncture (also called electropulse stimulation or 'E.P.S.') is preferable to hand stimulation in acupuncture anaesthesia. Electrical stimulation of the points may be carried out without the insertion of needles in patients who are hypersensitive to needles by using an electrode tip soaked in saline solution.

18 E.P.S. = Electro-pulse stimulation
S.I.A . = Stimulation induced analgesia (or anesthesia)
E.S.A. = Electro-stimulation analgesia (or anesthesia)

Three types of electrical apparatus are used in acupuncture practice :

1) Electrical pulse stimulators for administering therapy.

2) Acupuncture point detectors which locate the acupuncture points electrically by making use of the fact that these are points of lowered electrical resistance on the skin.

3) Dual-purpose instruments which combine the above functions. Electrical pulse stimulators are used to stimulate the acupuncture points by feeding them with a special type of electrical flux.

Direct current (D.C.) Galvanic and Faradic stimulation cannot be used for therapy as there is tendency to cause iontophoresis and cauterization of the tissues at the point of contact.

Alternating current (A.C.) is also not suitable as it causes much discomfort to the patient. It has been found that the best form of stimulation is to use a pulsatile (or 'pulsed') current generated by means of a transistorized or printed electronic circuit. Pulsed current can have many different wave-forms such as biphasic, square, biphasic spike, and sinusoidal; but the most widely used in electro-acupuncture is the biphasic spike. Stimulation with this wave-form can be delivered to the patient as either continuous, intermittent, or dense-disperse. The dense-disperse form is the most commonly used as the patient exhibits the least amount of sensory adaptation.

Many makes and models of electrical pulse stimulators are available, but they are all constructed on a common plan. The object is to deliver a minute pulsed current to the acupuncture points, and this current has to be adjustable in respect to three parameters : voltage, frequency, and intensity (current strength). The details regarding these variables are as follows:

a) **Voltage** must be adjustable from about 5 to 20 volts. The range of the voltage generally used for treatment is 5 to 10 Volts. The power source may be the mains supply or one to six dry cell batteries. Step-up transformers are used for getting the desired voltage. We do not recommend the mains supply as the source of power, as a breakdown of the transformer could have a disastrous effect on the patient.

b) **Frequency** must be adjustable according to requirements. For most forms of therapy, a low frequency of about 1 to 50 Hertz (i.e. 1 to 50 pulses per second) is sufficient. For acupuncture anaesthesia however, a higher frequency range (1000 to 2000 Hertz biphasic) is employed in the operative or painful area. In some models up to 30,000 Hertz can be delivered.[19]

c) ***Intensity*** (Current Strength) is generally very small-not more than a few micro-amps. The intensity must be adjustable so as not to cause discomfort to the patient. However, particularly in acupuncture anaesthesia, it should be sufficiently strong to induce the acupuncture sensation called 'deqi'.

During electrical pulse stimulation the above three variables must be regulated so that no discomfort is caused to the patient. Control knobs with calibration for fine tuning, these variables are provided on the instrument panel on all reliable models. Pilot lamps (or 'magic eyes') and loudspeakers (amplifiers) for audio-visual monitoring are available in some instruments. There are switches for selecting the waveforms; intermittent, dense-disperse, etc. Each instrument is also fitted with several output points from which there are sets of lead wires which can be connected to the inserted needles by means of fine wire and clips. One of the wires in each set of leads is an earth wire. By using different sets of leads. Several patients may be treated simultaneously with a single stimulator in therapy, (but not in anaesthesia.) An intelligent, co-operative patient can be taught to manipulate the controls himself during therapy.

Many portable transistorized models of Electro-Pulse Stimulators are available today. The most popular at our Institute is the Medicina Alternativa model manufactured in Sri Lanka. It is advisable

19 This is still experimental.

for the acupuncturist to use only reliable makes of these instruments because the use of unsafe machine has resulted in electrical burns, fractured needles, and other harmful effects. Transformer breakdown, in particular, may be lethal to the patient.

Contraindications to Electroacupuncture : In epilepsy and other convulsive states, electroacupuncture should not be used. It is also avoided in patients with cardiac disorders like auricular fibrillation and other conduction disorders. In all patients it is best to avoid electro-acupuncture at the points Baihui (Du 20.) and Neiguan (F. 6.) as cardiac irregularities and discomfort may occur. In high fever and in epileptics electroacupuncture is avoided. Electroacupuncture must not be carried out on any patient with a cardiac pacemaker. It is also contraindicated in infants, mentally ill, non co-operative patients, and those with excess Yang disorders particularly of the Heart, Pericardium, and the Brain.

When using an electrical stimulator, the patient should always he under the observation of an assistant or a fellow- patient because discomfort or other contingencies such as fainting may occasionally arise.

Acupuncture Point Detectors : These are instruments which have been designed to accurately locate the position of acupuncture points by making use of the fact that these are points of lowered electrical resistance on the skin. The positive electrode of the instrument is held by the patient in one hand while the negative electrode is used as a probe to explore the skin surface. Detection of an acupuncture point is indicated by hearing a higher-pitched sound from the vibrator. In the ear, these reactive points have been found to correspond to diseased areas of the body. In using the acupuncture point detector to diagnose disease, one must first take the whole clinical picture of the patient, the history, clinical examination, and the result of any special tests before arriving at a diagnosis. One must never rush into a rash diagnosis on the results of the ear-detector test alone.

Dual Purpose Instruments : The use of the Electro-Pulse Stimulators and Acupuncture Point Detectors as separate instruments has now been largely superseded by dual-purpose instruments which combine both functions in one unit. The Acupuncture Foundation of Sri Lanka recommends The Medicina Alternativa models, designed and manufactured in Sri Lanka with the latest generation of silicon chips. These models incorporate all the best features of the above instruments in tough, durable casings to withstand long clinical use. We have also carried out over 4,000 cases of major surgery using the latest larger Models for electro-anaesthesia.

The following guidelines are observed, when using electrical stimulation in therapy.

(1) Baihui (Du 20.) and Neiguan (P. 6.) should not be stimulated. Cardiac irregularities have been reported by stimulation of the latter point, headaches at the former point.

(2) Do not electrically stimulate the Dangerous Points.

(3) Electrical Stimulation should be avoided in epileptics, on patients suffering from convulsions, hypocalcaemia, high fevers or severe shock, and those wearing a cardiac pacemaker.

(4) If acupuncture has to be used on a pregnant patient, avoid using the stimulator as it greatly increases the possibility of an abortion. Especially avoid the abdominal and the lower limb points. (Acupuncture with electrical stimulation is being successfully carried out for the relief of pain during delivery.)

(5) Avoid electrical stimulation on patients who are over-anxious, mentally deficient, restless, or non-cooperative.

(6) Where a patient has an adverse response to stimulation such as fainting or excessive sweating, stimulation should be discontinued and the needles withdrawn immediately.

(7) When connecting a pair of leads from the stimulator to the needles, do not couple:

a) a yin and yang point ;

b) a tonification and a sedation point;

c) points on the two sides of the body especially in patients with cardiac irregularities or hypertension.

In carrying out surgery with acupuncture anaesthesia the leads are often connected so that the electricity crosses from one side to the other, especially in surgery of the midline areas. In such circumstances, the patient's vital functions must be continuously monitored.

8) Care should be taken so that the electrical setting is at zero before attaching-the leads to the needles. The current should then be increased gradually while watching the patient's expression for signs of discomfort. (Any sudden increase of the current may cause muscle spasms with the possibility of a fracture of the needle).

(9) Metal objects worn by the patient should be removed especially when electroacupuncture is to be used. (Metal fillings in teeth or metal internal prosthesis are not a contraindication.)

(10) It is a good practice to earth the patient.

(11) It is a good practice to electrically stimulate a proximal and distal point of the same channel with one pair of electrodes.

2. T.E.N.S.—Transcutaneous Electro-Neuro-Stimulation

T.C.N.S.—Transcutaneous Neuro-Stimulation:

Transcutaneous Neuro-Stimulation (T.C.N.S.) is a method of electro-analgesia which was developed in North America following the discovery by Wall and Sweet (1967), and Sweet and Wepsic (1968), that relief of pain can be obtained by electrical stimulation of the peripheral nerves. These developments were inspired by the technical advances in electroacupuncture. As in dorsal column stimulation, it is presumed that sensory-gate closure from stimulation of the large-diameter fast-conducting afferents occurs with this method. (Transcutaneous neuro-stimulation is often carried out in North America by physiotherapists and chiropracters without acknowledging its origin from acupuncture, as they do not have licences to practice acupuncture, which is an invasive type of medicine. This method is therefore labelled , "acupuncture through the back-door.")

Stimulation is applied through electrodes placed over the skin at certain points which lie on the course of the peripheral nerves. No acupuncture needles are inserted at these points which, by and large, correspond to classical acupuncture points. Although express acknowledgement of this fact is not often forthcoming. A bewildering array of instruments with complicated electronic circuitry add many eye-catching gadgets have appeared in the North American market for this purpose. The range of instrumentation offered is proliferating at an extraordinary rate. To add to the confusion, fantasic claims for this or that model are being made by competing manufacturers. It is extremely doubtful however whether all this sophisticated gadgetry is really necessary for obtaining the desired results. We have found that, what is most important in acupuncture, is the proper selection of points and the ability on the part of the acupuncturist to manipulate the needle correctly after tailoring the treatment to the needs of each individual patient. Moreover, manual techniques are far more effective than electrical stimulation. In a comparative study of acupuncture and transcutaneous stimulation in the treatment of low-back pain, it was found that pain relief greater than 33% was produced in 75% of the patients by acupuncture and only in 60% of the patients by electrical stimulation. The mean duration of pain relief was about 40 hours after acupuncture and 23 hours after electrical stimulation. In this study, acupuncture was carried out by the insertion of a needle into points U.B. 24, 26, and 62, with strong manual stimulation for 1 minute at each successive point. Transcutaneous stimulation was applied for 10 minutes at each of the same points in succession with an indifferent, electrode placed at a distant site (Melzack, R. and Fox, Elizabeth J.: *Transcutaneous Electrical Stimulation and Acupuncture: Comparison of Treatment for Low-Back Pain*, PAIN, 2, (1976) 141-148, Elsevier, North Holland, Amsterdam.)

In our experience, needle insertion followed by correct hand manipulation is still the best method of administering acupuncture therapy, the manipulation being done where there is a positive indication to do so. In a busy clinic however, many patients have to be put on the electro-stimulator as hand manipulation is time consuming.

3. Dorsal Column Stimulation:

This is a method of electroanalgesia which was developed by Norman Shealey and his co-workers at the Pain Rehibilitation Centre, La Crosse, Wisconsin, U.S.A. Details are described by Shealey in his paper *"Dorsal Column Electro- analgesia"* (HEADACHE 9: 99-102, 1969). The rationale of this technique is to bring about pain relief by direct stimulation of the dorsal column of the spinal cord (i.e. the tracts of Goll and Burdach), which consist almost entirely of large diameter fast conducting afferents. Stimulation applied to these fibres will result (according to the multipe gate-controi theory) in closure of the sensory gates at the brain-stem and thalamic levels. thereby preventing the pain impulses from reaching conscious awareness.[20]

Before dorsal column stimlation is performed, it is necessary to carry out a laminectomy to enable insertion of the platinum electrodes which are attached to a piece of silicon impregnated dacron. These electrodes are introduced subdurally into the spinal canal where they remain outside the arachnoid sheath. The electrode wires are then connected to a mini radio-receiver implanted subcutaneously in the subclavicular region. An external antenna serves to deliver the current whose frequency, pulse, width and voltage can be varied according to clinical requirements. In secondary cancer and certain other pain syndromes, such as phantom limb pain, this method is quite successful in many patients. Although it is a good method based on sound neurophysiological principles, dorsal column stimulation is an expensive procedure which involves surgery by a skilled neurosurgeon familiar with the problems of pain. Hence it is unsuitable for

20 Neurotransmitters are also involved.

general use. We have obtained equally good, if not better results, by the insertion of acupuncture needles paravertebrally at the Huatuojiaji (Ex. 21.). points corresponding to the affected segmental levels, combined with strong stimulation at Hegu (L.I. 4.), Xiangu (St. 43.) and other analgesic points. This has controlled the pain in the majority of our patients suffering from secondary carcinoma and other severe painful disorders. The acupuncture method is much simpler, safer, more economical, and effective than either dorsal column stimulation or transcutaneous electrical stimulation which is described below. The patient or an intelligent helper at home, may be taught to carry out electrostimulation of the acupuncture points without needling. In disorders like phantom limb pain, trigeminal neuralgia and herpes zoster, this procedure is extremely helpful.

4. Electroacupuncture According to Voll (EAV):

This is a method of electroacupuncture with an apparatus called the EAV—Dermatron developed by R. Voll of West Germany. It is used diagnostically as well as therapeutically. This method is based on the known fact that an acupuncture point has a higher electrical conductivity relative to the immediate surrounding skin area and that in conditions of disease there is usually a further decrease in the skin resistance of that point. In EAV, the normal range of skin resistance at each acupuncture point (referred to as its "energetic potential") is noted and taken as a reference base. Where the electrical conductivity of the skin has undergone a change, it is possible to detect it very accurately using the Dermatron. This is recognised as a pathological state indicating the disease or dysfunction of the Organ pertaining to that particular acupuncture point and therefore of a disequilibrium of the flow of vital energy in the related Channel. The equilibrium is restored by stimulating the specific acupuncture point or points using the Dermatron in a separate function. The main feature of the system therefore derives from the extreme sensitivity of this instrument in detecting changes in electrical conductivity of the acupuncture points, thus providing an extension of the traditional methods of diagnosis.

It is claimed that by using this system it would even be possible to indicate which part of an Organ and how much of it is affected, e.g., the exact location and size of a gastric ulcer. It is also claimed that the technique "can differentiate between acute, subacute and chronic inflammations, between intitial, progressed or final degeneration stages, and between simultaneous occurrence of inflammatory and degeneratiive organ processes."

Electroacupuncture, in general, is based on the now well established phenomenon that the electrical resistance of the skin is measurably lower at the acupuncture points, i.e., the acupuncture points conduct relatively more electric current than the surrounding skin. It is also established that the degree of electrical conductivity at each acupuncture point varies according to the pathological state of the related internal organ or other connected structures. If health is postulated as an energetic equilibrium and ill-health an energetic disequilibrium, it follows that with the aid of sensitive modern electronic devices, it should be possible to measure with reasonable accuracy the characteristics of electrical conductively at the acupuncture points and infer thereby the pathology attributable to any disequilibrium detected.

[21]EAV uses a specially designed electronic apparatus which allows the measurement of the minutest energetic reactions and the momentary potential of a pertaining organ as shown at the acupuncture points. It is therefore possible, not only to diagnose an illness, but also to detect the very inception of an illness; energetic alternations of organs before they develop into clinically manifest symptoms. The precise measurements in EAV are capable of determining the day and even the time of ovulation in women, or the changed pH values of the stomach after a meal. The accurate diagnosis possible with EAV, therefore, permits a greater emphasis on preventive medicine or early diagnosis.

The EAV meter is calibrated from 0 to 100. The position of 50 (the central position) indicates that the organ pertaining to the related acupuncture point is free of any pathology.

---

21 Similar instruments are employed in Moratherapy and Biotron therapy.

The advantages claimed for EAV over conventional acupuncture may be summarized as follows:

a) Early diagnosis (as the electrical conductivity at acupuncture points registers changes at the initial stages of a disease, even before it is externally manifested).

b) Accurate indication of the Organ or tissues diseased.

c) Indication of the stage to which any degeneration has occurred.

d) A painless and aseptic method of treatment, as the electrodes do not penetrate the skin.

In order to ascertain a diagnosis by the EAV method the following important working principles must be observed:

(1) **The diagnostic evaluation of the measurement criteria must be linked to pathological events. In practice, the following categories of measurements are determined:**

   a) The stable measured value, which remains constant for the entire measurement period.

   b) The initially measured maximum value decreases and settles at a lower value. This is referred to in EAV as indicator deflection and is of special significance in that it indicates disturbances of Organ function.

   c) A measured value which reaches the maximum slowly without any indicator deflection, indicating a preliminary stage of insufficiency.

   d) Maximum values above 90, reached rather quickly with subsequent indicator deflection, indicating a chemical intoxication.

As a rule, the deflection of the indicator occurs after the maximum value is reached in 1 to 3 seconds. In the case of a very slow indicator deflection, showing a disturbance of function which has already begun, the 3 second time period may be extended, e.g., an incipient odontogenic event localized at one of the 6 maxillary measurement points. The duration of the indicator deflection is related to the intensity and scope of the pathological process of the organ being measured. This is evaluated by making the acupuncture point measurement with a view to arriving at (i) the measured value of the point and (ii) the amount of the indicator deflection. Both these indices are expressed in terms of a narrow range of values.

(2) **The relationship of the individual acupuncture point to an Organ and its functional aspect must be established.**

The relationship of the individual acupuncture point to parts of organs in the large hollow organs and to tissue functions in the parenchymal organs must be tested. In smaller organs, the specific acupuncture points must be found in order to perniit a differential diagnosis with electrodiagnosis where non-specific pathological disturbances are produced by disease.

EAV gives four different measured values for the diagnosis of the large organs, both for the paired organs and the unpaired ones, distinguishing between the left and right halves of the unpaired organs. EAV can also differentiate precisely between acute, subacute, and chronic inflammations, between initial, advanced, or complete degeneration and between the simultaneous occurrence of inflammatory and degenerative changes in organs. For example, the four measurement points serve a diagnostic purpose with respect to the heart's (i) aortic valve, (ii) mitral valve, (iii) conduction system, and (iv) cardiac muscle, in addition to other points related to lymphatic drainage, the coronary vessels, the pericardium, cardiac muscle etc., other points show the tissue function of a parenchymas organ, such as the proteinase, nuclease, carbohydratase, or lipase ferment production in the pancreas.

Included in EAV are new acupuncture points and new vessels. (That author prefers to use the word vessel rather than meridian or channel as in EAV the energy conduits are somewhat different to those of traditional Chinese medicine.) From many years of clinical observation and measurment. Voll has discovered, for example, that the renal vessel (Kidney Channel) begins, on the inside of the little toe. Then continues to the traditional Chinese first point, Yonquan (K. I) and travels from there to the medial side of the foot. The new vessels according to EAV are as follows:

Lymph vessels (Ly)

Nervous or grey degeneration (ND)

Allergy and tissue degeneration (AL)

Parenchymatous and epithelial degeneration (PD)

Articular degeneration (AD)

Connective tissue degeneration (CT)

Skin vessels (S)

Fatty degeneration (FD)

Among the newly discovered important acupuncture points which are not known in classical acupuncture are the control measurement points. There are control points for all organs, including circulation, the endocrine system, all degenerative processes and the lymphatic system. By measuring these points it is possible to determine whether there is an inflammation with degeneration, or a degenerative pathology in the organ. This saves considerable diagnostic time. On the basis of the results of measurement from indicative points and control measurement points, the physician may take an abbreviated but well directed history from the patient, since the latter is often unaware which symptoms take priority in establishing a diagnosis. As a diagnostic method therefore, EAV is very helpful.

(3) The acupuncture point must be located in its precise topographic position.

Precise location of the acupuncture point to be measured is necessary because the correct deflection of the indicator is obtained only when the point is measured at its centre. Since the anatomical position of the point has to be determined by palpation prior to its precise location by electrical measurement, knowledge of the topographic position of acupuncture points is of great importance.

The inexact representations of acupuncture point positions in various charts and books on acupuncture have not helped the cause of acupuncture. That author has made over 100,000 measurements of acupuncture points, determining their exact locations on the body. Over 600 measurement points have been verified of which approximately 200 are outside the known points of classical acupuncture.

The above are the three main principles of EAV diagnostics.

In addition to diagnosis, EAV makes it possible to confirm every therapeutic success and every therapeutic failure. This is particularly useful in patients who respond on a delayed basis. Since the improvement in the measurement values has already indicated that there has been a change in the electrical potential and thus a return to the normal state. Thus, not only acupuncture but every other therapeutic method may be monitored, including drug therapy, irradiation, physiotherapy, hydrotherapy, homoeopathy, herbal therapy, rolfing and massage. The results of surgical procedures may also be monitored. For example, it is possible to clarify etiologically whether lymphostasis, irritation of serous membranes with tendency towards fibrosis or cicatrization are recent, or whether an area of irritation in a post-operative scar is the cause of the symptoms.

It must be remembered that clinical methods of investigation do not always provide confirmation of EAV diagnosis. This is because clinical diagnosis is positive only when the illness is manifest. X-ray diagnosis, for example is not an early, but a late, form of diagnosis, and the majority of laboratory diagnostic methods are positive only when the disease has already reached a critical level. It should, therefore, be the responsibility of the physician to make an early diagnosis whenever possible, so that, in accordance with the ancient principles of traditional Chinese medicine, the appropriate treatment may be applied as early as possible. EAV can therefore prevent many illnesses.

5. Ryodoraku (Nakatani):

Ryodoraku Is a Japanese variant of electroacupunture therapy. The measurements are carried out using a special electro-acupunctoscope. It is a diagnostic as well as a therapeutic method.

H. MAGNETISM (MAGNETOTHERAPY)

There are many designs of equipment where polarized magnetism is used in the treatment of a variety of disorders. This method is still experimental. It is said to be particularly useful in treating locomotor disorders and internal disorders, like migraine and peptic ulcer.

I. ANCILLIARY DRUGS

Ginseng:

Of the multitude of herbal medicines known to man, ginseng is certainly the most fascinating. It is the only plant which for thousands of years has been consistently regarded as a panacea or "cure-all". No other plant is used so widely in the Orient for such a variety of disorders. The Chinese, whose traditional medicine is, without doubt, one of the most sophisticated medical systems known, have pinned almost mystical hope on the miracle herb. For over 2000 years Oriental physicians have prescribed it as an essential tonic, a restorative and as a regular component of herbal therapy in the treatment of many serious illnesses. It is also the herbal medicine most often combined with acupuncture therapy. Although the Chinese, Koreans and Japanese have treasured the marvellous and mysterious ginseng root for centuries, it was dismissed by Western scientists-at least until very recently, as yet another inscrutable Oriental folly. The arousal of scientific curiosity in the West may indeed be attributed to the already established popularity of this herb originating from the interest taken in it by the natural food enthusiasts, the spiritually aware and Chinese scholars. It has since become a mainstay of the alternative life style.

Enthusiasts in Britain spend over £ 10 million on it each year, and an estimated six million Americans consume some 300 tons of it yearly. World trade in ginseng has surged from US $ 12.5 million in 1971 to US $ 125 million last year. Special pharmaceutical factories now turn out ginseng in tonic form, capsules and tablets. It is also available in teas, soft drinks, chewing gum and even soap. Even alco-

THE GINSENG PLANT

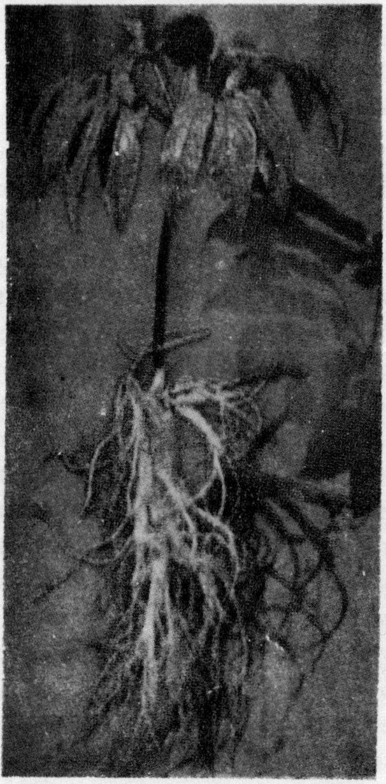

holic beverages are sold containing ginseng. For those who want a "double kick." Some New York bartenders offer a special cocktail laced with ginseng.

The natural system of classification of plants has kept the ginseng plant in the same family and genus ever since plants were named, even though systematics have changed continuously. The systematics of ginseng plants, according to Engler's natural system of classification is as follows:-

Phylum :	*Embryophyte*
Subphylum :	*Angiospermae*
Class :	*Dicotyledonocae*
Subclass :	*Anchichlamyeae*
Order :	*Umbellifloreae*
Family :	*Araliacece*
Genus :	*Panax*

The scientific name of the Oriental ginseng plant is Panax ginseng C. A. Meyer, who was a Russian, named the plant in 1843. Panax is from Latin and pan denotes all, axos means cure. Therefore Panax denotes **"cure all,"** and the word **"ginseng"** originated from the Chinese name for this plant. (Ginseng means "man-root" in Chinese, on a count of its remarkable human appearance.)

It has the following agricultural characteristics:

(1) It is a perennial plant which grows slowly. Its cultivation takes a long time, about five to six years from seeding to harvest.

(2) Ginseng must be raised in shady spots and must not be exposed to direct sunlight.

(3) Ginseng must be cultivated in virgin soil, for it is highly sensitive to soil quality. Once the soil has been used for ginseng, it must remain uncultivated for over 10 to 15 years before replantation.

(4) Ginseng grows slowly. Care should be taken not to damage its roots when it is cultivated. Damaged roots or uncertain seeds will not grow properly. Chemical fertilizers in strong concentrations should not be used. Ginseng is extremely vulnerable to insects and fungal diseases.

(5) The cultivation of ginseng needs facilities like covering, and the growth rate is slow. Therefore, it requires a considerable amount of capital and the return on the invested capital is very slow.

(6) The cultivation of ginseng is labour-intensive, because it is difficult to mechanize. It requires much experience and elaborate skill. Due to the sensitive characteristics of the ginseng plant, its large-scale cultivation is not feasible and its mass production to meet the heavy demand is impossible.

Its geographical distribution is limited mostly to between the 30th degree and the 48th degree North latitude, in East Asia.

The appearance of the Panax ginseng plant is quite unimpressive. The mature cultivated plant grows to about half a meter high, and has tiny purplish flowers which turn into clusters of bright red berries, each surrounded by five nearly serrated leaves. The real heart of the plant is its greyish white fleshy root. In the mature plant, the root grows to a length of about ten to fifteen centimeters and weighs on an average about 200 grams; and has usually two branching "thighs" that led early Chinese observers to call it the ginseng or "the man-root". The human-like form of its root has also earned it a veritable reputation of being an effective aphrodisiac.

Ginseng has held the esteem of the Chinese as the since omnipotent medical herb for more than 4000 years. China is not the only place where ginseng has been used since ancient times. The *Vedas*, or the ancient Indian scriptures, which reflect an oral teaching that may be 5000 years old have many hymns describing ways to attain health and fulfilment. One hymn describes ginseng as "the root which is dug from the earth and which strengthens the nerves." It continues: "the strength of the horse, the mule, the goat, combined with the strength of the bull, it bestows on the man who consumes it".

Ancient Chinese medical extracts describe its efficacy against fevers, impotence, malaria. worms, migraine, arthritis. insomnia, mental depression, loss of memory, the common cold , and countless other disorders. Chinese soldiers used it in battle for quick energy and to alleviate the effects of injuries. Chinese Emperors took it to prolong their life-spans.[22]

It is almost impossible to trace the time when ginseng was first found and used as a medicine. However, the Chinese use of ginseng and its mythology probably originated in the mountains of Manchuria. There is a Chinese tradition that ginseng was first found, and used medically, in the "Easterly Provinces" of Kirin, Shen-King and Heilung-Chiang. The Manchurian cedar forests could have provided the perfect environment necessary for the growth of ginseng, and for centuries this area has been known as China's ginseng belt. Although the discovery and utilization of the natural ginseng must have developed through long experience from prehistoric times. The history of ginseng can only be traced as far back as its written history.

The first description of ginseng as a miraculous tonic in the history of medicine appeared in a Chinese book of the **Chier Han** Era (B.C. 48-33) about 2,000 years ago. Among the many descriptions of the Sui Dynasty in the Chinese book entitled Han Yuan, there appear records of the production of ginseng on Mt. Ma-da San in Koryo (this might be the Mount Kai Ma Dai San in Korea at the present time). In the book Kuo Ching Poi Lu by a Buddhist author of the Sui Dynasty, there is a record of gingseng in Koryo. Also, in the book Ming I Pie Lu by Tao Hung King, we find a description of the dispatch of ginseng from Packehe (Po tsi), one of the Three Emperors of the Liang Dynasty of China. Before this, Koryo and the Wei Dynasty of China had already frequent trade exchanges and there are records of sending tributes of ginseng through emissaries from Koryo to China 92 times. From these records we may assume the ginseng of Koryo must have been sent to China regularly.

22 Ginseng and soyabean curd was a popular recipe.

In the book attributed to Shen Nung called the Pen Tsao Ching (The Book of Herbs), the fact that 11 kinds of herbal medicines were produced in Koroyo is noted. Of these medicines, ginseng and gold fragments are particularly mentioned in connection with the art of preparing "the elixir of life".

On April 12th 1711, Father Jarcous. a French Jesuit missionary priest, sent in a letter to another priest, a general account of his missions to India and China. The letter read as follows :

"From Peking, Dear Sir, I wish the peace of the lord be with you. In accordance with the order of the Emperor of China, we are making a survey to draw a map of the Tartarian area (northeastern area of China at the present day that is to say, the Manchurian area of the Koguryo era, 37 B.C.-668 A. D. Manchuria and the Liactung Peninsula then belonged to the territory of Korea). I acquired the opportunity to see the famous plant, ginseng which is not well known to Europe but is precious here in China. In July, 1709, we arrived at a village named Calca where Tartarians were living in the vicinity of 40 Ri (Ri is a Korean unit of distance, 40 Ri is about 16 Km) from the Chosen (Korea) Kingdom. One man among us brought four pieces of ginseng root in a basket that they picked from the nearby mountains. I am sending a detailed sketch of one root to you. The explanation of the picture will given at the end of this letter. Great medical scholars in China write many books about the effects of ginseng medicine."

This letter was published under the title "The descriptions of Tartarian ginseng" in the "Philosophical Transactions of the Royal Society of London, 1710,"

This publication reached another French priest, Father Francois Lafitan in Montreal, Canada. When he showed the picture of ginseng in the article to the Mohawk Indians, they immediately recognized it, went to the woods with the priest, and succeeded in finding ginseng there. Lafitan sent back a sample to France, and a botanist verified it in 1714 as the Ponex quinquefolium (American ginseng), a new strain belonging to the same Araliaceac family.Originally the Panax quinquefolium was found all the way from the rich, cool woods of Quebec and Manitoba southwards, almost reaching the Gulf of Mexico. When the Chinese heard about the new discovery they started importing North American ginseng, establishing a trade that is still flourishing today. But like wild ginseng elsewhere, the American variety is in danger of disappearing. The export of wild ginseng is now carefully controlled by the United States and Canada.

Ginseng was listed as an official drug in the United States Pharmacopoeia from 1840 to 1880, but thereafter this drug was deleted. At present, ginseng is only mentioned as an unofficial herbal plant Bulletin Number 89 of the U.S. Department of Agriculture Bureau of Plant Industry. The U.S. Food and Drug Administration now classifies it as a food additive for tea. Ginseng is not listed in most official Western Pharmacopoeias and many Western countries do not allow sellers to make any medicinal claims for it.

It is said that the Chinese character which represents ginseng appeared during the latter period of the Han Era around 2000 years ago. We do not know whether the ginseng used at that time was the same as the ginseng of today because there are no accurate descriptions. However, the book Shang Han-Lun by Chang Chung-Ching of the Han Dynasty describes the therapeutic effects of this plant.

Among the 113 ancient prescriptions recorded in that book, there are 21 prescriptions which contain ginseng. This ginseng is thought to be the Panax ginseng, because the description of the therapeutic indications of ginseng in medical prescriptions of later periods are the same as those in the Shang *Han-Lun.*

Garriques of U.S.A. in 1854, extracted from American ginseng (Panax quinquefolium) the saponin substance called panaquilon.

The Saito group in Japan, the U-Han group in Korea and the Elyakov group in the Soviet Union succeeded in separating thirteen kinds of saponins and found that these were contained in ginseng alone.

Trade links with China during the 17th century made ginseng the rage among the aristocracy of Europe. Ginseng was the most valuable cargo that travelled on the ancient silk route via the Brenner Pass to Europe.

Traditional Chinese and Korean physicians think of ginseng not only as a medicine which cures, but rather as a preventive. Administered regularly for a time, they are convinced that it will prevent a variety of disorders. Its great value, they believe, lies as a restorative to improve general health and help the body cure itself. Ginseng is believed to potentiate the immune mechanisms of the body.

To the Western scientific mind, such an hypothesis is hard to prove, since a controlled trial would involve monitoring the health of thousands of users and non-users of ginseng over several decades. Nonetheless, there has been much serious scientific work on the subject, and many international scientific conferences on ginseng have been held during the past few decades.

There have been a number of controlled scientific experiments to suggest that ginseng may be more than a "tonic". In 1948 a Soviet scientist, Israel Brekhman, administered small amounts of ginseng extract to Russian soldiers. He found that the men improved their time in cross-country runs by an average of six per cent. Later, Brekhman conducted similar studies with experimental mice, demonstrating that ginseng increased the stamina of the animals by 35 per cent in running and swimming tests.

In Bulgaria, Professor Petkov of the Sofia Institute of Specialized and Advanced Medical Training, observed the possible effects of ginseng on the brain. Petkov studied conditioned reflexes in rats fed with ginseng extract and also measured the electro-encephalographic activity of cats against those of control groups. In a third experiment, human volunteers were given strongly flavoured drinks, half of them contained ginseng extract, and then they were asked to respond to commands. Petkov concluded that ginseng improves learning ability, memory and physical performance.

Ginseng was taken by Russian astronauts to help them resist infections in their sealed space capsules. This protective use of the plant is precisely within the spirit of its traditional use as a preventive medicine.

Since the major researches of Brekhman and Petkov, scientists in more than a dozen other countries have been looking into the biological effects of ginseng. In independent studies carried out on Swedish students, on German patients, and on Russian telegraph operators, ginseng was reported to have increased energy and mental alertness. Although scientists do not agree on the benefits of ginseng or on how it works, it is most likely that ginseng probably operates via the endocrine and autonomic nervous systems. Some authorities hypothesize that the mechanism of its action is mainly a physiological one of causing homocostasis and in this respect there is a close parallelism to the acupuncture phenomenon.

The effects of Ginseng on Metabolism and Cell Division.

a) *Carbohydrate Metabolism:*

In 1959, Petkov reported that ginseng had an inhibitory effect on artificially induced hyperglycemia and a synergistic effect on insulin. Kimura and his associates (1967) confirmed the effect of ginseng on the reduction of ketone bodies and the lowering of blood sugar in alloxan diabetic mice and anti-insulin diabetic mice. Kimura and his associates assumed that ginseng would act more on the enzyme system involving glycogenesis in the body than on an oxidative enzyme system of carbohydrate metabolism. On the contrary, Oura and his co-workers (1972) found that when ginseng was administered to a normally raised animal group, ginseng extract had the effect of reducing glycogen in their livers more significantly than in those of a control group. However, they also found that when glucose was administered to an experimental group, ginseng extract facilitated the increase of glycogen formation. From such experiments they indicated that ginseng extract had contradictory effects to insulin.

b) *Lipid Metabolism:*

Nabm (1961) cytologically examined the effects of ginseng on the aorta, heart, coronary arteries and atherosclerotic livers of rabbits which suffered from hypercholesterolemia caused by prolonged administration of cholesterol. Atherosclerotic-like changes were noted less in the rabbits which were administered ginseng.

Yamanoto and his associates (1969) showed that ginseng decreased the lipid content of certain tissues like liver cells.

c) *Protein Metabolism:*

Oura and his associates (1971-1972) reported the effect of ginseng as accelerating the biosynthesis of RNA and protein. During the partial purification of ginseng extract, they obtained a fraction that mainly contained ginseng saponin of the protopanaxadiol system, and the fraction was named prostisol (protein synthesis stimulating factor). They reported that prostisol increased DNA-dependent RNA polymerase activity in liver nuclei, but it did not influence DNA synthesis. DNA, which was actively synthesized in nuclei, was transferred to the cytoplasm and accordingly facilitated the formation of polysomes, which had a high capacity of protein synthesis. When the ginseng extract was administered to rats for a long period, electron microscopic examination showed the distinctive development of rough endoplasmic reticulum of hepatocytes, to which a large amount of polysome was attached. Blood plasma protein and albumin synthesis were particularly accelerated and the synthesis of alpha, beta and gamma globulins were also enhanced by ginseng.

Han and his associates reported that panax saponin A (corresponding to ginsenoside, a ginseng saponin crystal) enhanced the incorporation of 14C leucine in protein in the livers and sera of mice, and the characteristic stimulating effect showed concomitant characteristics of the anti-inflammatory activity of this substance.

d) *Effect of Ginseng on Cell Division:*

From as tudy of radioactive iron metabolism, Oura and his associates (1972) observed that the incorporation of 59Fe into erythrocytes had been increased in ginseng-treated rats, indicating that ginseng enhanced the haemopoietic functions and iron metabolism in rats. Yamamoto and his associates (1969) reported that prostisol doubled the mitotic indices of the nucleated cells of bone marrow in rats. Mitotic indices were increased not only in both erythroid and myeloid rats, but also in blood reticulocytes, In vitro, addition of ginseng extract enhanced DNA synthesis in the nucleated cells of bone marrow, and mitotic indices were are also increased in both erythroid and myeloid, suggesting that the action of ginseng did not occur through the medium of erythra protein.

c) *Effect of Ginseng on the Immune Functions:*

Brekhman's adaptogenic theroy (1966) greatly encouraged the investigation of the ginseng saponins. Oura and his co- workers (1967) confirmed that adrencorticotropic hormones, such as cortisone, inhibited gamma globulin synthesis, while ginseng did not depress antibody synthesis, suggesting that an adrencorticotropic hormone-like substance was not present in ginseng. In 1970, Kim and his associates established that ginseng extract had a restorative action on the initial depletion of ascorbic acid content of the adrenal glands of stressed rats and that the effect on the stress mechanism was manifest in hypophysectomized animals, suggesting that ginseng acted on the peripheral site of the stress mechanism in response to stress. Choi and his associates (1972) found that the administration of ginseng extract protected the hepatic cells of animals from damage by carbon tetrachloride and X-ray irradiation. Han and his associates (1977) reported that ginseng removed the peroxyipids of hepatic cell membranes which were caused by acute alcoholism. They also reported that an antioxidant action was present in ginseng extract suggesting the presence of a phenolic compound in addition to ginseng saponins.

There are other unique features of ginseng which are important from the clinical point of view. It seems to be the only plant which can so clearly demonstrate the philosphy behind traditional healing and certainly no other has been the subject of such extensive scientific research yielding such puzzling and paradoxical conclusions.

THE GINSENG ROOT

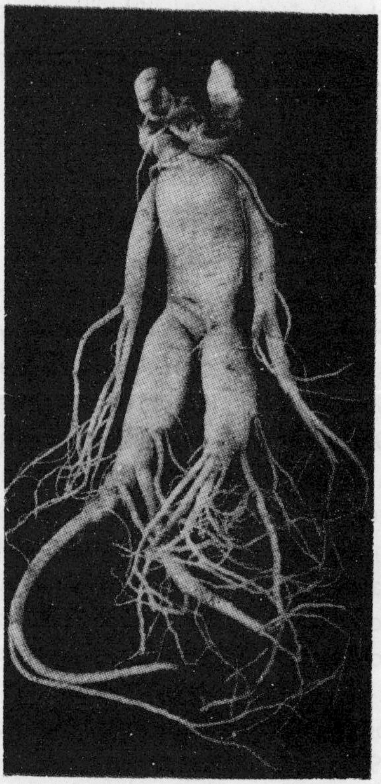

Note: The peculiar human appearance of the root.

Whatever the mechanisms of its actions are, the diversity of its effect may be due to its comparatively rich, wide-spectrum of chemical compounds which have been isolated, each having different physiological properties; some producing stimulating effects, while others being sedative in action.

The ancient claims for ginseng as a cure-all were based on wild specimens that have now virtually disappeared. Even today, the most prized ginseng grows wild only in the cold, rugged reaches of Manchuria in China and in certain parts of South Korea. It is said to be several times as potent and effective as its cultivated descendants, although there is no record of Western scientists putting it to a laboratory test because it is virtually impossible to obtain it in the West. Unfortunately, the wild ginseng of China and Korea, hunted assiduously for centuries, is now virtually extinct. In Korea only a small number of true wild ginseng plants remain. A 50 to 100 year old wild root can be worth, in unprocessed form, from U.S. $ 70 to 115 per gram. Wild ginseng grows on the heavily forested slopes. It takes about two years for the berries to germinate, but not until at least 20 years later will the roots be mature enough for harvesting.

A booming market in cultivated ginseng has taken up the slack. Korea, China and Japan have extensive ginseng cultivation programmes. The Russians, too, are producing excellent roots on many large state farms in Central Asia. In the United States, central Wisconsin has the well-drained soil ideal for growing the root and about 90 per cent of all U.S. cultivated ginseng grows there on a single 600 acre plot. Last year, American ginseng growers exported some 180 tons of ginseng, mostly to Hong Kong; from there much of it is distributed in processed form throughout East Asia.

However, it is generally accepted that high quality ginseng can only be grown in Korea. In fact, the cultivation of ginseng has been a feature of Korean agricultural life for over 500 years. Today about 56,000 Korean farmers are engaged in its cultivation. Total annual exports of Korean ginseng exceed U.S. $ 100 million, the main markets being Japan, Hong Kong, Taiwan and U.S.A.

IN ANCIENT CHINA TRADITIONAL MEDICINE, RELIGION, PHILOSOPHY, AND CULTURE, PRACTICES WERE CLOSELY ENMESHED WITH EACH OTHER

(From "Celestial Lancers" — Lu & Needham, 1980

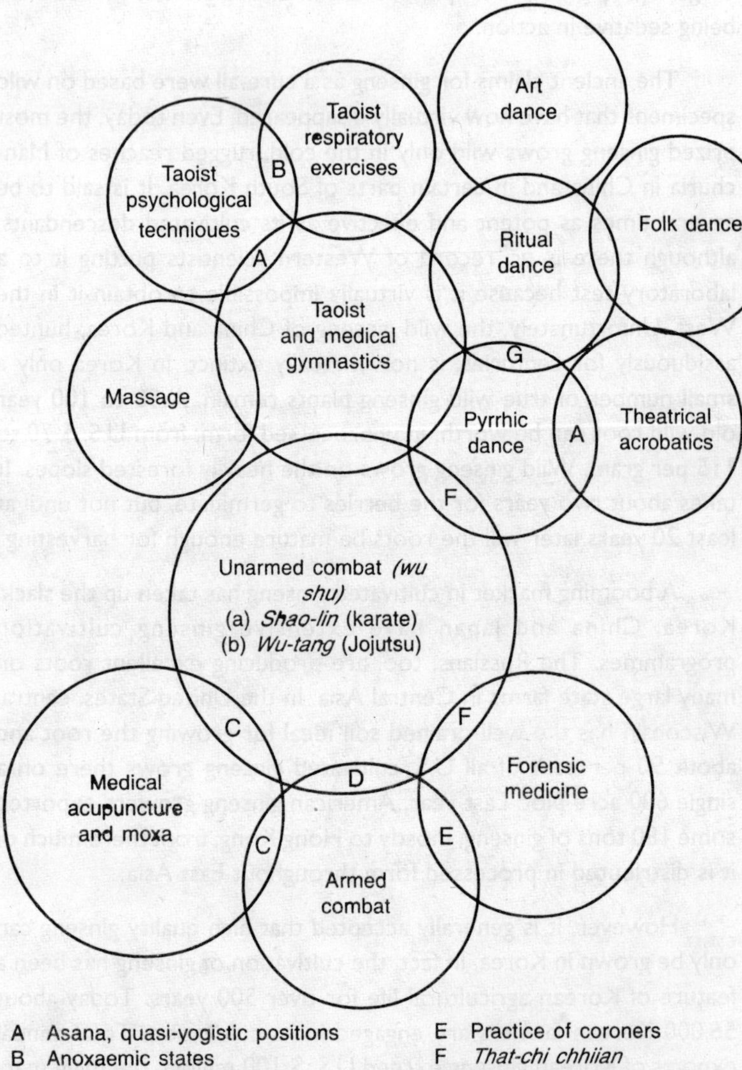

A Asana, quasi-yogistic positions
B Anoxaemic states
C Vital spots or danger points
D Spike-and-chain, thrown darts, etc.
E Practice of coroners
F *That-chi chhiian*
G Confucian temple dances

Chart to show the relationships between the many Chinese psycho-somatic practices.

The quality ginseng root is recognized by its color. When it is steamed before drying, it turns red, while the poorer quality root usually remains white. The market is however full of pitfalls for the inexperienced. There is a flourishing trade in "duplicate ginseng" even gnarled, dried carrots are passed off. The cultivated ginseng root is fleshy and fat, while the prized Manchurian variety is long and thin and "as springy as an angel's bosom" (in the ecstatic words of one ancient Chinese connoisseur.)

For centuries, the ancient Orientals pondered on the nature to ginseng and how it came to be. One tale from Kirin Province proclaimed that the plant was born one August night in the cedar forests, when lightning struck a mountain stream, which disappeared and became transformed into this root. In other words, all the five elements, namely, fire, earth, metal, water and wood are well balanced in the ginseng root making it a veritable panacea for all illnesses. This legend perhaps best sums up the exotic mystery of the ancient cure-all known as the ginseng.

J. MEDITATION, PSYCHOTHERAPY AND NUTRITION

(See diagram on Page No.816)

References:

Abstracts of Korean Ginseng studies (1978-1979), World wide collected bibliography Citations and Abstracts, The Research Institute, Office of Monopoly, Republic of Korean (1975).

Brakhman, I.I., Eleutheraococcus, Scientific and Clinical data (1969).

Breakhman, I.I., Annual Review of Pharm., Vol. 9, 419-430 (1969).

Bretchneider, Emilii Vasillevich, *Batanium Sinicum,* Botanical Investigations into the Materia Medica of the Ancient Chinese (1882).

Chang Chich Pin, *Ching Yao Ch'uan Shu,* Ming Dynasty.

Chang Chung Ching, *Shah-hun fum,* Hu Han Dynasty.

Daisha Vol. 10 (5), 83-147 (1973).

Diamond, E. Grey, *More than Herbs and Acupuncture* (1975).

Father Jartous, *The description of a Tartarian Plant called Ginseng; with an account of its virtues,* Royal Society of London, philosophical Transactions. 28-240 (1714).

Harding, A.R., *Ginseng and other Medicinal Plants,* A.R. Harding Pub. Co. (1972).

Harriman, Sarah, *The Book of Ginseng,* Pyramid Books (1974).

History of Ginseng in Japan, Nihon-ninjin hanbai-nogyok yodo-kumiairengokai (1968).

Hoetink, B., *Verhaal van hot Vergam van hot Jackt de Sperweer en van her* (Wedervaren der Schipbreukelingen op het Eiland Quel paert ep het Vasteland Van Korea (1653-1666) met eene. Beschrijving van dat Rijk door Hendrick Hamel, Den Haag (1920).

Hong, M.W., *Statistical Studies on the Formularies of Oriental Medicine, Statistical Analyses of Ginseng Prescriptions,* Korean Journal of Pharmacognosy, 3 (1972).

Hong, M. W., *Statistical Analyses of "Bang-yak-hab-pyon" Prescriptions.* Korean Journal of Pharmacognosy, 3 (1972).

Hong, M.W. *Origin of Ginseng, Korean Ginseng Science Symbosium,* Korean Society of Pharmacognosy (1974).

Immura A., *History of Ginseng,* Seoul, Korea.

Kim, J.Y., *Materials for Ginseng Markets in the United States,* Seoul, Korea (1973-1974).

Korean Ginseng Scl. *Symposium the Korean Society of Pharmacognosy* (1974).

Letters edit..tes et curieuses, scrites des Missions Ertangere, s Nouvelle edition, 26 Vols. Paris (1780-1783)/

Lowis, Walter H., and Memory P.F. Elvin Lewis, *Medical Botany Plants Affecting Man's Health,* Wiley-Interscience Publication (1977)

Li, Shih-chen, *Pents' ao Kang Mu* (1597).

Proceedings of International Ginseng Symposium, The Central Research Institute. Office of Monopoly. Republic of Korea (1974).

Shlbata, S., Tampakushits Kakusan Kpso 12, (1): 32-38 (1967).

Veninga Louise, The Ginseng Book, Big Trees Press, Felton, Calf. (1973).

■

ACUPUNCTURE ANALGESIA IN CHILDBIRTH

"*In pain thou shalt bring forth thy children*"

— *the Holy Bible*

Pain is an invariable accompaniment of childbirth. Parturition is considered a normal physiological process similar to micturition and defecation. Why women should experience pain during childbirth is therefore an enigma. Some psychologists believe that it is the civilized urban state that brings on the labor pains and that the incidence of pain during childbirth is less among primitive people. Other authorities have suggested that pains of childbirth are due to a drastic alteration of the entire mechanism of the pelvic floor during the evolution of the erect posture of the '*homo erectus*' and later the '*homo sapiens*'. The intense pains of labor are probably related to this change. The erect posture and the bipedal gait require a stronger pelvis and taut ligaments. With all the weight now being transmitted through the hips, these changes in structure in some way impede delivery. This may explain why voilent uterine contractions are necessary to expel the fetus. However, no single explanation is satisfactory, as the pains of labour seem to occur even in animals as well. Domestic animals seem to suffer more in this respect, thus making the picture even more complicated.

The benefits of using acupuncture during childbirth are two-fold:

I. TO THE MOTHER:

1. to expedite delivery,
2. to relieve the pain of childbirth,
3. to utilize the analgesic effects of acupuncture for manoeuvres such as episiotomy, suturing, removal of placenta and forceps deliveries, when indicated.

II. TO THE CHILD:

To deliver a child with the best chances of survival with the least toxic effect of drugs (with the highest possible Apgar scores).

Selection of Points:

Acupuncture points may be selected from the following:

A. Body Points:

(1) To promote contractions of the uterus:

Zhiyin (U.B. 67), Yanglingquan (G.B. 34).

(2) The two specific points which provide analgesia to the lower abdomen and the perineal area:

a) Neima (U. Ex.), or Sanyinjiao (Sp. 6.).

b) Zusanli (St. 36), or Weima (U. Ex.).

(3) Hegu (L.I. 4.) as a general analgesic point. Manual stimulation is used at this point.

(4) Baihui (Du 20.) as a sedative point.

(5) Jianjing (G.B. 21.) may also help to promote delivery of a postmature fetus.

B. Ear Points:

Uterus, Endocrine, Spleen, low-back, Shenmen Areas.

C. Scalp Areas :

Genital Area, Foot-Motor Sensory Area, Motor Area, Sensory Area.

Methods of Stimulation

The procedure is carried out as follows. A needle is first placed at Baihui (Du 20.) and the other selected needles are inserted on the left side, thus giving room for the accoucheur to work on the right side of the pregnant mother.

1. **Hand Manipulation:** The point Hegu (L.I. 4.) is manipulated by hand, the needle is held by the thumb, index and middle finger, and stimulation is performed to and fro, with lifting and thrusting movements, to produce acupuncture sensation or "deqi" (a feeling of soreness, numbness, distention, heaviness, and radiation of these sensations). The frequency of manipulation is maintained at about 100-200 per minute during the episodes of pain. The range of rotation is between 90 to 180 degrees and the depth of lifting and thrusting not more than 0.5 cm. The entire course of labor is aided by periodic manual rotation of the acupuncture needles to coincide with the onset of the pains.

2. **Electrical Pulse Stimulation:** The two needles placed in the (left) leg, are connected to an electric pulse stimulator. The frequency of the electrical pulse is adjusted to about 60-100 Hz. The pulsating current of a dense-disperse type is used. The intensities of stimulation, both manual and electrical, are gradually increased depending on the patient's sensitivity and tolerance to the stimulator, until the patient feels numbness soreness, heaviness and distention which makes the pains of labor. Ear points and Scalp points with electro-stimulation are added when the analgesia obtained at the body points is insufficient.

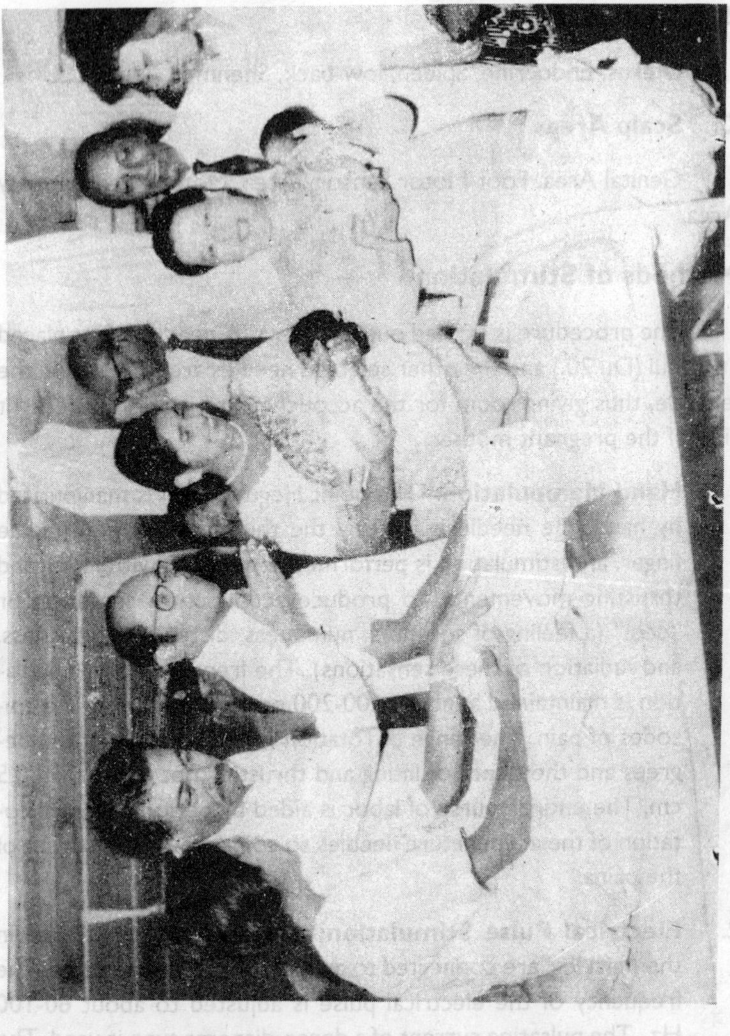

INSTITUTE OF ACUPUNCTURE, KALUBOWILA
Caesarean Section with Acupuncture Anaesthesia.
Mrs. D.P. 6th; Pregnancy: Twins.
June 1978.

Obstructed labor, Caesarean Section done under Acupuncture anaesthesia at Colombo South General Hospital. Bilateral Tubectomy. Operating time 23 minutes. Madam Chao Lan-hsiang and Madam Premadasa, wives of the Vice-Premier of the People's Republic of China and the Premier of Sri Lanka fondling the two children. Patient (Left) is seated on the bed 10 hours after delivery.

Usually 2000 Hertz stimulation is carried out at these points. The artificial rupture of membranes is carried out immediately after commencing the manual stimulation at Hegu (L.I. 4.). An oxytocin drip infusion is commenced following the rupture of the membranes.

Adjuvant Drugs:

The following groups of drugs may be used:

A. For the active management of labor

a) Oxytocin drip infusion is used commencing at the stage of labor. Artificial rupture of membranes and simultaneous oxytocin drip infusion in a concentration of 5 units in 500 ml. of 5% dextrose at the rate of 20 mL/Min is used in this method of active management of labor.

b) Syntometrine (0.5 mg of Ergometrine with 5 units of synthetic Oxytocin) may be given at the end of the second stage of labor.

B. For the relief of pain (if acupuncture analgesia is inadequate):

a) Pethedine-Meperidine I mg/kg where the relief pain is incomplete with acupuncture.

b) Local anaesthesia-Lignocaine 2% for local infiltration may be used in cases where the relief of pain is incomplete with the needles. In order to carry out episiotomy and suturing.

c) Inhalation analgesia-Where acupuncture analgesia is ineffective, or to carry out forceps deliveries, and manual removal of placenta, inhalation analgesia may be added. This is required in less than 5% of cases.

CHILDBIRTH WITH ACUPUNCTURE

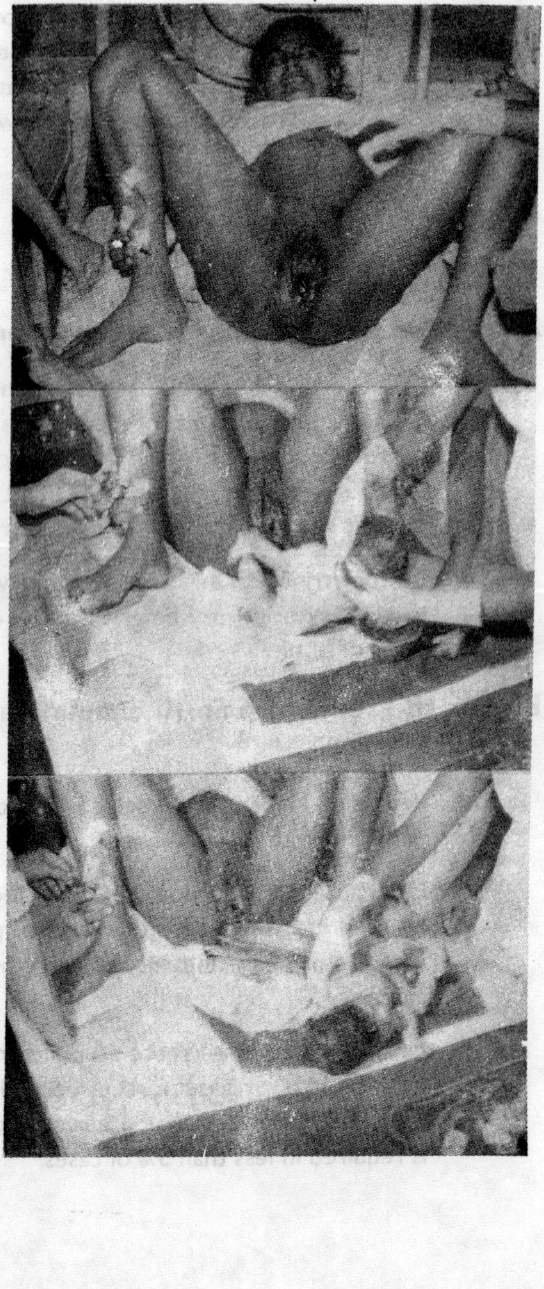

Patient bearing down Head is crowning

End of the second stage

Delivery completed

C. Other Drugs:

Other drugs are used on mothers who have complications like pre-eclamptic toxaemia or other accompanying disorders, where acupuncture is not able to satisfactorily allay the symptoms of these disorders.

At the Acupuncture Institute we have carried out a clinical trial on one hundred and ten pregnant mothers. Acupuncture analgesia to relieve the pain of childbirth was administered in this trial. It was effective in approximately 90% of the cases. The induction-delivery time interval was appreciably shortened (one third to about one fourth the time). The babies were born free of asphyxia. It is his observation that acupuncture analgesia, judiciously used together with oxytocin drip infusion, has a definite place in allaying the pain of childbirth expediting delivery and increasing the chances of a healthy off-spring being born.

It was concluded that the needling expedites labor by augmenting the natural "anti-pain mechanisms". Therefore, needling:

1) Relieves the pain of labor (to a satisfactory extent in about 90% of cases.)

2) Expedites the delivery.

Thus:

a) The necessity of giving large doses of analgesics to the mother is overcome thereby delivering the baby in a less toxic, drowsy state,

c) Shortening of the labor, which is also conducive to delivering a non-asphyxiated baby. According to our observations the Apgar scores of the babies delivered using acupuncture analgesia was much higher than a comparable group of babies whose mothers had orthodox sedative and analgesic drugs during the delivery.

ACUPUNCTURE ANAESTHESIA AT THE INSTITUTE OF ACUPUNCTURE COLOMBO SOUTH GOVERNMENT GENERAL HOSPITAL, KALUBOWILA

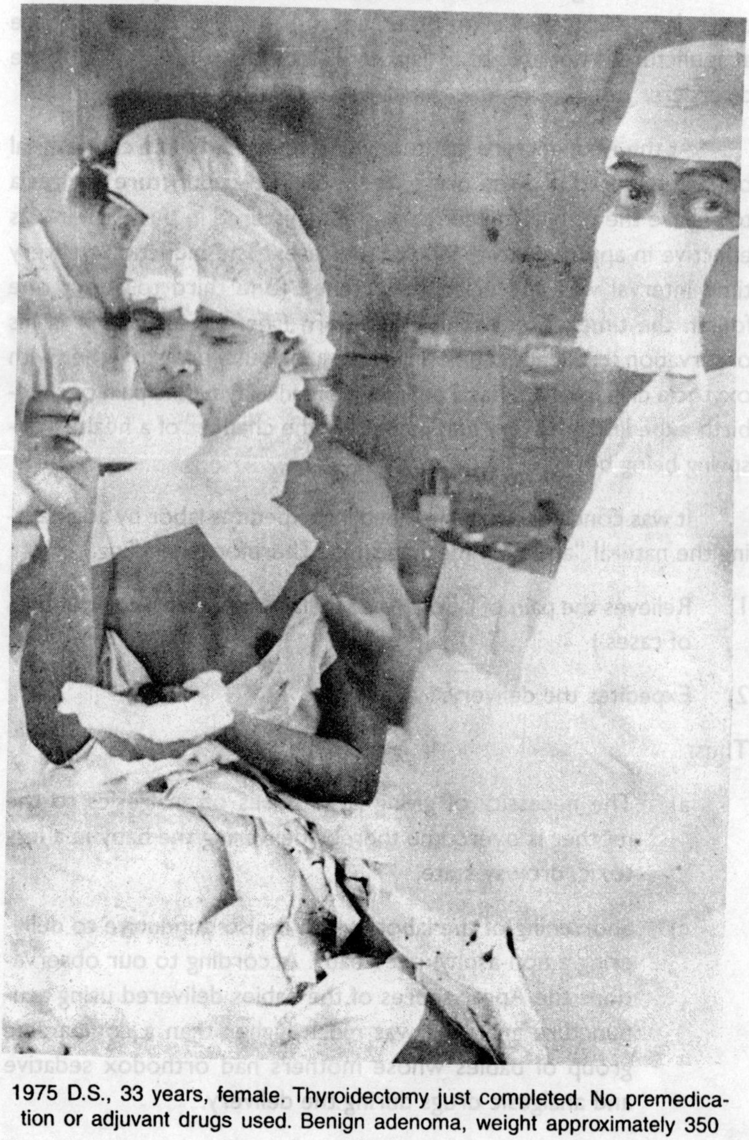

1975 D.S., 33 years, female. Thyroidectomy just completed. No premedication or adjuvant drugs used. Benign adenoma, weight approximately 350 grams.

Calmness and optimism can reduce the pain sensation and the response to pain. Furthermore, the active co-operation of the mother can be better solicited under acupuncture analgesia because she is not in a drowsy state. At the end of the delivery, the mother is more receptive to greet her new born and to appreciate the fruits of her labors as the climax of the pregnancy.

As no complicated apparatus is necessary, it could be used for home delivery and in the field. This method is especially suitable in the Third World as the cost benefit is high. The mother can co-operate during labor and the variations of the physiological functions are within normal limits.

A series of 296 Caresarean sections have been carried out at the Institute of Acupuncture, Kalubowila using acupuncture anaesthesia over a period of seven years. In 29 cases acupuncture was the only analgesic used. In the remaining cases a combination of drugs and acupuncture have been used (acuaesthesia). In two cases twins were delivered. Acupuncture anesthesia is also useful in forceps delivery and the manual removal of placenta. Where there is fetal distress there is a compelling reason to use acupuncture anaesthesia either alone or in combination with adjuvant drugs.

The use of homoeopuncture is extremely helpful during childbirth. (Aconite, Caulophyllum and Arnica are some of the common remedies used).

■

PROGNOSIS OF DISEASE WITH ACUPUNCTURE

"No medicine can cure old age or a withered flower"

–Ancient Chinese saying

Prognosis, the art of making predictions about the possible course and the final outcome of a disease, is one of the most hazardous exercises in the practice of clinical medicine. Not infrequently a patient, who has reached the point of no return according to the best medical opinion available, takes a one hundred and eighty degree turn and is *"recalled to life"*, to the astonishment of his physicians and relatives (no less the patient himself). Equally common are cases of people in seemingly bouyant health, whose fitness has just been confirmed by a battery of stringent tests, who suddenly drop dead of a heart attack, a stroke or other similar cause. It is therefore, not surprising that the experienced and astute physician is often content to give a "guarded prognosis," buttressed with many "ifs" and "buts", or even if possible, to avoid any prediction altogether. In the "average case", it is possible to give a reasonably accurate prognosis, or at least an informed guess, as to the probable outcome of the disease; qualified with a few possible complications that are likely to arise on the way to recovery.

Prognostication about the results of disease is a subject which seems to have baffled the traditional Chinese physicians even more than their Western counterparts. This is because in the classical texts there was no rule of thumb that enabled the predicting of the outcome of a particular disease. The ancient treatises gave many methods of assessing the gravity of a particular disease but were always vague as to the determination of the prognosis in a particular case, whereas Western medicine has now many technical parameters in the form of laboratory tests, E.C.G., X-ray, and other sensitive indicators to determine the gravity of an illness and to predict its subsequent course; the traditional physician had to rely mainly on his subjective assessment of the case, the rate of progress of alleviation or otherwise of the symptoms, and his own previous experience in similar cases. These methods, by and large, are not so helpful in arriving at a prognosis as the assessment of a patient by modern diagnostic aids.

However, in a majority of common diseases such as bronchial asthma, migraine, epilepsy, low backache, sciatica and the like, it is still the subjective feeling of the patient which remains, in the final analysis, the only indicator of progress of the illness. There are also numerous instances where the findings in special tests (e.g. the X-ray changes of cervical or lumbar spondylosis) are quite dissociated or incongruous with the gravity of the symptoms present. In view of these limitations, prognosis is a field where one could profitably combine the traditional methods of assessment with methods based on modern technology.

The leading indicators of prognosis as recognized by practising acupuncturists of today are as follows:

1) **The order of disappearance of symptoms:** When an illness is getting cured, the symptoms often disappear in the reverse order of their appearance. For example, when a severe asthmatic who is responding well to acupuncture complains of a sinusitis or a blocked nose, one should give a few additional needles for these latter problems. The patient complains of his sinusitis when the symptoms of his asthma are disappearing. The former symptoms predominate as the latter get cured. Again

in skin disorders, the patches to clear up first are generally those which appeared last. When using acupuncture, diseases may get cured from (a) the interior to exterior, (b) above downwards (c) periphery to centre, or (d) in the reverse order of the development of symptoms. These principles are similar to those of homoeopathy.[1]

2) **Age:** Younger people generally have a better prognosis than older people especially in rheumatoid, soft tissue, degenerative and vascular disorders. (Older persons however, generally speaking respond better to acupuncture anaesthesia.)

3) **Duration of the disease:** In general, all other things being equal. It is easier to cure a disease of short duration with acupuncture than one of long duration. It is curious to note that in some conditions of long duration like old cases of motor paralysis, where Western medicine can offer no hope of further Improvement, considerable progress is often seen with acupuncture treatment. Another example is aphasia following a stroke, where a good response to acupuncture is seen even when treated several years after the onset of the illness. Nearly 75% of the cases of frozen shoulder show immediate improvement, irrespective of the period of duration.

4) **Nature of the disease:** There are many diseases which respond well to acupuncture therapy although they are refractory to other methods of treatment. Hence the prognosis of a particular disease when acupuncture therapy is being used is independent of the prognosis of the same disease with drug therapy or when other modalities are used. As acupuncture gets assimilated into the mainstream of orthodox medicine, the section on prognosis in many standard medical textbooks will therefore have to be revised. For example, the cure rate of bronchial asthma with acupuncture treatment is about 60%.[2]

1 Hering's Law of Cure.

2 Using homoeopuncture about 75%.

5) **Duration of the treatment:** In many chronic painful disorders like trigeminal neuralgia, phantom limb and post-herpetic neuralgia, it may be necessary to persist with the therapy for some months before adequate relief is obtained. However, with the first few treatments the patient usually notices a favourable change in the quality, if not the quantity of pain. (In these very painful conditions one usually leaves the needles in situ for 45 minutes to one hour at each sitting and strong stimulation is used).

6) **Presence of complications:** In any disease, where the symptomatology is multiple and the complications many, the prognosis is usually less favourable.

7) **Malignant disease:** In malignant conditions the prognosis is bad. Acupuncture does not cure malignant disease. However, it is eminently suited for managing the secondary effects such as pain, cachexia, loss of appetite, sleeplessness and pyrexia. We have treated a large number of cases of inoperable carcinoma referred to us by the radio-therapists of the Cancer Hospital, Maharagama. We have found that acupuncture did relieve the pain considerably and help in making life tolerable for these patients. However, the final outcome was not influenced by this therapy.

(We have, however, seen 2 cases of acute lymphoblastic leukaemia where the marrow picture and the blood picture have been reported as normal after acupuncture. These cases are being followed up).

8) **Stimulation therapy:** In acute painful conditions strong stimulation at points like Hegu (L.I. 4.) helps to alleviate the symptoms considerably, and cuts short the duration of the disease, thereby improving the immediate prognosis. The stronger the stimulus up to a point, the better the relief of symptoms. The intensity of manual stimulation increases with:

a) the thickness of the needle.

b) the depth of penetration.

c) the amplitude and rate of rotation.

d) the length of time for which the needle is retained after stimulation.

e) repetition of the therapy at frequent intervals.

f) the number of points stimulated up to an optimum.

It should be noted that the stimulation has to be tailored to suit the individual case. Over stimulation may have adverse effects. The art of acupuncture implies the ability on the part of the physician to gauge the optimal stimulation required for each individual case and to exert the required manual dexterity to perform it correctly.

9) **Acute infections:** In acute or fulminating infections it is advisable to use antibiotics in preference to acupuncture, to bring the disorder under control. Concurrent or subsequent administration of acupuncture is helpful in cutting short the further course of the disease and the need for prolonged antibiotic therapy. Acupuncture alone has been reported by some Chinese workers to be effective in some acute conditions like acute appendicitis and malaria. In many chronic infections such as otitis media and chronic pyelitis where there has been no response to antibiotics, acupuncture is found to give good results.

10) **Surgery:** In cases where surgery has been previously carried out the response to acupuncture has, on the whole, been poor. In conditions like prolapsed intervertebral disc, deaf-mutism and Buerger's disease, it is best to try acupuncture before embarking on surgical procedures. In a large majority of these cases, surgery can be avoided altogether by the judicious and early use of acupuncture.

11) **Previous steroid therapy:** Where large doses of steroids have been administered over long periods (e.g. prednisolone in bronchial asthma) the prognosis with acupuncture therapy is not so hopeful as in untreated cases. However, it has been found possible to improve the results by judiciously cutting off the

requirements of steroids and by the use of special points such as Jianjing (G.B. 21.) and the Endocrine point of the ear, to overcome the drug withdrawal effects.

12) **Fainting:** This is one of the commonest complications with acupuncture therapy. It has, however, been noted that patients who react to the needles with fainting, generally at the first or early sittings, eventually show good recovery from their illness as they appear to be more responsive to the needle effect. The method of needling must be then changed to the non-retention method.

13) **Alarm Points:** As a disease gets better the relevant Alarm points become less tender. This is used as an index for the prognosis. In locomotor disorders similarly the Ah-Shi points become less tender.

14) **Electrical testing:** The electrical conductivity at the corresponding auricular points increases as the illness proceeds to a climax. Thereafter it slowly reverts to normal. By using a sensitive acupunctoscope (A.P.D.) it is possible to follow these changes to ascertain to the prognosis.

15) **The Pulse examination:** This is one of the best prognostic variables to those who are conversant with the technique. The disordered pulses progressively revert to normal as the disorder improves. It is claimed that long term prognosis of, and even the presence of latent disease, can be ascertained through pulse diagnosis by specialists in this art.

16) **Ear acupuncture:** The immediate prognosis in cases treated by ear acupuncture is usually better, especially, in disease of the internal organs. However, it is wise to consolidate the results by the use of body acupuncture points as well.

17) **Head Needling (Scalp Acupuncture):** This form of treatment gives good results in cerebro-vascular disorders, choreotremors, parkinsonism and similar neurological disorders. The long-term prognosis is even better when combined with body and ear acupuncture therapy.

18) **The accurate location of points:** This is the important determinant of success. Inaccuracy in location of points can only lead to indifferent results. Conversely, accuracy in location is the key to success.

19) **The manual dexterity of the acupuncturist:** Dexterity on the part of the acupuncturist both in the proper insertion and manipulation of the needles is a critical factor in the success of the therapy. This is all the more important when a strong stimulation is used. In the treatment of pain problems and motor paralysis it makes a substantial difference whether or not the technique of correct stimulation is applied in order to produce the desired degree of *deqi.*

20) **The correct selection of points:** Acupuncture points have highly specific therapeutic actions. The points or combination of points to be used have to be selected with a great deal of care. The points must be carefully selected, according to the principles laid down for the selection of points in order to obtain the best result.

21) **Combination of other therapeutic methods:** Combination with Aspirin to relieve chronic pain, with homoeopathic remedies in chronic disorders are helpful in obtaining relief.

22) **Rapport:** All medicine has a large subjective component. The establishment of a firm rapport between the patient and the healer is the most important step on the road to recovery.

■

AURICULOTHERAPY

Chinese Ear Acupuncture Therapy

"The ear is the place where all the channels meet"

— Huang Di Nei Jing, Ling Shu

Auriculotherapy is an historical form of acupuncture. Today it is being used widely, not only in the Orient, but it has also gained great popularity in the West. In France, the Nogier school of Ear Acupuncture is well known. In West Germany, the Munich Auriculotherapy Association counts over 3000 members.

Auriculotherapy may be defined as that branch of acupuncture which makes use of the external ear to diagnose as well as to treat illness. According to the Yellow Emperor's Classic of Internal Medicine "the ear is the place where all the channels meet". The relationships between organs, channels and points were described clearly in several of the ancient classics. There is historical evidence that in the Middle East and in North Africa, an ancient form of auriculotherapy, which in many respects was similar to that of Chinese auriculotherapy, existed and continues to be used up to the present day. According to some authorities the custom of wearing pierced earrings has more than an ornamental basis. Ear massage has been practised since ancient times both to tonify the body as well as to excite a person sexually.

The ear has a rich nerve supply derived from several spinal segments. In addition, branches of the vagus, glossopharyngeal, trigeminal, and facial nerves supply the ear. There is a rich blood supply from branches of several adjoining arteries, with both sympathetic and parasympathetic fibres running close to the blood vessels. As the nerves mentioned above spread out widely and have connections with all areas of the body including the internal organs, it is not surprising that any lesion, say for instance in the stomach, will exhibit changes in the collateral branch which supplies the ear. When a neurological representation of one part of the body occurs in any other part of the body such as the cortex, the thalamus, the cerebellum, the limbic system, the medulla oblongata, or the spinal cord, the different parts are represented in a very orderly arrangement. For example, in the motor cortex the contra-lateral half of the body is represented upside down in a very orderly arrangement (Penfield and Rasmussen). Similarly, the representation of the body and organs in the auricle is also upside down. Each of the billion cells of the body carries in the chromosomes a computer-memory-like representation of all the features of the human being. It is therefore not surprising that the ear carries the representation of the rest of the body, particularly in view of the fact that a number of collaterals of the nerves that supply the rest of the body innervate it. The external ear is looked upon by the acupuncturist of today as a "switch-board" for the rest of the body structures.

At the Institute of Physiology in Shanghai, it has been demonstrated in animal experiments that when an artificial lesion is caused in the stomach of an experimental rabbit, there is a fall of electrical resistance in the "stomach area" of both auricles. Such an artificial gastric ulcer can be created in an animal by injecting phenolphthalein under the submucosa. As the lesion heals, the electrical resistance reverts to normal. This effect cannot be demonstrated if the auricle is completely denervated or if a local anaesthetic is injected at the root of the auricle.

Since 1966, auriculotherapy has been widely used in all parts of the People's Republic of China both for therapy and anaesthesia. By and large, it is a more effective form of acupuncture therapy than body acupuncture in internal organ disorders. There are many acupuncture institutions in the West, particularly in West Germany and France, where only auriculotherapy is carried out. Paul Nogier of France has done much work to elucidate the problems of auriculotherapy. The modern revival of interest in this branch of acupuncture in the West is mainly due to his efforts. In our clinic at the Institute of Acupuncture, we practice mainly classical body acupuncture and reserve the ear only for those cases where there is an insufficient response. Auriculotherapy may be combined with either body acupuncture or Head-Needle Therapy where indicated. It is not combined with foot acupuncture as the latter is a yin form of acupuncture.

The external ear has an external (or yang) surface and an internal (or yin) surface also called the back of the auricle.

The distribution of auricular points on the yang surface simulates a fetus within the womb, with a head presentation (i.e., in an upside down position). The lobe represents the facial area, the antitragus the head, and the antihelix the trunk, as shown in the accompanying diagrams.

There are some 200 acupuncture points on the ear. The important points used frequently in therapy are described below (after the teachers at the Academies of Traditional Chinese Medicine, Peking, Shanlwhai and Nanking).

THE ANATOMY OF THE EAR

The ear is a skin-covered fibrocartilaginous plate moulded so that the concavities on its lateral aspect are convexities on its inner or cranial surface.

The anatomical parts of the external ear are as follows.-

A. THE LATERAL OR ANTERIOR SURFACE (YANG)

1. **Helix:** The prominent rim of the auricle.

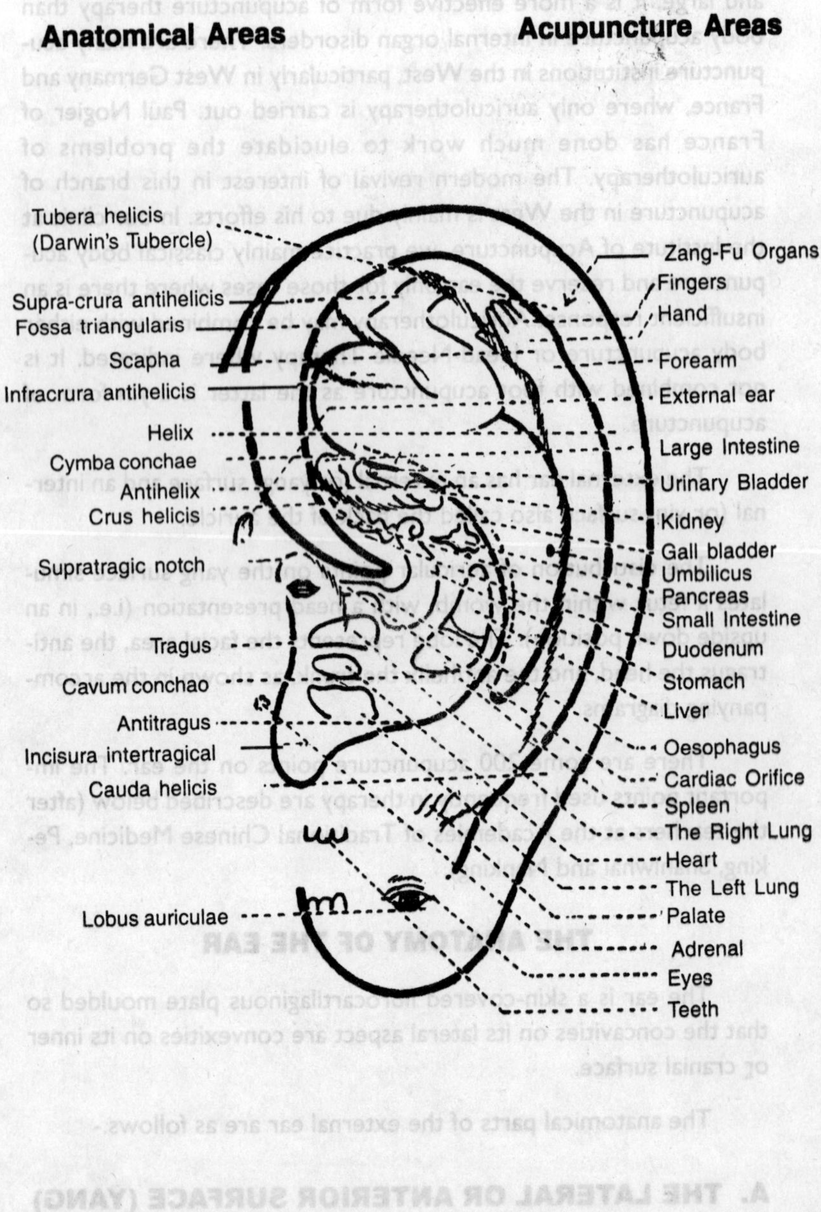
Anatomical Areas
Acupuncture Areas
Tubera helicis
(Darwin's Tubercle)
Supra-crura antihelicis
Fossa triangularis
Scapha
Infracrura antihelicis
Helix
Cymba conchae
Antihelix
Crus helicis
Supratragic notch
Tragus
Cavum conchao
Antitragus
Incisura intertragical
Cauda helicis
Lobus auriculae
Zang-Fu Organs
Fingers
Hand
Forearm
External ear
Large Intestine
Urinary Bladder
Kidney
Gall bladder
Umbilicus
Pancreas
Small Intestine
Duodenum
Stomach
Liver
Oesophagus
Cardiac Orifice
Spleen
The Right Lung
Heart
The Left Lung
Palate
Adrenal
Eyes
Teeth

2. **Helix crus:** The antero-inferior end of the helix, a horizontal prominence.

3. **Auricular tubercle** (Darwin's tubercle): A small tubercle at the posterior upper aspect of the helix.

4. **Helix cauda:** The inferior end of the helix at the junction of the helix and the lobule.

5. **Antihelix:** A curved prominence parallel to the vertical part of the helix. Its upper part branches out into the superior and-the inferior antibelix crus.

6. **Triangular fossa** (deltoid fossa): The depression between the two crura of the antihelix.

7. **Scapha:** The depression (groove) between the helix and the antihelix.

8. **Tragus:** A small curved flap at the front of the auricle covering the meatus.

9. **Supratragic notch:** The depression between the helix crus and the upper border of the tragus.

10. **Antitragus:** A small tubercle opposite the tragus and inferior to the antihelix.

11. **Intertragic notch:** The depression between the tragus and the antitragus.

12. **Lobule:** The lower part of the auricle where the cartilage is absent.

13. **Cymba conchae:** The concha superior to the helix crus.

14. **Cavum conchae:** The concha inferior to the helix crus.

15. **Orifice of the external auditory meatus:** The opening in the cavum conchae is shielded by the tragus.

THE ANATOMICAL AREAS

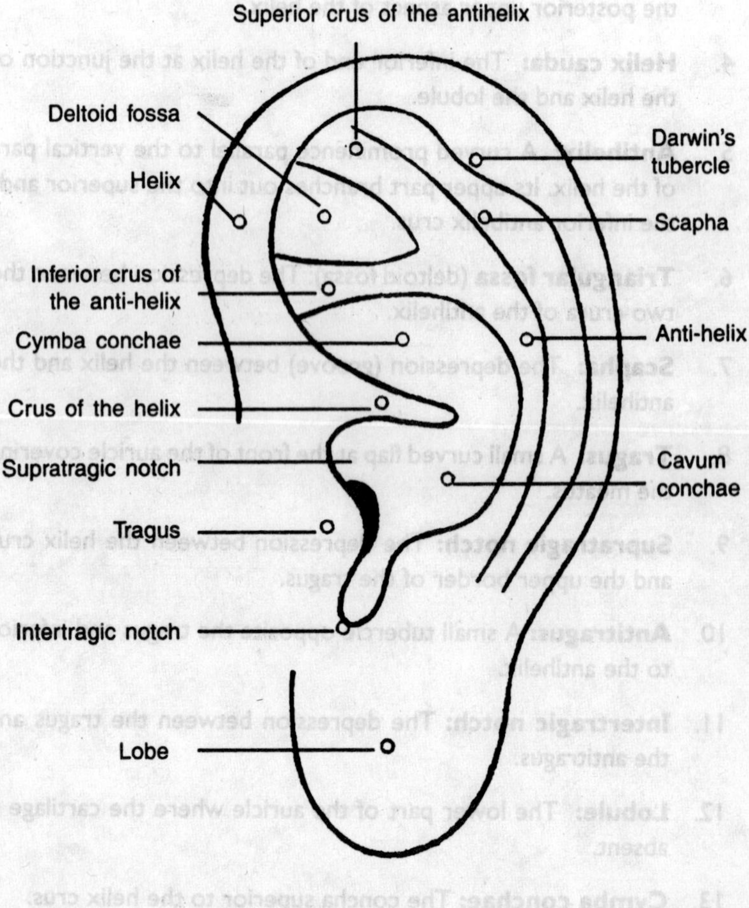

THE LATERAL SURFACE OF THE LEFT EXTERNAL EAR
(Yang surface)

B. THE MEDIAL, CRANIAL OR POSTERIOR SURFACE (YIN):

The medial surface faces the mastoid area.

The Anatomy: The lobe of the ear is without cartilage and may be freely hanging or attached to the side of the cheek. The helix or incurving margin curves down at the crus of the helix across the well of the conchae the rim of which is the anti- helix. The crus helix divides the conchae into the cymba and cavum. The antihelix divides into the superior and inferior crura forming the superior boundary of the triangular fossa. The helix forms the third side of the triangle. The tragus and the antitragus overhang the lower part of the conchae, with the intertragic notch placed between them. The supratragic notch lies above the tragus. The groove between the helix and the antihelix is the scapha.

The Nerve supply of the Ear : The ear is supplied by the following nerves:

Auriculo-temporal nerve.

Lesser occipital nerve.

Great auricular nerve.

Auricular branch of the vagus.

Auriculo-temporal branch of the trigeminal nerve.

Branches of the glosso-pharyngeal and facial.

Sympathetic and parasympathetic fibres.

The Blood Supply of the Ear:

Branches of middle meningeal artery.

Branch of the artery of the pterygoid canal.

Anterior tympanic artery.

Deep auricular artery.

Stylomastoid branch of the posterior auricular artery.

Auricular branches of the superficial auricular artery.

THE ANATOMICAL AREAS

Areas for backache:

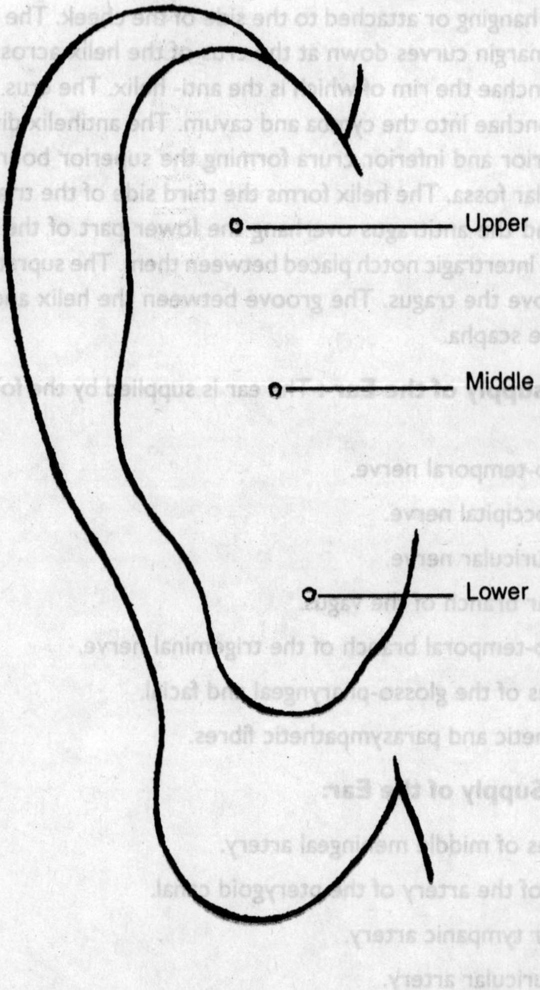

The posterior (medial) surface of the left external ear

COMMONLY USED AURICULAR AREAS AND POINTS

THE OUTER SURFACE OF THE AURICLE (YANG SURFACE)

The Ear Lobe:

The ear lobe represents the Face Area. The ear lobe can be divided with 3 horizontal lines and 2 vertical lines into 9 areas as shown in the diagram.

***AREA 1[1] and AREA 4[1]* :** Anaesthetic points for tooth extraction and analgesic points for toothache. Area 1 represents the *Teeth of the Lower Jaw* and Area 4 represents the *Teeth of the Upper Jaw.*

***AREA 2* :** The middle of this area represents the *Tongue*. The upper part of this area is the *Hard Palate* and the lower part the *Soft Palate.*

***AREA 3* :** Represents the jaws. In conformity with the position of the upside-down fetus, the position of the jaws is reversed. The upper border of Area 3 represents the *Lower Jaw* and the lower border of this area represents the *Upper Jaw.*

***AREA 5* :** This area is in the middle of ear lobe and represents the Eye. Also note that areas *Eye I and Eye II* on both sides of the intertragic notch represent the eye. Eye I is especially effective for astigmatism and Eye II for glaucoma.

***AREA 6** :** Representss the *Inner Ear.* It is useful in the treatment of inner ear disease; it can also be used in vertigo, dizziness, travel sickness, nausea, and vomiting of pregnancy. A press needle in this area is very helpful in such disorders.

***AREA 7 and AREA 9* :** Have no identifiable points.

***AREA 8* :** Represents the *Tonsils and Throat.*

Facio-Mandibular Area : This is an oval area lying between Areas 5 and 6 and extending a little beyond. This area is useful in the treatment of facial paralysis, trigeminal neuralgia and sinusitis.

---

1 The center of this area represents this point.

THE FETAL REPRESENTATION

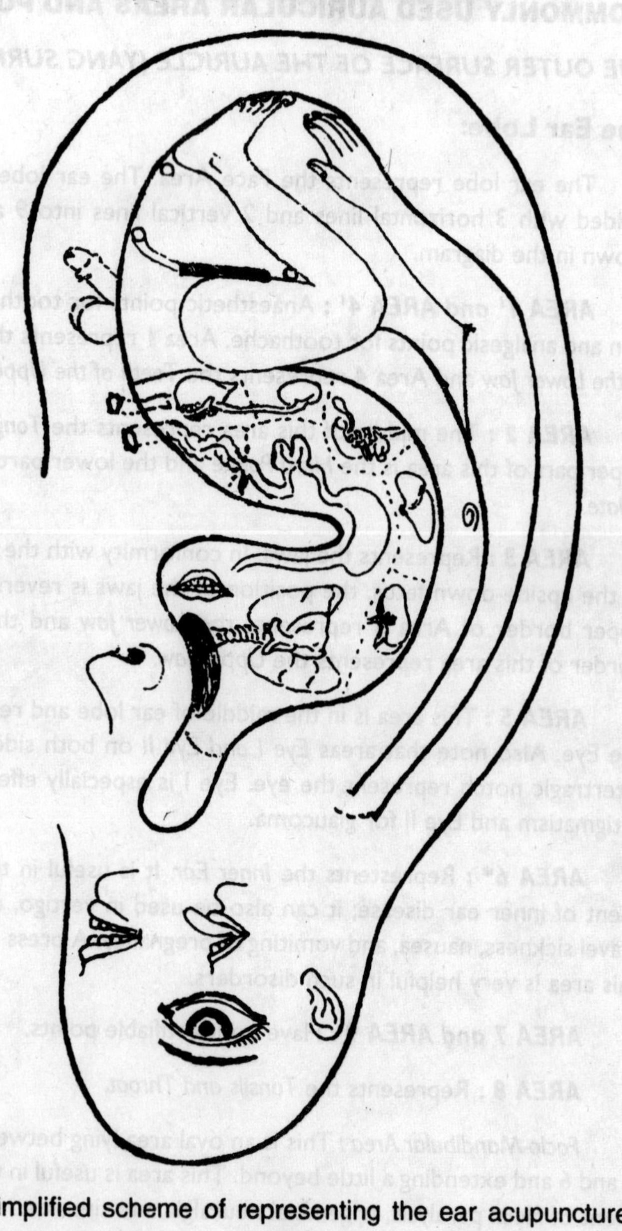

A simplified scheme of representing the ear acupuncture areas

The Tragus:

Represents the *Nose* and *Pharynx* Areas.

a) **Lateral Aspect :** At the center of the lateral aspect is the *External Nose Area.*

b) **Medical Aspect :** Just opposite the center of the external auditory meatus is the *Pharynx Area.* Below this point is the *Internal Nose Area.*

c) **Border of the Tragus :** On the free border of the tragus at the lowest part is the Adrenal Point. Between the adrenal point and the external nose area is the Hunger Point. This point is used for treating obesity.

The Antitragus:

Corresponds to the head region.

a) **Lateral aspect of antitragus:**

ForeheadArea: Junction of Area 2 of (lobe with) antitragus.

Occiput Area: Superior part of antitragus.

Parotid and Temporal areas:

Lies between the above two areas (Forehead and occiput).

b) **Free margin of the antitragus.**

Point Dingchuan : (Dingchuan in Chinese means "Soothing Asthma".)

This point is at the apex of the antitragus and is for soothing asthma. Needling this point in an acute bronchial asthmatic attack helps to control the asthmatic attack. A press needle in this position also helps to prevent attacks.

Brain Stem: Junction of the antitragus and antihelix.

Brain Point: Midpoint between the point Dingchuan and point Brain Stem. This point is also known as the *Encephalon point.*

c) **Medial aspect of Antitragus:** The Subcortex is situated on the medial wall of the antitragus.

Testis or Ovary: Lower part of Subcortex Area. This area is adjacent to the *Endocrine Area* located in the intertragic notch.

The Antihelix:

The antihelix corresponds to the *Trunk.* At the posterior end of the junction of the antihelix and antitragus is the *Neck Area.* The inferior crus of the antihelix corresponds to the *Gluteal Region* and *Thigh.* The superior crus of the antihelix corresponds to the lower extremity below the knee. In the antihelix the trunk and the leg are represented with the fetus facing posteriorly. Therefore the anterior margin of the antihelix represents the *Spine Area* (With the cervical, dorsal, lumbar and sacrococcygeal areas located from below upwards).

The Inferior Crus and Superior Crus of the Antihelix:

The posterior half of the inferior crus represents the *Buttock Area* with the *Hip Joint Area* on the superior border adjacent to this Area. The anterior half represents the *Lumbo-Sacral Plexus* and the *Sciatic Nerve Area.* The middle one third of the upper groove of this area is the *Constipation Area.* At the division of the antihelix into the superior and inferior crus is the *Knee Area.* The Leg *Area* is represented in the superior crus of the antihelix with the *Toe Area* uppermost.

The Helix:

The prominence on the helix at about the 2.00 o'clock position (left ear) is called Darwin's tubercle. It represents the *Zang-Fu Organs.* It may be used to treat internal Organ disorders as a homeostatic point.

The Crus of the Helix:

This represents the *Diaphragmatic Muscle.* The internal organs of the thorax are therefore represented inferior to the crus of the helix, and the abdominal organs are represented superior to the crus of the helix in the conchae. Similarly, the level of the crus helix divides the antihelix spine area into the *Cervical* and *Thoracic Spine Areas* below and the *Lumbar* and *Sacro-coccygeal Areas* above, in keeping with the representation of an upside-down fetus. The posterior borders of these two areas correspond respectively to the *Thoracic Wall* and the *Abdominal Wall Areas.*

The Scapha:

The scapha represents the upper limb. Just above the *Neck* point is the *Clavicle Area.* From this area upwards on the scapha, up to the level of the crus of the helix represents the *Shoulder Joint Area* and *Shoulder Area* respectively, (in that order). At the level of the inferior end of the inferior crus of the antihelix is the *Elbow Area.* At the level of the inferior end of the superior crus is the Wrist Area. The superior-most area of the Scapha is the Fingers Area. Between the Shoulder and Elbow area is the Upper Arm Area, between the Wrist and the Fingers is the Hand Area. The line of the Scapha continued downwards between the lobe and the antitragus is known as "The Line of Sound" It represents the auditory functions and is useful for treating deafness, tinnitus, vertigo and Meniere's disease.

The Triangular Fossa (Deltoid Fossa):

This is a triangular area bounded on the 3 sides by; side (1) the helix, side (2), superior crus of the antihelix (inferior border) and side (3), inferior crus of the antihelix (superior border). The most important and frequently used point in auriculotherapy is the *Point Ear Shenmen.* This point is located at the junction of the last 2 sides described above. This point has strong sedative and analgesic effects. It is the equivalent of Baihui (Du 20.) in body acupuncture. In addition it has a wide spectrum of physiological effects.

A line tangential to the same two sides which meets on the antihelix is known as the *Hot point.* This point is used in treating febrile illness. It is particularly effective and useful in treating fevers with toxic states in infants and children.

At the junction of side (1) and side (2) is the *Blood pressure Lowering Point (Hypertension Point)*.

On the middle 1/3rd of side (3) of the triangular fossa is the *Constipation Point*. Immediately lateral (posterior) to this area is the *Hip Joint Area*.

At the junction of side (1) and side (3) is the *Sympathetic Point*.

The midpoint of a line between the lowering of Blood Pressure Point and the Sympathetic Point is the *Uterus Point*. (In males this point represents the prostate gland and seminal vesical areas).

The Cavum Conchae:

The deepest point of the cavum conchae is the *Heart Area*. This is posterior to the external auditory meatus.

The posterior ½ of the line between the external auditory meatus and the heart area represents the *Trachea*. The two *Lung Areas* are superior and inferior to the heart area. The lower lung area represents the lung of the same side.

The area of the cavum conchae between the tragus and antitragus is divided into an upper half which is the area for the *Body Cavities* (*Sanjiao*) and a lower half, the *Endocrine Area*.

The area at the lower rim of the external auditory meatus represents the *Upper Abdominal Wall Area*. The area at the upper rim of the external auditory meatus represents the *Lower Abdominal Wall Area*.

The *Mouth Area* lies immediately superior and posterior to the external auditory meatus. Between the Mouth Area and lower border of the crus helix is another *Hunger Point* (named after Wou Wei-Ping[2] of Taipei. This point is also used extensively in western countries for the treatment of obesity).

The *Oesophagus Area* runs along the line from the mouth area

---

2 Wou Wei-Ping is a 63rd generation acupuncturist of an unbroken line of acupuncture practitioners.

to the Stomach Area just below the lower margin of the *Diaphragm*. Posterior to the area of the termination of the crus helix is the *Stomach Area*. Between the Stomach Area and the antihelix is the *Spleen Area*.

The Cymba Conchae:

The Stomach Area continues over into the cymba conchae above the upper border of the crus helix. The organs are represented from posterior to anterior in their usual order – *Duodenum, Small Intestine, Appendix* and *Large Intestine Areas*. On the helix immediately next to (in front of) the Large Intestine Area is the *Rectum*. Just above the representation of the gastrointestinal tract, are represented (in the cymba conchae) the rest of the intra-abdominal organs, in the following order: The *Liver, Gall bladder, Pancreas, Kidney, Urethra and Urinary Bladder*. The *Urethra* is situated on the helix at the level of the Urinary Bladder.

Note: The pancreas is represented only in the left ear and the gall bladder in the right ear, in the same position. The External Genitalia are represented in the helix just above the Urethra Area. Between the upper pole of the Kidney and the Small Intestine Areas is the *Ascites Point*. This point is used in eedema and ascites.

THE BACK OF THE AURICLE (YIN SURFACE)

There is a groove in the back of the ear (medial, surface) corresponding to the scapha. This is the Groove for Lowering Blood Pressure. The rest of this area is indistinctly divided into 3 areas known as the Upper, the Middle, and the lower Portions of the Back. These 3 areas correspond to the relevant areas of the back of the trunk and they are used for treating spinal disorders of the respective areas.

The auricular points described are those which are frequently used at the Academy of Traditional Chinese Medicine, Peking.

The points of the French School of Auricular Therapy as described by Paul Nogier vary in some detail, especially in the deltoid fossa area.

THE CLINICAL EXAMINATION OF THE EAR

(1) **Inspection :** All areas of the ear must be examined in good light. Certain skin changes such as excoriation, vesicle, and inflammed areas, may be seen. These are known as reaction points and often have some relation to the disorders of the internal organs or regions represented by these areas.

(2) **Tenderness (Palpation) :** Reaction points can be found by pressing the ear with the reverse end of an acupuncture needle or a match-stick.

(3) **Electro-Exploratory Technique :** With a suitable electrical detector, the entire ear must be explored in a set order. The skin resistance of an area may be lowered when there is a dysfunction of the corresponding organ. Overall, there is about a 90-95% concordance between the auricular reactions and various disorders. This is most accurate in internal organ disorders. The Five-Element relationship also holds good in auricular diagnosis (as well as in therapy).

RULES OF SELECTION OF POINTS IN AURICULOTHERAPY

(1) *Organ affected.*

e.g. Lung Area for bronchial asthma.

Stomach area for gastritis.

(2) *Coupled Organ.*

e.g. Large Intestine Area for bronchial asthma.

Spleen Area for gastritis.

(3) *Functions affected.*

e.g. Blood Pressure Lowering Point in hypertension.

Hunger Points for obesity.

(4) *According to the Theory of traditional Chinese medicine relationships.*

e.g. Liver Area in eye disease and musculotendinous disorders.

Lung Area in skin diseases and rhinitis.

Kidney Area in ear diseases, bone diseases and alopecia.

(5) *According to the Theory of the Five-Elements.*

e.g. Kidney Point for acute bronchial asthma.

(Water is the son of metal)

Kidney Point for anxiety syndromes.

(Water quenches fire)

(6) *Specific points for a disorder.*

e.g. Hot Point for fever.

Point Dingchuan for relieving asthma.

Constipation point for constipation.

Ascites Point for edema and ascites.

(7) *Points according to Western Medicine.*

e.g. Point Pancreas for diabetes mellitus.

Endocrine point for endocrine disorders.

Spleen for immune and digestive disorders.

(8) *Reactive points.*

Point selected (reactive points) in an individual case by:

a) Inspection.

b) Palpation.

c) Electrically reactive points.

(9) *Point Shenmen* : This point has a broad-spectrum action. It is the best sedative and analgesic point of the ear and is therefore invariably combined with other points in the treatment of most diseases.

(10) *Point Endocrine* : This area is often very useful when the patient has been on medication for a long period before commencing acupuncture. The point is particularly helpful in overcoming the

S — Shenmen

B.P.— Blood Pressure reducing

Symp.— Sympathetic

C — Constipation

H — Hotpoint

U — Urethra

A — Anus

O — Oedema and ascites

P — Pharynx

EN — External nose

IN — Internal nose

TA — Tragus

Ad — Adrenal

EI — Eye I

EII — Eye II

D — Dingchuan

Z-F — Zang-Fu area

FM — Facio-Mandibular area

U — Upper }
M — Middle } Backache area
L — Lower }

ACUPUNCTURE REGIONS OF THE EAR

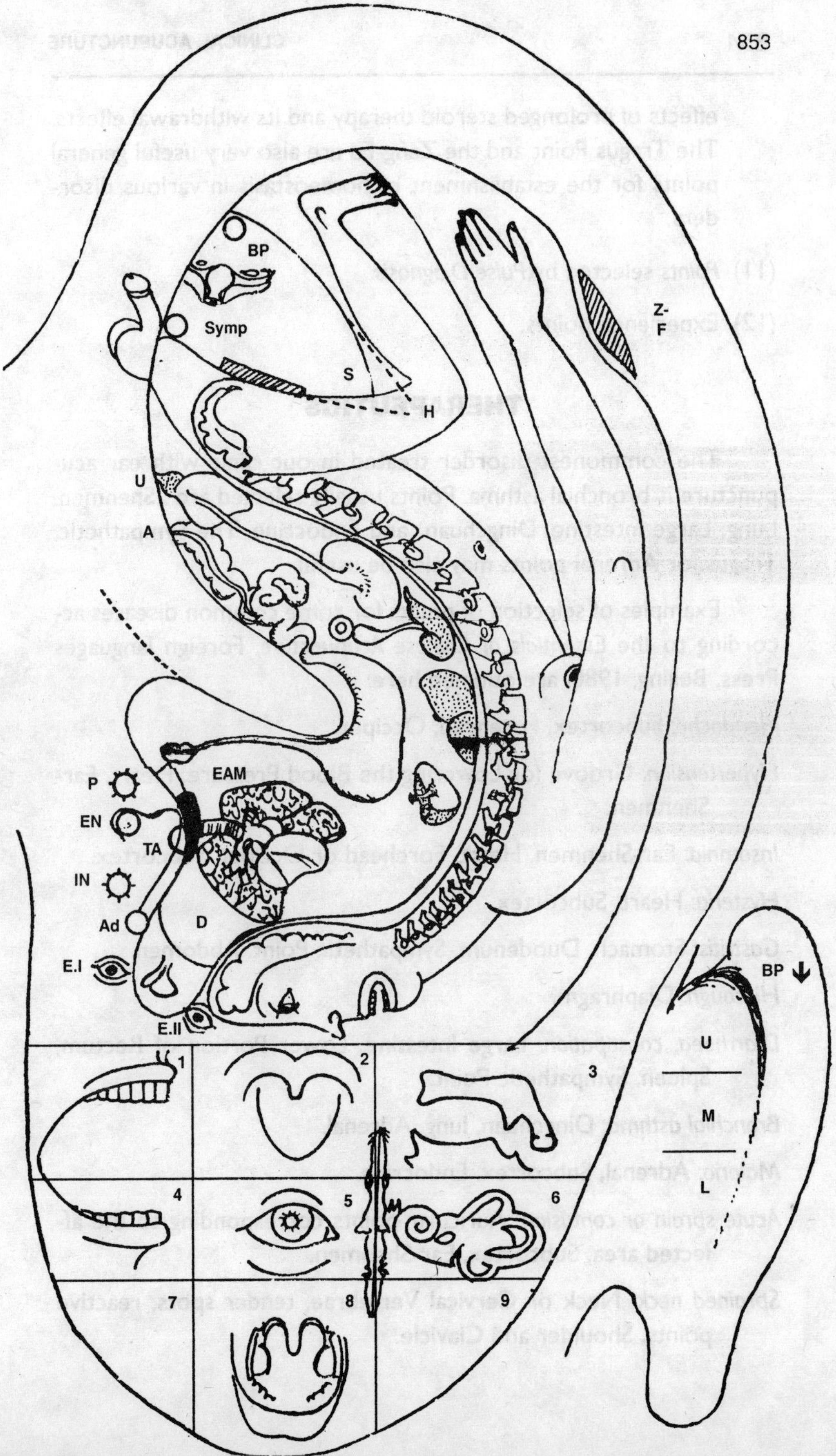

effects of prolonged steroid therapy and its withdrawal effects. The Tragus Point and the Zang-Fu are also very useful general points for the establishment of homeostasis in various disorders.

(11) *Points* selected by *Pulse Diagnosis.*

(12) Experience points.

THERAPEUTICS

The commonest disorder treated in our clinic with ear acupuncture is bronchial asthma. Points usually selected are : Shenmen. Lung, Large Intestine, Dingchuan and Endocrine. The Sympathetic, Tragus. or Adrenal points may also be useful.

Examples of selection of points for some common diseases according to the *Essentials of Chinese Acupuncture,* Foreign languages Press, Beijing, 1980, are outlined here:

Headache: Subcortex, Forehead, Occiput.

Hypertension: Groove for Lowering the Blood Pressure, Heart, Ear-Shenmen.

Insomnia: Ear-Shenmen, Heart, Forehead or Occiput, Subcortex.

Hysteria: Heart, Subcortex.

Gastritis: Stomach, Duodenum, Sympathetic Point. Abdomen.

Hiccough: Diaphragm.

Diarrhoea, constipation: Large Intestine, Lower Portion of Rectum, Spleen, Sympathetic Point.

Bronchial asthma: Dingchuan, lung. Adrenal.

Malaria: Adrenal, Subcortex, Endocrine.

Acute sprain or contusion: Auricular points corresponding to the affected area, Subcortex, Ear-Shenmen.

Sprained neck: Neck or Cervical Vertebrae, tender spots, reactive points, Shoulder and Clavicle.

Sciatica: Sciatic Nerve, Buttocks, Ear-Shenmen or Subcortex.

Acute orchitis: Testis, External Genitalia, Liver.

Post-operative analgesic points: Subcortex, Ear-Shenmen, auricular points corresponding to the operated region.

Dysmenorrhoea: Uterus, Endocrine, Liver.

Morning Sicknes: Area 6 of Lobe.

Enuresis, retention of urine: Urinary Bladder, Kidney, Urethra.

Herpes zoster: Auricular points corresponding to the affected areas, Adrenal.

Urticaria: Lung, Liver, Spleen.

Acute conjunctivitis: Ear, Liver, Ear apex.

Hordeolum: Eye, liver, Eye 1, Eye 2.

Acutepharyngitis: Pharynx area.

Impaired hearing: Internal Ear, Kidney.

THE PROCEDURES OF AURICULOTHERAPY

The most important steps to remember in performing auriculotherapy are:

(1) To clean the ear well before acupuncturing.

(2) Not to penetrate the cartilage when puncturing.

(3) To use short needles which have been properly cleaned and sterilized.

(4) Not to needle the inner (Yin) and outer (Yang) surfaces of the same ear, at the same sitting.

(5) Not to use hand manipulation of the needle to stimulate the ear points.

In the practice of Chinese auriculotherapy, steel single-spiral filiform needles are used. In the French School of Acupuncture, steel,

THE WESTERN NUMBERING SYSTEM OF AURICULAR POINTS

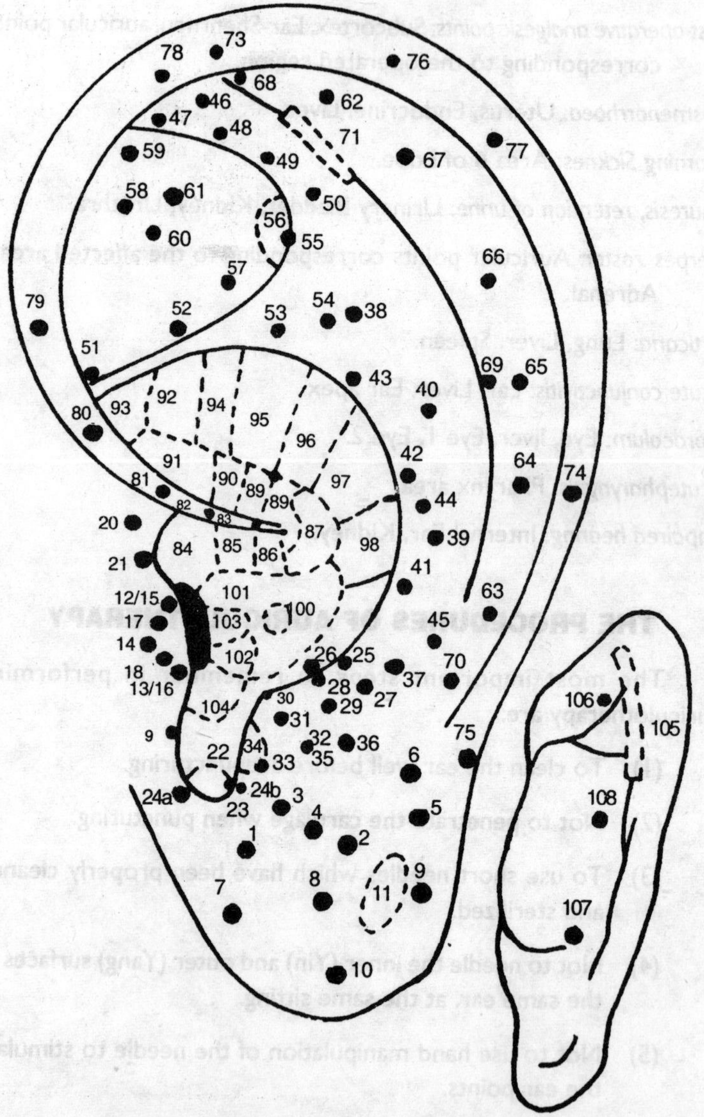

Diagram showing the numbering of ear acupuncture areas as designated by some western authors

gold, silver, and molybdenum needles are used. The order of placing the needles is generally immaterial in the former school, while the latter always lays great stress on the correct order of needle placement and their removal.

The needles may be inserted perpendicularly or obliquely. When inserted perpendicularly, the needles should hang by the skin and should not penetrate the cartilage, as this is relatively avascular and any injury or infection may have very serious consequences.

After insertion, the needles are left in place for about 20 to 30 minutes. If stimulation is desired electromanipulation is used. Hand stimulation is not carried out in our clinic as a rule, as it may cause traumatic damage to the cartilage. When there is distension or soreness felt at the site of the needle, the therapeutic result is usually said to be better.

The treatment is carried out daily or every other day for 7 to 10 days. Thereafter a 5 to 7 day rest-period is given and the patient is then reviewed.

The results obtained with auriculotherapy are generally better than with body acupuncture in internal organ disorders. It is often useful to combine both types of acupuncture for maximum response.

ACUPUNCTURE ANAESTHESIA USING AURICULOTHERAPY

Ear acupuncture is widely used for the extraction of teeth. The ear may also be used in general surgical procedures and for anaesthesia to relieve the pain of childbirth.

In childbirth as well as in abdominal surgery, it is our experience that the point Shenmen or the specific organ point of the ear, combined with electrostimulation of Renying (St. 9.) of the opposite side of the neck (or the same side), helps to alleviate the discomfort encountered on traction of the viscera. The mechanism of this action is probably due to the afferent sensations of the painful uterine contractions travelling to the brain via the vagus getting effectively

THE FETAL REPRESENTATION OF THE EAR ACUPUNCTURE AREAS

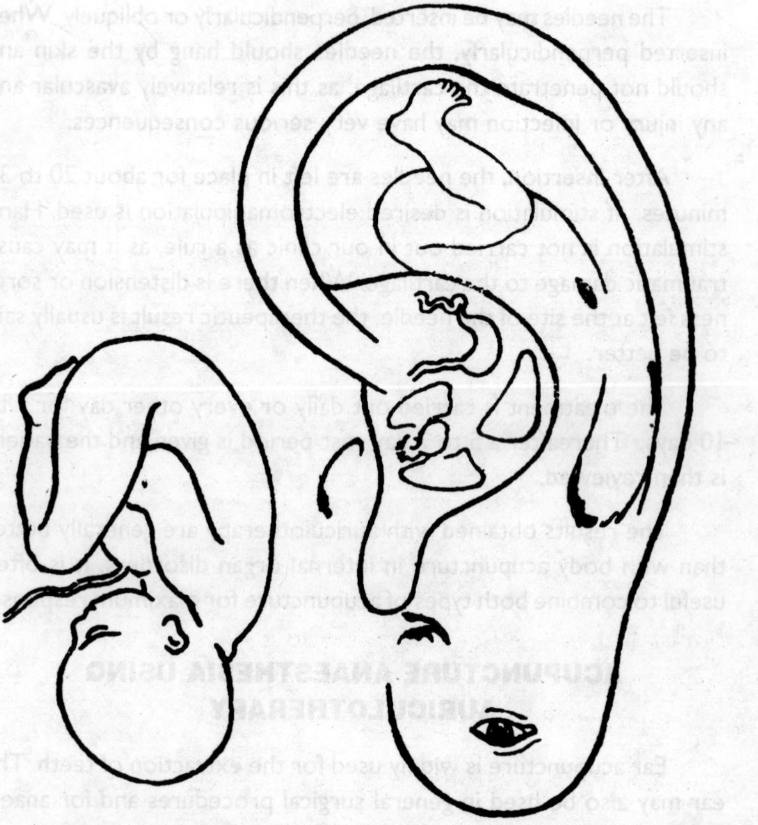

Note: The upside down representation.

blocked in childbirth. At the second stage (or during forceps delivery), a very high level of strong stimulation with high-frequency electro-stimulation (about 2000 Hertz) may be required. This procedure is extremely valuable when there is fetal distress.

Note: In many western auriculotherapy societies the ear acupuncture points are numbered. Unfortunately there is much divergence between the numbering adopted by the German schools and the North American auriculotherapists. In order to preserve some unity in practice, it is now considered more suitable to use the name of the regions and the names of the specific ear points, as described by the teachers, in the People's Republic of China.

■

THE INSTITUTE OF ACUPUNCTURE, COLOMBO SOUTH GOVERNMENT GENERAL HOSPITAL, KALUBOWILA, SRI LANKA.

HYSTERECTOMY USING ACUPUNCTURE ANAESTHESIA

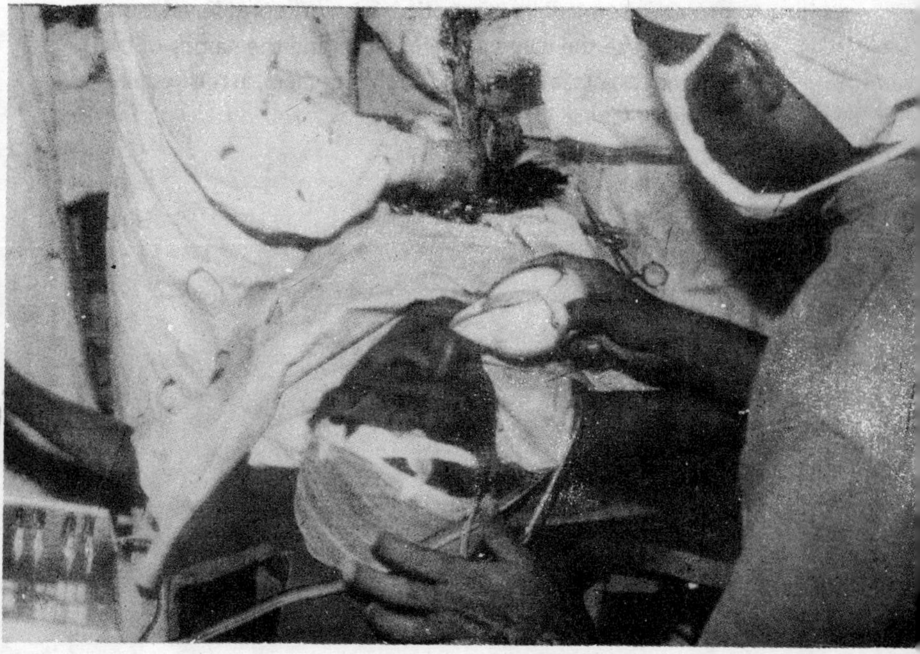

November 1975

Photo by the author

SCALP ACUPUNCTURE

Head Needle Therapy

The underlying principle behind scalp acupuncture is that specific areas of the brain cortex, which are functionally related to different organs and physiological functions, are represented topographically on the scalp. In most instances these areas of representation on the scalp are situated fairly close to the corresponding functional areas of the cerebral cortex, though not necessarily overlying them anatomically. This is because the scalp areas have been mapped out from empirical observation of the clinical responses to scalp acupuncture and not by a simple anatomical projection of the brain areas onto the scalp. The relationship between the brain areas and scalp acupuncture areas is electro- physiological rather than topographical.

There are 15 stimulation areas in scalp acupuncture. Although they are called "areas", they are in fact extremely narrow bands of varying length, and it is along these lines that the needles are inserted.

The locations of the 15 stimulation areas of scalp acupuncture and their therapeutic indications are as follows:

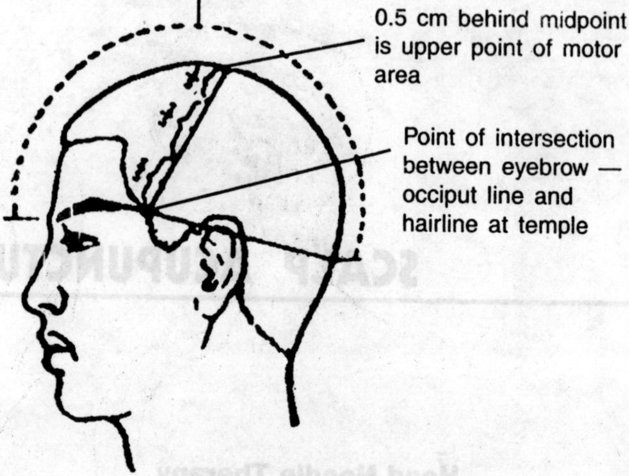

MOTOR AREA

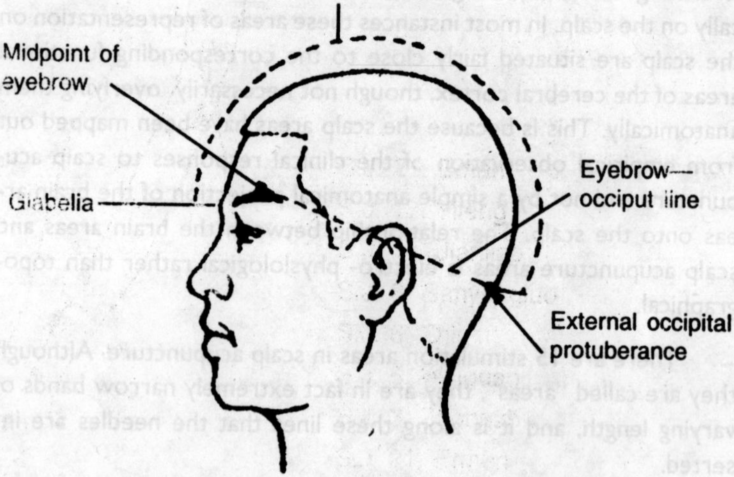

LINES OF REFERENCE

To perform scalp acupuncture (head needle therapy) effectively, the acupuncturist should locate the treatment areas with a great deal of accuracy. For this purpose there are four important lines of reference which must first be outlined on the surface of the scalp. These are:

(1) The *Antero-Posterior Midline* which is a straight line drawn in the sagittal plane, from the nasion (midpoint between the two eyebrows) to the lower edge of the external occipital protuberance.

(2) *The Supercilio: Occipital Line (Eyebrow* - Occiput Line) which is a straight line drawn obliquely backwards and downwards from the upper border of the midpoint of the eyebrow to the tip of the external occipital protuberance, on the lateral side of the head. There are therefore two such lines, one on each side of the head.

(3) The *Horizontal Line* on the back of the head at the level of the external occipital protuberance.

(4) The *Anterior Hair Line* which lies horizontally 3 cun above the eyebrows.

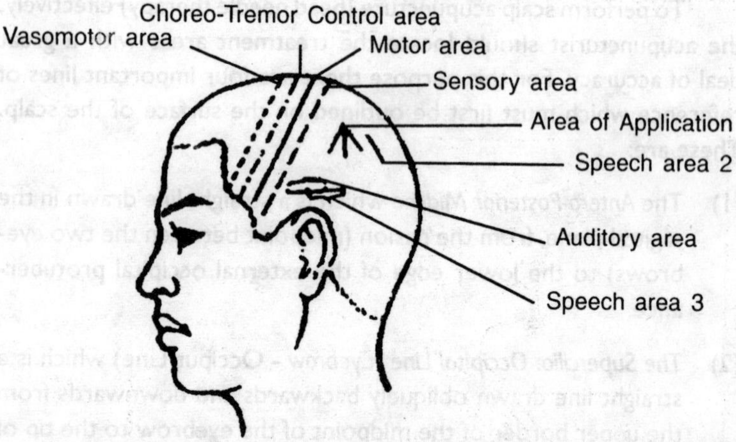

STIMULATION AREAS-SIDE VIEW

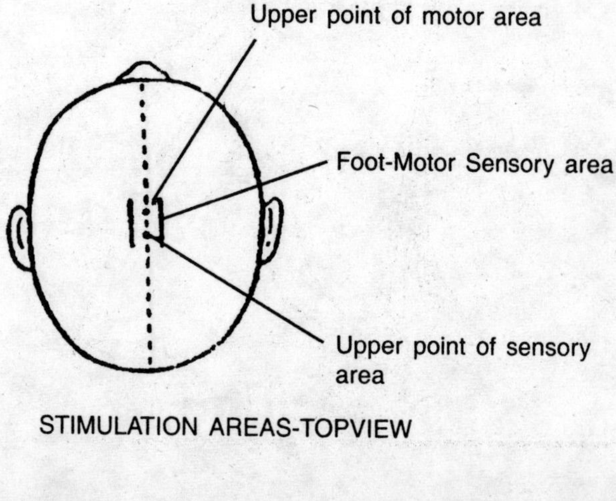

STIMULATION AREAS-TOPVIEW

AREA	LOCATION	INDICATIONS
Motor Area	A line connecting 2 points called the upper and lower points of the Motor Area. The upper point is situated on the antero-posterior midline. 0.5 cm behind its midpoint. The lower point of the Motor Area is the point in the temporal region where the supercilio-occipital line intersects the lateral hairline.	Motor paralysis of the contralateral side.
(a) Lower limb, head and trunk Area	Upper fifth of Motor Area.	Paralysis of contralateral lower limb.
(b) Upper limb Area	Second and third fifths of Motor Area.	Paralysis of contralateral upper limb.
(c) Facial Area (also called 1st Speech Area)	Lower two fifths of Motor Area.	Paralysis of face (opposite side), motor aphasia - dribbiling saliva, impaired speech.
2. Sensory Area	A line parallel to and 1.5 cm posterior to the Motor Area.	Sensory disorders of the contralateral side.
(a) Lower limb, head and trunk area	Upper fifth of Sensory Area.	Low back pain (opposite side), numbness or paraesthesia in that area, occipital headache, stiff neck.
(b) Upper Limb Area	Second and third fifths of Sensory Area.	Pain, numbness or paraesthesia of contralateral upper limb.
(c) Facial Area	Lower two fifths of Sensory Area.	Migraine, headache, trigeminal neuralgia, toothache (opposite side), arthritis of the temporo-mandibular joint.

3. Choreo-Tremor Control Area	Parallel to and 1.5 cm anterior to Motor Area.	Sydenham's chorea, parkinsonism, athetosis, tremors, palsy and related syndromes.
4. Vasomotor Area (also called Vasoconstriction Vasodilation Area)	Parallel to and 1.5 cm anterior to Choreo-Tremor Control Area.	Edema, hypertension, vascular disorders, Raynaud's disease, Burger's disease.
5. Foot-Motor Sensory Area	A line 3 cm long and parallel to the antero-posterior midline, its midpoint 1 cm lateral to midpoint of antero-posterior midline.	Paralysis pain or numbness of contralateral lower limb, acute lower back sprain, nocturnal enuresis.
6. Auditory Area (also called Vertigo-Auditory Area)	A horizontal line 4 cm ling, its midpoint 1.5 cm above the apex of the ear.	Deafness, tinnitus, vertigo, Meniere's syndrome.
7. Second Speech Area	A vertical line 3 cm long, parallel to the antero-posterior midline, its upper end 2 cm postero-inferior to the parietal tubercle.	Nominal aphasia
8. Third Speech Area	A horizontal line 4 cm long drawn posteriorly from the midpoint of the Auditory Area.	Sensory (receptive) aphasia.
9. Area of Application (Usage Area)	At the parietal tubercle three needles are inserted inferiorly, anteriorly and posteriorly to a length of 3 cm with 40 degree angles between them.	Apraxia.
10. Visual Area	A line 4 cm long drawn upwards and parallel to the antero-posterior midline from a point 1 cm lateral to the external occipital protuberance.	Cortical (central) blindness or visual disorders.

11. Balance Area (Equilibrium Area)	A line 4 cm long drawn downwards and parallel to the antero-posterior midline from a point at the level of the external occipital protuberance 3.5 cm[1] lateral to the midline.	Loss of balance due to cerebellum disorders.
12. Stomach Area (Gastric Area)	A line 2 cm long drawn directly backwards and parallel to the antero-posterior midline from a point on the anterior hairline vertically above the pupil of the eye.	Disorders of the upper abdomen and general malaise.
13. Thoracic Cavity Area	A line 4 cm long, parallel to the antero-posterior midline, with its midpoint at the anterior hairline, midway between the Stomach Area and the midline.	Chest pain, palpitation, shortness of breath, bronchial asthma.
14. Reproduction Area (Genital Area)	A line 4 cm[1] long, parallel to the antero-posterior midline, drawn directly backwards from the anterior hairline at the same distance laterally as that which separates the Stomach Area from the Thoracic Cavity Area.	Impotence, ejaculatio praecox, functional uterine haemorrhage. Aslo uded for surgery of prolapsed uterus combined with Foot-Motor Sensory Area.
15. Hepato-cystic Area (Liver and Gall bladder Area)	A line 2 cm long, extending anteriorly from the Stomach Area.	Pain or discomfort in the epigastrium and right hypochondrium, diseases of the liver and biliary system.

■

1 2 cm, according to the College of Traditional Medicine, Nanking.

LOCATIONS OF ALL ACUPUNCTURE POINTS OF THE 14 CHANNELS

I. The Lung Channel

Lu. 1. **Zhongfu:** At the level of the intercostal space between the 1st and 2nd ribs, 6 cun lateral to the midline, or 2 cun lateral to the nipple (mammary) line.

Lu. 2. **Yunmen:** At the inferior margin of the clavicle, between the pectoralis major and the deltoid muscles.

Lu. 3. **Tianfu:** 3 cun below the anterior end of the axillary crease at the lateral margin of the biceps brachii.

Lu. 4. **Xiabai:** 1 cum directly below Tianfu (Lu. 3.), on the radial side of the biceps brachii.

Lu. 5. **Chize:** At the elbow crease, on the lateral (radial) border of the tendon of the biceps muscle. (This tendon is better felt when the elbow is slightly flexed).

Lu. 6. **Kongzui:** 5 cun distal to Chize (Lu. 5.), on the line joining Chize (Lu. 5.) to Taiyuan (Lu. 9.).

Lu. 7. **Lieque:** When the index finger and the thumbs of both hands of the patient are crossed, this point is at the tip of the upper index finger. This point is best located by measuring 1.5 cun from the wrist-joint crease proximally on the outer (radial or lateral) border of the forearm.

Lu. 8. **Jingqu:** I cun directly proximal to Taiyuan Lu. 9.) at the medial margin of the radius.

Lu. 9. **Taiyuan:** At the outer (lateral) end of the wrist crease, on the lateral side of the radial artery. (Care has to be exercised when needling this point as it is located close to the radial artery).

Lu. 10. **Yuji:** On the palm, at the midpoint of the thenar eminence of the Ist metacarpus, on the border of the two colours of the skin.

Lu. 11. **Shaoshang:** 0.1 cun proximal to the lateral corner of the base of the nail of the thumb.

II. The Large Intestine Channel

L.I. 1. **Shangyang:** 0.1 cun proximal to the lateral (radial) corner of the base of the nail of the index finger.

L.I. 2. **Erjian:** In the depression distal to the 2nd metacarpophalangeal joint on the radial side.

L.I. 3. **Sanjian:** On the radial side of the index finger, in the depression proximal to the capitulum of the 2nd metacarpal bone.

L.I. 4. **Hegu:** In the web between the forefinger and the thumb on the dorsal (posterior) aspect of the hand.

(a) when the forefinger and the thumb are adducted, at the highest point of the muscles of the back of the hand;

(b) at the midpoint of a line drawn from the junction of the 1st and 2nd metacarpal bones to the middle point of the border of the web between them;

(c) place the distal-most crease of the thumb against the web of the opposite hand between thumb and forefinger; the point is on the latter hand where the tip of the former thumb (when it is flexed) then rests.

(d) at the middle of the 2nd metacarpal bone, on its radial border.

L.I. 5. **Yangxi:** On the radial aspect of the wrist, in the centre of the hollow formed when the thumb is well extended, between the tendons of the extensor pollicis longus and the extensor pollicis brevis. (This hollow is known as the "anatomical snuffbox".)

L.I. 6. **Pianli:** 3 cun proximal to Yangxi L.I. 5.), on the line joining Yangxi (L.I. 5.) and Quchi (L.I. 11.).

L.I. 7. **Wenliu:** 5 cun proximal to Yangxi (L.I. 5.), on the line joining Yangxi (L.I. 5.) and Quchi (L.I. 11.).

L.I. 8. **Xialian:** 4 cun distal to Quchi (L.I. 11.).

L.I. 9. **Shanglian:** 3 cun distal to Quchi (L.I. 11.).

L.I. 10. **Shousanli:** 2 cun distal to Quchi (L.I. 11.).

L.I. 11. **Quchi:** (a) At the lateral end of the elbow crease when the elbow is semiflexed. (b) Midway between Chize (Lu. 5.) and the lateral epicondyle of the humerus.

L.I. 12. **Zhouliao:** (a) With the arm extended, 2 cun proximal to Quchi (L.I. 11.). (b) With the elbow semiflexed, about 1 cun superolateral to Quchi (L.I. 11.) and supericr to the lateral epicondyle of the humerus on the medial border of the humerus.

L.I. 13. **Hand-Wuli:** 3 cun proximal to Quchi (L.I. 11.). on the line connecting Quchi (L.I. 11.) and Jianyu (L.I. 15.).

L.I. 14. **Binao:** On the lower border of deltoid muscle, on the line between Quchi (L.I. 11.) and Jianyu (L.I. 15.).

L.I. 15. **Jianyu:** In the anterior depression on the lateral border of the acromion process. The deltoid muscle has two prominent tendinous origins from the acromion. This point is situated in the anterior of these two depressions.

L.I. 16. **Jugu:** In the depression medial to the acromioclavicular joint.

L.I. 17. **Tianding:** 1 cun inferior to Neck-Futu (L.I. 18.), on the posterior border of the sternomastoid muscle.

L.I. 18. **Neck-Futu:** 3 cun lateral to the prominece of the thyroid cartilage (Adam's apple).

L.I. 19. **Nose-Heliao:** 0.5 cun lateral to the point Renzhong (Du 26.) on the side opposite to the origin of the Channel. (According to some authorities it is on the same side.)

L.I. 20. **Yingxiang:** At the midpoint of a horizontal line drawn between the outermost point of the ala nasi and the nasolabial groove.

III. The Stomach Channel

St. 1. **Chengqi:** Below the eyeball, at the midpoint of the lower margin of the orbit.

St. 2. **Sibai:** 0.7 cun below Chengqi, in the infraorbital foramen.

St. 3. **Juliao:** Directly below Sibai (St. 2.), at the level of the lower border of the ala nasi.

St. 4. **Dicang:** 0.4 cun lateral to the corner of the mouth.

St. 5. **Daying:** At the lowest point of the anterior border of the masseter muscle.

St. 6. **Jiache:** At the highest point of the masseter muscle felt on clenching the jaws.

St. 7. **Xiaguan:** In the depression at the lower border of the zygomatic arch. This point is located with the mouth closed.

St. 8. **Touwei:** 0.5 cun lateral to the corner of the anterior hairline, or 5 cun lateral to the midpoint of the anterior hairline.

St. 9. **Renying:** 1.5 cun lateral to the prominence of the thyroid cartilage (Adam's apple), on the anterior border of the sternomastoid muscle.

St. 10. **Shuitu:** Midway between Renying (St. 9.) and Qishe (St. 11.) on the anterior border of the sternomastoid muscle.

St. 11. **Qishe:** At the superior border of the sternal end of the clavicle, directly below Renying (St. 9.).

St. 12. **Quepen:** In the middle of the supraclavicular fossa, 4 cun lateral to the Ren Channel.

St. 13. **Qihu:** At the middle of the inferior border of the clavicle, 4 cun lateral to Xuanji (Ren 21.).

St. 14. **Kufang:** In the 1st intercostal space, 4 cun lateral to the Ren Channel.

St. 15. **Wuyi:** In the 2nd intercostal space, 4 cun lateral to the Ren Channel.

St. 16. **Yingchuang:** In the 3rd intercostal space, 4 cun lateral to the Ren Channel.

St. 17. **Ruzhong:** In the center of the nipple. (Acupuncture or moxibustion is prohibited at this point. It is used only as a landmark).

St. 18. **Rugen:** In the 5th intercostal space, one rib below the nipple.

St. 19. **Burong:** 6 cun above the umbilicus, 2 cun lateral to Juque (Ren 14.).

St. 20. **Chengman:** 5 cun above the umbilicus, 2 cun lateral to Shangwan (Ren 13.).

St. 21. **Liangmen:** 4 cun above the umbilicus, 2 cun lateral to Zhongwan (Ren 12.).

St. 22. **Guanmen:** 3 cun above the umbilicus, 2 cun lateral to Jiangli (Ren 11.).

St. 23. **Taiyi:** 2 cun above the umbilicus, 2 cun lateral to Xiawan (Ren 10.).

St. 24. **Huaroumen:** 1 cun above the umbilicus, 2 cun lateral to Shuifen (Ren 9.).

St. 25. **Tianshu:** 2 cun lateral to the center of the umbilicus.

St. 26. **Wailing:** 1 cun below the umbilicus, 2 cun lateral to Abdomen-Yinjiao (Ren 7.).

St. 27. **Daju:** 2 cun below the umbilicus, 2 cun lateral to Shimen (Ren 5.).

St. 28. **Shuidao:** 3 cun below the umbilicus, 2 cun lateral to Guanyuan (Ren 4.).

St. 29. **Guilai:** 4 cun below the umbilicus, 2 cun lateral to Zhongli (Ren 3.).

St. 30. **Qichong:** 5 cun below the umbilicus, 2 cun lateral to Qugu (Ren 2.).

St. 31. **Biguan:** At the meeting point of a vertical line drawn from the anterior superior iliac spine and a horizontal line drawn along the lower border of the pubic symphysis.

St. 32. **Femur-Futu:** (a) 6 cun proximal to the midpoint of the superior border of the patella. (According to some authorities it is 6 cun proximal to the supero-lateral border of the patella.) (b) With the patient seated, place the contralateral wrist-crease of the acupuncturist on the middle of the patient's knee-cap with the fingers of the acupuncturist along the front of the patient's thigh. The point is located at the tip of the acupuncturist's middle finger.

St. 33. **Yinshi:** 3 cun above the lateral end of the upper border of the patella, in the depression between the rectus femoris and vastus lateralis muscles.

St. 34. **Lianqiu:** 2 cun above the lateral end of the upper border of the patella.

St. 35. **Dubi:** In the depression (below the patella) lateral to the ligamentum patellae. This point is best located with the knee flexed.

St. 36. **Zusanli:** One finger breadth lateral to the inferior border of the tibial tuberosity, 3 cun distal to Dubi (St. 35.).

St. 37. **Shangjuxu:** 3 cun distal to Zusanli (St. 36.), one finger breadth lateral to the anterior border of the tibia.

St. 38. **Tiaokou:** 5 cun distal to Zusanli (St. 36.), one finger breadth lateral to the anterior border of the tibia.

St. 39. **Xiajuxu:** 3 cun distal to Shangjuxu (St. 37.)

St. 40. **Fenglong:** One finger breadth lateral to Tiaokou (St. 38.).

St. 41. **Jiexi:** One the front ankle crease midway between the lowest points (tips) of the two malleoli.

St. 42. **Chongyang:** 1.5 cun distal to Jiexi (St. 41.), at the highest point of the dorsum of the foot, in the depression between the 2nd and 3rd metatarsal bones and the cuneiform bone.

St. 43. **Xiangu:** In the depression immediately anterior to the bases of the 2nd and 3rd metatarsals.

St. 44. **Neiting:** 0.5 cun proximal to the margin of the web between the 2nd and 3rd toes.

St. 45. **Lidui:** 0.1 cun proximal to the lateral corner of the base of the 2nd toe nail.

IV. The Spleen Channel

SP. 1. **Yinbai:** 0.1 cun proximal to the medial corner of the base of the nail of the big toe.

Sp. 2. **Dadu:** On the medial aspect of the big toe. anterior and inferior to the Ist metatarso-phalangeal joint, at the border of the two colors of the skin.

Sp. 3. **Taibai:** Posterior and inferior to the head of the first metatarsal bone, at the border of the two colors of the skin.

Sp. 4. **Gongsun:** On the medial side of the foot, in the depression inferior to the base of the Ist metatarsal bone, at the border of the two colors of the skin.

Sp. 5. **Shangqiu:** (a) Draw a straight line along the anterior border and another along the inferior border of the medial malleolus. The point in where these two lines cross. (b) In the depression anterior to and slightly inferior to the medial malleolus.

Sp. 6. **Sanyinjiao:** 3 cun above the tip of the medial malleolus on the medial border of the tibia.

Sp. 7. **Lougu:** On the posterior border of the tibia. 3 cun proximal to Sanyinjiao (5p. 6.).

Sp. 8. **Diji:** On the posterior border of the tibia, 3 cun distal to Yinlingquan (Sp. 9.).

Sp. 9. **Yingingquan:** On the medial border of the tibial at the level of the inferior border of tie tibial tuberosity.

Sp. 10. **Xuehai:** (a) At the highest point of the vastus medialis muscle. (b) 2 cun proximal to the medial end of the upper border of the patella along the Channel. (c) Have the patient seated with his knees bent at right angles. The acupuncturist then places his right hand on the patient's left patella with the centre of his palm on the middle of the patella and his thumb resting on the inner surface of the thigh. The thumb should be held in a position midway between adduction and full abduction. The point will then lie at the tip of the thumb. (To use this method the acupuncturist's hands should have similar dimensions to those of the patient.)

Sp. 11. **Jimen:** 6 cun proximal to Xuehai (5p. 10.) on the medial aspect of the sartorius. (Avoid femoral artery).

Sp. 12. **Chongmen:** At the level of the upper border of the pubic symphysis, 3.5 cun lateral to Qugu (Ren 2.). on the lateral side of the femoral artery.

Sp. 13. **Fushe:** 0.7 cun proximal to Chongmen (5p. 12.), 4 cun lateral to the abdominal midline.

Sp. 14. **Fujie:** 1.3 cun distal to Daheng (5p. IS.), 4 cun lateral to the abdominal midline.

Sp. 15. **Daheng:** 4 cun lateral to the centre of the umbilicus.

Sp. 16. **Fuai:** 3 cun proximal to Daheng (Sp. 15.), 4 cun lateral to Jianli (Ren II.).

Sp. 17. **Shidou:** In the 5th intercostal space, 6 cun lateral to the abdominal midline or 2 cun lateral to the mammary line.

Sp. 18. **Tianxi:** In the 4th intercostal space, 6 cun lateral to the abdominal midline or 2 cun lateral to the nipple.

Sp. 19. **Xiongxiang:** In the 3rd intercostal space, 6 cun lateral to the midsternal line.

Sp. 20. **Zhourong:** In the 2nd intercostal space, 6 cun lateral to the midsternal line.

Sp. 21. **Dabao:** On the mid-axillary line, in the sixth intercostal space.

V. The Heart Channel

H. 1. **Jiquan:** At the center of the axilla.

H. 2. **Qingling:** 3 cun proximal to Shaohai (H. 3.).

H. 3. **Shaohai:** Midway between the medial end of the elbow crease and the medial epicondyle of the humerus when the elbow is fully flexed.

H. 4. **Lingdao:** 1.5 cun proximal to Shenmen (H. 7.) on the radial side of the tendon of the flexor carpi ulnaris.

H. 5. **Tongli:** 1 cun proximal to Shenmen (H. 7.) on the radial side of the tendon of the flexor carpi ulnaris.

H. 6. **Yinxi:** 0.5 cun proximal to Shenmen (H. 7.).

H. 7. **Shenmen:** At the wrist crease, on the radial side of the tendon of the flexor carpi ulnaris.

H. 8. **Shaofu:** On the palmar surface of the hand between the tips of the ring finger and the little finger on lightly clenching the first.

H. 9. **Shaochong:** 0.1 cun proximal to the radial corner of the base of the nail of the little finger.

VI. The Small Intestine Channel

S.I. 1. **Shaoze:** 0.1 cun proximal to the ulnar corner of the base of the nail of the little finger.

S.I. 2. **Qiangu:** At the medial end of the transverse crease of the metacarpophalangeal joint of the little finger, on the border of the two skin colours.

S.I. 3. **Houxi:** At the medial end of the main transverse crease of the palm, on the border of the two skin colours.

S.I. 4. **Hand-Wangu:** In the depression at the base of the 5th metacarpal bone, on the ulnar aspect of the palm.

S.I. 5. **Yanggu:** In the depression at the ulnar aspect of the wrist, distal to the styloid process of the ulna.

S.I. 6. **Yanglao:** On the back of the forearm in the depression proximal to the inferior radio-ulnar joint. This point is best located with the hand pronated.

S.I. 7. **Zhinzheng:** 5 cun proximal to the wrist, on the posterior border of the ulna.

S.I. 8. **Xiaohai:** Between the olecranon process of the ulna and the medial epicondyle of the humerus. It is best located with elbow joint flexed.

S.I. 9. **Jianzhen:** 1.0 cun superior to the highest point of the posterior axillary fold.

S.I. 10. **Naoshu:** Directly above Jianzhen (S.I. 9.), on the inferior border of the spine of the scapula.

S.I. 11. **Tianzong:** At the junction of the upper third and the lower two thirds of a line drawn between the inferior angle of the scapula and the inferior border of the spine of the scapula.

S.I. 12. **Bingfeng:** In the center of the suprascapular fossa, directly above Tianzong (S.I. 11.).

S.I. 13. **Quyuan:** At the medial end of the suprascapular fossa, midway between Naoshu (S.I. 10.) and the spinous process of the 2nd thoracic vertebra.

S.I. 14. **Jianwaishu:** 3 cun lateral to Taodao (Du 13.).

S.I. 15. **Zianzhongshu:** 2 cun lateral to Dazhui (Du 14.).

S.I. 16. **Tianchuang:** 0.5 cun posterosuperior to Neck-Futu (L.I. 18.) or the posterior border of the sternomastoid.

S.I. 17. **Tianrong:** In the depression on the anterior border of the sternomastoid at the level of the angle of the jaw.

S.I. 18. **Quanliao:** In the depression below the prominence of the maxillary bone on a vertical line drawn downwards from the outer canthus of the eye.

S.I. 19. **Tinggong:** In the depression felt between the tragus and the mandibular joint when the mouth is slightly open.

VII. The Urinary Bladder Channel

U.B. 1. **Jingming:** At the medial border of the orbit, 0.1 cun medial and superior to the inner canthus of the eye.

U. B. 2. **Zanzhu:** In the depression at the medial end of the eyebrow, directly above Jingming (U.B. 1.).

U.B. 3. **Meichong:** Directly above Zanzhu (U.B. 2.), 0.5 cun above the front hairline.

U.B. 4. **Ouchai:** 1.5 cun lateral to Shenting (Du 24.), 0.5 cun above the front hairline.

U.B. 5. **Wuchu:** 0.5 cun above Quchai (U.B. 4.).

U.B. 6. **Chengguang:** 1.5 cun posterior to Wuchu (U. B. S.).

U.B. 7. **Tongtian:** 1.5 cun posterior to Chengguang (U. B. 6.).

U.B. 8. **Luoque:** 1.5 cun posterior to Tongtian (U.8. 7.).

U.B. 9. **Yuzhen:** (On the lateral side of the upper border of the external occipital protuberance, 1.3 cun lateral to Naohu (Du 17.).

U,B. 10. **Tianzhu:** 0.5 cun above the posterior hairline, between the transverse processes of the Ist and 2nd cervical vertebrae, 1.3 cun lateral to Yamen (Du 15.).

U.B. 11. **Dashu:** 1.5 cun lateral to the lower border of the spinous process of the Ist thoracic vertebra.

U.B. 12. **Fengmen:** 1.5 cun lateral to the lower border of the spinous process of the 2nd thoracic vertebra.

U.B. 13. **Feishu:** 1.5 cun lateral to the lower border of the spinous process of the 3rd thoracic vertebra (at the level of the medial end of the spine of the scapula).

U.B. 14. **Jueyinshu:** 1.5 cun lateral to the lower border of the spinous process of the 4th thoracic vertebra

U.B. 15. **Xinshu:** 1.5 cun lateral to the lower border of the spinous process of the 5th thoracic vertebra.

U.B. 16. **Dusbu:** 1.5 cun lateral to the lower border of the spinous process of the 6th thoracic vertebra.

U.B. 17. **Geshu:** 1.5 cun lateral to the lower border of the spinous process of the 7th thoracic vertebra (at the level of the inferior angle of the scapula).

U.B. 18. **Ganshu:** 1.5 cun lateral to the lower border of the spinous process of the 9th thoracic vertebra.

U.B. 19. **Danshu:** 1.5 cun lateral to the lower border of the spinous process of the 10th thoracic vertebra.

U.B. 20. **Pishu:** 1.5 cun lateral to the lower border of the spinous process of the 11th thoracic vertebra.

U.B. 21. **Weishu:** 1.5 cun lateral to the lower border of the spinous process of the 12th thoracic vertebra.

U.B. 22. **Sanjiaoshu:** 1.5 cun lateral to the lower border of the spinous process of the 1st lumbar vertebra.

U.B. 23. **Shenshu:** 1.5 cun lateral to the lower border of the spinous process of the 2nd lumbar vertebra.

U.B. 24. **Qihaishu:** 1.5 cun lateral to the lower border of the spinous process of the 3rd lumbar vertebra.

U.B. 25. **Dachangshu:** 1.5 cun lateral to the lower border of the spinous process of the 4th lumbar vertebra.

U.B. 26. **Guanyuanshu:** 1.5 cun lateral to the lower border of the spinous process of the 5th lumbar vertebra.

U.B. 27. **Xiaochangshu:** 1.5 cun lateral to the back midline at the level of the 1st posterior sacral foramen.

U.B. 28. **Pangguanshu:** 1.5 cun lateral to the back midline at the level of the 2nd posterior sacral foramen,

U.B. 29. **Zhonglushu:** 1.5 cun lateral to the back midline, at the level of the 3rd posterior sacral foramen.

U.B. 30. **Baihuanshu:** 1.5 cun lateral to, the back midline, at the level of the 4th posterior sacral foramen.

U.B. 31. **Shangliao:** On the 1st posterior sacral foramen, midway between the posterior superior iliac spine and the back midline.

U.B. 32. **Ciliao:** On the 2nd posterior sacral foramen.

U.B. 33. **Zhongliao:** On the 3rd posterior sacral foramen, midway between Zhonglushu (U.B. 29.) and the back midline.

U.B. 34. **Xialiao:** On the 4th posterior sacral foramen, midway between Baihuanshu (U.B. 30.) and the back midline.

U.B. 35. **Huiyang:** 0.5 cun lateral to the back midline, at the level of the tip of the coccyx.

U.B. 36. **Chengfu:** At the midpoint of the gluteal fold.

U.B. 37. **Yinmen:** (a) At the midpoint of a line joining Chengfu (U.B. 36.) and Weizhong (U.B. 40.). (b) 6 cun distal to Chengfu (U.B. 36.).

U.B. 38. **Fuxi:** 1 cun proximal to Weiyang (U.B. 39.), on the medial side of the tendon of the biceps femoris.

U.B. 39. **Weiyang:** Lateral to Weizhong (U.B. 40.), on the medial side of the tendon of the biceps femoris.

U.B. 40. **Weizhong:** At the midpoint of the popliteal transverse crease.

U.B. 41. **Fufen:** 3 cun lateral to the lower border of the spinous process of the 2nd thoracic vertebra.

U.B. 42. **Pohu:** 3 cun lateral to the lower border of the spinous process of the 3rd thoracic vertebra (level with the medial end of the spine of the scapula).

U.B. 43. **Gaohunag:** 3 cun lateral to the lower border of the spinous process of the 4th thoracic vertebra.

U.B. 44. **Shentang:** 3 cun lateral to the lower border of the spinous process of the 5th thoracic vertebra.

U.B. 45. **Yixi:** 3 cun lateral to the lower border of the spinous process of the 6th thoracic vertebra.

U.B. 46. **Geguan:** 3 cun lateral to the lower border of the spinous process of the 7th thoracic vertebra (at the level of the inferior angle of the scapula).

U.B. 47. **Hunmen:** 3 cun lateral to the lower border of the spinous process of the 9th thoracic vertebra.

U.B. 48. **Yanggang:** 3 cun lateral to the lower border of the spinous process of the 10th thoracic vertebra.

U.B. 49. **Yishe:** 3 cun lateral to the lower border of the spinous process of the 11th thoracic vertebra.

U.B. 50. **Weicang:** 3 cun lateral to the lower border of the spinous process of the 12th thoracic vertebra.

U.B. 51. **Huangmen:** 3 cun lateral to the lower border of the spinous process of the 1st lumbar vertebra.

U.B. 52. **Zhishi:** 3 cun lateral to the lower border of the spinous process of the 2nd lumbar vertebra.

U.B. 53. **Baohuang:** 3 cun lateral to the back midline, at the same level as the 2nd sacral foramen.

U.B. 54. **Zhibian:** 3 cun lateral to the back midline, at the same level as the 4th sacral foramen.

U.B. 55. **Heyang:** 2 cun directly below Weizhong (U.B. 40.), on a line connecting it to Chengshan (U.B. 57.).

U.B. 56. **Chengjin:** In the centre of the belly of the gastrocnemius muscle, midway between Heyang (U.B. 55.) and Chengshan (U.B. 57.)

U.B. 57. **Chengshan:** (a) At the level where the two bellies of the gastrocnemius unite to form the tendo-Achilles, 8 cun distal to Weizhong (U.B. 40.). (b) Half way between Weizhong (U.B. 40.) and the ankle joint.

U.B. 58. **Feiyang:** 7 cun proximal to Kunlun (U.B. 60.), an the posterior border of the fibula, about 1 cun inferior and lateral to Chengshan (U.B. 57.), on the lateral aspect of the gastrocnemius.

U. B. 59. **Fuyang:** 3 cun proximal to Kunlun (U.B. 60.).

U.B. 60. **Kunlun:** Midway between the tip of the lateral malleolus and the lateral border of the tendo-Achilles.

U.B. 61. **Pushen:** 1.5 cun distal to Kunlun (U.B. 60.), in the depression of the calcaneum at the border of the two colors of the skin.

U.B. 62. **Shenmai:** 0.5 cun inferior to the tip of the lateral malleolus.

U.B. 63. **Jinmen:** In the depression posterior to the tuberosity of the 5th metatarsal bone.

U.B. 64. **Jinggu:** In the depression inferior to the tuberosity of the 5th metatarsal bone, at the border of the two colors of the skin.

U.B. 65. **Shugu:** In the depression postero-inferior to the head of the 5th metatarsal bone, at the border of the two colours of the skin.

U.B. 66. **Foot-Tonggu:** In the depression antero-inferior to the 5th metatarso-phalangeal joint.

U.B. 67. **Zhiyin:** 0.1 cun proximal to the lateral corner of the base of the nail of the little toe.

VIII. The Kidney Channel

K. 1. **Yongquan:** In the sole of the foot, on a line drawn posteriorly between the 2nd and 3rd toes, in the depression formed between the anterior one-third and posterior two-third parts of the sole, which is specially prominent when the toes are Plantar-flexed.

K. 2. **Rangu:** In the depression on the lower border of the tuberosity of the navicular bone.

K. 3. **Taixi:** Midway between the tip of the medial malleolus and the medial border of the tendo-Achilles.

K. 4. **Dazhong:** In the depression medial to the attachment to the tendo calcaneus, 0.5 cun inferior to and slightly posterior to Taixi (K. 3.).

K. 5. **Shuiquan:** 1.0 cun distal to Taixi (K. 3.), in the depression anterior and superior to the medial side of the tuberosity of the calcaneum.

K. 6. **Zhaohai:** In the depression 1.0 cun distal to the tip of the medial malleolus.

K. 7. **Fuliu:** 2 cun proximal to Taixi (K. 3.), on the anterior border of the tendo Achilles.

K. 8. **Jiaoxin:** 0.5 cun anterior to Fuliu (K. 7,).

K. 9. **Zhubin:** 5 cun proximal to Taixi (K. 3.), and 2 cun posterior to the medial border of the tibia, at the inferior end of the medial belly of the gastrocnemius.

K. 10. **Yingu:** At the Popliteal crease, on the medial border of semitendinosus tendon.

K. 11. **Hengzu:** On the superior border of the pubic symphysis, 0.5 cun lateral to Qugu (Ren 2.).

K. 12. **Dahe:** 0.5 cun lateral to Zhongji (Ren 3.), 1 cun above Henggu (K. 11.), and 4 cun below the umbilicus.

K. 13. **Qixue:** 0.5 cun lateral to Guanyuan (Ren 4.), 2 cun above Henggu (K. 11.), and 3 cun below the, umbilicus.

K. 14. **Siman:** 0.5 cun lateral to Shimen (Ren S.), 3 cun above Henggu (K. 11.), and 2 cun below the umbilicus.

K. 15. **Abdomen – Zhongzhu:** 0.5 cun lateral to Abdomen-Yinjiao (Ren 7.), 1.0 cun below the umbilicus.

K. 16. **Huangshu:** 0.5 cun lateral to the umbilicus.

K. 17. **Shangqu:** 0.5 cun lateral to Xiawan (Ren l0), 2 cun above the umbilicus.

K. 18. **Shiguan:** 0.5 cun lateral to Jianli (Ren ll.), 3 cun above the umbilicus.

K. 19. **Yindu:** 0.5 cun lateral to Zhongwan (Ren 12.). 4 cun above the umbilicus

K. 20. **Abdomen-Tonggu:** 0.5 cun lateral to Shangwan (Ren 13.), 5 cun above the umbilicus.

K. 21. **Youmen:** 0.5 cun lateral to Jugue[1] (Ren 14.), 6 cun above the umbilicus.

K. 22. **Bulang:** In the 5th intercostal space, 2 cun lateral to the Ren Channel.

K. 23. **Shenfeng:** In the 4th intercostal space, 2 cun lateral to the Ren Channel.

K. 24. **Lingxu:** In the 3rd intercostal space, 2 cun lateral to the Ren Channel.

K. 25. **Shencang:** In the 2nd intercostal space, 2 cun lateral to the Ren Channel.

K. 26. **Yuzhong:** In the Ist intercostal space, 2 cun lateral to the Ren Channel.

K. 27. **Shufu:** In the depression between the lower border of the clavicle and the 1st rib, 2 cun lateral to the Ren Channel.

IX. The Pericardium Channel

P. 1. **Tianchi:** In the intercostal space, 1 cun lateral to the nipple or 5 cun lateral to the front midline.

P. 2. **Tianquan:** 2 cun distal to the top of the anterior axillary fold, between the two heads of the biceps brachi muscle.

P. 3. **Quze:** In the anti-cubital crease, on the medial (ulnar) border of the biceps tendon.

P. 4. **Ximen:** 5 cun proximal to the midpoint of the anterior wrist crease, between the tendons of the palmaris longus and the flexor carpi radials muscles.

P. 5. **Jianshi:** 3 cun proximal to the midpoint of the anterior wrist crease, between the tendons of the palmaris longus and the flexor carpi radialis muscles.

p. 6. **Neiguan:** 2 cun proximal to the midpoint of the anterior wrist crease, between the tendons of the palmaris longus and the flexor carpi radialis muscles.

1 Also written *'Jujue'*

P. 7. **Daling:** At the midpoint of the anterior wrist crease, between the tendons of the palmaris longus and the flexor carpi radialis muscles.

P. 8. **Laogong:** On the palmar surface, between the tips of the 3rd (middle) and 4th (ring) fingers when they touch the central region of the palm on lightly clenching the fist.

P. 9. **Zhongchong:** At the midpoint of the tip of the middle finger. (According to some authorities, this point is located 0.1 cun proximal to the radial corner of the base of the nail of the middle finger).

X. The Sanjiao Channel

S.J. 1. **Guanchong:** 0.1 cun proximal to the ulna corner of the base of the nail of the 4th ring finger.

S.J. 2. **Yemen:** 0.5 cun proximal to the margin of the web between the 4th and 5th fingers.

S.J. 3. **Zhongzhu:** On the dorsum of the hand, in the depression between the heads of the 4th and 5th metacarpal bones.

S.J. 4. **Yangchi:** At the wrist joint, in the depression lateral to the tendon of the extensor digitorum muscle.

S.J. 5. **Waiguan:** 2 cun proximal to the midpoint of the dorsal transverse crease of the wrist, between the radius and the ulna.

S.J. 6. **Zhigou:** 1.0 cun proximal to Waiguan (S.J. 5.).

S.J. 7. **Huizong:** 3 cun proximal to the wrist, 1 finger breadth lateral to Zhigou (S.J.. 6.).

5.J. 8. **Sanyangluo:** 1.0 cun proximal to Zhigou (S.J. 6).

S.J. 9. **Sidu:** Between the ulna and the radius, 5. cun distal to the point of the elbow (olecranon).

S.J. 10. **Tianjing:** With the elbow flexed, this point is located in the depression 1.0 cun proximal to the point of the elbow (olecranon).

S.J. 11. **Qinglengyuan:** 1.0 cun proximal to Tianjing SJ.10.).

S.J. 12. **Xiaoluo:** Midway between Qinglengyuan (S.J. 11.) and Naohui (S.J. 13.).

S.J. 13. **Naohui:** 3 cun distal to Jianliao (S.J. 14.), at the posterior margin of the deltoid muscle.

S.J. 14. **Jianliao:** With the arm abducted to a horizontal position, in the posterior depression of the origin of the deltoid muscle from the lateral border of the acromion.

S.J. 15. **Tianliao:** On the superior angle of the scapula, midway between the tip of the acromion and Dazhui (Du 14.); 1.0 cun posterior and inferior to Jianjing (G.B. 21.).

S.J. 16. **Tianyou:** Posterior and inferior to the mastoid process, on the posterior border of the sternomastoid, in level with Tianzhu (U.B. 10.) and the angle of the jaw.

S.J. 17. **Yifeng:** At the highest point of the depression behind the ear lobe, between the angle of the jaw and the mastoid process.

S.J. 18. **Qimai:** At the center of the mastoid process.

S.J. 19. **Luxi:** 1.0 cun above Qimai (S.J. 18.).

S.J. 20. **Jiaosun:** On the scalp, at the level of the apex of the ear when it is gently pulled forwards.

S.J. 21. **Ermen:** In the depression in front of the supratragic notch. It is easier to locate this point with the mouth slightly open.

S.J. 22. **Ear-Heliao:** Anterior and superior to Ermen (S.J. 21.), at the level of the root of the auricle, on the posterior border of the hairline of the temple.

S.J. 23. **Sizhukong:** In the depression at the lateral end of the eyebrow.

XI. The Gall bladder Channel

G.B. 1. **Tongziliao:** 0.5 cun lateral to the outer canthus of the eye.

G.B. 2. **Tinghui:** In the depression immediately in front of the intertragic notch when the mouth is open.

G.B. 3. **Shanguan:** On the midpoint of the superior margin of the zygomatic arch, directly superior to Xiaguan (St. 7,).

G.B. 4. **Hanyan:** Within the lateral hairline 1/4th the distance from Touwei (St. S.) to Qubin (G.B. 7.).

G.B. 5. **Xuanlu:** Within the lateral hairline, midway between Touwei (St. 8.) and Qubin (G.B. 7.).

G.B. 6. **Xuanli:** Within the lateral hairline, midway between Xuanlu (G.B. S.) and Qubin (G.B. 7.).

G.B. 7. **Gubin:** Within the hairline, finger breadth anterior to Jiaosun (S.J. 20.).

G.B. 8. **Shuaigu:** Directly above the apex of the ear, 1.5 cun above the hairline.

G.B. 9. **Tianchong:** 0.5 cun posterior to Shuaigu (G.B.8.).

G.B.10. **Fubai:** 1.0 cun postero-inferior to Tianchong (G.B. 9.), on the superior part of the mastoid process

G.B.11. **Head-Qiaoyin:** 1.0 cun below Fubai (G.B. 10,), posterior and superior to the mastoid process.

G.B.12. **Head-Wangu:** In the depression posterior and inferior to the mastoid process, 0.7 cun below Qiaoyin (G.B. 11.) and level with Fengfu (Du 16.).

G.B.13. **Benshen:** 0.5 cun within the anterior hairline, 3 cun lateral to Shenting (Du 24.).

G.B.14. **Yangbai:** 1.0 cun superior to the midpoint of the eyebrow.

G.B.15. **Head-Linqi:** (a) 0.5 cun within the anterior hairline, directly above Yangbai (G.B. 14.). (b) Midway between Shenting (Du 24.) and Touwei (St. 8.).

G.B.16. **Muchuang:** 1.5 cun posterior to Head-Linqi (G.B. 15.).

G.B.17. **Zhengying:** 1.5 cun posterior to Muchuang (G.B. 16.).

G.B.18. **Chengling:** 1.5 cun posterior to Zhengying (G.B. 17.).

G.B.19. **Naokong:** Directly above Fengchi (G.B. 20.), level with Naohu (Du 17.) on the back of the head.

G.B.20. **Fengchi:** In the depression immediately inferior and medial to the mastoid process, between the orgins of the trapezius and sterno-mastoid muscles.

G.B.21. **Jianjing:** Midway between Dazhi (Du 14.) and Jianyu (L.I. 15.), at the highest point of the shoulder.

G.B.22. **Yuanye:** On the midaxillary line 3 cun below the axilla, in the 5th intercostal space.

G.B.23. **Zhejin:** 1.0 cun anterior to Yuanye (G.B. 22.), in the 5th intercostal space.

G.B.24. **Riyue:** On the nipple line, in the 7th intercostal space (directly below Qimen (Liv. 14.) which lies in the 6th intercostal space).

G.B.25. **Jingmen:** At the tip of the free end of the 12th rib.

G.B.26. **Daimai:** At the level of the umbilicus, on a vertical line drawn from the midpoint between the free ends of the 11th and 12th ribs. (According to some authorities it is directly below the free end of the 11th rib Zhangmen (Liv. 13.), at the level of the umbilicus.)

G.B.27. **Wushu:** In front of the anterior superior iliac spine in the lateral aspect of the abdomen, at the same horizontal level with Guanyuan (Ren 4.).

G.B.28. **Weidao:** 0.5 cun anterior and inferior to Wushu (G.B.) 27.

G.B.29. **Femur-Juliao:** At the midpoint of a line connecting the anterior superior iliac spine and the greater trochanter of the femur. This point is best located in the lateral recumbent position.

G.B.30. **Huantiao:** At the junction of the outer third with the medial two-thirds of a line connecting the highest point of the greater trochanter of the femur and the hiatus of the sacrum (sarcococcygeal junction). This point is best located in the prone or lateral recumbent positions.

G.B.31. **Fengshi:** (a) On the lateral aspect of the thigh, 7 cun proximal to the transverse popliteal crease, on the groove between the vastus lateralis and biceps femoris muscles. (b) With the patient standing erect with his hands on the lateral aspect of his thighs, this point lies at the tip of his middle finger.

G.B.32. **Femur-Zhongdu:** 2 cun distal to Fengshi (G.B. 31.), between the vastus lateralis and biceps femoris muscles.

G.B.33. **Xiyangguan:** Lateral to the knee joint, in the depression above the lateral epicondyle of the femur, between the bone and the biceps femoris tendon. This point is best located with the knee flexed.

G.B.34. **Yanglingquan:** (a) In the depression anterior and inferior to the head of the fibula. (b) At the meeting point of two straight lines, one drawn vertically on the anterior margin of the head of the fibula, the other horizontally at the neck of the fibula.

G.B.35. **Yangjiao:** 7 cun proximal to the tip of the lateral malleolus, on the posterior border of the fibula.

G.B.36. **Waiqiu:** 7 cun proximal to the tip of the lateral malleolus, on the anterior border of the fibula.

G.B.37. **Guangming:** 5 cun promimal to the tip of the lateral malleolus, on the anterior border of the fibula.

G.B.38. **Yangfu:** 4 cun proximal to the lateral malleolus, on the anterior border of the fibula.

G.B.39. **Xuanzhong:** 3 cun proximal to the tip of the lateral malleolus, on the posterior border of the fibula.

G.B.40. **Qiuxu:** At the meeting point of two straight lines, one drawn vertically on the anterior border of the lateral malleolus, the other horizontally on its inferior border.

G.B.41. **Foot-Linqi:** In the derpression immediately distal to the junction of the bases of the 4th and 5th metatarsals.

G.B.42. **Diwuhui:** 1.0 cun proximal to Xiaxi (G.B. 43.)

G.B.43. **Xiaxi:** 0.5 cun proximal to the margin of the web between the 4th and 5th toes.

G.B.44. **Foot-Qiaoyin:** 0.1 cun proximal to the lateral corner of the base of the nail of the 4th toe.

XII. The Liver Channel

Liv. 1. **Dadun:** On the big toe, between the lateral corner of the nail and the interphalangeal joint.

Liv. 2. **Xingjian:** 0.5 cun proximal to the margin of the web between the big toe and the 2nd toe.

Liv. 3. **Taichong:** 2 cun proximal to the margin of the web between the Ist and 2nd toes.

Liv. 4. **Zhongfeng:** In the medial aspect of the ankle. in the depression on the medial side of the tendon of the tibialis anterior muscle, midway between Shangqiu (Sp. 5.) and Jiexi (St. 41.).

Liv. 5. **Ligou:** 5 cun superior to the tip on the medial malleolus, one finger breadth anterior to the medial border of the tibia.

Liv. 6. **Foot-Zhongdu:** 7 cun superior to the tip of the medial malleolus, one finger breadth anterior to the medial border of the tibia.

Liv. 7. **Xiguan:** 1.0 cun posterior to Yiniingquan (Sp.9.).

Liv. 8. **Ququan:** In the transverse crease of the knee joint, at the medial border of the semimembranous tendon. This point is better located at the medial end of the popliteal crease when the knee is fully flexed.

Liv. 9. **Yinbao:** Between the vastus medialis and sartorius muscles. 4 cun superior to the medial epicondyle of the femur.

Liv. 10. **Femur-Wuli:** 3 cun inferior to Qichong (St.30.), on the medial aspect of the thigh.

Liv. 11. **Yinlian:** 2 cun inferior to Qichong (St. 30.), on the medial aspect of the thigh.

Liv. 12. **Jimai:** 2.5 cun lateral to the centre of the pubic symphysis.

Liv. 13. **Zhangmen:** At the free end of the 11th rib.

Liv. 14. **Qimen:** Vertically below the nipple, in the intercostal space between the 6th and 7th ribs.

XIII. The Du Channel

Du. 1. **Changqiang:** Midway between the tip of the coccyx and the anus. This point is best located with the patient in the prone position.

Du. 2. **Yaoshu:** On the back midline, at the sacral hiatus.

Du. 3. **Yaoyangguan:** On the back midline, between the dorsal spines of the 4th and 5th lumbar vertebrae (at the level of the upper border of the iliac crests).

Du. 4. **Mingmen:** On the back midline, between the dorsal spines of the 2nd and 3rd lumbar vertebrae (at the level of the lower border of the rib cage).

Du. 5. **Xuanshu:** On the back midline, between the dorsal spines of the 1st and 2nd lumbar vertebrae.

Du. 6. **Jizhong:** On the back midline, between the dorsal spines of the 11th and 12th thoracic vertebrae.

Du. 7. **Zhongshu:** On the back midline, between the dorsal spines of the 10th and 11th thoracic vertebrae.

Du. 8. **Jinsuo:** On the back midline, between the dorsal spines of the 9th and 10th thoracic vertebrae.

Du. 9. **Zhiyang:** On the back midline, between the dorsal spines of the 7th and 8th thoracic vertebrae (at the level of the inferior angle of the scapula).

Du. 10. **Lingtai:** On the back midline, between the dorsal spines of the 6th and 7th thoracic vertebrae.

Du. 11. **Shendao:** On the back midline between the dorsal spines of the 5th and 6th thoracic vertebrae.

Du. 12. **Shenzhu:** On the back midline, between the dorsal spines of the 3rd and 4th thoracic vertebrae.

Du. 13. **Taodao:** On the back midline, between the dorsal spines of the 1st and 2nd thoracic vertebrae.

Du. 14. **Dazhui:** On the back midline, between the dorsal spines of the 7th cervical (vertebra prominents) and the 1st thoracic vertebrae.

Du. 15. **Yamen:** (a) At the nape of the neck on the midline, between the dorsal spines of the 1st and 2nd cervical vertebrae. (b) On the midline, 0.5 cun above the posterior hairline. (c) On the midline, 3.5 cun above the posterior hairline. (c) On the midline, 3.5 cun above the spinous process of the 7th cervical vertebra when the head is held erect.

Du. 16. **Fengfu:** (a) At the nape of the neck on the midline, in the depression directly below the occipital protuberance. (b) On the midline, 1.0 cun above the posterior hairline. (c) On the midline, 4 cun above the vertebra prominents.

Du. 17. **Naohu:** On the superior border of the occipital protuberance, 1.5 cun superior to Fengfu (Du 16.).

Du. 18. **Qiangjian:** On the back of the head, on the midline, 1.5 cun superior to Naohu (Du 17.). midway between Fengfu (Du 16.) and Baihui (Du 20.).

Du. 19. **Houding:** On the back of the head, on the midline, 1.5 cun superior to Qiangjian (Du 18.).

Du. 20. **Baihui:** (a) Draw a straight line from the lowest point of the ear lobe to the apex of the auricle and extend this line upwards on the scalp till it intersects the midline. The point lies at this intersection. (b) On the vertex of the skull, 5 cun behind the anterior hairline, on the midline (c) 8 cun above and behind the glabella, on the midline. (d) 7 cun above the posterior hairline, on the midline. (e) 10 cun above the vertebra prominents, on the midline.

Du 21. **Qianding:** 1.5 Cun superior to Baihui (Du 20.).

Du 22. **Xinhui:** (a) 3 cun anterior to Baihui Du 20.). (b) 2 cun Posterior to the anterior hairline

Du 23. **Shangxing:** 1.0 cun Posterior to the midpoint of the anterior hairline.

Du 24. **Shenting:** 0.5 cun Posterior to the midpoint of the anterior hairline.

Du 25. **Suliao:** At the tip of the nose.

Du 26. **Renzhong:** At the junction of the upper third and lower two-thirds of the philtrum of the upper lip on the midline.

Du 27. **Duiduan:** At the junction of the philtrum, with the upper lip on the midline.

Du 28. **Mouth-Yinjiao:** At the midpoint of the frenulum of the upper lip.

XIV. The Ren Channel

Ren 1. **Huiyin:** In the center to the perineum.

Ren 2. **Qugu:** Immediately above the Midpoint of the superior border of the public symphysis.

Ren 3. **Zhongji:** On the front midline, 4 cun below the umbilicus, 1 cun above Qugu (Ren 2.).

Ren 4. **Guanyuan:** On the front midline, 3 cun below the umbilicus, 2 cun above Qugu (Ren 2.).

Ren 5. **Shimen:** On the front midline, 2 cun below the umbilicus.

Ren 6. **Qihai:** On the front midline, 1.5 cun below the umbilicus.

Ren 7. **Abdomen-Yinjiao:** In the front midline, 1 cun below the umbilicus.

Ren 8. **Shenque:** In the center of the umbilicus. (Forbidden for acupuncture. Moxibustion only).

Ren 9. **Shuifen:** On the front midline, 1.0 cun above the umbilicus.

Ren10. **Xiawan:** On the front midline, 2 cun above the umbilicus.

Ren11. **Jianli:** On the front midline, 3 cun above the umbilicus.

Ren12. **Zhongwan:** (a) On the front midline, midway between the xyphoid process and the umbilicus. (b) On the front midline, 4 cun above the umbilicus.

Ren13. **Shangwan:** On the front midline, 5 cun above the umbilicus.

Ren14. **Juque:**[2] On the front midline, 6 cun above the umbilicus.

Ren15. **Jiuwei:** On the front midline, 7 cun above the umbilicus, just below the xyphoid process. (Locate the point in the supine position with the arms abducted).

2 Also spelt jujue

Ren16. **Zhongting:** On the midline of the sternum, at the level of the 5th intercostal space.

Ren17. **Shanzhong:** On the midline of the sternum, midway between the two nipples at the level of the intercostal space.

Ren18. **Yutang:** On the midline of the sternum, at the level of the 3rd intercostal space.

Ren19. **Chest-Zigong:** On the midline of the sternum, at the level of the 2nd intercostal space.

Ren20. **Huagai:** On the midline of the sternum, at the level of the 1st intercostal space.

Ren21. **Xuanji:** On the midline of the sternum, midway between Tiantu (Ren 22.) and Huagai (Ren 20.).

Ren22. **Tiantu:** At the center of the suprasternal fossa 0.5 cun above the sternal notch.

Ren23. **Lianquan:** On the midline of the neck, midway between the upper border of the cricoid cartilage and the lower border of the mandible.

Ren24. **Chengjiang:** In the depression in the center of the mentolabial groove.

APPENDIX OF UNNUMBERED EXTRAORDINARY ACUPUNCTURE POINTS

The points described here are less frequently used in the People's Republic of China. They are from a later publication.

Weiguanxiashu:

Location: 1.5 cun lateral to the lower border of the spinous process of the 8th thoracic vertebra.

Indications: Vomiting, abdominal pain.

Puncture: 0.5-0.7 cun obliquely. Moxibustion is applicable.

[1]**Yaoyan:**

Location: In the depression lateral to the interspace between the spinous processes of the 4th and 5th lumbar vertebrae. The point is located in the prone position.

Indications: Pulmonary tuberculosis, irregular menstruation, backache.

Puncture: Perpendicularly 0.5 – 1.0 cun. Moxibustion is applicable.

Shiqizhui (17th Vertebra):

Location: In the depression below the spinous process of the 5th lumbar vertebra.

Indications: Backache.

Puncture: Perpendicularly 0.5 – 1.0 cun. Moxibustion is applicable.

Abdomen-Zigong:

Location: 4 cun below the umbilicus, 3 cun lateral to Zhongji (Ren 3.).

Indications: Prolapse of the uterus, irregular menstruation.

Puncture: Perpendicularly 1.0 – 1.5 cun. Moxibustion is applicable.

1 Many authorities state that this is Dachangshu (U.B. 25.)

Jianqian (Also known as Jianneiling):

Location: When the arm is adducted, the point is midway between the end of the anterior axillary fold and Jianyu (L.I. 15.).

Indications: Pain in the shoulder and arm, paralysis of the upper extremities.

Puncture: Perendicularly 0.6 – 1.0 cun. Moxibustion is applicable.

Zhongquan:

Location: On the dorsum of the wrist, radial to the tendon of the extensor digitorum communis, in the depression between Yangchi (S.J. 4.) Yangxi (L.I. 5.).

Indications: Arthritis of the wrist, stifling feeling in the chest, haematemesis, gastric pain.

Puncture: Perpendicularly 0.3 – 0.5 cun. Moxibustion is applicable.

Sifeng:

Location: On the palmar surface, in the transverse creases of the proximal interphalangeal joints of the index, middle, ring and little fingers.

Indications: Rheumatoid arthritis, polyneuropathy, malnutrition and malabsorption syndromes in children.

Puncture: Prick with a three-edged needle and squeeze out a small amount of viscous yellowish fluid.

As these are new points they are in Pinyin spelling only.

Index of the Acupuncture Points and their English Equivalents

A

Abdomen-Tonggu (K. 20.)	*Connecting Valley on the Abdomen*
Abdomen-Yinjiao (Ren 7.).	*Junction of Yin*
Abbomen-Zhongzhu (K. 15.).	*Middle (Energy) Flow*
Anmian I (Extra 8.).	*Peaceful Sleep I*
Animain II (Extra 9.).	*Peaceful Sleep II*

B

Bafeng (Extra 36.).	*Eight Winds*
Baihuanshu (U.B. 30.)	*White Circle's Hollow*[1]
Baihui (Du 20.).	*Hundred meetings*
Baohuang (U.B. 53.).	*Placenta and Vitals*
Baxie (Extra 28.).	*Eight Evils*
Benshen (G.B. 13.).	*Original Spirit*
Bientao (U. Ex.).	*Tonsil*
Biguan (St. 31.).	*Hip's Hinge*
Binao (L.I. 14.).	*Arm and Scapula*
Bingfeng (S.I. 12.).	*Holding Wind*
Bipay (U.Ex.).	*Specific for Heart*
Bulang (K. 22.).	*Stepping Corridor*
Burong (St. 19.).	*Uncontainable*

C

Changqiang (Du 1.).	*Long Strength*
Chengfu (U.B. 36.).	*Receive Support*
Chengguang (U.B. 6.).	*Support Light*
Chengjiang (Ren 24.).	*Contain Fluid*

Chengjin (U.B. 56.).	*Support Sinews*
Chengling (G.B. 18.).	*Support the Spirit*
Chengman (St. 20.).	*Support Fullness*
Chengqi (St. 1.).	*Contain the Tears*
Chengshan (U.B. 57.).	*Support the Mountain*
Chest-Zigong (Ren 19.).	*Purple Palace*
Chize (Lu. 5.).	*Cubit Marsh*
Chongmen (Sp. 12.).	*Pouring Door*
Chongyang (St. 42.).	*Pouring Yang*
Ciliao (U.B. 32.).	*Second Seam*
Dabao (Sp. 21.).	*Big Wrapping*
Dachangshu (U.B. 25.).	*Large Intestine's Hollow*
Dadu (Sp. 2.).	*Big Metropolis*
Dadun (Liv. 1.).	*Great Honesty*
Dahe (K. 12.).	*Great Clarity*
Daheng (Sp. 15.).	*Big Horizontal*
Daimai (G.B. 26.).	*Girdle Vessel*
Daju (St. 27.).	*The Great*
Daling (P. 7.).	*Big Tomb*
Dannang (Extra 35.).	*Gall bladder Orifice*
Danshu (U.B. 19.).	*Gall bladder's Hollow**
Dashu (U.B. 11.).	*Big Shuttle*
Daying (St. 5.).	*Big Welcome*
Dazhong (K. 4.).	*Big Goblet*
Dazhui (Du 14.).	*Big Vertebra*
Dicang (St. 4.).	*Earth Granary*
Diji (Sp. 8.).	*Earth's Mechanism*
Dingchan or Chienshi (U.Ex.).	*Soothing the Sprain*
Dingchuan (Extra 17.).	*Soothing Asthma*
Diwuhui (G.B. 42.).	*Ground's Fifth Meeting*
Dubi (St. 35.).	*Nose of Calf*

Duiduan (Du. 27.).	*Exchange Terminus*
Dushu (U.B. 16.).	*Governing Hollow**

E

Ear-Heliao (S.J. 22.).	*Harmony's Seam*
Erjian (L.I. 2.).	*Between Two*
Ermen (S.J. 21.).	*Ear's Door*

F

Feishu (U.B. 13.).	*Lung's Hollow*
Feiyang (U.B. 58.).	*Soaring*
Femur-Futu (St. 32.).	*Hidden Rabbit*
Femur-Juliao (G.B. 29.).	*Stationary Seam*
Femur-Wuli (Liv. 10.).	*Five Measures*
Femur-Zhongdu (G.B. 32.)	*Middle Ditch*
Fengchi (G.B. 20.).	*Pool of Wind*
Fengfu (du 16.).	*Wind's Dwelling*
Fengling (St. 40.).	*Abundance and Prosperity*
Fengmen (U.B. 12.).	*Wind's Door*
Fengshi (G.B. 31.).	*Wind's Market*
Foot-Linqi (G.B. 41.).	*Nine Tears*
Foot-Qiaoyin (G.B. 44.).	*Yin Cavity*
Foot-Tonggu (U.B. 66.).	*Connecting Valley*
Foot-Zhongdu (Liv. 6.).	*Middle Metropolis*
Fuai (Sp. 16.).	*Abdomen's Sorrow*
Fubai (G.B. 10.).	*Floating White*
Fufen (U.B. 41.).	*Appended Part*
Fujie (Sp. 14.).	*Abdomen's Knot*
Fuliu (K. 7.).	*Returning Column*
Fushe (Sp. 13.).	*Dwelling*
Fuxi (U.B. 38.).	*Floating Xi*
Fuyang (U.B. 59.).	*Tarsal Yang*

G

Ganshu (U.B. 18.). *Liver's Hollow**
Gaohuangshu (U.B. 43.). *Vital's Hollow**
Geguan (U.B. 46.). *Diaphragm's Hinge*
Geshu (U.B. 17.). *Diaphragm's Hollow**
Gongsun (Sp. 4.). *Grandfather's Grandson*
Guanchong (S.J. 1.). *Gate's Pouring*
Guangming (G.B. 37.). *Bright Light*
Guanmen (St. 22.). *Gate*
Guanyuan (Ren 4.). *Hinge at the Source*
Guanyuanshu (U.B. 26.). *Hinge of the Source Locus*
Guilai (St. 29.). *Return (of Energy)*

H

Hand-Wangu (S.I. 4.). *Wrist Bone*
Hand-Wuli (L.I. 13.). *Five Measures*
Hand-zhongzhu (S.J. 3.). *Middle Island*
Hanyan (G.B. 4.). *Jaw's Dislike*
Head-Linqi (B.B. 15.). *Near Tears*
Head-Qiaoyin (G.B. 11.). *Yin Cavity*
Head-Wangu (G.B. 12.). *Finished Bone*
Heding (Extra 31). *Crane's Top*
Hegu (L.I. 4.). *Adjoining Valleys*
Henggu (K. 11.). *Horizontal Bone*
Heyang (U.B. 55.). *Confluence of Yang*
Houding (Du. 19.). *Behind Top*
Houxi (S.I. 3.). *Back Creek*
Huagi (Ren 20.). *Lustrous Cover*
Huangmen (U.B. 51.). *Vital's Door*
Huangshu (K. 16.). *Vital's Hollow**
Huantiao (G.B. 30.). *Encircling Leap*

Huaroumen (St. 24.).	*Door of Slippery Flesh*
Huatuojiaji (Extra 21.).	*Huatuo's Lining of the Spine*
Huiyang (U.B. 35.).	*Meeting of the Yang*
Huiyin (Ren 1.).	*Perineum (Yin point)*
Huizong (S.J. 7.).	*Meeting of the Clan*
Hunmen (U.B. 47.).	*Soul's Door*

J

Jiache (St. 6.).	*Jaw's Vehicle*
Jiachengjang (Extra 5.).	*Containing Fluid*
Jianjing (G.B. 21.).	*Shoulder Well*
Jianli (Ren 11.).	*Establish Measure*
Jianliao (S.J. 14.).	*Shoulder Seam*
Jian-Nie-Ling (U. Ex.).	*Shoulder's Inner Tomb*
Jianshi (P. 5.).	*Intermediary*
Jianwaishu (S.I. 14.).	*Shoulder's Outer Hollow**
Jianyu (L.I. 15.).	*Shoulder Bone*
Jianzhen (S.I. 9.).	*Shoulder Chastity*
Jianzhongshu (S.I. 15.).	*Mid-Shoulder Hollow**
jiaosun (S.J. 20.).	*Angle of Regeneration*
Jiaoxin (K. 8.).	*Communicate Belief*
Jiexi (St. 41.).	*Release Stream*
Jimai (Liv. 12.).	*Urgent Pulse*
Jimen (Sp. 11.).	*Basket's Door*
Jinggu (U.B. 64.).	*Capital Bone*
Jingmen (G.B. 25.).	*Capital's Door*
Jingming (U.B. 1.).	*Eyes Bright*
Jingqu (Lu. 8.).	*Across the Ditch*
Jinjin, Yuye (Extra. 10.).	*Golden Fluid, Jade Fluid*
Jinmen (U.B. 63.).	*GoldenDoor*
Jinsuo (Du 8.).	*Sinew's Shrinking*

Jiquan (H. 1.).	*Summit's Spring*
Jiuwei (Ren 15.).	*Wild Pigeion's Tail*
Jizhong (Du 6.).	*Middle of the Spine*
Juegu (See Xuanzhong).	
Jueyinshu (U.B. 14.).	*Absolute Yin Hollow**
Juliao (St. 3.).	*Great Seam*
Jugu (L.I. 16.).	*Great Bone*
Juque** (Ren 14.).	*Great Palace*

K

Kongzui (Lu. 6.).	*Opening Maximum*
Kufang (St. 14.).	*Storehouse*
Kunlun (U.B. 60.).	*Kunlun Mountans*

L

Lanwei (Extra. 33.).	*Appendix (point)*
Laogong (P. 8.).	*Labour's Palace*
Liangmen (St. 21.).	*Door of the Beam*
Liangqiu (St. 34.).	*Ridge Mound*
Lianquan (Ren 23.).	*Modest Spring*
Lidui (St. 45.).	*Strict Exchange*
Lieque (Lu. 7.).	*Broken Sequence*
Ligou (Liv. 5.).	*Worm-eater's Groove*
Lingdao (H. 4.).	*Spirit's Path*
Lingtai (Du 10.).	*Spirit's Platform*
Lingxu (K. 24.).	*Spirit's Ruins*
Lougu (Sp. 7.).	*Seeping Valley*
Luoque (U.B. 8.).	*Decline*
Luxi (S.J. 19.).	*Skull's Rest*

** = Also spelt Jujue.

M

Meichong (U.B. 3.).	*Eyebrow's Pouring*
Mingmen (Du 4.).	*Life's Door*
Mouth-Yinjiao (Du. 28.).	*Gum's (Yin) Junction*
Muchuang (G.B. 16.).	*Vision's Window*

N

Naohu (Du 17.).	*Brain's Household*
Naohui (S.I. 13.).	*Shoulder's Meeting*
Naokong (G.B. 19.).	*Brain Cavity*
Naoshu (S.I. 10.).	*Scapula Hollow*
Neck-Futu (L.I. 18.).	*Support the Prominence*
Neiguan (P. 6.).	*Inner Gate*
Neima (U. Ex.).	*Medical anesthetic*
Neiting (St. 44.).	*Inner Court*
Nose-Heliao (L.I. 19.).	*Grain Seam*
Nose-Juliao (St. 3.).	*Great Seam*

P

Pangguanshu (U.B. 28.).	*Bladder's Hollow*
Pianli (L.I. 6.).	*Partial Order**
Pishu (U.B.20.).	*Spleen Hollow**
Pohu (U.B. 42.).	*Soul's Household*
Posterior-Tinggong (U. Ex.).	*Posterior Palace of Hearing*
Pushen (U.B. 61.).	*Serve and Consult*

Q

Qianding (Du 21.).	*Before Top*
Qianjian (Du 18.).	*Between Strength*
Qiangu (S.I. 2.).	*Forward Valley*
Qichong (St. 30.).	*Pouring of Qi*

Qihai (Ren 6.). *Sea of Qi*
Qihaishu (U.B. 23.). *Sea of Qi Hollow**
Qihu (St. 13.). *Qi's Household*
Qimai (S.J. 18.). *Feeding the Vessels*
Qimen (Liv. 14.). *Expectation's Door*
Qinglengyuan (S.J. 11.). *Cooling Gulf*
Qingling (H. 2.). *Youthful Spirit*
Qishe (St. 11.). *Qi's Residence*
Qihou (Extra. 4.). *Behind the Ball*
Qiuxu (G.B. 40.). *Mound of Ruins*
Qixue (K. 13.). *Qi's Orifice*
Quanliao (S.I. 18.). *Cheek Seam*
Qubin (G.B. 7.). *Crook of the Temple*
Quchai (U.B. 4.). *Discrepancy*
Quchi (L.I. 11.). *Crooked Pool*
Quepen (St. 12.). *Empty Basin*
Qugu (Ren 2.). *Crooked Bone*
Ququan (Liv. 8.). *Crooked Spring*
Quyuan (S.I. 13.). *Crooked Wall*
Quze (P. 3.). *Crooked March*

R

Rangu (K. 2.). *Burning Valley*
Renying (St. 9.). *Man's Welcome*
Renzhong (Du 26.). *Philtrum*
Riyue (G.B. 24.). *Sun and Moon*
Rugen (St. 18.). *Breast's Root*
Ruzhong (St. 17.). *Middle of the Breat*

S

Sanjian (L.I. 3.). *Between Three*

Sanjiaoshu (U.B. 22.).	*Triple Burner's Hollow**
Sanyanglulo (S.J. 8.).	*Three Yang Connection point*
Sanyinjiao (Sp. 6.).	*Three Yin Junction*
Shangguan (G.B. 3.).	*Upper Hinge*
Shangjuxu (St. 37.).	*Upper Void*
Shanglian (L.I. 9.).	*Upper Integrity*
Shangliao (U.B. 31.).	*Upper Seam*
Shangqiu (Sp. 5.).	*Mound of Commerce*
Shangqu (K. 17.).	*Trade's Bend*
Shanwan (Ren 13.).	*Upper Cavity*
Shangxing (Du 23.).	*Upper Star*
Shangyang (L.I. 1.).	*Trade Yang*
Shanzhong (Ren 17.).	*Penetrating Odour*
Shaochong (H. 9.).	*Lesser Pouring*
Shaofu (H. 8.).	*Lesser Residence*
Shaohai (H. 3.).	*Lesser Sea*
Shaoshang (Lu. 11.).	*Lesser Merchant*
Shaoxe (S.I. 1.).	*Lesser Marsh*
Shencang (K. 25.).	*Spirit's Storage*
Shendao (Du 11.).	*Spirit's Path*
Shenfeng (K. 23.).	*Spirit's Seal*
Shenmai (U.B. 62.).	*Extending Vessel*
Shenmen (H. 7.).	*Spirit's Door*
Shenque or Qizhone (Ren 8.).	*Middle of the Navel*
Shenshu (U.B. 23.).	*Kidney's Hollow**
Shentang (U.B. 44.).	*Spirit's Hall*
Shenting (Du. 24.).	*Spirit's Abode*
Shenzhu (Du 12.).	*Body's Pillar*
Shidou (Sp. 17.).	*Food's Cavity*
Shiguan (K. 18.).	*Stone Hinge*
Shimen (Ren 5.).	*Stone Door*

Shousanli (L.I. 10.).	*Arm's Three Measures*
Shuaigu (G.B. 8.).	*Leading to the Valley*
Shufu (K. 27.).	*Hollow Residence*
Shugu (U.B. 65.).	*Restraining Bone*
Shuidao (St. 28.).	*Waterway*
Shuifen (Ren 9.).	*Water Part*
Shuigou (See Renzhong).	
Shuiquan (K. 5.).	*Spring*
Shuitu (St. 10.).	*Water Prominence*
Sibai (St. 2.).	*Four Whites*
Sidu (S.J. 9.).	*Four Ditches*
Siman (K. 14.).	*Four Full*
Sishencong (Extra. 6.).	*Four Intelligences*
Sizhukong (S.J. 23.).	*Silken Bamboo Hollow*
Suliao (Du 25.).	*Plain Seam*

T

Taibai (Sp. 3.).	*Most White*
Taichong (Liv. 3.).	*Great Pouring*
Taixi (K. 3.).	*Great Creek*
Taiyang (Extra. 2.).	*Sun*
Taiyi (St. 23.).	*Great Yi*
Taiyuan (Lu. 9.).	*Great Abyss*
Taner or Naoshang (U. Ex.).	*Above the Scapula*
Taodao (Du 13.).	*Way of Happiness*
Tianchi (P. 1.).	*Heaven's Pool*
Tianchong (G.B. 9.).	*Heaven's Pouring*
Tianchuang (S.I. 16.).	*Heaven's Window*
Tianding (L.I. 17.).	*Heaven's Vessel*
Tianfu (Lu. 3.).	*Heaven's Residence*
Tianjing (S.J. 10.).	*Heaven's Well*

Tianliao (S.J. 15.).	*Heaven's Seam*
Tianquan (P. 2.).	*Heaven's Spring*
Tianrong (S.I. 17.).	*Heaven's Contents*
Tianshu (St. 25.).	*Heaven's Axis*
Tiantu (Ren 22.).	*Heaven's Prominence*
Tianxi (Sp. 18.).	*Heaven's Stream*
Tianyou (S.J. 16.).	*Heaven's Window*
Tianzhu (U.B. 10.).	*Heaven's Pillar*
Tianzong (S.I. 11.).	*Heaven's Ancestor*
Tiaokou (St. 38.).	*Line's Opening*
Tinggong (S.I. 19.).	*Palace of Hearing*
Tinghui (G.B. 2.).	*Confluence of Hearing*
Tongli (H. 5.).	*Reaching the Measure*
Tongtian (U.B. 7.).	*Reaching Heaven*
Tongziliao (G.B. 1.).	*Pupil Seam*
Touwei (St. 8.).	*Head Support*
Tunzhong (U. Ex.).	*Middle of the Buttock*

W

Waiguan (S.J. 5.).	*Outer Gate*
Wailing (St. 26.).	*Outer Tomb*
Waiqiu (G.B. 36.).	*Outer Mound*
Weicang (U.B. 50.).	*Stomach's Storehouse*
Weidao (G.B. 28.).	*Maintain the Way*
Weima (U. Ex.).	*Lateral Anaesthetic*
Weishu (U.B. 21.).	*Stomach's Hollow**
Weiyang (U.B. 39.).	*Commission the Yang*
Weizhong (U.B. 40.).	*Commission the Middle*
Wenliu (L.I. 7.).	*Warm Slide*
Wuchu (U.B. 5.).	*Five Places*
Wushu (G.B.27.).	*Five Pivots*
Wuyi (St. 15.).	*Room Screen*

X

Xiabai (Lu. 4.). *Gallantry*
Xiaguan (St. 7.). *Lower Hinges*
Xiajuxu (St. 39.). *Lower Void*
Xialian (L.I. 8.). *Lower Integrity*
Xialiao (U.B. 34.). *Lower Seam*
Xiangu (St. 43.). *Sinking Valley*
Xiaochangshu (U.B. 27.). *Small Intestine's Hollow**
Xiaohai (S.I. 8.). *Small Sea*
Xiaoluo (S.J. 12.). *Meting Luo River*
Xiawan (Ren 10.). *Lower Cavity*
Xiaxi (G.B. 43.). *Gallantry's Stream*
Yia-Yifeng (U. Ex.). *Below Yifeng*
Xiguan (Liv. 7.). *Knee's Hinge*
Ximen (P. 4.). *Gate of the Crevice*
Xingjian (Liv. 2.). *Walk Between*
Xinhui (Du 22.). *Fontanelle's Meeting*
Xinshu (U.B.15.). *Heart's Hollow**
Xiongxiang (St. 19.). *Chest Home*
Xiyan (Extra. 32.). *Eyes of the Knee*
Xiyangguan (G.B. 33.). *Knee's Young Hinge*
Xuanji (Ren 21.). *North Star*
Xuanli (G.B. 6.). *Suspended Millimeter*
Xuanlu (G.B. 5.). *Suspended Skull*
Xuanshu (Du. 5.). *Suspended Axis*
Xuanzhong (G.B. 39.). *Suspended Time*
Xuehai (Sp. 10.). *Sea of Blood*

Y

Yamen (Du 15.). *Door of Muteness*
Yangbai (G.B. 14.). *Yang White*
Yangchi (S.J. 4.). *Pool of Yang*
Yangju (G.B. 38.). *Yang's Help*

Yanggang (U.B. 48.).	*Yang's Parameter*
Yanggu (S.I. 5.).	*Valley of Yang*
Yangjiao (G.B. 35.).	*Yang's Intersection*
Yanglao (S.I. 6.).	*Nourish the Old*
Yanglingquan (G.B. 34.).	*Yang Tomb Spring*
Yangxi (L.I. 5.).	*Yang Creek*
Yaoshu (Du. 2.).	*Lower Back's Hollow**
Yaoyan (U. Ex.).	*Waist's Eye*
Yaoyangguan (Du. 3.).	*Lumbar Yang's Hinge*
Yemen (S.J. 2.).	*Fluid's Door*
Yifeng (S.J. 17.).	*Shielding Wind*
Yiming (Extra. 7.).	*Shielding Brightness*
Yinbai (Sp. 1.).	*Hidden White*
Yinbao (Liv. 9.).	*Yin's Wrapping*
Yindu (K. 19.).	*Yin's Metropolis*
Yingchuang (St. 16.).	*Breast's Window*
Yingu (K. 10.).	*Yin's Valley*
Yingxiang (L.I. 20.).	*Welcome Fragrance*
Yinlian (Liv. 11.).	*Yin's Modesty*
Yinlingquan (St. 9.).	*Yin Tomb Spring*
Yinmen (U.B. 37.).	*Door of Abundance*
Yinshi (St. 33.).	*Yin's Market*
Yintang (Extra. 1.).	*Seal Hall*
Yinxi (H. 6.).	*Yin Perverse*
Yishe (U.B. 49.).	*Will's Residence*
Yixi (U.B. 45.).	*Surprise*
Yongquan (K. 1.).	*Gushing Spring*
Youmen (K. 21.).	*Secluded Door (Pylorus)*
Yuanye (G.B. 22.).	*Gulf's Fluids*
Yuji (Lu. 10.).	*Fish Border*
Yunmen (Lu. 2.).	*Cloud's Door*
Yutang (Ren 18.).	*Jade Court*
Yuyao (Extra. 3.).	*Fish Waist*

Yuzhen (U.B. 9.).	*Jade Pillow*
Yuzhong (K. 26.).	*Amid Elegance*

Z

Zanzhu (U.B. 2.).	*Gathered Bamboo*
Zhangmen (Liv. 13.).	*System's Door*
Zhaohai (K. 6.).	*Shining Sea*
Zhejin (G.B. 23.).	*Flank's Sinews*
Zhengyirg (G.B. 17.).	*Upright Encampment*
Zhibian (U.B. 54.).	*Order's Edge*
Zhigou (S.J. 6.).	*Branch Ditch*
Zhishi (U.B. 52.).	*Will's Dwelling*
Zhiyang (Du 9.).	*Reaching Yang*
Zhiyin (U.B. 67.).	*End of Yin*
Zhizheng (S.I. 7.).	*Branch of Uprightness*
Zhongchong (P. 9.).	*Middle Pouring*
Zhongfeng (Liv. 4.).	*Middle Seal*
Zhongfu (Lu. 1.).	*Central Residence*
Zhongji (Ren 3.).	*Middle Summit*
Znongliao (U.B. 33.).	*Middle Seam*
Zhonglushu (U.B. 29.).	*Mid-Spine Hollow**
Zhongshu (Du. 7.).	*Middle Axis*
Zhongting (Ren 16.).	*Middle Hall*
Zhongwan (Ren 12.).	*Middle Cavity*
Zhouliao (L.I. 12.).	*Elbow Seam*
Zhourong (Sp. 20.).	*Encircling Glory*
Zhubin (K. 9.).	*House Guest*
Zusanli (St.36.).	*Three Measures on the Leg*

* Hollow, opening or direct communication.

GLOSSARY OF COMMON TERMS USED IN ACUPUNCTURE PRACTICE

Acupuncture analgesia: Abolition or dulling of pain sensation by the use of acupuncture, also called "acupuncture anaesthesia" when used for surgical operations. The Chinese name for this is "*Chen-Ma*", which means "Needle-Anaesthesia".

Acupuncture Points: Points on the body surface discovered by the ancient physicians which, on puncturing, heating or applying pressure, cure or relieve the symptoms of disease. Modern research has shown that there is a lowered electrical resistance at the majority of traditional points and, perhaps, even biological differences, such as increased oxygen consumption.

Acupunctoscope: (Also called Acupuncture Point Detector and Stimulator.) A multi-purpose electronic instrument which (a) detects acupuncture points using the phenomenon of lowered electrical resistance at these points, and (b) generates a pulsed electric current to stimulate the acupuncture point (with or without needles).

Acupuncturist: A practitioner of acupuncture and allied healing arts who practices in conformity with the laws and traditions pertaining to these arts, irrespective of whether he is qualified or not in unrelated systems of medicine.

Ah-Shi points: Tender points on the body surface. These points are not necessarily on a Channel. Needling these points at the correct depth and stimulating them seems to break up the pathology at the local areas and bring relief. Ah-Shi in Chinese means "Oh-Yes", this being the verbal reaction of the patient who is instructed to indicate to the acupuncturist the presence of these points when the latter is palpating. These points correspond to the "locus dolendi" of the medicine of medieval Europe.

Alarm points: Acupuncture points which become tender when there is disease in the pertaining Organ.

Acupuncture: The injection of distilled water or drugs at acupuncture points for the purpose of creating further stimulation. This is a form of point injection therapy. (See Point-injection therapy).

Artemisia vulgaris: Botanical name for the plant from which the moxa used for moxibustion is obtained.

Auriculotherapy: An ancient method of using the external ear to diagnose and treat illness. Every part of the body has functional representation on the ear, and the locations of these points have been charted with a great deal of accurary. The ear points selected for treatment can also be detected and treated by using the acupunctoscope.

Bu method: Reinforcing method of applying needle stimulation to an acupuncture point to increase the vital energy (Qi). This is also known as the tonification method of stimulation and is used in Xu diseases. (Opposite of Xie method).

Channels or Meridians: (Jing). Lines drawn more or less vertically on the body surface connecting acupuncture points having similar therapeutic properties. There are 14 main Channels of which 12 are paired (bilateral) and 2 are unpaired (midline). Vital energy (Qi) flows in these Channels in an orderly cyclic sequence.

Collaterals: (Luo). Branches of Channels which connect one Channel to another in order to balance the flow of vital energy.

Confluent points: Certain points situated in the extremities and belonging to the Twelve Paired Channels which effect connections with the Eight Extraordinary Channels. They can be used to treat diseases related to the Twelve Paired Channels as well as the Eight Extraordinary Channels.

Cun: The unit of measurement used for locating acupuncture points. A cun is the distance between the interphalangeal creases of the middle finger of the patient; it is also the breadth of the thumb at the level where it is widest. A cun may be rendered in English as a "body inch" I cun-10 fen.

Cunometer: An instrument to measure cuns.

Cupping: A techniqe of traditional Chinese medicine where suction is applied to diseased parts of the body using ceramic glass or bamboo cups in order to increase the regional circulation and thereby promote healing. In very ancient times the horns of animals were used for this purpose.

Deqi: The subjective sensation felt by a person who is needled, also referred to as the "acupuncture sensation". It is described as being a combination of numbness, heaviness, soreness, distension, and the radiation of one or more of these sensations. It is believed that better therapeutic success is obtained when "deqi" is elicited, particularly in acupuncture anaesthesia. The sensation felt by the acupuncturist due to local musclespasms around the needle in also called deqi.

Diseases: (types of): According to traditional Chinese medicine, diseases are broadly divisible into two types: a) "Shi" diseases in which there is hyperactivity such as in acute conditions, and b) "Xu" diseases in which there is hypofunction such as in chronic conditions.

Diseases: (causative factors of Sieqi). According to traditional Chinese medicine, diseases are caused by either intrinsic or extrinsic factors. a) Intrinsic factors are emotional states like joy, anger, obsession, sorrow, horror, anxiety, surprise and shock. These intrinsic or "endogenous" factors initially produce alterations have effects on the flow of vital energy in the Channels. The manifestation of these changes is disease. b) Extrinsic factors refer to "exogenous" causes originating in the external environment. These include climatic factors like cold, warmth, damp and wind. Bacterial infection and environment pollution also belong to this category. Usually, it is the Channels that are first attacked by these extrinsic factors; later the internal Organs become diseased.

Distal points: Acupuncture points situated distal to the elbow (in case of the upper limb) and distal to the lines (in case of the lower limb). These points have therapeutic effects on diseases in the specific proximal areas to which they are related.

Electrical pulse stimulation: see **Acupunctoscope.**

Embedding therapy: A recently developed technique in which sterile catgut is surgically implanted at one or more acupuncture points in order to give prolonged stimulation. Dermal needles and press needles are also embedded in the skin to provide continuous stimulation between treatment sessions. These therapies are very useful in chronic or resistant conditions like bronchial asthma, trigeminal neuralgia, migraine, and the pain of secondary cancer.

Endorphins: These are the body's own opiates which are released on acupuncture needling. It takes about half an hour maximal release of these and other chemicals after needling.

Extraordinary Channels: Channels other than the 12 Organ Channels are called Extraordinary Channels. There are 8 such Channels including the Ren and Du Channels (the midline Channels).

Extraordinary points: Acupuncture points which were discovered after the known (classical) points were placed in the Channels and numbered about two thousand years ago. While the majority of the Extraordinary points fall outside the Channels, some lie in the path of a Channel and some even coincide with regular points.

Fen: One tenth of a cun.

Filiform needle: This is the common type of stainless steel needle used in acupuncture practice today.

Five Elements: (Wu-Hsing). According to the ancient Chinese philosophy the Universe is made up of the five Elements; these are Wood, Fire, Earth, Metal and Water. Man being a part of nature is therefore made of the same Elements and is subject to the same universal laws which govern the interactions between these Elements. The central thesis of traditional Chinese medicine is the relationship of these Five Elements to one another as applied to the body in health and disease. According to the ancient classic, the Huang Di Nei Jing, the Five Element system is a symbolism which encompasses all natural phenomena as well as man. It should not therefore be interpreted in a literal or restrictive sense.

Five Shu points: On each of the Twelve Channels there are five acupuncture points, one for each of the Five Elements. These points which are situated distal to the elbow and distal to the knee are known as the Five Shu points. Each of these points has special therapeutic properties based on its relationship to its particular Element.

Gate-Control Theory of Pain: According to this theory which was proposed by R. Melzack and P.D. Wall in 1965, our subjective awareness of pain cannot be explained on the basis of simple telephone-like circuits as formerly believed, but is subject to considerable modulation by means of a functional "gate" situated in the substantia gelatinosa of the spinal cord. Under normal circumstances the pain impulses get through this gate quite easily, and pain is felt. But when, as in acupuncture anaesthesia, a second stream of (non-painful) impulses is set up and made to converge on this gate, there is an overcrowding, a competitive inhibition of the pain impulses and finally a jamming or closing of the gate. This is the most popular of the neurological theories which have been proposed to explain acupuncture analgesia. According to some researchers there may be other gates at the thalamus or even at higher levels as the substantia gelatinosa is present only in the spinal cord and is therefore incapable of modulating the pain impulses from the head and neck regions. This is called the "Multiple Gate theory".

Head Needle therapy: (Scalp Acupuncture). A form of acupunture therapy which uses certain areas of the scalp to treat diseases. It is based on the principle that there is a functional representation on the scalp of many body areas and functions. This is a modern discovery made by medical workers in the People's Republic of China during the Cultural Revolution (1965-1970). This form of acupuncture has been very successfully used for anaesthetic purposes as well.

Homoeopuncture: The puncturing of acupunture points after dipping the needle in specific homoeopathic remedy.

Hot Needling: The rapid insertion and withdrawal of a heated silver alloy needle into certain pathological enlargements like cysts, "ganglions", solitary nodules and benign enlargements of the thyroid gland. This is another example of how traditional methods are being used today to provide highly effective methods of treatment in the People's Republic of China.

Huang Di Nei Jing: (Yellow Emperor's Classic of Internal Medicine). This is the name of the most highly regarded book on traditional Chinese medicine, and is said to be the oldest extant medical book in the world. Although tradition ascribes its authorship to the Emperor Huang Di (2696 – 2591 B. C.), scholars today believe that it is a compilation of the then-extant medical knowledge by Li Chu-Kuo around the year 26 A. D. However, some parts of the book certainly data back to the third century B.C. and others are possibly even older. The book takes the form of a conversation between the Yellow Emperor (Huang Di) and his court physician Chi Po. They discuss the relationship between Man and Nature, the five Elements, the medical importance of Yin and Yang and the causes and cures for illness, including the principles of acupuncture and moxibustion.

Husband – Wife Law: This is one of the Laws of traditional Chinese acupuncture. This Law is intimately related to the traditional method of pulse diagnosis certain aspects of the relationships between the pulses and their pertaining Organs and Channels. The Twelve Channels and their pertaining Organs are represented by twelve pulse positions, six on each wrist. The Organs and Channels represented by the pulse positions on the left wrist are called "husband" and they are said to dominate the Organs and Channels represented by the corresponding pulse positions of the right wrist which are called "wife".

Conversely, the Organs and Channels represented by the positions on the right wrist (wife) are said to endanger those represented on the corresponding positions of the left wrist (husband). Thus the husband dominates the wife and the endangers the husband (perhaps in retaliation for the husband's domineering attitude!). Needling of a Channel that corresponds to a "husband" pulse affects the Channel and Organ corresponding to a "wife" pulse and vice-versa. These picturesquely named relationships are scrupulously observed in traditional Chinese acupuncture based on pulse diagnosis.

Influential points: This is a group of eight points, each of which affects certain specific tissue disorders, e.g., blood, tendon, bone, marrow, the blood vessels, respiratory functions, "hollow" and 'solid" organs.

Interior-exterior relationship of Channels: Each of the Yin Channels has a special relationship (both functionally and positionally) with one of the Yang Channels which is referred to as the interior-exterior relationship of the Channels. There are six pairs of Channels having this relationship. These pairs of Channels are called "Coupled Channels" Thus we have the coupled sequence of Lung-Large Intestine; Stomach-Spleen; Heart-Small-Intestine; Urinary Bladder-Kidney; Pericardium-Sanjiao; Gall Bladder-Liver. The interior-exterior relationship of the Coupled Channels is clearly seen by their disposition on the opposite aspects of the limbs; the Yin Channels run along the medial (interior) aspect of the extremities, and the Yang Channels run along the "lateral" aspect of the extremities. Functionally, too, these interior-exteriorly related Coupled Channels are under the governance of one of the five Elements, e.g., the Lung and Large Intestine Channels both belong to the Element Metal. These relationships have an important bearing on the diagnosis and treatment of diseases according to the principle of traditional Chinese medicine.

Jing-Luo: This is the Chinese term for the system of Channels and collaterals. The postulation of their existence is called the "Jing-Luo theory". This is one of the basic concepts on which the theory and practice of acupuncture is built.

Jing-Well points: The extreme points of the Channels located on the fingers and toes. They are used mainly in the treatment of acute emergencies like shock, coma and cardiorespiratory depression. The point Renzhong (Du 26.), the last skin point on the Du Channel, is one of the more useful points for this purpose.

Jing-Qi: The vital energy flowing in the Channels.

Ko cycle: ("subjugative cycle", or "Five Point Star cycle"). This is a Five Element relationship where each Element in turn subjugates another in a definite order. The sequence of subjugation is Fire-Metal-wood-Earth-Water. This may be understood as Fire melting Metal, Metal (an axe) cutting Wood (trees); Wood (trees) overlying the Earth, the Earth stopping Water, and Water putting out Fire. These symbolic relationships are imputed to the five sets of paired Organs and are used for the purposes of diagnosis and for selection of acupuncture points in traditional Chinese medicine.

Laser therapy: A new method of acupuncture therapy using a laser-beam instead of needle to stimulate the acupuncture points.

Laws of Acupuncture: This refers to the Four Laws of traditional Chinese acupuncture which form the basis of the diagnosis and selection of points. These Four Laws are: 1) the Mother-Son Law; 2) the Noon-Midnight Law; 3) the Husband-Wife Law; and 4) the Theory of the Five Elements.

Luo-Connecting points: Acupuncture points where connections exist between interior-exterior related Yin and Yang Channels. There is a Luo-Connecting point on each of the Fourteen Channels, the (Spleen Channel has two such points), making a total of 15 Luo-Connecting points.

Manipulation of the needle: The art of moving the needle after insertion in order to cause further stimulation at the acupuncture points. Three chief methods used are: I) rotation; ii) lifting and thrusting; and iii) a combination of rotation and lifting and thrusting. The art of manipulation is best learnt under the guidance of a trained acupuncturist. The same effects may be obtained electrically. This is known as electrostimulation of a point.

Midline Channels: These are the two unpaired Channels, the Ren and Du Channels.

Mother-Son Law: This is one of the Four Laws of traditional Chinese acupuncture. In the sequence of the flow of vital energy (Qi) in the Twelve Paired Channels, a Channel is called "mother" in its relationship to the Channel which immediately succeeds it, the latter being called the "son". The sequence of energy is as follows: Lung—Large Intestine.—Stomach—Spleen—Heart—Small Intestine—Urinary Bladder—Kidney—Pericardium—Sanjiao—Gall Bladder—Liver and back to—Lung. If the flow of vital energy is blocked or hindered from circulating freely, an abnormal surplus may develop in one Channel; a corresponding deficiency in the Channel which succeeds it; and perhaps in other Channels as well. This is disease, and the whole organism may be affected. In order to restore the balance, the Channel which is deficient is strengthened by stimulating it so that it draws more energy from the Channel which precedes it, i.e., the mother, (just as a son is nourished by his mother). The same principle applies to the flow of vital energy between the internal Organs in accordance with the Theory of the Five Elements.

Motor Gate Theory: A neurophysiological explanation of the phenomenon of late motor recovery in paralytic disorders following the use of acupuncture.

Moxibustion: A method of Chinese medicine where disease is treated by directly or indirectly heating the acupuncture points by burning "moxas" made from the dried leaves of the plant artemesia vulgaris. "Mogusa" (pronounced "moxa") is the Japanese name of this plant which means "burning herb".

Mu points: There are certain acupuncture points on the front of the trunk which often become painful or tender when there is disease of the pertaining Organ. This phenomenon is useful diagnostically as well as therapeutically. These points are included in the category of what are known as "Alarm points" and are often used in combination with a similar set of Alarm points on the back of the trunk (the "Shu points" lying on the Urinary Bladder Channel) in the treatment of disease.

Noon-Midnight Law: (Also known as the Midday-Midnight Law) Vital energy (Qi) flows through the Twelve Channels to make a complete cycle every 24 hour. The tide of energy passes through each Channel therefore in a two hour period. Diseases due to a deficiency of a particular Channel are said to be most responsive to treatment by acupuncture at the commencement of this two hour period, as advantage may be taken of the force of the entering tide of energy. It is also believed that by treating a Channel, an effect is registered in the Channel which lies diametrically opposite to it on the so-called "Organ Clock".

Organ Clock: The diurnal rhythm of bio-energy flow as depicted on the organ clock. These clocks were beautifully made with ornamentally marked animal signs representing the twelve hours, one for each of the Twelve Organ Channels. The relationships of the Noon-Midnight Law could be easily read on this clock.

Paired Channels: (Organ Channels). Channels which are bilateral (i.e. present on both sides of the body) are known as Paired Channels. There are twelve Paired Channels, each pair corresponding to one of the twelve internal Organs, and for this reason they are also known as the Organ Channels. The term Paired Channels should not be confused with the term Coupled Channels which refers to pairs of Channels having an exterior-interior relationship with one another, e.g., the Lung and the Large Intestine Channels.

Pertaining Organ: The specific internal Organ to which each of the Twelve Paired Channels is connected and from which the name of the Channel is in fact derived. For example, the pertaining Organ of the Lung Channel is the Lung.

Physiological effects of acupuncture: 1) Analgesia, 2) Sedation. 3) Homeostasis. 4) Enhancement of the immune mechanisms. 5) Motor recovery.

Plum Blossom needle: This is a composite needle consisting of 5 or 7 small points mounted side by side in a holder attached to a long handle. It is also known as the "Five Star needle" or "Seven Star needle" depending on the number of points it carries; and it is sometimes called the "cutaneous needle". It is used to treat young children and old and debilitated persons where the insertion of needles is impractical or inadvisable. The method is to tap the skin surface of the area being treated; the tapping being light, medium or heavy according to the disease condition, the patient's constitution and the area being treated. Tapping is performed along the course of the Channels according to their therapeutic properties and those of the points on them, particularly the points of the Urinary Bladder Channel on the back of the trunk which treat the related internal Organs. It is especially effective in soft tissue disorders and certain skin diseases like neurodermatitis where the tapping is performed on the affected area.

Point-injection therapy: A form of acupuncture therapy recently developed in the People's Republic of China where certain substances like distilled water, vitamins, analgesics and placental extracts are injected into acupuncture points, thus providing both physical and chemical stimulation of the acupuncture point.

Press needle: (Embedding needle). A small needle which is plastered onto the skin at an acupuncture point in order to give continuous stimulation between treatment sessions. The ear is a commonly used site for press needles.

Prismatic needle: see under "Three-edged needle".

P.S.C.: Propagated Sensation along the Channels, or the phenomenon of the radiation of acupuncture sensations along a Channel.

Pulse diagnosis: The traditional diagnostic using the radial pulses of both arms. Each pulse is divided into three segments, each segment having a deep and a superficial pulse. Thus there are a total of twelve pulses, six on each wrist. Each of these twelve pulses is related to a specific internal Organ. A disease of an internal Organ is reflected in the corresponding pulse. Pulse diagnosis is a subjective art which can obviously be acquired only after years of training under a traditional acupuncturist who is thoroughly conversant with its practice. Even in the People's Republic of China there are very few adepts of this art today. (Hence it is advisable to be wary of the claims of those who say they are practicing pulse diagnosis after attending a few week-end courses in acupuncture.)

Qi: The Chinese term for the primal energy which pervades the entire Universe. As applied to the human organism, it refers mainly to the energy circulating in the Channels (Jing-Qi). As in the Universe, so in the human body, Qi influences the interaction of Yin and Yang and the relationship between the Five Elements. Disease therefore is due to the inadequate circulation or lack of Qi, or its imbalance within the organism. The body carries a certain amount of Qi as birth; it is depleted by the daily activities of living; it is augmented by the intake of food and air. The absence of Qi is death.

Regular Channels: The Channels which are commonly or regularly used in the practice of body acupuncture. There are 14 Regular Channels comprising the Twelve Paired Channels and the Two Unpaired Midline Channels called the Ren and Du Channels. The 14 Regular Channels are often simply called "the Fourteen Channels".

Sheng cycle: ("Generative cycle"). This is a Five Element relationship where each Element in turn generates or creates another Element in a definite order. The generative sequence is Fire—Earth—Metal—Water—Wood. This may be understood as Fire resulting in ashes or Earth, the Earth containing and bringing forth Metal, Metal generating Water (this is not easily explainable), Water producing Wood by means of plant growth, and Wood making Fire. These symbolic relationships are imputed to the five sets of paired Organs and are used for the purposes of diagnosis and selection of points in traditional Chinese medicine.

Shi diseases: Generally, the acute diseases, e.g., toothache, an acute attack of bronchial asthma or, in terms of traditional Chinese medicine, diseases of an "excessive activity". In such diseases, the "Xie" or reducing (sedation) method of needle manipulation is used, i.e., where the stimulation is strong or forceful.

Sieqi: The Chinese term for disease factors which may be extrinsic or intrinsic. See under "Diseases" (causative factors)

Stimulation: The activation of an acupuncture point by the precise manipulation of the needle in order to achieve certain effects, mainly tonification by applying the "Bu" method of stimulation and sedation by applying the "Xie" method. Stimulation can also be obtained electrically.

Swift insertion of needles: The art of inserting needles with the swiftest possible speed. By using this method the pain the felt on inserting is considerably reduced or even eliminated. (In contradistinction to this, the Chinese barefoot doctors employ a slow insertion method.)

Three-edged needle: (Prismatic needle). A needle which is used to cause bleeding as a form of therapy in certain diseases. It is used with a quick pricking method at the Jing-Well points in treating conditions like shock, coma and cardiorespiratory depression, and with the slow pricking method at points like Chize (Lu. 5.) and Weizhong (U.B. 40.) in treating certain chronic conditions.

Un-numbered Extraordinary points: Recently discovered acupuncture points. Some of them are said to be highly effective for certain disorders, but these claims await confirmation. (Meanwhile they will remain un-numbered.)

Wu-Hsing: The Chinese term for the Five Elements.

Xi-Cleft point: A point which has the specific property of being able to treat acute diseases of the pertaining Organ and its

Channel. For example, the point Liangqiu (St. 34.) is effective in treating acute stomach disorders like acute gastroenteritis, vomiting, nausea, morning sickness. Altogether there are 16 such points—one for each of the Twelve Paired Channels, and one each in four of the Extraordinary Channels: Yinwel, Yangwel, Yinchiao and Yangchiao.

Xie method: The reducing method of applying needle stimulation of an acupuncture point to disperse an excess of vital energy (Qi). This is also known as the sedation method of stimulation and is used in Shi diseases. (Opposite of the Bu method).

Xu diseases: Generally the chronic diseases, or in terms traditional Chinese medicine, diseases of a "deficient activity" nature. In such diseases the "Bu" or reinforcing (tonification) method of needle manipulation is used, i.e., where the stimulation is mild.

Yin-Yang: These are the negative and positive factors in the Universe which activate Qi or vital energy. The term is also used to denote the relativity of all phenomena and of all concepts of the human mind. The Chinese ideograph for Yang depicts the sunny side of the hill while the symbol for Yin shows the harder side of the hill. The Qi in the human organism is also categorized into Yin and Yang according to the nature of the energy flow through each Channel. By inserting needles specific acupuncture points it is possible to restore any imbalance in the Yin-Yang nature of the energy flow, or in other words, to restore homeostasis. This is the basis of all acupuncture therapy.

Yuan-Source point: A point on each of the Twelve Channels located near the wrist or ankle which helps to treat chronic or subacute disorders of that Channel or its pertaining Organ.

Zang-Fu Theory: The division of the 12 Organs into Zang ("solid") Organs and Fu ("hollow") Organs. The Zang Organs are Yin in nature while the Fu Organs are Yang. There are 6 Zang and 6 Fu Organs. Each Zang Organ is coupled to a Fu Organ and each set of Zang-Fu Organs belongs to one of the Five Elements:-

Spleen (Zang) and Stomach (Fu) belong to the Element Earth; Lung (Zang) and Large Intestine (Fu) belong to the Element Metal;

Kidney (Zang) and Urinary Bladder (Fu) belong to the Element Water; Liver (Zang) and Gall bladder (Fu) belong to the Element Wood; Heart (Zang) and Small intestine (Fu) belong to the Element Fire; Pericardium (Zang) and Sanjiao (Fu) also belong to the Element Fire.

■

APPENDIX I

APPENDIX ON COMPLICATIONS

ACUPUNCTURE NEEDLES AS A CAUSE OF BACTERIAL ENDOCARDITIS: Reported by D.B. Jefferys. et al. *British Medical Journal Vol.* 287, 30th July 1983:—

The incidence of infective endocarditis has remained unchanged over the past 40 years. Acupuncture is cited as a possible new way of inducing endocarditis in "at risk" patient. The authors report the development of bacterial endocarditis after insertion and manipulation of acupuncture needles.

The case described was a 57 year old woman with a prosthetic Starr-Edwards valve in the mitral position. She presented with a 10-day history of symptoms suggestive of endocarditis; a diagnosis which was confirmed following furuher investigations and blood cultures. Treatment with antibiotics was started and full recovery is reported. Eighteen days before presentation, acupuncture needles has been inserted in both ears, in an effort to stop her smoking. These needles has remained *in situ* for one week and had then been replaced by a second set, after which she had complained of irrititation and discharge from the skin around the needle.

The authors discuss the advisability of antibiotic prophylaxis on patients with cardiac lesions who wish to have acupuncture therapy.

CIRCADIAN RHYTHMS:

The pineal gland is an endocrine organ which affects the brain and behavior. Since the discovery of the pineal hormone melatonin 20 years ago, the pineal gland has become an important tool in studying neurotransmitters, receptors and circadian rhythms.

Melatonin production is influenced by the light-dark cycle and is inhibited by light. Its secretion pattern display a circadian rhythm, with the lowest concentration during the day and peak levels at about 2 a.m. Due to this fluctuation, melatonin can serve as a marker for biological rhythms.

Results from recent studies of depressive patients show a disturbance in melatonin secretion. These patients had significantly lower melatonon levels at 2 a.m. than did normal controls. The disturbances in melatonin secretion did not normalize, even when the patients underwent clinical remission. Also, disturbances were evident in subjects with a long disease history, but at the time of the testing were free of clinical symptoms. Depressive patients also suppress nocturnal melatonin more readily in response to light than normal subjects. Furthermore, patients with low melatonin levels show a higher frequency of relatives displaying clinical manifestations. These results suggest that melatonin levels indicate a predisposition to depression.

Discovering etiological markers, such as melatonin patterns, brings the clinical researcher closer to discovering better ways of treating specific depressive disorders.

Patients may get worse with acupuncture treatment if their biological rhythms are not congruent; or they may result in a bizarre responses to acupuncture therapy.

Radioimmunoassay allows melatonin to be measured after their extraction from serum, saliva and urine. The sensitive assay (2 pg/ml) is based on a specific rabbit anti-melatonin antiserum and a Bolton-Hunter iodinated melatonin-tracer, with a pre-incubation and a solid phase separation. Melatonin levels in depressive patients may show a shift in melatonin rhythm, the peak of the circadian rhythm occurring too early or too late. Abnormal serum melatonin concentrations have also been found in schizophrenic patients. Changes in melatonin synthesis have been observed in cancer patients. In women with mammary-carcinoma, decreased melatonin concentrations in serum and urine were found at night, whereas normal values were obtained during the day. In men with prostatic carcinoma, too, the nocturnal serum melatonin concentrations are lower than normal.

MELATONIN RADIO IMMUNOASSAY

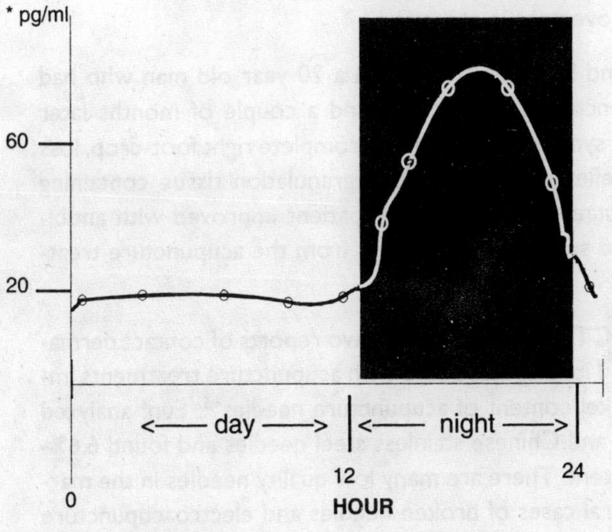

day/night rhythm

SPINAL CORD INJURY: Shiraishi and co-worker's report a case of a 30 year old man who had received the "*okibari*" procedure for migraine headaches in which about 20 acupuncture needles were inserted in the cervical and occipital areas and then cut off at the skin surface to be retained permanently. Six months later he fell on some staires striking the back of his neck and within six hours he had

1 pg/ml= picograms per milliliter.

developed a cervical myelopathy, with right hand and left leg weakness and loss of pain and temperature sensation on the right side below the level of[2] C 4. Computerized tomography revealed that one of the needles had pierced the spinal cord at the level of* C 2. It was removed surgically but the patients neurological symptoms were largely unchanged, even after one year.

Kondo et al[2] present a 62 year old woman who developed loss of pain and temperature sensation on the right side two years after acupuncture treatment for a stiff neck. Two years later, a broken acupuncture needle was found penetrating the spinal cord at the level of the C1-C2 interspace. Surgical removal was followed by moderate improvement in sensation.

Hadden and Swanson[3] report on a 20 year old man who had received acupuncture for back pain and a couple of months later developed root symptoms (including a complete right foot-drop, loss of ankle jerk reflexes, and a positive granulation tissue containing *Staphylococcus aureus* organisms. The patient improved with antibiotic therapy and surgical infection was from the acupuncture treatments received.

CONTACT DERMATITIS: Two reports of contact dermatitis with marked itching associated with acupuncture treatments implicated the nickel content of acupuncture needles[4,5]. Eun[6] analyzed several Korean and Chinese stainless steel needles and found 6.6%-8.5% nickel content. There are many low quality needles in the market today. Several cases of broken needles and electroacupuncture burns due to sub-standard needles have been reported. Local reaction may occur due to the alcohol rubbed on skin or due to strands of cotton-wool penerating the tissues with the needle.

INFECTIONS:

Hepatitis B: Boxall[7] reported 29 serologically proven cases of hepatitis B traced to an acupuncture clinic in Birmingham, England.

---

2 C= Cervical

The acupuncturist used hollow syringe-type needles which accumulate blood (and virus) more easily within the shaft than solid needles. Apparently, the needles were reused without even being cleaned between patients.

Four cases of hepatitis B were reported and traced to acupuncture treatment received at a chiropractic clinic in Florida in 1980.[8] During the period when hepatitis was spread, the clinic had not been sterilizing their needles by autoclave (as they had done on other occasions); but were soaking them in a 1:750 solution of benzalkonium chloride.

Staphylococcal Sepsis: Two cases of fatal staphylococcal sepsis were reported by Pierik[9]. Both of these after acupuncture therapy for arthritis; and in both cases joint aspirates and blood cultures grew hemolytic *Staphylococcus aureus.*

AIDS and Acupuncture: There exist no reported cases of acupuncture transmission of the virus HTLV III (Human T Lymphotropic Virus type III) which is the etiological agent in the Acquired Immune Deficiency Syndrome (AIDS)[10]. In addition, no association of AIDS due to acupuncture is reported (by accidental puncture).

The higher incidence in intravenous drug abusers via shared needles highlights the potential for acupuncture to spread AIDS through inadequate needle cleanliness.

The Center for Disease Control[3] has published guidelines for those who provide dental care to patients with AIDS.[11] These include: wearing gloves, mask and protective eyewear when performing dental or oral surgical procedures; and sterilizing all instruments coming into contact with patients. For acupuncturists we would adapt those recommendations to include wearing gloves, mask and gown (as for hepatitis B), and sterilizing all needles. Protective eyewear is probably not necessary. Further, we prefer disposable needles or at least needles isolated to the exclusive use of the patient with AIDS

---

3 Washington D.C., U.S.A.

or suspected AIDS. Davis and Knapp have outlined additional recommendations for dentists.[12]

The existence of devastating infections diseases, some of which we are only beginning to understand, dictates caustion in the practice of acupuncture. Careful attention to hand-washing, skin cleanliness and the use of sterilized disposable needles are recommended. When disposable needles are not available, it must be kept in mind that needles require cleaning prior to sterilization.

Plum blossom needles and other non-metal devices must be sterilized using a gas such as ethylene oxide at lower temperatures for longer periods. Immune compromised patients (e.g. those with AIDS, diabetes mellitus, those on steroid medications or cancer chemotherapeutic agents, etc.) require special attention to skin disinfection and disposable or exclusive-use needles; and in some cases wearing sterile gloves may be appropriate.

RADIATION:

Patients who have been exposed to radiation respond poorly to acupuncture. They are also more prone to needle injury. (Moxibustion is claimed to neutralize some of the radiation effects. Reports from Hiroshima and Nagasaki after the atomic bomb seem to support this view).

REFERENCES:

1. **Shiraishi S. Goto I. Kuroiwa Y. et *al:*** Spinal cord injury as a complication of acupuncture. *Neurology.* Aug. 1979, 29: 1180-1182.

2. **Kondo A. Tsunemaro K. Ishikawa J. et *al:*** Injury to the spinal cord produced by acupuncture needle. *Surg Neurol.* Feb. 1979, 11: 155-156.

3. **Hadden W. A. Swanson A. J. G.:** Spinal infection caused by acupuncture mimicking a prolapsed intervertebral disc. *J. Bone Joint Surg.* Apr. 1982, 64-A (4): 624-626.

4. **Romaguera C. Grimalt F:** Contact dermatitis from a permanent acupuncture needle. *Contect Derm.* May, 1981. 7(3): 156-157.

5. **Romaguera C. Grimalt F:** Nickel dermatitis from acupuncture needles. *Contact* Derm. May, 1979, 5 (3): 195.

6. **Eun H. C:** Nickel in acupuncture needles. *Contact Derm.* Nov. 1981. 7 (6): 334.

7. **Boxall E. H.:** Acupuncture hepatitis in the West Midlands. 1977. *J. Med Virol.* 1978, 2: 377-379.

8. **Hepatitis B associated with acupuncture**: Florida. *Morbidity Mortality Weekly Rep. Jan.* 16, 1981, 30 (l): 1-3.

9. **Pierik M. G.:** Fatal staphylococcal septicemia following acupuncture: Report of two cases. *RI Med. J.* Jun. 1982, 65: 251 – 253.

10. **Masur H. Macher A. M.:** Acquired immune deficiency syndrome (AIDS). in mandell, Douglas, Bennett: *Principles and Practice of Infections Diseases.* New York, John Wiley & Sons. 1985 pp 1670-1673.

11. **Acquired immune deficiency syndrome (AIDS):** Precautions for healthcare workers and allied professionals. *Morbidity Mortality Weekly Rep.* Sept. 2, 1983. 32 (34): 450-451.

12. **Davis D. R. Knapp J. F.:** The significance of AIDS to dentists and dental practice. *J Prosthetic Dentistry.* Nov. 1984, 52 (5): 736-738.

■

APPENDIX II

TAI YUN – THE GREAT 60 YEAR CHINESE CALENDAR

"Medicine is subtle and no one knows most of its secrets. The way of Medicine is so vast and its scope is as immeasurable as the height of Heavens and the depths of the four seas.

—Su Wen, Chapter 78

The Great 60 Year Cycle is based on the concepts of the ten 'Celestial Stems' and the twelve 'Terrestrial Branches'. It is based on ideas formulated by the mathematician-philosopher Ching Fang (circa 45. B. C.) and others, and was integrated into the I Ching during the Hun period, and by the tenth centrury it was fully discussed and accepted in all the important medical classics and intimately related with the practice of medical horoscopy, diagnosis, therapy and prognosis[1].

These concepts are based on the premise that all human affairs are affected by and related to cosmic and planetary influences. The celestial stems and terrestrial branches describe the prevailing extrinsic influences on the human organism at any given period, and the manner in which the intrinsic energies of the living body respond to them.

An organism is affected spiritually, emotionally, physically and

1 The Yellow Emperor's Classic mentions these rhythms in depth.

aesthetically by climatic and other extrinsic changes which alter its specific hourly, daily, lunar, monthly, seasonal and yearly inborn rhythms. Every person has his or her own particular cycle. Every living organism and each cell has its own rhythm. These are activated at the moment of conception, and manifest as positive and negative (sine wave like) phases of activity throughout life.

The daily organismic rhythm is well-known as the circadian cycle, the body's biological clock. Traditional acupuncture describes the ebb and flow of Yin and Yang energies. Yang is most active in the morning and reaches its maximum at noon; then a slow change into Yin, which maximizes at midnight and reverts slowly back to Yang by morning. The 24 hour cycle of energy, with the energy peak in the Lungs between 3 to 5 a.m. and progressing through the twelve channels in a regular order through the day is known as the Noon-Midnight Law or the Organ Clock.

Modern research has parallels to this in that hormones, enzymes and the activity of the immune system follow parallel rhythmic patterns. Corticosterone and plasma ACTH[2] peak at noon, fall off during the afternoon to a minimum at midnight, and then slowly rises again. They operate in this manner by positive and negative feedback mechanisms and, also, *via* biochemical modulators. The phenomenon of 'jet-lag', occurs when the circadian rhythms are disturbed. This is a physiological dysrhythmia. The secretion, of melatonin by the pineal gland is said to follow a diurnal rhythm.

The Chinese observations of the rhythmic effects of the moon have been summed up with extraordinary clarity by Yen Su's Hai Chao Tu Lun (circa 1030 A.D.) as follows:

"Tao's forces breathe in and out. The sky, following these forces expands and contracts, while the tide going and coming in the seas follows the sky and flows and ebbs. The sun is the mother of the double Yang, and Yin is born of Yang, the whole is subject to the sun; and since the moon is the essence of the Yin, and water is also Yin,

2 ACTH = Adrenocorticotrophic hormone.

the tide follows the motions of the moon as well. For this reason, following the sun and responding to the moon, (corresponding to the motions of the Yin and yet subject to the Yang), the tide is at its highest at new and full moon, contracts as the moon waxes or wanes, being at its lowest at the first and last quarter, and grows just before full and new moon. This is the reason why there are major and minor tides.".

The monthly (lunar) rhythms have a relationship to certain diseases, mood changes, menstruation and pregnancy. Seasonal biological variations are based on the 5-Element relationships, such as the increased activity of the liver in the spring, the heart in the summer, the spleen in the long summer, the lungs in the autumn and the kidneys in the winter. Variations in pulse qualities associated with seasonal changes also takes place. These are physiological variations.

The effects of the extrinsic rhythms of the universe continuously modify the state of the individual's own rhythms at any particular time. The response to treatment may, therefore, vary correspondingly.

This is why the effects from treatment will vary from day to day and from patient to patient. The same patient may respond more readily on some days than on others.

The overall dominant cosmic influence on a person is the specific year within the Chinese 60 year cycle; next the seasonal influence affects everyone and everything. The influence of the specific day and time of day on the individual is integrated with the yearly and seasonal influences.

The over-riding cosmic influences are the ten celestial stems. They are the influences of Heaven upon Earth; they are Yang by nature. The energies with which they interact are called the twelve Terrestrial Branches, which are Yin by nature.

The Chinese names of the ten Celestial Sterms and the twelve Terrestrial Branches are:

10 Celestial Stems	12 Terrestrial Branches	
Jia	Zi	(Rat)
Yi	Chou	(Ox)
Bing	Yin	(Tiger)
Ding	Mao	(Hare)
Wu	Chen	(Dragon)
Ji	Si	(Snake)
Geng	Wu	(Horse)
Xin	Wei	(Sheep)
Ren	Shen	(Monkey)
Gui	Yu	(Rooster)
	Xu	(Dog)
	Hai	(Pig)

When Buddhism first came to China during the reign of Emperor Ashoka of India. it integrated with Taoism and Confucianism. According to Neo-Taostic legend, as the Lord Buddha lay dying he summoned all the animals. The first twelve to arrive being, in order of appearance, the Rat, Ox, Tiger, Hare, Dragon, Snake, Horse, Sheep, Monkey, Rooster, Dog and Pig. As a reward they were immortalized in the 12 terrestrial branches.

In the Great 60 Year Cycle the Stems and Branches are both combined to form years. They give the overall quality of life of that year.

The Stems are the celestial energies, and the Branches are the reacting energies of the earth; each year being characterized by the combination of the two.

The present cycle commenced with a Jia Zi year in 1984.

THE PRESENT GRAT SIXITY YEAR CYCLE
(Commenced 1984)

				Jia E	Yi M	Bing Wa	Ding Wo	Wu F	Ji E	Geng M	Shin Wa	Ren Wo	Gui F
Rat	Zi	Shao Yin	F Emperor	1984		1996		2008		2020		2032	
Ox	Chou	Tai Yin	E		1985		1997		2009		2021		2033
Tiger	Yin	Shao Yang	F Minister	2034		1986		1998		2010		2022	
Hare	Mao	Yang Mind	M		2035		1987		1999		2011		2023
Dragon	Chen	Tai Yang	Wa	2024		2036		1988		2000		2012	
Snake	Si	Jueh Yin	Wo		2025		2037		1989		2001		2013
Horse	Wu	Shao Yin	F Emperor	2014		2026		2038		1990		2002	
Sheep	Wei	Tai Yin	E		2015		2027		2039		1991		2003
Monkey	Shen	Shao Yang	F Minister	2004		2016		2028		2040		1992	
Rooster	Yu	Yang Ming	M		2005		2017		2029		2041		1993
Dog	Xu	Tai Yang	Wa	1994		2006		2018		2030		2042	
Pig	Hai	Jueh Yin	Wo		1995		2007		2019		2031		2041

12 Branches from Earth F - Fire; E - Earth; M - Metal; Wa - Water; Wo - Wood.

The Celestial Stems determine the directions, and the Terrestrial Branches the Qi energies. The Yang of Heaven is the basic motivating force while the Yin Branches of Earth are the resultant energies springing from that motivation. The basic energetic force pattern of the specific year is, therefore, determined mainly by the Celestial Stem of that year.

In the monthly cycle, the stems are the days and the branches are the twelve divisions of the 24 hours, (corresponding to the 12 visceral channels and internal organs[3]).

Man possesses the consciousness to ponder about himself and about his environment. Looking inwards the ancient sages discovered the Tao within; looking outwards, they perceived the firmament (skies) and the manifestation of the Tao throughout the whole universe. Ancient man realized that he and the Tao were one.

Looking into the heavens above, the ancient Chinese astronomers perceived a fixed, "immovable" star – the Polestar. This was the center of the Tao. Throughout the year, the other constellations moved majestically in various directions. During their progress the climatic changes through the seasons, and the changes in the Yin Yang balance (which is the essence of the Tao) occurred. Once in every sixty years the Moon, the Earth, the Sun and the Pole star are in alignment, and then the Chinese calender commences again.

By measuring the length of the shadows cast by the sun, the solstices were determined. The movements of the stars by night determined the sidereal year in ancient China. These were very precise methods of determining the exact beginnings of the different seasons. The solstices and equinoxes marked the middle of the seasons. The Chinese astronomers even observed the comet Halley two centuries before Christ.

The Chinese New Year is celebreated on the appearance of the second new moon after the winter solstice, and occurs between 21st January and 19th February of the Gregorian (modern) calendar[4].

3 The Organ Clock.

4 The Buddhist (Sri Lanka), the Hindu, the Jewish and the Moslem calendars are also still in use among the respective religious and ethnic groups.

The months of the year have specific names of an animal to exemplify its nature and the character of that month.

These are also the names of the twelve Terrestrial Branches.

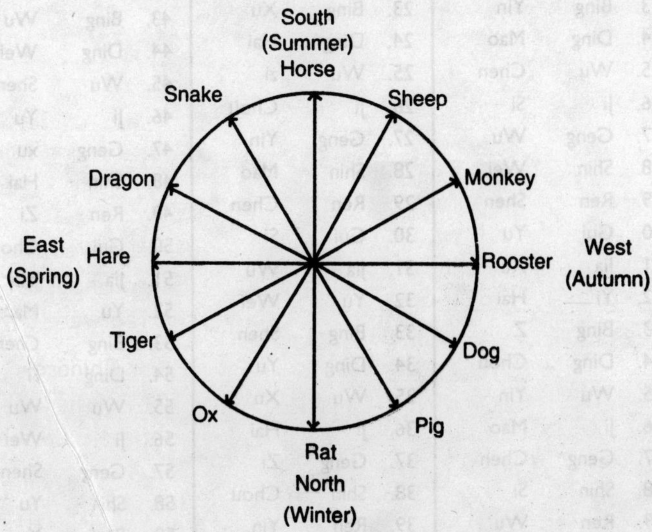

Man is the resultant of the constant interaction of the energies of Heaven and Earth. Just as there are inherent biological rhythms within man responding to daily and yearly rhythms, so the interplay between the Celestial Stems and the Terrestrial Branches occurs on a constantly varying spectrum. There is the daily effect upon the channel varying spectrum. There is the daily effect upon the channel and Organ energies in the 24-hour cycle. There is also a seasonal effect *via* the cycle of the months.

By serially pairing, we arrive at the following names of each of the 60 years in a cycle:

NAMES OF THE 60 YEARS OF A CYCLE

Stem	Branch	Stem	Branch	Stem	Branch
1. Jia	Zi	21. Jia	Shen	41. Jia	Chen
2. Yi	Chou	22. Yu	Yu	42. Yi	Si
3. Bing	Yin	23. Bing	Xu	43. Bing	Wu
4. Ding	Mao	24. Ding	Hai	44. Ding	Wei
5. Wu	Chen	25. Wu	zi	45. Wu	Shen
6. Ji	Si	26. Ji	Chou	46. Ji	Yu
7. Geng	Wu	27. Geng	Yin	47. Geng	xu
8. Shin	Wei	28. Shin	Mao	48. Shin	Hai
9. Ren	Shen	29. Ren	Chen	49. Ren	Zi
10. Gui	Yu	30. Gui	Si	50. Gui	Chou
11. Jia	Xu	31. Jia	Wu	51. Jia	Yin
12. Yi	Hai	32. Yu	Wei	52. Yu	Mao
13. Bing	Z	33. Bing	Shen	53. Bing	Chen
14. Ding	Chou	34. Ding	Yu	54. Ding	Si
15. Wu	Yin	35. Wu	Xu	55. Wu	Wu
16. Ji	Mao	36. Ji	Hai	56. Ji	Wei
17. Geng	Chen	37. Geng	Zi	57. Geng	Shen
18. Shin	Si	38. Shin	Chou	58. Shin	Yu
19. Ren	Wu	39. Ren	Yin	59. Ren	Xu
20. Gui	Wei	40. Gui	Mao	60. Gui	Hai

Sixty combinations occur before The Great 60 Year Cycle repeats itself. This Great Cycle of Sixty deals with the yearly influence. The more detailed characteristics of the year are the environmental influences of the stems and branches of the 5 elements, such as:

Stems:

Wood is Wind	- Is pliable, bends and straightens.
Fire is Heat	- Burns and ascends.
Earth is Humid	- Receives the seeds and gives the crops.
Metal is Dryness	- Responds to the hand of the worker and takes different forms.
Water is Damp	- Crops grow.

Branches:

Jueh Yin	- Wood	- Wind
Shao Yin	- Fire (Emperor)	- Fire
Tai Yin	- Earth	- Dampness
Shao Yang	- Fire (Minister)	- Heat
Yang Ming	- Metal	- Dryness
Tai Yang	- Water	- Cold

The resultant effect is always dependent upon the integration between the Heaven and Earth influences. Although the Stems are the celestial motivating movements, they are also the recipients of the earthly energies. Although, the Branches are the resultant energies of earth, they are also the recipients of the celestial energies. The permutation and combination determines the resultant. One can, therefore, determine the basic character of any particular time of the year on any person with regard to health and disease, fortunes and misfortunes, by summating the Stem and Branch energies.

Heaven is Yang and Earth is Yin, and harmony on earth is the result of the balance between the two forces. If the energy of Heaven should predominate there will be Yang-type disorders; if that of the earth is in excess, then the disorders will be most likely of a Yin-type.

Favourable influences are either identicals or Mother/Son relationships. Unfavourable are Reverse Sheng (Where the Son is strong and the Mother weak), Ko, or Wu (reverse Ko)[1] cycle combinations.

Where there is a deficiency, its specific quality would tend to be affected by those of the preceding and succeeding years. It may also suffer from a weakness on the Ko cycle effect; for example, a weakness of Fire would render it likely to be attacked by the cold of Water, and the year would be cold with little growth. There may be floods, hurricanes, tornadoes and genitourinary disorders, in those who are susceptible.

1 Wu is a serious pathological state, usually incurable.

The 60 Year Tai Yun or the Great Cycle determines basic underlying characteristics for the whole year, but these are modified to a considerable extent by the effects of the seasons, the so called, Chu Yun.

The energies of the five seasons of the year in the 5-Element cycle starts with the Wood of Spring. They then follow an alternative Yang-Yin pattern:

EFFECTS OF SEASONS (CHU YUN)

Yin of Yang	Season	Element	Celestial stems
Yang	Spring	Wood	Jia
Yin			Yin
Yang	Summer	Fire	Bing
Yin			Ding
Yang	Long	Earth	Wu
Yin	Summer		Ji
Yang	Autumn	Metal	Geng
Yin			Xin
Yang	Winter	Water	Ren
Yin			Gui

These are known as 'Host' energies and are unchangeable, being the basic seasonal influences, but they are superimposed upon the fundamental yearly energies and the resultant effects are known as the 'Guest' energies.

The year is governed by the unchanging Great Cycle aspect of that year, and if this is placed in the center one can then assemble around it the seasonal influences.

As with the Great 60 Year Cycle, the ten Celestial Stems of the annual cycle are in their turn balanced by the twelve Terrestrial

SEASONAL INFLUENCES

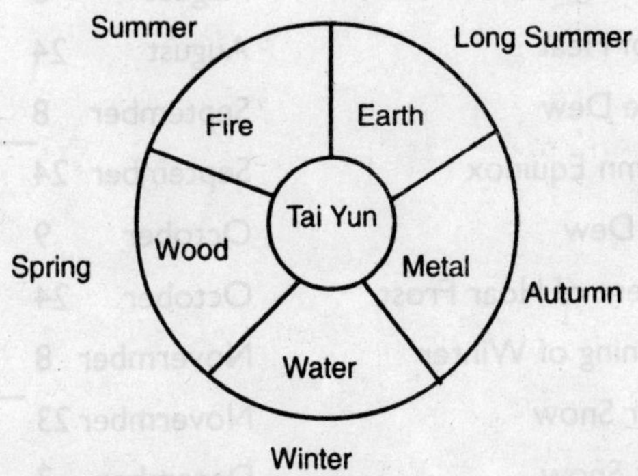

Branches, and these reflect the effect of the celestial movements on the seasonal energies. They are linked to the heavenly cycles by the division of the year into twenty-four 'fortnightly' periods.

Seasonal Variations	Date of Commencement & Divisions		
1. Great Cold	January	21	
2. Beginning of Spring	February	5	I
3. The Rains	February	20	
4. Awakening from Hibernation	March	7	
5. Spring Equinox	March	22	
6. Clear and Bright (weather)	April	6	II Rising
7. Rain on the Grains	April	21	
8. Beginning of Summer	May	6	
9. Lesser Fullness (of grain)	May	22	
10. Grain in Ear	June	7	III
11. Summer Solstice	June	22	

12.	Lesser Heat	July	8	Peak
13.	Great Heat	July	24	
14.	Beginning of Autumn	August	8	
15.	End of Heat	August	24	IV
16.	White Dew	September	8	
17.	Autumn Equinox	September	24	
18.	Cold Dew	October	9	
19.	Descent of Hoar Frost	October	24	V Declining
20.	Beginning of Winter	Novermber	8	
21.	Lesser Snow	Novermber	23	
22.	Great Snow	December	7	
23.	Winter Solstice	December	22	VI
24.	Lesser Cold	January	6	

These twenty-four periods may be sub-divided into groups of six correlating with the seasonal influences:

Division	Chiao	
I	Jueh Yin	Wood (Wind)
II	Shao Yin	Fire Emperor (Fire)
III	Shao Yang	Fire Minister (Heat)
IV	Tai Yin	Earth (Humidity)
V	Yang Ming	Metal (Dryness)
VI	Yai Yang	Water (Cold)

There are the Host energies of the Terrestrial Branches.

The quality of an year will depend upon the relative balance between the Stems and Branches and the interplay between the Guest and Host energies. The good Host should always be mindful of the wishes of the Guest, and provide the basic amenities on which the Guest may thrive in his domain.

For harmony in the household, the welfare of the Guest should take priority. Harmony between Guest and Host is essential for food health. If the Host is Water energy and the Guest energy Fire, then on the Ko cycle the Host will have friction with the Guest and disharmony will ensue. If the Guest checks the Host, (this is called 'Torment of Heaven') imbalance results and a tendency to meteorological disturbances and inclement weather will ensue in that year. Extrinsic causes of disease will operate on those who are susceptible.

Favourable combinations are where Host and Guest are in a Mother-Son relationship. Here one feeds the other on the Sheng cycle. If they should be both of the same sign it is not particularly unfavourable, but the prevailing conditions are likely to be exaggerated and possibly extreme. Excess disorders are likely. Allergies may also result.

The efficacy of the acupuncture points themselves depend upon the circadian rhythms and the body's daily responses, the actual hourly changes which take place in the ebb and flow of the channel energy.

One techinique of treatment is to reinforce or reduce the energy when it is flowing at its peak hours in a channel, using the specific Horary point.

Animal (Organ)	Hours (Branches)
Zi	23.00-01.00 Hours
Chou	01.00-03.00 Hours
Yin	03.00-05.00 Hours
Mao	05.00-07.00 Hours
Chen	07.00-09.00 Hours
Si	09.00-11.00 Hours
Wu	11.00-13.00 Hours
Wei	13.00-15.00 Hours

Host should be mother and Guest the son (not vice-versa)

Shen	15.00-17.00	Hours
Yu	17.00-19.00	Hours
Xu	19.00-21.00	Hours
Hai	21.00-23.00	Hours

The acupuncturist could also make use of the "opening times" of the 66 command points. (These times are different to the Horary points and times).

The times when the 66 command points are 'open' are named:

Lu11 - Shin-Mao	H9 - Ding-Wei	P9 - Chia-Yu
Lu10 - Ji-Wei	H8 - Yee-Hai	P8 - Ping-Wei
Lu9 - Ding-Hai Shin-Wei	H7 - Chia-Mao Ding-Hai	P7 - Wu-Si Chia-Mao
Lu8 - Ping-Mao	H4 - Shin-Yu	P5 - Geng-Mao
Lu5 - Chia-Wei	H3 - Geng-Chou	P3 - Ren-Chou
LI1 - Geng-Chen	SI1 - Ping-Shen	SJ1 - Gui-Tzu
LI2 - Wo-Shen	SI2 - Yee-Tzu	SJ2 - Yee-Shen
LI3 - Ding-Tzu	SI3 - Ren-Wu	SJ3 - Ding-Wu
LI4 - Geng-Shen	SI4 - Ding-Tzu	SJ4 - Ren-Wu
LI5 - Yee-Chen	SI5 - Geng-Shu	SJ6 - Ji-Chen
LI11 - Ren-Shu	SI8 - Ji-Yin	SJ10 - Shin-Yin
St45 - Wo-Wu	UB67 - Ren-Yin	GB44 - Chia-Shu
St44 - Ping-Shu	UB66 - Geng-Wu	GB43 - Ren-Chen
St43 - Yee-Yin	UB65 - Wu-Shu	GB41 - Geng-Shen
St42 - Wu-Shu	UB64 - Ren-Wu	GB40 - Yee-Yin
St41 - Ren-Shen	UB60 - Ding-Yin	GB38 - Ji-Tzu
St36 - Shin-Tzu	UB54 - Yee-Wu	GB34 - Ding-Chen
Sp1 - Ji-Si	K1 - Gui-Hai	Liv1 - Yee-Yu
Sp2 - Ding-Yu	K2 - Gui-Hai	Liv2 - Chia-Chou
Sp3 - Ping-Chou Ji-Yu	K3 - Ji-Yu Chia-Mao	Liv3 - Shin-Wei Ping-Chou
Sp5 - Chia-Si	K7 - wu-Chou	Liv4 - Ji-Hai
Sp9 - Shin-Hai	K10 - Ping-Si	Liv8 - Wu-Mao

A CHINESE HOROSCOPE

THE YUN QI HSUEH COMPUTER

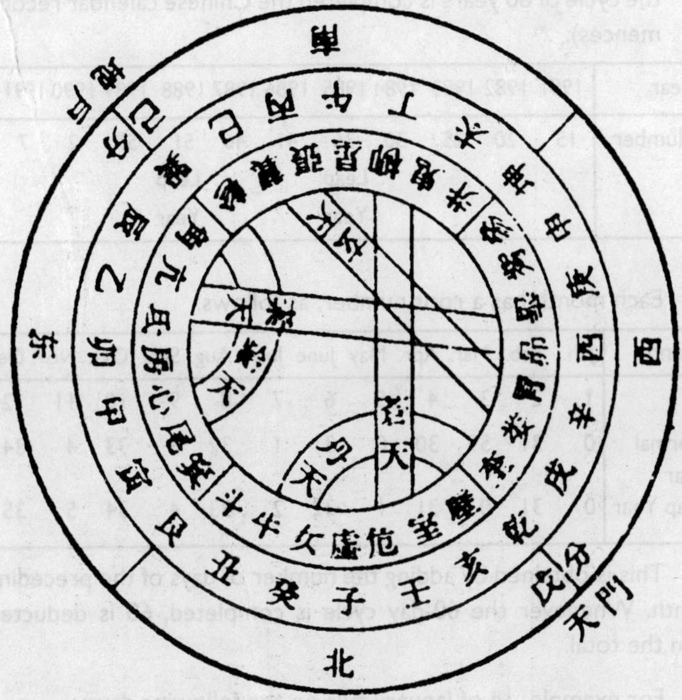

Example of a diagram in the complicated medieval computus for determining optimal times for acupuncture and moxa in accordance with the recurrent cyclical changes in the human body (circadian rhythms) and the recurrent celestial-terrestial permutations and combinations. This was the doctrine of *wu yun liu chhi,* the cyclical changes of the Five Elements and the Six Qi.

— **After Joseph Needham.**

In relation to the current (Gregorian) calendar the Chinese calendar may be worked out as follows:

(a) Each year has a 'root number' for the Stem and Branch of that year. This number increases by a factor of 5 for each year, except for a year, following a Leap Year, when 6 is added. (When the cycle of 60 years is completed the Chinese calendar recommences).

Year	1981	1982	1983	1984	1985	1986	1987	1988	1989	1990	1991
Number	15	20	25	30	36 Leap Year	41	46	51 Leap Year	57	2	7

(b) Each month has a root number, as follows:

Month	Jan.	Feb.	Mar.	Apr.	May	June	July	Aug.	Sep.	Oct.	Nov.	Dec
	1	2	3	4	5	6	7	8	9	10	11	12
Normal Year	0	31	59	30	0	31	1	32	3	33	4	34
Leap Year	0	31	0	31	1	32	2	33	4	34	5	35

This is obtained by adding the number of days of the preceding month. Whenever the 60-day cycle is completed, 60 is deducted from the total.

For example, 1st of January falls on the following days:

	Year		Day	(Number)
	1987	January 1st	Geng-Shu	(47)
Leap Year	1988	"	Yee-Mao	(52)
	1989	"	Shin-Yu	(58)
	1990	"	Ping-Yin	(3)
	1991	"	Shin-Wei	(8)
Leap Year	1992	"	Ping-Tzu	(13)

	1993	"	Ren-Wu	(19)
	1994	"	Ding-Hai	(24)
	1995	"	Ren-Shen	(29)
Leap Year	1996	"	Ding-Yu	(34)
	1997	"	Gui-Mao	(40)
	1998	"	Wo-Shen	(45)
	1999	"	Gui-Chou	(50)
Leap Year	2000	"	Wu-Wu	(55)
	2001	"	Chia-Tzu	(1)
	2002	"	Ji-Si	(6)
	2003	"	Chia-Shu	(11)
	2004	"	Ji-Mao	(16)

To assess the effect of external energies upon a patient, one needs to elucidate more about the individual himself. The innate strengths and weaknesses will determine the strength and degree of the response to therapy. These innate weaknesses, otherwise, may be ascertained to a great extent by a study of the astrological make-up. In ancient China, the casting of a horoscope would be considered essential before treatment in any major illness, or of an important patient like the Emperor or a War-Lord, even in a minor illness.

The horoscope is based upon several cycles of energy. The descending order of importance of the cycles of energy are:

1. Sex of the person
2. Year of birth (Stem)
3. Animal Sign of the day of birth and the day of treatment (Branch)
4. Hour of birth
5. Month of birth
6. Country (region) of birth (latitude, longitude)
7. Birth dates of parents.
8. Significant birthmarks
9. Physical deformities
10. Influences from siblings, teachers, friends, enemies

Each year of the Great 60 Year Cycle comes under the rulership of both a Stem and a Branch – the branch gives the governing 'animal' of the year, the Stem the 5-element component. The Branches repeat in a 12-yearly cycle. The person born during each of those years is likely to possess the basic personality characteristics assigned to that particular animal and also the associated 5-element component governing that branch, in that particular year.

Animal	Year[1]
Rat	1912 1924 1936 1948 1960 1972 1984 1996 2008
Ox	1913 1925 1937 1949 1961 1973 1985 1997 2009
Tiger	1914 1926 1938 1950 1962 1974 1986 1998 2010
Hare	1915 1927 1939 1951 1963 1975 1987 1999 2011
Dragon	1916 1927 1940 1952 1964 1976 1988 2000 2012
Snake	1917 1928 1941 1953 1965 1977 1989 2001 2013
Horse	1918 1929 1942 1954 1966 1978 1990 2002 2014
Sheep	1919 1930 1943 1955 1967 1979 1991 2003 2015
Monkey	1920 1931 1944 1956 1968 1980 1992 2004 2016
Rooster	1921 1932 1945 1957 1969 1981 1993 2005 2017
Dog	1922 1933 1946 1958 1970 1982 1994 2006 2018
Pig	1923 1934 1947 1959 1971 1983 1995 2007 2019

With regard to the personal relationship with the healer and the effects of therapy are concerned, there are certain harmonious and inharmonious combinations:

The animals may be in compatible and incompatible groups, as follows:

The triad of Horse, Tiger and Dog seek to serve humanity, are extrovert, impulsive and idealistic. The Sheep, Hare and Pig are aesthetic types, guided by their emotions. They rely on others for leadership, but can tune into their environment and become flexible in

1 Year of birth of a person.

THE TRIANGLES

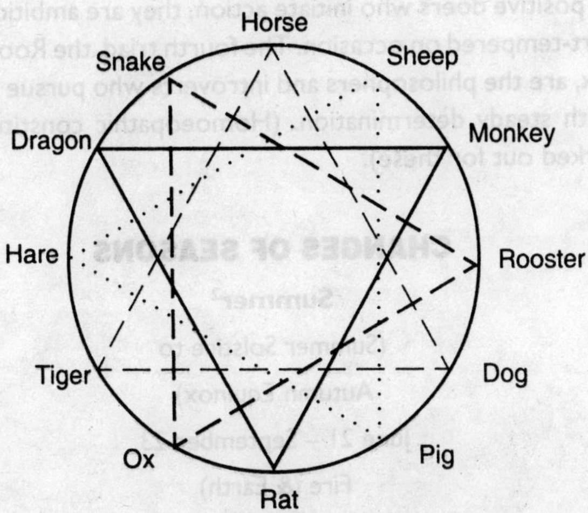

The Four Affinity Triangles (Compatible Groups)

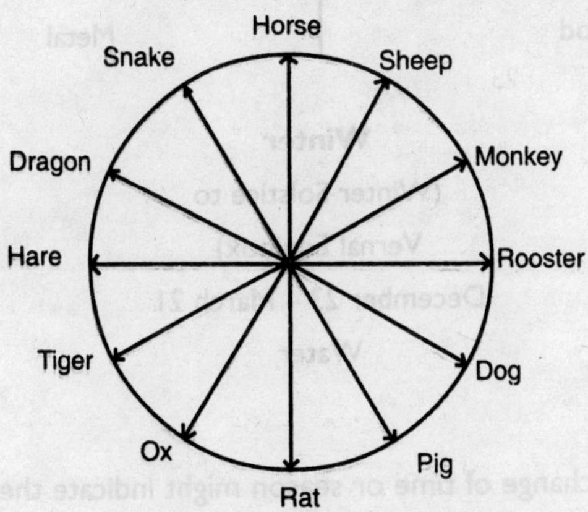

Triangles of Incompatible Groups

their behavior. The Monkey, Dragon and Rat are always restless; always positive doers who initiate action, they are ambitious and can be short-tempered on occasion. The fourth triad, the Rooster, Snake and Ox, are the philosophers and introverts who pursue their theories with steady determination. (Homoeopathic constitutions may be worked out for these).

CHANGES OF SEASONS

Summer[2]
(Summer Solstice to
Autumn Equinox)
June 21 – September 23
Fire (& Earth)

Spring
(Vernal Equinox to
Summer Solstice)
March 21 – June 21
Wood

Autumn
(Autumnal Equinox to
Winter Solstice)
September 23 – December 23
Metal

Winter
(Winter Solstice to
Vernal Equinox)
December 23 – March 21
Water

Birth at change of time or season might indicate the necessity for consideration of either or both the adjacent elements.

2 The late (hot) summer is the Earth element. This is also called the long summer.

Each year has a dominant Qi depending on what year in the 60 year cycle it is. If it is a Yang one the year is said to be superabundant (thai kuo); if it is a Yin one it is said to be insufficient (pu chi). For example, if the year of the series was a Yang one, and therefore dominant, at the same time there was also a 'visiting circumambulator' from the celestial stems, and this was important because it was believed to dictate the pulses of the patient and hence the acupuncture treatment (or moxibustion) which it was appropriate to administer, as guided by the final resultant energy disturbance.

Within each year the months were divided into six periods (pu) each characterized by one or other of the forms of Yin and Yang and of the medical-meteorological Qi. All these relationships were inscribed in a discoidal horoscope[3] of much complexity specific for each person, from which it was possible to infer what the meteorological conditions of a particular time of year are expected to be, and hence, what illnesses were to be foreseen, and what prognostications followed. However, as with all human affairs, all too often the weather failed to correspond with this rather arbitrary prediction system, and in this case some of the technical terms already encountered were used in a different sense. If the factual phenomena went beyond the theoretical deductions (e.g. hotter or colder, rainier or drier) the situation was called 'over-vigorous' (sheng or thai kuo); if it failed to come up to expectations it was termed 'weak' or 'failing' (shuai or pu chi). Similarly, the term Phing Qi was used for the situations in which the meteorological conditions transpired exactly as expected from the predicted cyclical sequences.

Chapter 69 of the Su Wen states that, "If in a given year Wood is super-abundant, the wind will be roving, reckless and rampant, the Earth element will be damaged and, hence, the Spleen will be subject to heteropathies; the people will suffer from diarrhoea with flatulence, their appetites will decrease and they may be depressed and listless, with a distension of the abdomen and weak extremities. On the other hand, if in a given year the Wood is insufficient, the dryness Qi will be on the ascendant, the life giving Qi may fail to resonate

3 Yun Qi Hsuch.

with the season; plant growth will be retarded, and everything will the season; frustrated and dried up. The people will have excessive appetite, without gaining weight; there will be pains in the thorax and lower abdomen, with flatulence and another type of diarrhoea or constipation, (or alternating diarrhoea and constipation)."

Such was the complex algorithm by which the learned physicians of the Sung Dynasty decided exactly when and where to apply their acupuncture, moxibustion and other therapies.

This system presents at first sight a certain similarity with the medical astrology of the European middle ages, but the likeness does not go very far, as the latter was not based on observations of the rhythms of nature. The theories of the Chinese circumambulators (celestial stems) were based on more or less regular seasonal phenomena and the rhythms of climate and weather, and in a way they have much more to do with the prediction of health, disease and epidemics. It was from these systems that the ancient learned Chinese physicians could draw conclusions about the ideal times for applying acupuncture or moxa to individual patients. The aim of the whole complex exercise was the counter-balancing of the abnormal quality or quantity of Qi which was causing the pathological disturbance against the normal external macrocosmic Qi, which varied according to the double hour, the day, the month, the season and the year.

These conceps were applied meticulously in Sung and Yuan times to the whole of medicine, herbal therapy as well which, according to some of the classics, played an even more important part than acupuncture or moxibustion.

The Yun Qi Hsueh computus was a daunting edifice of a priori systematization, described by some modern authorities as by far the weakest link discerned in the correspondence system of Chinese medicine[4]. The computus book considerable notice of geographical longitude, latitude and altitude, but it was based on a body of meteorological knowledge essentially medieval in character. Indeed the great

4 The other is pulse diagnosis

medical historian Li Thao has gone so far as to maintain that its dogmatism inhibited the further progress of Chinese traditional medicine after the Sung Dynasty; it tended to be the delight of men who were better academic scholars (contemplative Taoists) than practicing physicians, and encouraged proto-scientific, theory-making rather than clinical case study, astute observation at the bed side and clinical recording. At the same time, psychological factors can never be forgotten where medicine is concerned, and so complex a system, with its many diagrams and confident predictions, could have great psychological back-up to many rural physicians working in trying conditions of inclement weather, abject poverty and plague. Not only so, but the patients themselves would have been very impressed with the good therapeutic results, if only by suggestion, all the more because the advent of printing was contemporaneous with the Yun Qi Hsueh and brought it widely to public knowledge. Clearly no description of the history of acupuncture could omit some account of it, especially since it is still in use to this day by a number of traditional Chinese physicians (and by all Chinese astrologists).

Its period of doctrinal dominane came to an end, however, in the latter part of the Ming Dynasty. When men such as Wang Chi (1522 to 1567 A.D.) and Chang Chien-Pin (1563 to 1640 A.D.) criticized it severely, as being too dogmatic and overtly mechanical. The former deplored its mechanical application by physicians numerologically inclined, without any real understanding of the environmental background of epidemiology; and the later felt that in his own legalistic use of it he had sometimes been like a frog surveying the universe from the bottom of muddy well. Both considered, however, that when fully understood and judiciously applied the system could still be a sensible guide to a pragmatic clinical practice, while reinforcing the psychosomatic parameters to elicit the cure.

Just how right the old Chinese bio-medical observers were in visualizing regular cyclic changes in the function and composition of living bodies, especially those of human beings, can best be appreciated by those who are familiar with the researches of the last couple of decades on biological time keeping'. It has been established beyond doubt that there are a great number of inbuilt rhythms in organisms of all the phyla of the animal kingdom, and beyond that, in many plant forms also; biological clocks, as it were which given motion, rest and sleep, feeding and excretion, the chemical composition and the internal relations of tissue fluids, glands and other organs. The long known phenomena of plant photoperoidism is a manifestation of such inbuilt rhythms. These may be of almost any length of time, but among the commonest are those which repeat every twenty-four hours, and these are called diurnal or circadian rhythms.

One reason for the great contemporary relevance of this is a development of which the old Chinese physicians could never have dreamt of, the growth of rapid and world-wide air travel (and space travel). Many human psychophysiological rhythms are upset by the sudden transpositions which these impose.

Some of the observations which form the stimuli for these rhythms are as old as the pre-Socratic and Warring States periods, but so far all the resources of modern science have not sufficed to solve the basic problem and two contrasting views have now crystallized. The 'exogenous' view is that rhythmic geophysical forces provide living organisms with informational inputs which regulate the timing of their recurrent regulating processes. The endogenous view is that organisms possess internal, autonomous biological clocks, not immediately dependent on the external world, and constituting an inbuilt self-timing mechanism. One can see that the insistence of the ancient Chinese physicians on the rhythmic character of physiological and pathological phenomena, both diurnal, monthly and annual, brought them clearly into the mainstream of human knowledge of this strange microcosm-macrocosm relationship out of which the universal Yin-Yang philosophy arose.

Among the most interesting of oscillations, from our present point of view, are those which are to be seen in the pathological states of human beings. Every organ has its own cycle. Other interesting phenomena are those of migration of birds and mammals, swarming in invertebrates, hibernation in mammals, and reproductive cycles in many phyla.

From all this it is clear that the traditional Taosistic idea of 'circulations of the Qi' profoundly affecting human beings in health and disease was a very justifiable one. Of all ancient cultures, China was by far the most, 'circulation-minded'. The apparent diurnal revolution of the heavens was very familiar, and the planetary revolution periods were sufficiently well known at quite an early date. There was also the annual rhythms of the seasons. If this was taking place in the macrocosm, why should one hesitate to accept the conclusion, strongly indicated as it was by millennia of clinical experience, that the microcosm was the theatre of rhythms too. The natural ovulation and menstruation rhythms would always have given an incontestable paradigm.

Conclusions could obviously be drawn from the patient's genethliacal horoscope, and the specific influences of planets and zodiacal constellations on organs and parts of the human body was a commonplace belief, while the state of the heaven at the time of the onset of the illness would naturally matter. Although the zodiacal signs rotated and the planets came and went was known in Europe, it does not appear that Western astrology suggested any rhythms intrinsic to the person (patient) himself. Although medieval European medicine was also deeply enmeshed with astrology, its concepts were far removed from geophysical natural rhythms of the universe. This the Chinese system took cognizance of and the therapist, whether applying acupuncture, moxibustion or pharmacy, took great care to find and make use fo the optimum, acceptable time for such medication. Unfortunately lacking the methods of modern science, Chinese physicians constructed an arbitrary and numerological, almost glyphomantic scheme, from the flow of double-hours, days and months, expressed by the five elements, the two sets of cyclical characters (ten and twelve), branches and stems and the twenty-eight lunar mansions. The system was so complicated as to lead one to suspect that when a physician was choosing a suitable time to apply acupuncture he did so rather on the basis of his acquired experience inherited from previous generations of researchers and also, acquired by himself in the course of his practice, finding good reasons for his action afterwards from the complex interplay of the chronorhaphic symbols to justify the plan of his therapeutics.

SOME COMMON WESTERN MEDICAL (ALLOPATHIC) DISORDERS WITH THEIR TRADITIONAL CHINESE AND HOMOEOPATHIC EQUIVALENTS

HEADACHES

TRADITIONAL CHINESE DIAGNOSIS	*Signs & Symptoms*	*Tongue*	*Pulse*	*HOMOEOPATHY*
Cold and Wind	Sudden headache that feels tight and radiates to neck and back; fear of cold accompanied by slight fever; no thirst.	Thin, white coating.	Tight and floating.	*Apis mellifica.*
Hot Wind	Sudden headache, with splitting pain; aversion to cold; high fever; red face; thirst; sore throat.	Thin, yellow coating.	Floating and rapid.	*Aconitum napellus.*
Damp Wind	Sudden headache that feels heavy and full; intermittent fever; stiff joints; pressure in chest; no thirst; sticky tongue.	Greasy, white coating.	Floating and slippery.	*Gelsemium sempervirens.*
Constrained Liver Qi	One sided headache; flanks are distended; melancholy; nausea.	White coating.	Wiry.	*Pulsatilla nigricans.*

TRADITIONAL CHINESE DIAGNOSIS	*Signs & Symptoms*	*Tongue*	*Pulse*	*HOMOEOPATHY*
Liver Fire Blazing Upwards	One sided splitting headache; irritability; angers easily; bitter taste in mouth; scanty, dark urine; constipation; red eyes.	Red or yellow coating.	Wiry and rapid.	*Bryonia alba.*
Aberrant Liver Yang Ascending	One sided headache that radiates to top of head; vertigo; tinnitus.	Red, thin, dry coating.	Wiry.	*Belladonna atropa, Nux vomica.*
Deficient Spleen Qi	Slight headache; shiny white face; fatigue; spontaneous sweating; poor appetite.	Pale white coating.	Empty.	*Hydrastis canadensis.*
Deficient Blood	Slight on-and-off-again headache; luster-less face; palpitations; impaired vision; insomnia.	Pale, white coating.	Thin and soft.	*Ferrum phosphoricum.*
Turbid Mucus	Headache accompanied by heaviness and vertigo; bloated chest; vomiting of sputum.	Greasy, pasty, white coating.	Slippery.	*Bryonia alba, Nux vomica.*
Deficient Kidney Yin	Headache accompanied by an empty feeling in the head; vertigo; tinnitus; soreness in the lower back and knees; leucorrhea.	Red, peeled, dry coating.	Thin and rapid.	*Phosphorus.*

TRADITIONAL CHINESE DIAGNOSIS	*Signs & Symptoms*	*Tongue*	*Pulse*	*HOMOEOPATHY*
Deficient Qi	Shiny white face; cold limbs; edema.	Pale, swollen, moist, scanty coating.	Frail and soft.	*Natrium muriaticum*[1].
Congealed Blood	Chronic headache with sharp and stabbing pain in a fixed location	Purplish darkish coating or red spots on tongue.	Choppy.	*Lachesis.*

CEREBRO-VASCULAR ACCIDENTS - STROKES

Wind Mucus Obstructing Meridians, Liver Yang	Slow onset; mouth and eyes are askew; slurred speech; numb or trembling limbs; hemiplegia; vertigo; head is heavy and painful; excess saliva; sudden loss of consciousness or sudden collapse.	Greasy, white coating.	Wiry and slippery.	*Opium.*
Fire Mucus Suddenly Collapsing, Liver Fire Blazing	Sudden collapse; unconsciousness; clenched teeth; clenched palms; tremors; hot body; red face; snoring; throat rattling; headache; vomiting; scanty, dark urine; constipation.	Greasy, yellow coating.	Wiry, slippery, and full.	*Opium.*

[1] Or constitutional remedy.

TRADITIONAL CHINESE DIAGNOSIS	*Signs & Symptoms*	*Tongue*	*Pulse*	*HOMOEOPATHY*
Cold Mucus Obstructing	Sudden collapse; tremors; slurred speech; headaches; vertigo; nausea; hemiplegia; pale face, purple lips.	Pale, puffy, darkish coating.	Sinking and wiry.	*Camphora officinalis.*
Yin and Yang Collapsing	Open eyes and mouth; unconsciousness; pale face; slightly red cheeks; cold sweat; flaccidity.	Tremulous, pale.	Sinking, rapid and thin or hidden.	*Veratrum album.*
Deficient Qi, Congealed Blood	Hemiplegia; slurred speech; numb limbs; sore body; no strength, fatigue; sallow or pale face.	Pale, white coating.	Sinking and choppy.	*Causticum.*
Deficient Liver Yin and Deficient Kidney Yin	Hemiplegia; emaciation; sore or numb body; vertigo; insomnia; red cheeks; dry mouth; night sweats; anger; scanty, dark urine; constipation.	Red coating.	Wiry.	*Pyrogenium.*

INSOMNIA, ANXIETY, ENDOGENOUS DEPRESSION

TRADITIONAL CHINESE DIAGNOSIS	*Signs & Symptoms*	*Tongue*	*Pulse*	*HOMOEOPATHY*
Deficient Blood and Deficient Spleen Qi	Insomnia; palpitations; forgetfulness; lethargy; food is tasteless, poor appetite; pale face.	Pale coating.	Thin or empty.	*Coffea cruda.*
Heart and Kidney not in Balance (or Deficient Heart Yin and Deficient Kidney Yin)	Insomnia and irritability; palpitations; forgetfulness; night sweats; tinnitus; vertigo; lumbago; anxiety.	Red coating.	Rapid and thin.	*Sulphur.*
Deficient Heart Qi and Gall-bladder Qi	Insomnia; awakens easily with fright; nightmares; timidity.	Pale coating.	Wiry and thin.	*Lycopodium clavatum, Phosphorus.*
Stomach not Harmonized	Insomnia; distended epigastrium; belching; abdominal discomfort; defecation is not smooth; excessive sweating.	Greasy.	Slippery.	*Argentum nitricum, Nux vomica.*
Liver Fire and Gall-bladder Fire	Insomnia; headache; vertigo; sore flanks; anger; bitter taste.	Red coated.	Wiry and strong.	*Bryonia alba.*

TINNITUS, VERTIGO

TRADITIONAL CHINESE DIAGNOSIS	*Signs & Symptoms*	*Tongue*	*Pulse*	*HOMOEOPATHY*
Deficient Qi and Deficient Blood	Vertigo; tinnitus (exacerbated by exertion); lethargy; pale face; shortness of breath; insomnia.	Pale white coating.	Thin and frail.	*Chininum sulphuricum, Phosphorus.*
Deficient Kidney Yin	Vertigo, tinnitus; poor memory; low back is sore and weak; palms and soles are warm.	Reddish coating.	Thin and rapid.	*Sulphur.*
Deficient Kidney Yang	Vertigo; tinnitus; Spirit is very low; back is sore and weak; cold limbs; impotence; sterility.	Pale, moist coating.	Imperceptible.	*Lycopodium clavatum.*
Liver Wind	Vertigo; tinnitus; angers easily; disorder is often related to emotions; headache; sometimes vomiting; bitter taste in the mouth; dry throat; numb limbs.	Red, scanty coating.	Wiry.	*Chamomilla.*
Turbid Mucus in Excess	Vertigo; tinnitus; head feels heavy like a rock; head seems to be spinning; fatigue; no appetite; vomiting.	Greasy.	Slippery.	*China officinalis*[2].

[2] Cinchona officinalis.

EPILEPSY, SPASMS, TREMORS OR CONVULSIONS

Spasms, tremors or convulsions are usually related to Wind and may be of either external or internal origin (excess sputum).

TRADITIONAL CHINESE DIAGNOSIS	*Signs & Symptoms*	*Tongue*	*Pulse*	*HOMOEOPATHY*
External Wind; Pernicious Influences Collecting in Channels	Headache; neck and back tremors; sometimes tetany; fear of cold; fever; sore limbs and body; clear Spirit.	Variable.	Floating and tight.	*Nux vomica.*
Extreme Heat Generating Wind	High fever; sometimes coma, tremors and spasms in limbs; mouth tightly closed.	Red coating.	Wiry and fast.	*Belladonna atropa.*
Deficient Blood Generating Wind	Vertigo; fatigue; spasms; tremors; palpitations.	Pale coating.	Fragile and soft.	*Gelsemium sempervirens.*
Deficient Yin Generating Wind	Disorder injures Yin; tremor in limbs; warm palms and soles.	Red coating, little coating.	Thin and rapid.	*Sulphur.*
Excess Sputum Obstructing and Generating Wind	Thin body; spasms; headache with pain in a fixed location; epilepsy.	Darkish coating with red and purple spots.	Choppy and soft.	*Argentum nitricum*[3].

[3] Constitutional remedy or aetiological remedy (e.g. Arnica montana in head injury).

THE COMMON COLD (CORYZA), RHINITIS

TRADITIONAL CHINESE DIAGNOSIS	*Signs & Symptoms*	*Tongue*	*Pulse*	*HOMOEOPATHY*
Wind Cold, Pernicious Influence	Low fever; severe chills; no perspiration; sore limbs; stuffed or running nose; itching throat; cough with clear or white phlegm.	Thin, white coating.	Floating and tight.	*Gelsemium sempervirens*[4].
Wind Heat, Pernicious Influence.	High fever; slight chills; headache; sweats; dry or sore throat; thirst; cough with thick yellow phlegm; dark urine.	Thin, yellow coating.	Floating and rapid.	*Bryonia alba.*
Wind Cold with Dampness, Pernicious Influence	Wind Cold signs; head feels swollen, like a balloon; heavy, tired limbs; sore, heavy joints.	Greasy, white coating.	Soggy and slow.	*Gelsemium sempervirens.*
Summer Heat, Dampness, Pernicious Influence	Wind Heat signs; nausea; diarrhea; great thirst; irritability; profuse sweat; occurs in hot season.	Greasy, yellow coating.	Soggy and rapid.	*Gemsemium sempervirens.*
Dryness, Pernicious Influence	Wind Heat signs; dry nose; cracked lips; dry cough with no phlegm.	Red, dry coating.	Floating thin and rapid.	*Natrium muriaticum.*

[4] Allium sativum at the onset.

EPISTAXIS (NOSE-BLEED)

TRADITIONAL CHINESE DIAGNOSIS	*Signs & Symptoms*	*Tongue*	*Pulse*	*HOMOEOPATHY*
Lung Heat Injuring Meridians	Epistaxis; fever; cough; little phlegm; dry mouth.	Red, yellow coating.	Floating and rapid.	*Pulsatilla nigricans.*
Stomach, Fire Rebelling Upwards	Epistaxis; dry mouth; bad breath; irritability; constipation.	Red, yellow coating.	Slippery and flooding.	*Phosphorus, Sulphur.*
Liver, Fire, Ascending	Epistaxis; vertigo; headache; red eyes; bitter taste in mouth; irritability; quickness to anger.	Red, yellow coating.	Wiry and rapid.	*Nux vomica.*
Deficient Yin Empty Fire	Epistaxis; vertigo; red eyes; dry throat; tinnitus; irritability; insomnia.	Thin red coating.	Thin and rapid, with little strength.	*Phosphorus.*

SHOCK, COLLAPSE, DEHYDRATION, SUNSTROKE

Excess Dryness and Heat in Lungs and Stomach	Dry mouth and throat; desire to drink; hot body; perspiration; slight or no fear of cold; aversion to heat; full abdomen; constipation.	Red coating.	Full and rapid or floating.	*Bryonia alba.*

TRADITIONAL CHINESE DIAGNOSIS	*Signs & Symptoms*	*Tongue*	*Pulse*	*HOMOEOPATHY*
Deficient Yin	Thirst but little desire to drink; warm palms and soles; insomnia; afternoon fever; night sweats.	Reddish, no coating.	Thin and rapid.	*Arsenicum album.*
Deficient Spleen Qi and Dampness Accumulation	Thirst but no desire to drink, or a desire for hot fluids; tired limbs; heavy head and body; loose stools.	Pale, greasy, scanty coating.	Empty or soggy.	*Arsenicum album.*
Kidney Yang Insufficient to Transform Water	Thirst but no desire to drink, or vomiting after drinking; aversion to cold; fatigue; cold limbs.	Swollen, pale, scanty coating.	Fragile.	*Arsenicum album, Bryonia alb.*
Dryness and Mucus Excess	Thirst but no desire to drink, or vomiting after drinking; excess saliva, distended abdomen; difficult, scanty or incomplete urination.	Greasy, white coating.	Slippery, soft.	*Mercurius.*
Congealed Blood	Thirst; irritability; desire to gargle water but no desire to swallow; other signs of Congealed Blood.	Darkish, purple coating.	Choppy and rapid.	*Opium.*

HYPERTHYROIDISM - HYPOTHYROIDISM

TRADITIONAL CHINESE DIAGNOSIS	*Signs & Symptoms*	*Tongue*	*Pulse*	*HOMOEOPATHY*
Constrained Liver Qi	Painful chest and flanks; anxiety; irritability; quickness to anger; menstrual irregularities; mild swelling in the neck.	Thin, white coating.	Wiry.	*Bryonia alba.*
Liver Fire Blazing and Heart Fire Ascending	Protruding eyes; fear of light; red face; quickness to anger; irritability; tremors of tongue and hands; increased appetite; dry mouth; palpitations.	Red coating.	Wiry and rapid with force.	*Belladonna atropa, Iodium.*
Deficient Heart Yin	Insomnia; irritability; palpitations; night sweats; dry mouth.	Reddish, thin coating.	Thin and rapid.	*Pulsatilla nigricans.*
Mucus, Dampness Obstructing Neck	Soft swelling of the neck; feeling of pressure in chest; nausea; vomiting; watery stool; (this pattern often merges with one of the above three).	Thin, greasy coating.	Soggy or slippery.	*Natrium muriaticum.*
Deficient Liver Yin and Deficient Kidney Yin	Vertigo; headache; spots before eyes; tinnitus; palpitations; night sweats; irritability; afternoon temperature; dry throat; sore low back and knees.	Red, scanty coating.	Sinking, wiry, thin, and rapid.	*Phosphorus, Iodium.*

TRADITIONAL CHINESE DIAGNOSIS	*Signs & Symptoms*	*Tongue*	*Pulse*	*HOMOEOPATHY*
Deficient Kidney Yang	Vertigo; tinnitus, loss of hearing; bright white face; knees are sore and weak; fear of cold; watery stools; impotence.	Swollen, pale accretions.	Frail.	*Mercurius, Nitricum acidum.*

BRONCHITIS, BRONCHIAL ASTHMA, EMPHYSEMA

TRADITIONAL CHINESE DIAGNOSIS	*Signs & Symptoms*	*Tongue*	*Pulse*	*HOMOEOPATHY*
Deficient Lung Yin	Dry cough; dry mouth and throat; red cheeks; other Deficient Yin signs.	Red, scanty coating.	Thin and rapid.	*Ferrum metallicum.*
Deficient Lung Qi	Weak cough usually associated with asthma; frequent colds; spontaneous sweating; other Deficient Qi signs.	Pale, moist coating.	Empty or frail.	*Silicea.*
Mucus and Dampness Hindering the Lungs	Cough with copious white expectoration; distended chest and epigastrium; no appetite; fatigue; symptoms often occur with Deficient or Damp Spleen Signs.	Greasy, white coating.	Soggy or slippery.	*Lycopodium clavatum.*
Mucus Heat Collecting in Lungs	Cough with copious, thick, yellow expectoration; sometimes phlegm has foul smell; other signs of Heat.	Greasy, yellow coating.	Slippery and rapid.	*Chelidonium majus, Mercurius.*

TRADITIONAL CHINESE DIAGNOSIS	*Signs & Symptoms*	*Tongue*	*Pulse*	*HOMOEOPATHY*
Liver Fire Invading Lungs	Sputtering, sporadic cough; cough causes flanks to be painful; dry throat; red face; other Liver disharmony signs.	Thin, dry, yellow coating.	Wiry and rapid.	*Pulsatilla nigricans, Nux vomica.*
Deficient Kidney Yang Unable to Absorb Lung Qi	Usually there has been a long history of illness; exhalation is easier than inhalation; asthma; exertion exacerbates symptoms; sore low back; fear of cold; dark face.	Pale, swollen, moist coating.	Frail.	*Mercurius.*

PNEUMONIA, PLEURISY

Wind Heat Invading Lungs	Sudden chills and fever; headache; sore throat; cough; chest pain; small quantity of thick phlegm; dry mouth.	Thin, white or thin, yellow coating.	Floating.	*Pulsatilla nigricans.*
Heat Obstructing Lung Qi	High fever; red face; sweating but no reduction of fever, or little sweat; thirst and desire to drink; coughing of thick yellow phlegm, sometimes with blood; coarse respiration; asthma, chest pain.	Red, yellow coating.	Rapid and slippery.	*Belladonna atropa.*

TRADITIONAL CHINESE DIAGNOSIS	*Signs & Symptoms*	*Tongue*	*Pulse*	*HOMOEOPATHY*
Deficient Lung Qi and Deficient Lung Yin	Usually occurs during recovery period after a high fever; dry cough; little phlegm; afternoon fever; exhausted Spirit; no desire to speak; irritability; quickness to anger; scanty urine; constipation.	Red or scarlet or yellow peeled coating.	Deep, thin and rapid.	*Lycopodium clavatum.*
Excess Heat Collapsing into Yin	High fever; cough; chest pain; coughing of phlegm with blood or foul mucus; dry throat; dry mouth but no desire to drink; Spirit is sometimes delirious; convulsions; red face; irritability; occasional coma.	Scarlet or dry grayish coating.	Sinking, wiry, thin and rapid.	*Pulsatilla nigricans.*
Collapsed Qi	Shallow respiration; cyanosis; gray-white face; no fever or suddenly resolving fever; cold limbs; cold sweat; muddled Spirit.	Pale coating.	Frail and weak.	*Carbo vegetabilis.*

PNEUMONITIS DUE TO HEART, LIVER OR KIDNEY DISORDERS

TRADITIONAL CHINESE DIAGNOSIS	*Signs & Symptoms*	*Tongue*	*Pulse*	*HOMOEOPATHY*
External Heat Invading Lungs	Chest and flanks are painful and sore; cough; asthma; yellow or rust coloured phlegm; fever; chills.	Yellow red tip.	Floating and rapid.	*Rhus toxicodendron.*
External Dryness, Scorching Lungs	Hot body; painful chest; cough; little phlegm; thirst.	Red, dry coating.	Rapid.	*Belladonna atropa, Arsenicum album.*
Mucus Obstructing the Chest	Flanks are painful and distended; frothy cough with phlegm and saliva; cough aggravates pain; sometimes fever; no thirst.	Greasy, white coating.	Wiry and slippery.	*Arsenicum album, Pulsatilla nigricans.*
Deficient Heart Yang with Congealed Heart Blood	Sporadic chest pain; sometimes stabbing pain; fixed pain; pressure in chest.	Darkish coating or red spots.	Choppy.	*Phosphorus.*
Deficient Heart Yang with Mucus Dampness Obstructing Lungs	Chest is distended, sore and painful; pain radiates to shoulder; cough with phlegm; shortness of breath or asthma.	Pale, greasy, white coating.	Slippery.	*Crotalus cascavella.*

TRADITIONAL CHINESE DIAGNOSIS	*Signs & Symptoms*	*Tongue*	*Pulse*	*HOMOEOPATHY*
Damp Heat of Liver and Gall-bladder	Painful flanks; distended epigastrium; feeling of distress in chest; nausea; yellow urine; fever; jaundice.	Red, greasy, yellow coating.	Wiry and rapid.	*Lycopodium clavatum*, *Nux vomica*.
Constrained Liver Qi	Distended and painful flanks; impatience or quickness to anger; emotional stress increases pain; chest feels uncomfortable; little desire to drink.	Thin, white or yellow coating.	Wiry.	*Staphysagria*.
Congealed Liver Blood	Stabbing loin pain in fixed position; palpable mass under rib cage.	Purple, darkish coating.	Wiry and choppy.	*Lachesis*, *Petroleum*.
Deficient Liver Yin and Deficient Kidney Yin	Loin has slight dull pain or soreness; dry mouth; irritability; vertigo; low back pain.	Red, scanty coating.	Wiry and thin.	*Bryonia alba*.

HEMOPTYSIS (LUNG ABSCESS)

TRADITIONAL CHINESE DIAGNOSIS	*Signs & Symptoms*	*Tongue*	*Pulse*	*HOMOEOPATHY*
Wind and Heat Dryness, Pernicious Sieqi Injuring Lungs	Fever; dry mouth; dry nose; sore throat; coughing of phlegm with blood; chest pain.	Red, yellow coating.	Floating and rapid.	*Phosphorus.*
Deficient Yin Empty Fire Injuring Lungs	Dry cough; bloody phlegm; afternoon low fever; no physical strength; cough is worse at night.	Red, scanty coating.	Thin and rapid.	*Pulsatilla nigricans.*
Liver Fire Invading Lungs	Chest and flank pain; coughing of phlegm with blood or coughing of pure blood; irritability; anger; constipation; dark urine.	Red, thin, yellow coating.	Wiry and rapid.	*Bryonia alba.*
Congealed Blood Obstructing Chest	Cough; coughing of phlegm with blood or of bloody foam; piercing chest pain; heart palpitations.	Darkish or red spots on tongue.	Intermittent or wiry and slow or choppy.	*Pulsatilla nigricans.*

ESSENTIAL HYPERTENSION

TRADITIONAL CHINESE DIAGNOSIS	*Signs & Symptoms*	*Tongue*	*Pulse*	*HOMOEOPATHY*
Liver Fire Blazing	Vertigo; headache; painful, red eyes; red face; quickness to anger; irritability severe constipation; dark, scanty urine.	Red or scarlet-yellow coating.	Wiry and full or rapid.	*Belladonna atropa.*
Turbid Mucus Obstructing Middle Burner (Spleen)	Vertigo; head feels heavy as if in a vice; poor appetite; nausea; chest and epigastrium feel pressure; numb limbs.	Thick, greasy coating.	Soggy or slippery.	*Gelsemium sempervirens, Nux vomica.*
Aberrant Liver Yang Ascending	Vertigo; tinnitus; blurred vision; palpitations; insomnia; bitter taste in mouth.	Reddish, yellow coating.	Wiry.	*China officinalis.*

CORONARY ARTERY DISEASE (ARTERIOSCLEROSIS, ATHEROSCLEROSIS)

Turbid Mucus Obstructing Heart	Pain or feeling of pressure in chest; pain sometimes radiates down Heart Channel; left shoulder is sore or numb; coughing of phlegm; no appetite; conditions often seen in obese people.	Pale, greasy coating.	Slippery and wiry or soggy and moderate.	*Rhus toxicodendron.*

TRADITIONAL CHINESE DIAGNOSIS	*Signs & Symptoms*	*Tongue*	*Pulse*	*HOMOEOPATHY*
Congealed Heart Blood	Intermittent stabbing pain in heart or chest; palpitations; shortness of breath; chest feels oppressed.	Darkish red or purple coating.	Sinking, choppy.	*Phosphorus*, *Mercurius.*
Deficient Heart Yang	No pain, or patient has recovered from acute pain; fear of cold; fatigue; spontaneous sweating; puffy, grayish white face; palpitations or empty feeling in chest; clear, copious urine.	Pale, white coating.	Frail, slow or empty.	*Sepia.*
Deficient Heart Yin	No pain, or patient has recovered from acute pain; flushed face (especially cheeks); sweats; thirst but no desire to drink.	Red tip of tongue with little coating.	Thin and rapid.	*Rhus toxicodendron.*
Deficient Liver Yin and Deficient Kidney Yin	Vertigo; tinnitus; headache; numb limbs; weak low back and knees; dry mouth; night sweats; hot palms and soles; constipation.	Red, scanty coating.	Thin, wiry or rapid.	*Sulphuricum acidum*, *Lycopodium clavatum.*

CARDIAC INSUFFICIENCY (CARDIAC FAILURE), COR PULMONALE[5]

TRADITIONAL CHINESE DIAGNOSIS	*Signs & Symptoms*	*Tongue*	*Pulse*	*HOMOEOPATHY*
Deficient Heart Qi and Deficient Spleen Qi	Palpitation and shortness of breath after exertion; fatigue; ashen, pale face; spontaneous sweating; little appetite; watery stools.	Pale, thin, white coating.	Thin or frail and knotted.	*Arsenicum album.*
Deficient Heart Yang and Deficient Kidney Yang	Palpitations; asthma; face, eyelids and four limbs are swollen; ashen, white face; sweat on forehead; scanty urine; cold limbs.	Swollen, pale, white coating.	Thin and frail or knotted or intermittent.	*Digitalis purpurea.*
Deficient Heart Yang and Congealed Heart Blood	Palpitations; hurried breath; darkish face; purplish lips; painful flanks; lower limbs are slightly swollen; coughing with blood; scanty urine	Purple, darkish or purple coating with red spots.	Thin and choppy or knotted or intermittent.	*China officinalis.*
Deficient Kidney Yang, with Water Radiating to Lungs	Asthma; urgent breathing; saliva and phlegm or even a great amount of foaming phlegm from nose; gray-white face; very cold limbs; copious, cold perspiration; fear; irritability.	Pale, greasy, white coating.	Intermittent.	*Lycopodium clavatum.*

[5] Also ischemic heart disease.

CARDIAC AND RENAL FAILURE (UREMIA)

TRADITIONAL CHINESE DIAGNOSIS	*Signs & Symptoms*	*Tongue*	*Pulse*	*HOMOEOPATHY*
Deficient Heart Qi and Deficient Lung Qi	Palpitations; shortness of breath; weak cough, asthma; spontaneous sweating.	Pale.	Frail, soft.	*Calcarea carbonica.*
Deficient Heart Blood and Deficient Spleen Qi	Palpitations; insomnia; loss of appetite; abdominal distention; loose stools; lethargy; pale, sallow complexion; menstrual blood is pale and excessive, or amenorrhea.	Pale, thin.	Empty.	*China officinalis.*
Heart and Kidney lose Communication (Heart Yin and Kidney Yin both Deficient)	Palpitations; insomnia; irritability; forgetfulness; vertigo; tinnitus; dry throat; sore back; nocturnal emissions; afternoon fever; night sweats.	Reddish, dry, scanty coating.	Thin, rapid, sinking.	*Phosphorus.*
Heart Yang and Kidney Yang both Deficient	Palpitations; cold appearance; edema; scanty urine.	Pale, swollen, moist, white coating.	Sinking and feeble.	*Arsenicum album, China officinalis.*

TRADITIONAL CHINESE DIAGNOSIS	*Signs & Symptoms*	*Tongue*	*Pulse*	*HOMOEOPATHY*
Lung Yin and Kidney Yin both Deficient	Cough with little mucus; mucus with blood; mouth and throat dry; voice low or hoarse; lower back and limbs sore and weak; night sweats; red cheeks; afternoon fever; sterility.	Red, scanty coating.	Rapid.	*Pulsatilla nigrigans.*

NAUSEA, VOMITING (INCLUDING MORNING SICKNESS[6])

Vomiting is usually Stomach Qi in rebellion and can be the result of Stomach Disharmonies alone or other Disharmonies that affect the Stomach and Spleen.

External Cold Wind Invading Stomach	Acute onset of vomiting; nausea accompanied by fever and fear of cold; head and body ache; distended chest and abdomen; diarrhea.	White coating.	Tight.	*Nux vomica.*
External Heat or Summer Heat Invading Stomach	Acute onset of vomiting; nausea accompanied by fever; thirst; irritability diarrhea.	Red-yellow coating.	Rapid and wiry or soggy.	*Bryonia alba.*

[6] Including hyperemesis gravidarum.

TRADITIONAL CHINESE DIAGNOSIS	*Signs & Symptoms*	*Tongue*	*Pulse*	*HOMOEOPATHY*
Mucus Obstructing Stomach	Vomiting; chest is uncomfortable; no desire to drink; vertigo.	Greasy, white coating.	Slippery.	*Pulsatilla nigricans.*
Liver Invading Stomach	Vomiting; food matter appears in vomitus; sour taste in mouth; distended chest and flanks; condition is often pregnancy related.	Thin, white coating.	Wiry.	*Nux vomica.*
Heat Generating Liver Wind which Invades Stomach	Projectile vomiting; high fever; headache; stiff neck; convulsion in limbs; tetany.	Red or scarlet coating.	Wiry and rapid.	*Belladonna atropa.*
Deficient Stomach Yin	Occasional vomiting; dry mouth; hunger but no desire to eat; other Deficient Yin signs.	Red coating.	Thin and rapid.	*Pulsatilla nigricans.*
Deficient Spleen and Stomach Qi	Vomiting, especially after even slight overeating; unpredictable vomiting that is chronic; fatigue; watery stools; pale, white face.	Pale coating.	Empty.	*Nux vomica.*

TRADITIONAL CHINESE DIAGNOSIS	*Signs & Symptoms*	*Tongue*	*Pulse*	*HOMOEOPATHY*
Stagnant Food (Stagnant Food Vecomes Sieqi)	Vomiting of sour, rotten food; much relief after vomiting; abdomen is full, sore and distended after eating; constipation or diarrhea.	Greasy coating.	Slippery and full.	*Nux vomica.*
Worms Invading Stomach	Vomiting of worms; vomiting of clear fluid, saliva or yellow-green fluid after eating; sore abdomen; discomfort is occasional.	Thick coating.	Variable.	*Cina*[7].

ACUTE GASTRITIS

Stomach Fire Blazing	Thirst; excessive drinking; excessive appetite; bad breath; gums swollen and painful; burning sensation in epigastrium.	Red coating.	Flooding, or rapid and full.	*Constitutional remedy.*
Deficient Stomach Qi	Dry mouth and lips; no appetite; dry vomit or belching; constipation.	Peeled, reddish coating.	Thin and rapid.	*Pulsatilla nigricans.*

[7] Cina was used as a vermifuge in western medicine.

TRADITIONAL CHINESE DIAGNOSIS	*Signs & Symptoms*	*Tongue*	*Pulse*	*HOMOEOPATHY*
Stagnant Stomach Qi	Epigastrium is distended and painful; pain often extends to sides; pain often extends to sides; pain is often related to emotions; belching; sour taste in mouth.	Darkish coating.	Wiry and deep.	*Nux vomica.*
Congealed Blood in Stomach	Stabbing, piercing pain in epigastrium distention; touch aggravation pain; black or dark stools; darkish face.	Darker areas with red dots; thin yellow coating.	Wiry and choppy.	*Arsenicum album.*
Deficient Cold in Stomach	Slight, persistent pain in epigastrium; discomfort relieved by warmth, eating and touching.	Pale, moist, white coating.	Deep or moderate without strength.	*Magnesium phosphoricum.*

CHRONIC GASTRITIS, ANOREXIA

Liver Invading Spleen and Stomach	Distended epigastrium and abdomen; no appetite; belching; soreness; stools pass uncomfortably.	Thin coating.	Wiry.	*Nux vomica.*

TRADITIONAL CHINESE DIAGNOSIS	*Signs & Symptoms*	*Tongue*	*Pulse*	*HOMOEOPATHY*
Deficient Cold in Spleen and Stomach	Stomach discomfort relieved by cold and pressure; distention; no appetite; vomiting of clear liquid.	Pale, sticky, thin, white coating.	Slow and empty.	*Phosphorus, Natrium muriaticum.*
Dampness Distressing Spleen	Nausea; vomiting; no thirst; persistent distention; scanty urine.	Greasy, white coating.	Soggy.	*Pusatilla nigricans.*

GASTROENTERITIS, DIARRHEA

Damp Heat	Acute onset; stools are yellow and seem to be dissolved in fluid; foul smell; anus is hot; scanty, dark urine; abdominal pain; bitter taste in mouth; dry mouth; fever; vomiting.	Yellow, greasy coating.	Soggy and rapid.	*Arsenicum album, Pulsatilla nigricans.*
Damp Cold	Usually acute onset; watery stool; defecation is uncomfortable; abdominal pain; intestinal rumbling; heat relieves pain; chest and epigastrium feel oppressed; symptoms are sometimes accompanied by External Cold Wind Pernicious Influences.	Greasy, white coating.	Soggy.	*Sulphur.*

TRADITIONAL CHINESE DIAGNOSIS	*Signs & Symptoms*	*Tongue*	*Pulse*	*HOMOEOPATHY*
Stagnant Food	Sticky stools offensive and foul; epigastrium and abdomen are distended and resist pressure; greater comfort after defecation; sour belching.	Greasy coating.	Slippery.	*Nux vomica.*
Deficient Spleen Qi	Watery stools, usually chronic; undigested food in stool; distention; no appetite; desire for heat and touch; fear of cold; lethargy.	Pale, white coating.	Frail and thin.	*Arsenicum album.*
Deficient Kidney Yang	Need to defecate at early hours; sparse, watery stools; all four limbs are cold; desire for heat; symptoms found especially in the elderly; other Kidney disorders.	Pale coating.	Deep and thin.	*Nux vomica.*
Constrained Liver	Related to emotions; sudden need to defecate, accompanied by pain; patient is more comfortable after defecation; distended chest and loins; quickness to anger; irritability; belching.	Thin coating.	Wiry and small.	*Nux vomica.*

ACUTE ABDOMINAL PAIN (ACUTE ABDOMEN)

Abdominal pain may appear in Disharmonies of the Liver, Gall-bladder, Spleen, Stomach, Kidney, Large and Small Intestines, Bladder and Uterus. This list summarizes some common presentations.

TRADITIONAL CHINESE DIAGNOSIS	*Signs & Symptoms*	*Tongue*	*Pulse*	*HOMOEOPATHY*
Cold Obstructing Abdomen	Sudden, urgent, severe pain; warmth relieves and cold aggravates pain; no thirst; clear urine.	Pale, white coating.	Deep and tight.	*Magnesium phosphoricum.*
Cold Obstructing Liver Meridian	Urgent cold pain in groin; pain radiates to testicles.	White coating.	Deep and wiry.	*Pulsatilla nigricans.*
Heat Constructing the Abdomen	Painful and distended abdomen; warm body and abdomen; vomiting; constipation; yellow, scanty urine; irritability.	Yellow coating.	Rapid and full.	*Chelidonium majus.*
Damp Heat in Liver and Gall-bladder	Usually upper right quadrant of body is sore; pain; nausea; vomiting; food is repulsive; jaundice sometimes.	Greasy, yellow coating.	Wiry and rapid.	*Sulphur.*
Damp Heat in Stomach and Intestines	Pain in abdomen accompanied by diarrhea with pus or blood; patient feels heavy and worse after defecation; burning anus; fever; scanty, dark urine.	Greasy, yellow coating.	Slippery and rapid.	*Sulphur.*

TRADITIONAL CHINESE DIAGNOSIS	Signs & Symptoms	Tongue	Pulse	HOMOEOPATHY
Intestinal Sieqi[8]	Abdomen (especially lower right quadrant) is sore and painful; abdomen resists touch; right foot tends to curl up; sometimes accompanied by fever; vomiting.	Greasy, yellow coating.	Rapid and deep.	*Colocynthis*[9].
Damp Heat in Bladder	Acute pain in lower abdomen that sometimes radiates to lower back; burning urination that is painful and rough, may contain blood or granules.	Yellow, thin coating.	Rapid and slow.	*Lycopodium clavatum, Cantharis vesicatoria.*

CHRONIC ABDOMINAL PAIN

Constrained Liver Qi	Distended epigastrium and abdomen; distended flanks; patient resists touch; passing gas relieves pain; disorder is emotionally related.	Thin coating.	Wiry.	*Chelidonium majus.*

[8] Acute appendicitis.
[9] Hepar sulphuris calcareum or Silicea may also help.

TRADITIONAL CHINESE DIAGNOSIS	*Signs & Symptoms*	*Tongue*	*Pulse*	*HOMOEOPATHY*
Congealed Blood in Abdomen	Sharp, stabbing abdominal pain that radiates to sides; pain is located in a fixed position, or palpable mass.	Purplish tongue.	Choppy.	*Arsenicum album, Lycopodium clavatum.*
Deficient Cold Sieqi	Slight, dull abdominal pain; patient desires heat and touching; loose stools; lethargy.	Pale, white coating.	Frail, soft.	*Magnesium phosphoricum.*
Stagnant Food Sieqi	Distended abdomen; soreness; pain that resists touch; patient is repelled by food; belching of sour, rotten material; eating aggravates pain; diarrhea relieves pain.	Greasy coating.	Slippery or deep and full.	*Colchicum autumnale, Nux vomica.*
Worm Infestation	Intermittent abdominal pain, sometimes very severe, often clusters around navel or to one side; sometimes vomiting of worms; emaciation; peculiar eating prejudices (pica); lips or cheeks have tiny white dots.	Thick coating.	Variable.	*Cina.*

ENTERITIS—UPPER BOWEL DISORDERS

TRADITIONAL CHINESE DIAGNOSIS	*Signs & Symptoms*	*Tongue*	*Pulse*	*HOMOEOPATHY*
Deficient Cold of Small Intestine	Slight, persistent discomfort in lower abdomen; gurgling noises in abdomen; watery stools.	Pale, thin, white coating.	Empty.	*Pulsatilla nigricans.*
Stagnant Qi of Small Intestine	Excruciating pain in groin and hypogastrium often extending to low back; one testicle descends further down.	White coating.	Deep and wiry or deep and tight.	*Colocynthis, Lycopodium clavatum.*
Excess Heat of Small Intestines	Irritability; cold sores in mouth; sore throat; urination is frequent and even painful, with dark urine; lower abdomen feels full.	Red, dry, yellow coating.	Rapid and slippery	*Nitricum acidum, Lycopodium clavatum.*
Obstructed Qi of Small Intestine	Violent pains in abdomen; constipation no gas passes; possible vomiting of fecal material.	Greasy, yellow coating.	Wiry and full.	*Sulphur, Podophyllum peltatum.*

COLITIS (ACUTE OR CHRONIC)—LARGE BOWEL DISORDERS

TRADITIONAL CHINESE DIAGNOSIS	*Signs & Symptoms*	*Tongue*	*Pulse*	*HOMOEOPATHY*
Damp Heat Invading Large Intestine	Urgent need to defecate, intensifies after defecation; stool has pus or blood; burning anus; often accompanied by fever.	Red, greasy, yellow coating.	Slippery and rapid.	*Arsenicum album, Mercurius corrosivus*
Exhausted Fluid of Large Intestine Disorder	Constipation; dry stools; often associated with post-partum.	Red, dry coating.	Thin.	*Bryonia alba, Natrium muriaticum*
Cold Dampness in Large Intestine	Rumbling in intestines; abdomen sometimes painful; diarrhea; clear urine.	Moist, greasy, white coating.	Deep and slippery.	*Pulsatilla nigricans.*
Deficient Qi of Large Intestine	Chronic diarrhea; slight persistent lower abdominal discomfort; rumbling in intestines; pressure relieves discomfort; cold limbs; tired Shen[10].	Pale, white coating.	Frail.	*Colocynthis.*

[10] Spirit.

CONSTIPATION (HEMORRHOIDS)

TRADITIONAL CHINESE DIAGNOSIS	*Signs & Symptoms*	*Tongue*	*Pulse*	*HOMOEOPATHY*
Dry Heat Collecting Internally	Constipation; dry stools; offensive breath; distended abdomen; scanty, dark urine.	Thin yellow coating.	Slippery and full.	*Nitricum acidum, Arsenicum album, Natrium muriaticum*[11].
Stagnant Qi	Constipation; distended chest and flanks; no appetite; belching; unproductive desire to defecate; hemorrhoids.	Thin, greasy coating.	Wiry and deep.	*Nux vomica.*
Deficient Blood	Constipation; vertigo; palpitation; face, lips and nails are lustreless, white.	White coating.	Thin.	*Ferrum metallicum.*
Cold Obstructing the Qi	Constipation; slight abdominal discomfort; pressure and warmth relieves pain; clear, copious urine; cold limbs.	White coating.	Deep and slow.	*Magnesium phosphoricum.*
Deficient Qi	Constipation; fatigue; spontaneous sweating; patient becomes more tired after defecation; stool is not dry; hemorrhoids.	Pale and swollen.	Empty.	*Arsenicum album, Hamamelis virginica.*

Note: Constipation is often associated with Lung, Nose and Skin disorders. Constipation alone is often a sign of Heat and Excess and points to a Disharmony in the Large Intestine. As a presenting symptoms it appears in various other disorders.

[11] Also Nux vomica.

MELENA (& HEMORRHOIDS)

TRADITIONAL CHINESE DIAGNOSIS	*Signs & Symptoms*	*Tongue*	*Pulse*	*HOMOEOPATHY*
Heat Entering Large Intestine	Fresh red blood in stools; blood is passed before stools. Other Heat signs.	Yellow coating.	Rapid.	*Phosphorus.*
Deficient Cold with Blood in Stools	Darkish blood in stools; blood is passed after stool; cold limbs; sallow face; tired Shen.	Pale, white coating.	Sinking and thin.	*Carbo vegetabilis.*

ACUTE (INFECTIVE) HEPATITIS

Constrained Liver Qi and Congealed Blood	Piercing, fixed flank pain; palpable mass under ribs; darkish face; distended epigastrium and abdomen.	Darkish coating or coating with red or purple spots.	Wiry and choppy.	*China officinalis, Lachesis.*
Liver Invading Spleen	Chest feels pressure; distention; belching; passing gas; little appetite; nausea; diarrhea; slight flank discomfort.	Thick coating.	Wiry and soggy.	*Lycopodium clavatum, Phosphorus.*
Deficient Liver Yin	Slight flank pain; vertigo; irritability; fatigue; warm palms and soles; low fever.	Red, dry coating.	Wiry and thin.	*Sulphur, Lycopodium clavatum.*

TRADITIONAL CHINESE DIAGNOSIS	*Signs & Symptoms*	*Tongue*	*Pulse*	*HOMOEOPATHY*
Deficient Spleen Qi	Fatigue; bright white face; no appetite; distended abdomen; slight flank pain; watery stools.	Pale, white coating.	Empty.	*Arsenicum album.*

TOXIC HEPATITIS

TRADITIONAL CHINESE DIAGNOSIS	*Signs & Symptoms*	*Tongue*	*Pulse*	*HOMOEOPATHY*
Damp Heat in Spleen and Gall-bladder	Sore, painful flanks; jaundice; no appetite; fatigue; distended abdomen; patient is repelled by greasy food; scanty, dark urine; watery stools; possible fever.	Greasy, yellow coating.	Slippery and rapid.	*Nux vomica.*
Heat Toxicity	Acute, rapid onset; jaundice; high fever; irritability; delirium; bleeding; skin rashes.	Scarlet, thick, greasy, yellow or black coating.	Wiry and rapid.	*Belladonna atropa.*
Constrained Liver Qi	Distended, painful flanks, chest feels pressure; no appetite; nausea; belching.	Thin coating.	Wiry.	*Nux vomica.*

CHRONIC HEPATITIS (CIRRHOSIS) - ALCOHOLIC HEPATITIS[12]

TRADITIONAL CHINESE DIAGNOSIS	*Signs & Symptoms*	*Tongue*	*Pulse*	*HOMOEOPATHY*
Heat Poison in Liver and Gall-bladder	Irregular fever; jaundice; dark urine; bleeding from various orifices e.g., nose or anus.	Greasy, yellow coating.	Wiry and rapid.	*Nux vomica.*
Congealed Liver Blood	Liver becomes enlarged and painful; pain in fixed regions; darkish face.	Grey coating.	Choppy.	*Arsenicum album, Lycopodium clavatum, Phosphorus.*
Liver Invading Spleen	Distended and painful right flank; full epigastrium; distended abdomen; ascites; no appetite.	Greasy, white coating.	Wiry.	*Pulsatilla nigricans.*
Deficient Spleen Yang and Deficient Kidney Yang	Progressive emaciation; low Spirit; darkish face; day and night perspiration; no appetite; watery stools.	Pale, dry, white coating.	Frail.	*Arsenicum album.*

LIVER AND KIDNEY FAILURE (UREMIA)

Deficient Liver Yin and Deficient Kidney Yin	Vertigo; headaches; spots before eyes; forgetfulness; tinnitus; dry mouth and throat; flank pain; lower back and limbs are sore, weak; hot palms and soles; red cheeks; menses irregular or reduced.	Red with little coating.	Thin and rapid.	*Phosphorus, Sulphur.*

[12] Also toxic hepatitis, amoebic hepatitis.

CHOLECYSTITIS (ACUTE & CHRONIC)

TRADITIONAL CHINESE DIAGNOSIS	*Signs & Symptoms*	*Tongue*	*Pulse*	*HOMOEOPATHY*
Excess Gall-bladder Heat	Flank and chest are painful and distended; bitter taste in mouth; vomits bitter fluid; patient angers easily.	Red, yellow coating.	Wiry, rapid and full.	*Nux vomica.*
Damp Heat in both Gall-bladder and liver	Jaundice (Yang type with bright yellow colour); painful flanks; scanty, dark urine; fever; nausea; vomiting.	Greasy, yellow coating.	Wiry, rapid and slippery.	*Sepia, Plumbum metallicum.*
Deficient Gall-bladder Heat	Vertigo; easily frightened; timidity; indescision; unclear vision; annoyance at petty things.	Thin, white coating.	Wiry and thin.	*Calcarea carbonica, Sulphur.*

HEPATIC CHOLANGITIS

Constrained Liver Qi	Colicky pain in the loins; bitter taste and dry mouth; no appetite; nausea; distended epigastrium and abdomen; constipation or diarrhea.	Normal.	Wiry.	*Bryonia alba.*

TRADITIONAL CHINESE DIAGNOSIS	*Signs & Symptoms*	*Tongue*	*Pulse*	*HOMOEOPATHY*
Liver Fire and Gall-bladder Fire	Severe pain in flanks and epigastrium that radiates to shoulder; intermittent fever and chills; dry mouth and throat; distention; nausea; constipation.	Cracked, yellow coating.	Wiry and rapid.	*Chelidonium majus, Mercurius solubilis.*
Damp Heat in Liver and Spleen	Loin pain; distended epigastrium and abdomen; distention; heaviness; fatigue; fever; nausea; no appetite; thirst but no desire to drink; jaundice; constipation or diarrhea.	Red, greasy coating.	Slippery, rapid and wiry.	*Lycopodium clavatum.*

ACUTE PANCREATITIS

Constrained Liver Qi	Soreness in upper abdomen; connects to chest and flanks; bitter taste and dry mouth; vomiting; sometimes heat flushes and then chills; frustration.	Thin, white or yellow coating.	Wiry.	*Nux vomica, Pulsatilla nigricans.*

TRADITIONAL CHINESE DIAGNOSIS	*Signs & Symptoms*	*Tongue*	*Pulse*	*HOMOEOPATHY*
Damp Heat in Spleen, Stomach, and Liver	Left upper abdomen feels painful and full; no appetite; thirst but no desire to drink; jaundice; fever; pain that sometimes radiates to back and shoulder; dark urine; constipation; pain resists touch.	Greasy, yellow coating.	Wiry, slippery and rapid.	*Spongia tosta.*
Excess Fire in Liver and Gallbladder	Painful upper abdomen; pain that resists touch or stabbing pain that radiates to back; nausea; vomiting; bitter taste in mouth; fever; irritability; thirst; constipation; scanty, dark urine.	Red, yellow coating.	Floating, rapid, wiry and full.	*Bryonia alba.*

SUBACUTE & CHRONIC PANCREATITIS

This follows acute pancreatitis. The presentation is similar with less pain. It is known as Chronic Spleen Sieqi. The homoeopathic remedies are: Pulsatilla nigricans, Lycopodium clavatum, Carbo vegetabilis and Nux vomica.

DIABETES MELLITUS

There are two distinct ideograms in Chinese for diabetes; the traditional medical name, *xiao-ke,* which means "wasting and thirsting," and the scientific term *tangniaobing,* which means "sugar urine illness". Discussions of diabetes by its traditional name appears in all the earliest texts, including the *Nei Jing.* Traditionally, it is divided into three types: upper, middle and lower jiao. Each type lays disproportionate emphasis on the three main symptoms - thirst, hunger and excessive urination. Deficient Yin is usually associated with all three types. Also, a traditional diagnosis of "wasting and thirsting" may include illness besides diabetes mellitus.

TRADITIONAL CHINESE DIAGNOSIS	*Signs & Symptoms*	*Tongue*	*Pulse*	*HOMOEOPATHY*
Lung Fire (Upper Diabetes)	Severe thirst; drinking of large quantities of water; dry mouth.	Red-yellow coating.	Floating and rapid.	*Bryonia alba, Phosphorus.*
Stomach Fire (Middle Diabetes)	Large appetite and excessive eating; thinness; constipation; polyneuropathy.	Red-yellow coating.	Rapid.	*Iodium, Natrium muriaticum.*
Kidney Fire (Lower Diabetes)	Frequent, copious urination; cloudy urine (as if greasy); progressive weight loss; dizziness; blurred vision; sore back, sometimes accompanied by ulceration on skin or itching; vaginal itching; impotence.	Red coating.	Thin and sinking.	*Mercurius solubilis, Phosphorus.*

GENITO-URINARY DISORDERS

TRADITIONAL CHINESE DIAGNOSIS	*Signs & Symptoms*	*Tongue*	*Pulse*	*HOMOEOPATHY*
Damp Cold	Low back feels cold; bending is difficult; patient desires a heating pad; pain becomes severe when weather is cold or damp.	Greasy, white coating.	Deep and slippery.	*Rhus toxicodendron.*
Damp Heat	Low back is sore and feels heavy; scanty, dark urine.	Greasy, yellow coating.	Slippery and wiry.	*Mercurius solubilis, Phosphorus.*
Damp Heat Filling Bladder	(a) Stabbing back pain; frequent, burning and painful urination; bitter taste in mouth.	Yellow coating.	Rapid and wiry.	*Bryonia alba.*
	(b) Intermittent, severe back pain; pain radiates to groin; frequent, painful urination, often with blood, or urine has calculi; difficulty of passing urine.	Yellow coating[13].	Rapid and wiry.	*Cantharis vesicatoria.*
Dry Cold	Low back is sore after exertion; all four limbs are tired; rest relieves pain; no other unusual signs.	Thin, white coating[13].	Moderate.	*Bryonia alba.*

[13] Flabby tongue.

TRADITIONAL CHINESE DIAGNOSIS	*Signs & Symptoms*	*Tongue*	*Pulse*	*HOMOEOPATHY*
Congealed Blood	Stabbing back pain at fixed point; pressure visibly increases discomfort; movement is difficult; pain is worse at night.	Darkish coating.	Choppy.	*Plumbum metallicum.*
Deficient Kidney Yang	Dull, aching, weak back; back and knees are without strength; patient cannot tolerate physical labour; bright white face; cold limbs; frequent urination at night.	Pale coating.	Frail.	*Natrium muriaticum, Rhus toxicodendron.*
Deficient Kidney Yin	Back is sore, weak and painful; legs are without strength; vertigo; tinnitus; insomnia.	Red coating.	Rapid and thin.	*Nux vomica, Sulphur.*

AMENORRHEA

Deficient Blood and Qi	Menstrual loss over a period of time gradually diminishes until there is none; watery leucorrhea; acrid odor; sallow face; fatigue, no Spirit; limbs are without strength; vertigo; palpitations.	Thin, white coating.	Sinking and thin, or empty.	*Natrium muriaticum.*

TRADITIONAL CHINESE DIAGNOSIS	*Signs & Symptoms*	*Tongue*	*Pulse*	*HOMOEOPATHY*
Stagnant Qi Congealed Blood	Amenorrhea seems related to emotional stress; menses suddenly cease; distended breasts and flanks; sallow face; headache.	Darkish or purple tongue.	Wiry or choppy.	*Zincum metallicum.*
Deficient Liver Yin and Deficient Kidney Yin	Gradual ceasing of menses; weight loss; patient feels hot; afternoon fever; dry skin; dark face; lower back and legs are weak; vertigo, tinnitus; dry mouth, constipation.	Red or scarlet, scanty coating.	Thin and slightly rapid.	*Pulsatilla nigricans.*
Mucus Dampness Obstructing Menses flow	Slight discomfort in lower abdomen; abdomen feels full but soft; much leucorrhea; vertigo; nausea; no taste in mouth; no appetite; distended breasts; condition is usually found in overweight women.	Greasy, white coating.	Slippery.	*Graphites, Silicea.*

DYSMENORRHEA (PMT[14] SYNDROME)

TRADITIONAL CHINESE DIAGNOSIS	*Signs & Symptoms*	*Tongue*	*Pulse*	*HOMOEOPATHY*
Stagnant Qi, Congealed Blood	Before or during menses lower abdomen is distended or painful and resists touch; menses flow unevenly; blood is darkish and has clots; passing of clots reduces discomfort; distended breasts.	Purple, dark or normal coating.	Wiry or choppy.	*Belladonna atropa, Lachesis, Lycopodium clavatum, Sulphur.*
Cold Damp Obstructing Menses	Before or during menses, lower abdomen is painful and cold; heat relieves pain; menstrual flow is not smooth; blood is dark coloured, thin and watery with clots.	Pale material; moist coating.	Sinking, tight or slow.	*Magnesium phosphoricum.*
Deficient Blood and Qi	Persistent dull soreness in abdomen during or after menses; pressure relli-eves pain; pale face; fatigue; no desire to speak; small amount of pale blood.	Pale material; white coating.	Empty or thin.	*Sepia.*

[14] PMT - Pre-menstrual tension.

ABNORMAL UTERINE BLEEDING

TRADITIONAL CHINESE DIAGNOSIS	*Signs & Symptoms*	*Tongue*	*Pulse*	*HOMOEOPATHY*
Heat in Blood	Heavy bleeding; bright red blood; increased the breasts and flanks are distended; flushed face; dry mouth; irritability.	Red tongue.	Rapid and full.	*Phosphorus.*
Deficient Spleen Qi Unable to Govern Blood	Heavy bleeding; pale, thin blood; puffy face; pale bright face; no Spirit; no appetite; watery stools.	Pale, thin, white coating.	Empty.	*China officinalis, Calcarea carbonica, Phosphorus.*
Stagnant Qi Congealed Blood	Constant slight bleeding or sudden heavy bleeding; distended flanks; distended lower abdomen; purple or dark blood clots; passing of clots reduces discomfort; dark face.	Darkish colour of tongue.	Sinking and wiry or choppy.	*China officinalis.*
Deficient Liver Yin and Deficient Kidney Yin	Menses occurs early; small amount of blood; pale or purple blood; vertigo; tinnitus; spots before eyes; sore back; insomnia; dry mouth.	Red, scarlet and small, glossy tongue.	Rapid, thin and wiry.	*China officinalis.*

PELVIC INFLAMMATORY DISORDERS

TRADITIONAL CHINESE DIAGNOSIS	*Signs & Symptoms*	*Tongue*	*Pulse*	*HOMOEOPATHY*
Fire Heat, Toxins Collecting in Lower Burner	Acute onset; fever; painful lower abdomen; pain resists touch; yellow, thick and foul smelling leucorrhea; low back pain; frequent urination; no appetite; nausea; dry mouth; constipation.	Red, yellow coating.	Wiry and rapid.	*Nux vomica.*
Stagnant Qi and Congealed Blood in Lower Burner	Painful lower abdomen and hypogastrium; abdomen has falling sensation or stabbing pain; low back pain; leucorrhea; sometimes palpable mass in hypogastrium.	Pale, dark, white coating or red dots.	Wiry and choppy.	*Nux vomica.*
Deficient Qi and Deficient Kidney Qi	Clear leucorrhea; sore low back; distended lower abdomen that feels worse after exertion or intercourse; fatigue; swollen lower limbs; vertigo; fear of cold; no appetite; frequent urination; watery stools.	Pale, white coating.	Frail and soggy.	*Calcarea carbonica, Causticum.*

GENITO-URINARY INFECTIONS

TRADITIONAL CHINESE DIAGNOSIS	*Signs & Symptoms*	*Tongue*	*Pulse*	*HOMOEOPATHY*
Damp Heat Filling Bladder (Lower Burner Damp Heat)	Frequent, urgent and painful urination; dry mouth or thirst or fever, backache or blood in urine.	Red, greasy coating.	Slippery and rapid.	*Belladonna atropa, Cantharis vesicatoria.*
Deficient Kidney Yin with Residual Damp Heat	Frequent, urgent, painful urination; scanty urine; warm palms and soles; dizziness; dry mouth; low fever, sometimes intermittent.	Red coating, greasy at root of tongue.	Thin and rapid.	*Lycopodium clavatum.*
Deficient Qi and Deficient Yin with Residual Damp Heat	Fatigue; vertigo; white face; no appetite; frequent, urgent and reduced urination; slight pain; some swelling; sore low back.	Normal.	Empty.	*China officinalis.*
Deficient Spleen and Deficient Kidney	Fatigue; no appetite; swollen limbs; cold back; frequent urination with slight discomfort.	Thin, white coating.	Frail.	*Silicea.*

ACUTE AND CHRONIC GLOMERULO-NEPHRITIS

TRADITIONAL CHINESE DIAGNOSIS	*Signs & Symptoms*	*Tongue*	*Pulse*	*HOMOEOPATHY*
Wind and Water in Conflict (Pernicious Influence Invading Lungs)	Acute onset; at beginning, eyelids and face are swollen; headaches; fever; fear of drafts; red, swollen, painful throat, or cough; urination is reduced; dark red urine; condition may progress to entire body with oedema.	Thin, yellow coating.	Floating, rapid.	*Belladonna atropa, Hepar sulphuris calcareum.*
Damp Heat Causing Sieqi	Whole body is swollen, skin is shiny; scanty urine sometimes blood in urine; frequent and urgent urination; headache; vertigo; bitter taste in mouth; constipation.	Greasy, yellow coating.	Wiry, slippery, full.	*Apis mellifica, Bryonia alba.*
Deficient Spleen Yang and Deficient Kidney Yang	Swollen body; bright pale face; no appetite; tired Spirit; scanty urine; sometimes no urination; rapid breathing; vertigo; nausea; vomiting.	Pale, white coating.	Soggy or frail.	*Digitalis rotundifolia.*
Dampness Distressing Spleen	Yellow skin; fatigue; no appetite; vomitting; whole body is swollen.	Greasy, white coating.	Sinking, slippery.	*Arsenicum album.*

TRADITIONAL CHINESE DIAGNOSIS	*Signs & Symptoms*	*Tongue*	*Pulse*	*HOMOEOPATHY*
Deficient Spleen Yang	Lower limbs are swollen; chronic intermittent oedema; sallow face; fatigue; distended chest and abdomen; no appetite; watery stools.	Pale, white coating.	Soggy, empty or slow.	*Natrium muriaticum.*
Deficient Spleen Yang and Deficient Kidney Yang	Chronic symptoms; reduced urination; swollen abdomen; oedema in lower body; bright pale face; fear of cold; cold limbs; no taste in mouth; sore low back; watery stools.	Pale, swollen, moist tongue.	Frail.	*Constitutional remedy.*
Deficient Liver Yin and Deficient Kidney Yin	Headache; vertigo; afternoon fever; red cheeks; night sweats; tinnitus; dry throat; insomnia; lumbago; irritability; dark, scanty urine; slight or no oedema.	Reddish, dry coating.	Thin and rapid.	*Lachesis, Pulsatilla nigricans.*

CYSTITIS, PYELITIS, PROSTATITIS (RENAL LITHIASIS)

Damp Heat Seeping Downwards into Bladder	Frequent, urgent, painful urination; fever; thirst; dry mouth; backache.	Red, greasy coating.	Wiry and rapid or slippery and Rapid.	*Cantharis vesicatoria, Berberis vulgaris.*

TRADITIONAL CHINESE DIAGNOSIS	*Signs & Symptoms*	*Tongue*	*Pulse*	*HOMOEOPATHY*
Damp Heat Accumulating and Crystallizing in Bladder	Urine occasionally contains sand-like deposits; difficult urination or sudden urine obstruction; occasional violent stabbing pain in lower groin or back; occasional blood in urine; calculi.	Normal coating.	Rapid.	*Lycopodium clavatum.*
Turbid Damp Heat Obstructing Bladder	Urine contains deposits.	Red, greasy coating.	Soggy and rapid.	*Sepia.*
Deficient Bladder Qi	Incontinence or frequent urination or bed wetting.	Moist, white coating.	Deep and frail.	*Sepia.*

INCONTINENCE OF URINE

Hear Violates Lungs, Obstructing Water's Descent	Dribbling urination; acute onset; dry throat; irritability; thirst; cough.	Thin, yellow coating	Rapid.	*Bryonia alba.*
Damp Heat Obstructing Middle Burner	Dribbling, cloudy urination; epigastrium feels full; distended abdomen; thirst but no desire to drink.	Greasy coating.	Soggy and slippery.	*Mercurius solubilis.*

TRADITIONAL CHINESE DIAGNOSIS	*Signs & Symptoms*	*Tongue*	*Pulse*	*HOMOEOPATHY*
Deficient Middle Burner (Spleen) Qi	Clear, dribbling urination; lethargy; chronic Deficient Spleen signs.	Pale coating.	Soggy and weak.	*Gelsemium sempervirens, Natrium muriaticum.*
Weak Life Gate Fire	Dribbling urination; no strength in elimination; bright pale face; painful lower back is cold; knees are without strength.	Pale coating.	Frail (especially proximal position).	*Phosphoricum acidum.*
Bladder Heat Collecting.	Dribbling, often painful urination; painful hypogastrium.	Red coating.	Rapid and slippery.	*Cantharis vesicatoria.*
Bladder Obstructed	Dribbling urination or thread-like urine; pain in hypogastrium.	Dark purple coating.	Choppy.	*Mercurius solubilis.*

HEMATURIA

Damp Heat Radiating Downwards into bladder	Bloody urine; frequent and painful urination; thirst; low back pain.	Red, greasy, yellow coating.	Wiry and rapid, or slippery and rapid.	*Cantharis vesicatoria.*

TRADITIONAL CHINESE DIAGNOSIS	*Signs & Symptoms*	*Tongue*	*Pulse*	*HOMOEOPATHY*
Small Intestine Fire Excess	Bloody urine; urine feels hot when passed; dark urine; painful urination; irritability; dry mouth; tongue ulceration.	Yellow coating.	Rapid.	*Apis mellifica.*
Spleen and Kid-neys Exhausted	Frequent urination with pale red blood; poor appetite; no Spirit, fatigue; sallow face; soreness in lower back; vertigo; tinnitus.	Pale, white coating.	Empty or frail.	*Sepia.*

EDEMA, ASCITES

TRADITIONAL CHINESE DIAGNOSIS	*Signs & Symptoms*	*Tongue*	*Pulse*	*HOMOEOPATHY*
External Influe-nce with Lung Qi not Circulating	Fever; fear of drafts; headache; coughing; sore throat; swollen, puffy face; eventually entire body swells; scanty urination.	Thin, white coating.	Tight and floating.	*Hepar sulphuris calcareum.*
Spleen Losing Transforming Ability	Sallow face; distended epigastrium; no appetite; watery stools; scanty urine; all four limbs are cold.	Pale, moist coating.	Sinking, moderate, or empty.	*Digitalis, Arsenicum album.*

TRADITIONAL CHINESE DIAGNOSIS	*Signs & Symptoms*	*Tongue*	*Pulse*	*HOMOEOPATHY*
Kidney Yang Exhausted	Whole body is swollen, especially below waist; lower back is sore and heavy; scanty urine; all four limbs are cold; fear of cold; no Spirit; dark face.	Swollen, pale, white coating.	Frail.	*Lycopodium clavatum.*

FEVERS, INFECTIONS

Exterior Wind Cold	Fever; aversion to cold; headache or body ache; sometimes coughing; sometimes running or stuffed nose; no thirst.	Thin, white coating.	Floating and tight or floating and moderate.	*Belladonna atropa, Pyrogenium.*
Exterior Wind Heat	Fever; slight aversion to cold; headache; thirst; sore throat; sometimes cough with yellow phlegm.	Tip of the tongue is red; slightly yellow coating.	Floating and rapid.	*Rhus toxicodendron.*
External Cold and Interior Deficient Yang Simultaneously	Very slight fever; acute onset; desire for more clothing; desire for sleep; great aversion to cold.	Pale, moist coating.	Feeble.	*Nux vomica.*

TRADITIONAL CHINESE DIAGNOSIS	*Signs & Symptoms*	*Tongue*	*Pulse*	*HOMOEOPATHY*
Sieqi Influence in Shao Yang Stage[15]	Fever and chills are alternating (i.e., not simultaneous); no appetite.	Thin and white or yellow and white coating.	Wiry.	*Calcarea carbonica.*
Sieqi Influence in Yang Ming Stage[16]	Mild fever; aversion to food; red face; perspiration.	Red, dry, yellow coating.	Flooding with strength or slippery and rapid.	*Bryonia alba.*
Deficient Yin	Chronic low afternoon fever; warm palms and soles; insomnia; night sweats; red cheeks.	Reddish, thin coating.	Thin and rapid.	*Sulphur.*
Deficient Qi	Chronic low fever especially in mornings; spontaneous sweating; fear of draft; fatigue; pale face.	Pale, thin, white coating.	Frail.	*Nux vomica.*
Congealed Blood	Chronic low fever; no thirst, or thirst but no desire to drink; stabbing, fixed pain; hemorrhages.	Dark purple coating or red pimples on surface.	Choppy.	*Nux vomica, Tuberculinum.*

[15] Shao Yang - Sanjiao and Gall-bladder.
[16] Yang Ming - Large Intestine and Stomach.

INFESTATIONS & INFECTIONS OF INTERNAL ORGANS

TRADITIONAL CHINESE DIAGNOSIS	*Signs & Symptoms*	*Tongue*	*Pulse*	*HOMOEOPATHY*
Deficient Lung Qi and Deficient Kidney Yang, Kidney unable to Absorb Qi	Asthma (especially exhalation easy, inhalation difficult); shortness of breath; exertion worsens the condition; no Spirit; low voice; spontaneous sweating; cold limbs.	Pale, moist, swollen tongue.	Frail or empty.	*Calcarea carbonica.*
Deficient Spleen Qi and Deficient Lung Qi	Shortness of breath; cough; asthma accompanied by copious, thin, white phlegm; reduced appetite; loose stools; oedema.	Pale with white coating.	Empty.	*Arsenicum album.*
Deficient Spleen Qi and Deficient Kidney Yang	Cold appearance; bright pale complexion; lower back and limbs are cold and sore; loose stools with undigested food; oedema; difficulty in urination; ascites.	Pale, moist, swollen, with white coating.	Frail and especially sinking.	*Pulsatilla nigricans.*
Liver Invading Spleen	Chest and flanks are distended and sore; emotional frustration, moodiness, or anger; reduced appetite; distended abdomen; loose stools; passing flatus.	Dark or normal, white coating.	Wiry, taut.	*Ignatia amara.*

TRADITIONAL CHINESE DIAGNOSIS	*Signs & Symptoms*	*Tongue*	*Pulse*	*HOMOEOPATHY*
Liver Fire Invading Lungs	Burning pain in chest and flanks; irritability and quick anger; vertigo; red eyes; bitter taste in mouth; serial coughing; coughing of blood.	Red tongue with thin, yellow coating.	Wiry and rapid.	*Nux vomica.*

ANEMIA

TRADITIONAL CHINESE DIAGNOSIS	*Signs & Symptoms*	*Tongue*	*Pulse*	*HOMOEOPATHY*
Deficient Qi and Deficient Blood of Heart and Spleen	Pale or sallow face; pale lips and fingernails; vertigo; fatigue; palpitations; tinnitus; no appetite; watery stools; late menses with pale blood.	Pale, white coating.	Empty, frail or thin.	*China officinalis*[17], *Ferrum phosphoricum.*
Dampness Distressing Spleen	Sallow, yellow face; swollen body; vertigo; no appetite; no taste in the mouth; nausea; distended abdomen; heavy, tired limbs; watery stools.	Pale, greasy, white coating.	Soggy, slippery or thin.	*Sepia*[17].
Deficient Liver Yin and Deficient Kidney Yin	Face lacks brightness; red cheeks, especially in afternoon; low fever; dry mouth vertigo; tinnitus; bleeding gums.	Red or scarlet coating.	Sinking, thin and rapid.	*Ferrum metallicum*[17].

[17] Tissue salts are helpful.

TRADITIONAL CHINESE DIAGNOSIS	*Signs & Symptoms*	*Tongue*	*Pulse*	*HOMOEOPATHY*
Deficient Spleen Yang and Deficient Kidney Yang	Pale face; pale lips and fingernails; vertigo; spots before eyes; tired Spirit; tinnitus; lower limbs are weak; no appetite; no taste in mouth; watery stool; swollen lower limbs; sometimes amenorrhea.	Pale, swollen white coating.	Frail.	*China officinalis*[18].

LOCOMOTOR DISORDERS (Bi & Wei SYNDROMES)

Wind Obstructing Channels	Sore, painful joints; pain changes location; sometimes accompanied by fever; chills.	White coating.	Floating.	*Pulsatilla nigricans.*
Cold Obstructing Channels	Painful joints; fixed pain; movement aggravates pain; heat relieves pain; cold weather aggravates pain.	White coating.	Tight.	*Bryonia alba.*
Dampness Obstructing Channels	Joints are sore and feel heavy; discomfort; fixed pain; numb limbs; damp weather aggravates pain.	Greasy coating.	Soggy.	*Rhus toxicodendron.*

[18] Tissue salts are helpful.

TRADITIONAL CHINESE DIAGNOSIS	*Signs & Symptoms*	*Tongue*	*Pulse*	*HOMOEOPATHY*
Wind Cold and Dampness Obstructing Chennels	Combinations of the above, worse with cold.	Greasy coating.	Soggy.	*Dulcamara.*
Wind Heat Obstructing Chennals	Sore joints; difficult movement; fever; thirst.	Red-yellow coating.	Floating and rapid.	*Bryonia alba.*
Damp Heat Obstructing Channels	Fever; thirst; swollen and painful joints; red eruptions on skin.	Red, greasy coating.	Rapid and slippery.	*Sulphur.*

CHINESE LANGUAGE

UNLIKE most modern languages, Chinese does not have a phonetic alphabet. Instead, Chinese uses "pictographs", generally referred to as "characters" or "ideograms". These symbolize objects and actions and contain little or no indication how they are to be pronounced.

The pitches or "tones" of spoken Chinese present another difficulty to the novice. With its tens of thousands of characters. Chinese has some 400 syllables, with which to pronounce them. As a result, a single sound may represent more than 100 different written characters. Tones and the use of compounds multiply the number of available word-sounds. For example, Putonghaua, the national dialect, has four separate tones. Cantonese has the most, with nine.

TONE. The tone or pitch can completely change a syllable's denotation. For instance, the sound "mah" is represented by several different Chinese characters. Pronounced in putonghua's first tone, mā (māh), means "mother"; in the second tone, mă (máh), means "numb" or "hemp". In the third tone, mă (măh), it is "horse", and in the fourth, ma (ṃàh), it means "to scold".

One can never learn tones from a book. One has to hear and imitate then hundreds of times before grasping their subtle tonal variations. Nevertheless, a very general guide for the sound "mah" in the four tones of putonghua is as follows; The first tone is pronounced at a level, fairly high pitch: ma (mah). The second tone rises from the middle register to the level of the first tone: ma (máh). In the third tone, the voice dips and rises-the dip is low and rather elongated and the rise is somewhat quicker: ma (măh). The fourth tone begins high and falls to a low pitch, very abruptly and definitely: mà (màh).

DIALECTS. Written Chinese is uniform throughout China, but the spoken language varies from region to region, and sometimes even from village to village. China has eight major dialect groups. The Beijing dialect and closely related pronounciations are mainly found in the northeastern and southwestern regions of China. Since 1949, Beijing dialect has been the basis of the national dialect and is spoken today by 70 per cent of China's Chinese-speaking population. As the official dialect of the People's Republic, it is used in government and commercial circles, on radio and TV broadcasts, and is taught in schools throughout the country. Outside China it's often referred to as "Mandarin".

PINYIN ROMANIZATION: There are two and sometimes three different spellings in English for the same word. The latest phonetic system of romanizing Chinese sounds is Pinyin, meaning "phonetic transcription". Earlier Chinese words were transliterated in the Wade-Giles or Yale system, which is why peking now seems strange as Beijing, and Mo Tse-tung as Mao Zedong. These two names are at least more or less recognizable. The name we know for the huge southern city of Canton bears no resemblance whatsoever to it new rendering-"Guangzhou".

Since 1958, Pinyin has been the officially endorsed system in China, and Western media are increasingly adopting pinyin.

PINYIN ALPHABET PRONOUNCIATION GUIDE

(Letters in parenthesis are equivalents used a traditional Wade-Giles spellings)

a (a)	Vowel as in *far*
b (p)	Consonant as in *be*
c (ts)	Consonant as in *its*
ch (ch)	Consonant as in *ip* strongly aspirated

d (t)	Consonant as in *do*
e (e)	Vowel as in *her*
F (f)	Consonant as in *foot*
g (k)	Consonant as in *go*
h (h)	Cosonant as in *her* : strongly aspirated
i (i)	Vowel as in *eat* or as in *sir* (when in syllables beginning with c. ch. r. s. sh. z and ch.)
j (ch)	Consonant as in *jeep*
k (k)	Consonant as in *kind,* strongly aspirated
l (l)	Consonant as in *land*
m (m)	Consonant as in *me*
o (o)	Vowel as in *law*
p (p)	Consonant as in *par :* strongly aspirated
q (ch)	Consonant as in *cheek*
r (j)	Consonant as in *right* or pronounced as z in *azure*
s (s. ss. sz.)	Consonant as in *sister*
sh (sh)	Consonant as in *shore*
t (t)	Consonant as in *top* : strongly aspirated
u (u)	Vowel as in *too*; also as in French *tu* or the German Munchen
v (v)	Consonant used only to produce foreign words, national minority words, and local dialects
w (w)	Semi-vowel in syllables beginning with u when not preceded by consonants, as in *want*
x (hs)	Consonant as in *she*
y	Semi-vowel in syllables beginning with i or u when not preceded by consonants, as in *yef.*
z (ts. tz)	Consonant as in *zero*
zh (ch)	Consonant as in *jump.*

SOME COMMON IDEOGRAMS AND THEIR MEANINGS

阿是	a-shi	Is there, Oh yes
秉	bing	to grasp, to hold (a handful of corn)
白	bai	White, clear, bright, to notify, simple, empty
百	bai	One hundred, many, all
不	bu	no, not
藏	cáng	to hide, to store, to preserve to put
肠	cháng	intestine, viscera, the inner part
冲	chõng	to rinse, to pour out, to foliate, to flow over, young, the impulse
	chõng	vigorous, full of energy
窗	chuãng	window
大	dà	big, window, whole, very, important
带	dai	belt, area, to carry to take along, band (wrapping)
胆	dăn	bile, valour, the inside of an object
地	di	earth, country, place
督	dû	to monitor, to lead
都	dû	capital metropolis, all beautiful, noble
二	èr	two, both
耳	ěr	ear, lateral, handle
肺	feì	lung

风	feñg	wind, hearsay, custom, conduct
封	feñg	to close, to seal, to envelope
府	fŭ	magistrate, office, house, palace, storeroom
肝	gān	liver
谷	gŭ	valley, gorge, difficult, congested, to nourish
骨	gŭ	bone, character, framework, structure, scaffolding
关	gŭan	to close, to bar, interrelation
海	haì	ocean, sea
寒	hán	coldness, celd front. poverty, poor
后	hoù	behind, backwards, after, later
户	hù	door, openine, family
华	húa	opulent, china, chinese, beautiful, colourful, glory
会	hui	union, to gather, to be able, community
疾	jí	disease, haite, annoying
极	jí	summit, top, upper, end
脊	jí	spine, back, peak, fish-bone, ridge
夹	jía	grasp, press, punch, to carry (to have on one's person)
肩	jiān	shoulder, to carry
交	jiāo	to associate, to cross, mutual, to unite
金	jiñ	gold, golden, metal, money
经	jiñg	to pass through, warp (of a fabric), to rule to lead
京	jiñg	the capital, big, numerous, Beijing
井	jiñg	well, pit. order, system
厥	júe	nobody else but, he, she, it, his, her, that one.

孔	kong	whole, very, passage, big, cavity
髎	liáo	cleft of a bone, cleft of a joint
陵	líng	hill, tomb, tomb of the emperor
门	mén	door, opening, family
明	ming	bright, shining, open, clear, mind, tomorrow
脉	mai	pulse, vessel, artery, vein, line, beat of the pulse
脑	năo	brain, mind
内	nei	inner, inside, in
脾	pi	spleen, stomach, mood, essence.
前	qian	anterior, in front, earlier, deceased
泉	quán	well, money, wealth
曲	qŭ	curved, bent, angle, curve injustice
人	rén	man, people, person
任	rén	responsible for, office, to appoint, to let
容	ròng	contents, face, to suffer
三	sān	three, often
少	shăo	little, seldom
上	shàng	upper, on top, above peak, best, former, the authorities
商	shàng	consult, merchant, trade, indicator of a water-clock, two tones of the five note musical scale
申	shēn	notify, to inform a superior
肾	shèn	kidney
神	shén	spirit, soul, god, godly, effective
水	shŭi	water, liquid, fluid
市	shi	town, market, village, to buy, to trade

四	si	four, roundabout, everywhere
石	shi	stone, stony, rock, barren, useless
俞	shù	transport, point, point of transport
太	tài	very, supreme, sublime, greatest
太阳	tài yańg	greatest yang, sun
天	tiān	heaven, heavenly, day, nature, weather
庭	tíng	hall, yard, house, courtyard, family
听	tiñg	to hear, to listen, to inquire, to understand
通	toñg	to pass through, circulation, complete, generally
脘	wăn	cavity of the stomach, channel in the body
胃	wèi	stomach
五	wũi	five
郄	xì	border, cleft, separation, gap
膝	xī	knee, lap
溪	xī	stream, mountain stream
心	xīn	heart, the inside, middle, center
星	xiñg	star, spark, sparsely
虚	xū	empty, wrong, modest, not genuine, pretence
血	xue	blood, bloody, related by blood
小	xiaō	small, young
墟	xū	old grave, ruin, wasteland
腰	yaō	kidney*, hip, cross, sacral region, loin, isthmus
哑	Yă	hoarse

* genital functions

液	yè	juice, discharge, fluid, liquid
医	yī	doctor, to heal, medicine
鱼	yú	fish, fishlike
玉	yù	jade, precious, sublime, gems
元	yúan	the begining, primordial, leader, great
泽	zé	pond, swamp, shining, benefit
渚	zhŭ	small island, sand bank
注	zhù	injection
椎	zhūi	spine, hammer, to hammer, wooden club
中	zhoñg	middle, inside, in, mediator, Chinese
中国	zhōng guo	realm of the middle, China
竹	zhú	bamboo

CORRESPONDENCES OF THE 5 ELEMENTS

五行归类表 wú xing guī leí biǎō

THE BODY 人体

Element	Solid Organs	Hollow Organs	Sense Organs	Body tissues	Emotions	Tastes
	脏	腑	官	体	情志	味
	zang	tu	guan	u	qing zhi	wei
Wood	Liver	Gall bladder	Eye	Muscles	Anger	Sour
木	肝	胆	目	筋	怒	酸
mu	gan	dan	mu	jin	nu	suan
Fire	Heart	Small Intestine	Tongue	Blood vessels	Joy	Bitter
火	心	小肠	舌	脉	喜	苦
huo	xin	chang	she	mai	xi	ku
Earth	Spleen	Stomach	Mouth	Soft Tissue (flesh)	Anxiety	Sweet
土	脾	胃	口	肉	思	甘
fu	pi	wei	kou	rou	si	gan
Metal	Lung	Large intestine	Nose	Skin	Sadness	Pungent
金	肺	大肠	鼻	皮毛	悲忧	辛
jin	fei	da chang	bi	pimao	ben you	xin
Water	Kidney	Urinary Bladder	Ear	Bone Cartilage	Fear	Salty
水	肾	膀胱	耳	骨	惊恐	咸
shui	shen	pang-guan	er	gu	jing kong	xian

NATURE

自然界

S. Seasons	Climate	Stages of development	Colors	Cardinal point	Planets	Sounds	Heavenly stems (tribes)
季节 ji jie	气候 qi hou	生长 zhang	颜 yan	方位 wei	星 xing	音 yin	天干 tiangan
Spring 春 chun	Wind 风 feng	Birth 生 sheng	Green 青 qing	East 东 dong	Jupiter 木星 xing	角 jue	甲乙 jia yi
Early Summer 夏 xia	Heat 热 re	Growth 长 chang	Red 赤 chi	South 南 nan	Mars 火星 huo xing	徵 zheng	丙丁 bing ding
Late Summer 长夏 chang chun	Humidity 湿 shi	Reproduction 化 hua	Yellow 黄 huang	Middle 中 zhong	Saturn 土星 tuxing	宫 gong	戊己 wu ji
Autumn 秋 qiu	Dry 燥 zao	Harvest 收 shou	White 白 bai	West 西 xi	Venus 金星 xing	商 shang	庚辛 geng xin
Winter 冬 dong	Cold 寒 han	Storage 藏 cang	Black 黑 hei	North 北 bei	Mercury 水星 xing	羽 yu	壬癸 ren gui

HEALTH CARE/MEDICINE

English	Pinyin (Chinese Pronunciation)	Chinese Characters
Medicine	Yao (yuo)	药
Pharmacy	Yaodian (yun dee-en)	药店
Where can I find medicine?	nali you yao (nah-lee yo yao)	哪里有药
Aspirin	Asipilin (ah-suh-pee-leen)	阿斯匹林
I have a cold.	wo shangfengle (waw shahng fung-hih)	我伤风了
I don't feel well.	wo bu shufu (waw yo boo shoo-foo)	我不舒服
I am ill.	wo youbing (waw yo-bing)	我有病
Please call a doctor.	qing yisheng lai (ching yee-shung lye)	请医生来
Dentist	Yayi (yah-yee)	牙医
Hospital	yiyuan (yee yoo-en)	医院
Headache	touteng (toe-tuhng)	头痛
Toothache	yateng (yah-tuhng)	牙痛
Dizziness	touyun (toe yew-win)	头晕
Diarrhea	xiedu (shee-eh doo)	泻肚
Stomach sickness	weibing (way-bing)	胃病
Stomach pain	weiteng (way tuhng)	胃痛
It hurts me here.	wo zheli teng (waw juh-lee tuhng)	我这里痛

NUMBERS

One	yi (yee)	一
Two	er (are)	二
Three	san (san)	三
Four	si (suh)	四
Five	wu (woo)	五
Six	liu (lee-oh)	六
Seven	qi (chee)	七
Eight	ba (bah)	八
Nine	jiu (jee-oh)	九
Ten	shi (shir)	十
Eleven	shiyi (shir-yee)	十一
Twelve	shier (shit-are)	十二
Thirteen	shisan (shir-san)	十三
Fourteen	shisi (shir-suh)	十四
Twenty	ershi (are-shir)	二十
Thirty	sanshi (san-shir)	三十
One hundred	yibai (yee-bye)	一百
One thousand	yiqian (yee-chee-en)	一千

Index I

LIST OF ILLUSTRATIONS AND TABLES

A

Acupuncture areas of the ear 838, 844, 852
Acupuncture equipment, traditional xii
Acupuncture needles 36, 37
Alalrm points 444, 446
Alarm points Front (Mu) 276
Anatomy of the ear 838, 840, 842
Ancillary techniques of acupuncture 754

B

Back-Shu points, anatomy 192
Back-Shu points 461, 462
Baihui (Du 20.), localisation of 264
Bronze figure xiii

C

Cerebral palsy 470
Chest wall, front points 238
Chinese cultural interrelationships 814
Chronic rhinitis 468
Command points 458
Confluent points 452, 453
Cun 40

D

Dangerous points of the orbit 144
Directions of insertions 54
Disease management 358
Distal points (6 important) 112, 120, 122, 124, 125
Distal points, proximal target areas 112

E

Ear, points around the 240, 288
Ear points, numbering system 856
Ear, representation of the foetus 858
Electro-acupuncture stimulation 786
Elephant, acupuncture points 2
Energy circulation 422
Energy flow in Ren and Du Channels 268
Energy levels 418
Enkephalin 28

F

Finger measurements 40
Five Elements and bio-physical processes 324
Five Elements and the Universe 323
Five Element relationships 318, 320
Foot points 244, 294

G

Gate Control Theory 25
Great Law of Bu-Xie 61, 433

H

Head Needle therapy areas, 862, 864
Head points 284, 862
He-Sea points 459
Horary points 341
Huang Di Nei Jing 8, 10
Huatuo Jiajo (Ex 21) 462

L

Ling Shu 8
Lower back points 240, 260
Luo-connecting points 449

M

Mother and Son points 460
Motor Gate Theory 24
Moxa Plant, names of 776
Mu Front points 276

N

Needle Insertion, methods 54
Needles, traditional 6

O

Organ Clock, 358, 340, 418, 463

P

Paralysis of limbs 461
Patella, points around the 154
Patients at the Institute of Acupuncture, Kalubowila 471
Postures for Acupuncture 38
Proportional measurements 48
Pulse positions 396, 398, 380

R

Rhinitis and Chronic bronchial asthma 469
Rhinitis, chronic 468

S

Scalp points 284, 862, 864, 794
Sedative & tranquilizing points 221
Selection of points 852
Summary of acupuncture 33
System of Channels 112

T

Tongue diagnosis 410

U

Upper limb points, posterior aspect 228

Y

Yin and Yang excesses 424, 426
Yuan-Source points 448

Z

Zang-fu relationships 98
Zang-Fu-Theory 328
Zang Organs and Emotions, Sounds, Fluids, 330

■

Index II

CLINICAL ACUPUNCTURE

A

Abdominal distension 193, 204, 449, 453, 515, 534, 733
Abdominal pain 156, 335, 641, 689, 694, 735
Achilles tendinitis 198, 586
Acne 590
Acupressure 62, 137, 198, 267, 467, 754, 758
Acupunctoscope 51, 915, 918
Acupuncture 337, 770
Acupuncture analgesia 823, 915
Acupuncture point 790, 799
Acupuncture point detector 788
Acupuncture points 30, 108, 137, 211, 657, 672, 678, 682, 818, 833, 898, 916, 918, 922
Acupuncture practice 915
Acupuncturist 72, 74, 645, 915
Acute coryza 501
Acute diarrhea 641
Acute infections 831
Acute mastitis 738
Addiction 80
Adnexitis 563
Agalactia 568
Ah-Shi points 5, 63, 67, 181, 383, 407, 443, 465, 483, 484, 488, 489, 533, 535, 565, 566, 573, 574, 575, 576, 577, 578, 579, 580, 584, 595, 759, 760, 777, 832, 915
AIDS and Acupuncture 935
Alarm points 5, 51, 188, 246, 428, 443, 444, 465, 494, 542, 832, 916, 924
Allergic rhinitis 502
Alopecia areata 597
Amebiasis 536
Amebic 537
Amebic hepatitis 543
Amenorrhea 559, 719
Anal fissure 539
Analgesia 440, 817, 925
Anatomy of acupuncture 87, 89, 91, 93
Anatomy of the ear 837
Ancillary techniques of acupuncture 754
Ancilliary 85
Ancilliary drugs 801
Angina pectoris 173, 219, 521, 640
Angioneurotic edema 592
Ankle 579
Ankle Disorders 243, 586
Ankylosing Spondylitis 576
Anterior Hair Line 863
Anterior surface 837
Antero-Posterior Midline 863
Anuria 554
Anxiety 678
Aphasia 173, 277, 647

Apoplexy 265, 645. 646
Appendicitis 534, 642
Arrhythmias 81, 513, 514, 680
Artemisia 773, 775, 916
Artemisia vulgaris 775, 776
Ascites 515, 546, 702, 849
Asthma 672
Astigmatism 609
Auricular areas and points 843
Auriculotherapy 850, 855, 857, 916
Auscultation 361, 368
Autonomic nervous system 498

B

Back of the auricle 849
Backache 575
Bacterial endocarditis 931
Bed wetting 557
Behaviour disorders 631
Bell's palsy 486
Biliary colic 546, 642
Bipay 298
Bleeding 73
Bleeding Therapy 760
Blepharitis 608
Blood disorders 523
Blood Supply of the Ear 841
Body Points 818
Bradycardia 516
Bronchial asthma 509, 639
Bronchitis 507
Bu method 916
Bu-xie 432
Bulbar palsy 493

C

Calf Muscles 586
Cardiac asthma 515
Cardiac disorders 513
Cardiovascular disorders 513
Care of the needles 45
Carpal joints 578
Cataract 611
Cervicitis 563
Channels or meridians 916
Chemical methods 44
Chinese calendar 939
Chinese metaphysics 348
Chize 121
Chorea 482
Chronic cough 669
Chuang tzu 311
Circadian rhythms 932
Circulation of energy in the du and ren channels 281
Circulation of energy in the gall bladder 246
Circulation of energy in the heart 174
Circulation of energy in the kidney 212
Circulation of energy in the large intestine 140
Circulation of energy in the liver 253
Circulation of energy in the lung 130
Circulation of energy in the small intestine 185
Circulation of energy in the spleen 168
Circulation of energy in the stomach 158

Circulation of energy in the urinary bladder 202
Cirrhosis of the liver 545
Cold 376
Collapse 514
Collaterals 916
Common cold 501, 667
Confluent points 916
Conjunctivitis 608
Constipation 539
Contact dermatitis 934
Contraindications 770, 790
Coronary insufficiency 640
Cough 508
Cryopuncture 777
Cunometer 917
Cupping 688, 769, 917
Cystitis 556

D

Damp-heat in the Urinary Bladder 202
Dampness 377
Deafness 601, 743
Deep channels 116
Deficient kidney yang 709
Depressive and manic mental disorders 681
Depth and direction 58
Deqi 917
Dermatitis 595
Detached retina 610
Diabetes mellitus 619
Diagnostic evaluation 797
Diarrhea 537, 691
Dingchan 299
Diplopia 609
Direct moxibustion 773
Disappearance of symptoms 828
Diseases of the nervous system 477
Disorders of the knee joint 585
Disturbance in the urinary bladder functions 202
Divergent channels 116
Dizziness 518, 657
Dorsal column stimulation 794
Dorsal region 574
Dryness 377
Du channel 255, 893
Dual Purpose Instruments 791
Duodenal ulcer 532
Duration of the disease 829
Duration of the treatment 830
Dysentery 537, 693
Dysmenorrhea 560, 721
Dysmenorrhea 643
Dyspepsia 533
Dysphagia 528
Dyspnea 515

E

Ear acupuncture 832
Ear acupuncture points 652, 660, 675, 688, 701, 705, 709, 710, 718, 723, 725, 728, 735, 741, 745, 747, 750, 754
Ear Acupuncture Therapy 835
Ear diagnosis 407
Ear disorders 601, 639
Ear Lobe 843
Ear Points 819
Edema 515
Effects of acupuncture 925
Electrical Pulse Stimulation 819

Electrical pulse stimulation 918
Electrical testing 832
Electro-acupuncture 755
Electro-acupuncture 78, 795
Electrotherapy 755
Embedding Needle Therapy 763, 918
Emergency Measures 635
Encephalitis 485
Endocrine disorders 615
Endorphins 918
Energy circulation in the pericardium 221
Energy circulation in the sanjiao 232
Enuresis 557
Epigastric pain 686
Epilepsy 630
Epileptic attack 636
Epistaxis 503, 749
Erysipelas 594
Excess extrinsic lung disorder 667
Excess of heart 678
Excessive – deficient 383
Exogenous heat 736, 746
Exterior – Interior 380
Exterior Cold 381
Exterior Deficiency 381
Exterior Excess 381
Exterior Hot 381
Extraordinary Channels 918
Extraordinary organs 95
Extraordinary points 283
Extrinsic excess heat disorder 663
Extrinsic humid heat and damp disorder 665
Eye disorders 607, 638

F

Facial hemispasm 486
Facial paralysis 486, 660
Fainting 73, 832
febrile fit 636
Febrile fits 630
Filiform needle 918
Fire imbalance 717
Five zang organs6 91
Flatulence 534
Focal epilepsy 479
Frontal headache 637
Fu organs 93, 328
Functional uterine bleeding 561
Furuncle 737
Furunculosis 590

G

Gall bladdar Channel 233, 247, 334, 889
Gall Bladder 94, 116, 329
Gastric ulcer 532
Gastritis 531, 640, 683
Gastro-enteritis 641
Gate-Control Theory of Pain 919
Genitourinary disorders 551
Ginseng 801, 809, 810, 811
Glaucoma 612
Glossitis 527
Goiter 618, 740
Grand mal 478
Gynecological disorders 559
Gynecomastia 617

H

Habit spasms 482
Hand manipulation 819

Hay fever 502
He-sea point 457
Head needle therapy 832, 920
Headache 482, 518
Heart 91
Heart and small intestines 104
Heart channel 115, 169, 175, 333, 877
Heart dysfunctions 681
Heat 376
Heat disorder 734
Heat stroke 636
Hematuria 554
Hemiparesis 490
Hemiplegia 490
Hemorrhoids 539
Hepatitis 543, 934
Herpes zoster 595
Hiatus hernia 529
Hiccough 515, 530, 640
Hiccup 530
High fever 638
Hoarse voice 506
Homoeopuncture 920
Horary points 459.
Hordeolum 608
Horizontal Line 863
Hot needle therapy 772, 920
Hot-cold 382
Husband – wife law 343, 920
Hydrotherapy 755, 770
Hyperemesis 566
Hypochondrium 697
Hypogonadism 616
Hypotension 517
Hysteria 623
Hysterical attack 636

I

I ching 346
Indigestion 533
Infantile convulsions 630, 730
Infantile diarrhea 732
Infection 77
Influential points 921
Insertion of the needle 55
Insomnia 484, 675
Inspection 361, 363
Intercostal neuralgia 574
Interior cold 382
Interior hot 382
Interior-exterior relationship of channels 921
Intermediate channels 116
Intestinal colic 538
Intestinal colic 641
Intestinal parasitosis 536
Irregular menstruation 559

J

Jacksonian fits 479
Jaundice 696
Jianneiling 298
Jing-river point 457
Jing-well point 456, 922

K

Kidney 92, 329
Kidney and urinary bladder 699
Kidney channel 115, 207, 212, 334, 884
Kidney dysfunctions 657
Kidneys and urinary bladder 105
Knee 579

L

Labyrinthitis 604
Lactation deficiency 568
Language and semantic problems 355
Large intestine 93, 133
Large intestine channel 115, 140, 333
Large intestine organ 140
Laryngitis 506
Laser beam therapy 779, 922
Leucoderma 596
Leucorrhea 562, 725
Lifting and thrusting 60
Liver 92, 329
Liver and gall bladder 109, 746
Liver channel 116, 234, 254, 334, 892
Locating acupuncture points 47
Location of points 833
Locomotor disorders 571, 711
Low back pain 699
Lung 92
Lung channel 115, 117, 333, 869
Lung deficiency 669
Lungs and large intestines 102
Lying down position: 46
Lymphangitis 593, 737

M

Magnetotherapy 801
Malaria 665
Malignant disease 830
Malposition of the fetus 566
Management of labor 821
Manipulation 661
Manipulation of the needle 923
Manual dexterity of the acupuncturist 833
Masculinization 617
Mastitis 568
Mechanical methods 754, 758
Medial aspect of antitragus 846
Meniere's disease 485, 604
Meningitis 485
Menorrhagia 561, 723
Mental depression 625
Metabolism 809, 810
Metatarsalgia 587
Methods of puncture 55
Methods of stimulation 819
Midday-midnight law 339
Moist heat 43
Morning sickness5 727
Mother-son law 337, 923
Motor neurone disease 497
Moxibustion 772, 923
Mumps 734
Muscular dystrophies 497
Myopathies 497
Myopia 609

N

Nature of the disease 829
Nausea 530, 683
Nausea 515
Nausea, vomiting 641
Needle therapy 861
Needling sensations 63
Neima 299
Nephritis 552
Nerve supply of the ear 841
Nettle rash 592
Neurasthenia 623
Neurasthenia 516

Neuro-stimulation 792
Neuropraxia 497
Night blindness 613
Nocturnal enuresis 557, 631, 704
Nose bleeding 503
Nose disorders 605
Nose disorders 639

O

Obesity of endocrine origin 620
Obstetric disorders 566
Occipital headache 638
Oligomenorrhea 559
Oliguria 554
Ophthalmoplegia 612
Optic nerve atrophy 610
Organ gall bladder 247
Organ heart 175
Organ kidney 212
Organ liver 254
Organ small intestine 185
Organ spleen 168
Organ stomach 159
Organ urinary bladder 202
Osteoarthritis 585
Osteoarthritis of hip 585

P

Palpation 362, 373, 850
Palpitation 514, 678
Pancreatitis 548
Paralysis 714
Paraparesis 494
Paraplegia 494
Parietal headache 637
Parkinsonism 481
Pelvic inflammations 563
Penetration puncture 766
Peptic ulcer 532, 683
Percussion 361
Pericardium 91
Pericardium and sanjiao 107
Pericardium channel 115, 215, 334, 886
Periosteal acupuncture 759
Peripheral vascular disorders 520
Pertussis 508
Petit mal 478
Piles 539
Plum blossom needle 925
Plum-blossom tapping 762
Point-injection therapy 925
Points for the different syndromes 685
Posterior surface 841
Posterior-tinggong 298
Posture of the patient during acupuncture 46
Presence of complications 830
Press needle 925
Prismatic needle 925
Prognosis of disease 827
Prolapse of the rectum 540
Pruritus vulvae 565
Psoriasis 598
Psychiatric disorders 621
Psychomotor (temporal lobe) epilepsy 480
Pulse diagnosis 386, 926
Pulse examination 832
Pyelitis 552
Pyelonephritis 552
Pyrexias 632

Q

Qi 102, 319, 415, 416, 741
Qi Flow 90

R

Radiant heat 777
Radiation 44, 936
Rapport 833
Reflexotherapy 765
Regular channels 926
Relaxation therapy 765
Ren channel 271, 896
Renal colic 555, 642
Renal failure 516
Repetitive fits 630
Respiratory disorders 501
Retaining of the acupuncture needle 59
Retention of urine 556
Retinitis 610
Rheumatic heart disease 516
Rhinitis 747
Rhinorrhea 747

S

Sacroiliac joints 578
Salpingitis 563
Sanjiao channel 91, 223
Sanjiao channel 115, 334, 887
Scalp areas 819
Schizophrenia 624
Sciatica 642
Selection of points 833
Sense organs 95
Serum hepatitis 543
Severe headache 636
Sheng cycle 926
Shi diseases 927
Shock 514, 638
Shu-Stream point 457
Sieqi 423, 927
Sinusitis 504, 747
Sitting position: 46
Skin disorders 589
Small intestine 93
Small intestine channel 115, 117, 185, 333, 878
Sonopuncture 787
Sore throat 752
Sound therapy 787
Spastic paralysis 482
Spinal cord injury 933
Spleen 92
Spleen and stomach 103
Spleen channel 115, 161, 168, 333, 875
Splenomegaly 550
Sprain and strain 741
Sprain of pectoral muscles 574
Squint 609
Staphylococcal sepsis 935
Sterilization and disinfection of needles 42
Steroid therapy 831
Stimulation 830, 927
Stimulation with the needle 60
Stomach 93, 143
Stomach channel 115, 159, 333, 872
Stomatitis 527
Strabismus 609
Strong stimulation technique 767
Stye 608
Summer heat 377
Sunstroke 663
Supercilio: Occipital line 863

Superficial channels 115
Surgery 831
Surgical suture embedding therapy 759
Swift insertion of needles 927
Symdromes of the small intestine 185
Syncope 651
Syndromes of the gall bladder 247
Syndromes of the heart 175
Syndromes of the kidney 212
Syndromes of the large intestine 140
Syndromes of the liver 254
Syndromes of the lung 131
Syndromes of the pericardium 221
Syndromes of the san jiao 232
Syndromes of the spleen 168
Syndromes of the stomach 159
Syndromes of the urinary bladder 202

T

Taner 299
Tao 306
Techniques of acupuncture 757
Temporal areas 845
Temporal headache 637
The acupuncture needles 35
Theory of jing-luo 332
Theory of the five elements 321
Theory of yin and yang 301
Theory of zang-fu 327
Therapeutic methods 833
Thermal burns of the eye 608
Three-edged needle 927
Tic doloureux 488
Tics 482
Tinnitus 603, 743
Tinnitus 518
Tissues 94
Tongue diagnosis 408
Tonification & sedation 61
Tonsillitis 504
Toothache 528, 750
Toxic excess heat 737
Tracheitis 506
Tragus 845
Traumatic chest pain 574
Traumatic disorders of hip 585
Travel sickness 485, 604
Trigeminal neuralgia 488, 656
Trigger finger 584
Tunzhong 299

U

Ulcers of the skin 590
Un-numbered extraordinary points 927
Un-numberedextraordinary points 297
Upper 15
Urethritis 556
Urinary bladder 94, 329
Urinary bladder channel 115, 202, 204, 334, 879
Urinary bladderchannel 187
Urticaria 592, 735
Uterovaginal prolapse 563
Uterus and ovaries 565

V

Vaginitis 563
Vascular disorders 517
Vertical headache 638

Vertigo 485, 604, 657
Vertigo 518
Vital energy 319, 415
Vitiligo 596
Vomiting 530, 683
Vomiting 515

W

Warts 591
Wei syndrome 660
Weima 300
Whooping cough 508
Wind 376
Windstrokes 645, 646
Wu-hsing 927

X

Xi-Cleft point 927
Xia-Yifeng 298
Xie method 928
Xu disease 432, 928

Y

Yang excess 653, 656
Yangwei 453
Yaoyang 299
Yin (zang) and yang 100
Yin excess 651
Yin-yang 384, 928
Yinwei 453
Yuan-source point 928
Yung-spring point9 456

Z

Zang organs 94, 328
Zang—fu functions 94, 99
Zang-fu 111
Zang-fu theory 328
Zang-fu theory 928
Zhongfu 119

■